Aesthetic Surgery for Men

Keith Jeffords
Ernest K. Manders
William G. Austen, Jr.
Editors

Aesthetic Surgery for Men

A Comprehensive Clinical Guide

Springer

Editors
Keith Jeffords
Private Practice
Paramount Plastic Surgery
Smyrna, GA, USA

Ernest K. Manders
Department of Plastic Surgery
University of Pittsburgh
Pittsburgh, PA, USA

William G. Austen, Jr.
Harvard Medical School, Plastic Surgery
Massachusetts General Hospital
Boston, MA, USA

ISBN 978-3-032-03839-5 ISBN 978-3-032-03840-1 (eBook)
https://doi.org/10.1007/978-3-032-03840-1

This Springer imprint is published by the registered company Springer Nature Switzerland AG
The registered company address is: Gewerbestrasse 11, 6330 Cham, Switzerland

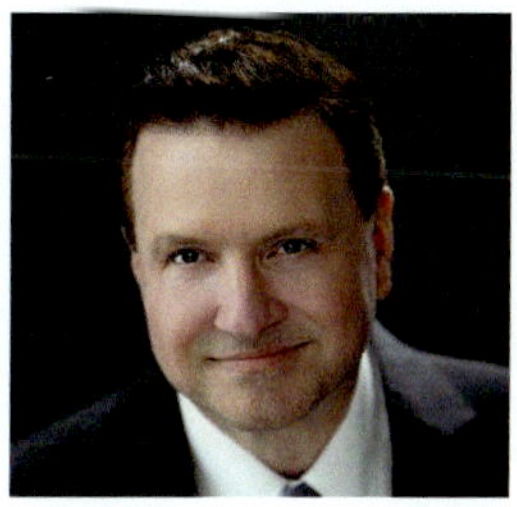

This volume is dedicated to the memory of our dear friend and colleague Dr. Keith Jeffords. Keith suddenly passed away on November 6, 2024. It was Keith who conceived of the need for this book. He recognized that male aesthetic surgical care has been neglected. Through his teaching in North America, South America, and Europe, he has assembled a group of authors who as valued friends and colleagues have contributed to this book. He will be lovingly remembered as a faithful friend, a trusted colleague, and as a loyal University of Pittsburgh alumnus.

In a biographical note, Keith graduated with a dental degree from Emory University in 1988. He next trained as a Clinical Fellow in General Dentistry at Harvard. Training in Maxillofacial Surgery at Jackson Memorial Hospital in Miami followed. He then earned an MD at Eastern Virginia Medical School in 1995 and started General Surgery. From there he moved to training in Plastic Surgery at the University of Pittsburgh. After graduation he started a private practice in Atlanta area and soon became recognized for his care for male patients. About half of his aesthetic patients were men. Among several special skills were his treatments of gynecomastia and his expertise in hair restoration. While a busy plastic surgeon, he was a member of the Atlanta Symphony Chorus for 30 years. He was very proud of his many Grammy Awards earned as a part of the Chorus. He had a great sense of humor and a prodigious knowledge of European history. He was kind and caring. His friends, family, and patients alike will greatly miss him.

Contents

1 Introduction: Why Men and Refuting SIMON

Ernest K. Manders

Why not men? Writers from *Gulliver's Travels* to *Star Trek* have used the motif of a foreigner assessing the conventional to show us a rational view of customs we take for granted. Ask yourself if a critical observer of our society would assess the need for aesthetic surgery as being any different for men as opposed to women. The critical word here is *need*, of course. Consider need to represent a personal desire felt by an individual, something desired to enhance that person's life through better self-image and expanded opportunities. Would the observer report a difference? Perhaps in an earlier era of our history, but today, the visitor would likely ask "Why not men, too?"

There has been a bias even among those of us in plastic surgery against having men as patients. I recall the teaching in my residency that every young man who came to the office requesting a rhinoplasty have a compulsory psychiatric consultation. This is far from common practice today. Although some young male patients may indeed benefit from such a consultation preoperatively, it is unlikely that all male patients seeking nasal surgery would benefit in a significant way. Indeed, this is a practice pattern that has gone the way of the dodo!

Drs. Gorney and Martello gave us an acronym that gained a momentum of perhaps greater force than deserved [1]. SIMON (single immature male overly expectant narcissistic) has entered the lexicon of plastic surgery risks. Recently Dr. Bulstrode, Waterhouse, and Forrester have amplified this to SLAP-SIMON for the young male who "still lives at parents" [2]. These warnings join those regarding men and women with body dysmorphic disorder. We all need to be on our toes, whatever the gender of the patient before us. However, there is a sea change going on in which well-balanced, emotionally healthy men are seeking aesthetic procedures to improve their lives. Whereas a male patient visiting a plastic surgeon four decades ago may have signaled an underlying psychiatric disquiet, today the norms of our population have changed and individuals enjoying good mental health are seeking surgery for improved appearance and self-confidence.

1.1 Why Does Appearance Matter?

We are all taught "Don't judge a book by its cover." But we do, all day, each day, as we live our lives in social environments. This judgment is a type of pattern recognition that has evolved within us as a species to help us cope with the world in which we live [3]. We are tasked with identifying those among us who are fit, sick, safe, and dangerous. Identification of attribute cues in facial appearance happens in seconds and guides

E. K. Manders (✉)
Department of Plastic Surgery, University of Pittsburgh, Pittsburgh, PA, USA
e-mail: mandersek@upmc.edu

K. Jeffords et al. (eds.), *Aesthetic Surgery for Men*, https://doi.org/10.1007/978-3-032-03840-1_1

our thoughts and behavior. As all plastic surgeons know, appearance does count. One reason for this is the "attractiveness halo" which leads attractive people to be judged positively on a host of other dimensions without objective evidence to support the impressions [4]. This has a profound effect from business to the criminal justice system to elections. The attractive man or woman is imbued through the halo effect with positive attributes like intelligence, health, and being socially adept, powerful, and sexually responsive. Looking good can provide both deserved and undeserved opportunities. Our patients want to have an appearance, both facially and in body form, that makes them confident and which confers attractiveness to anyone who holds them for however briefly in their gaze. They want opportunities in life. Aesthetic surgery cannot change fundamental personality flaws, but it can provide opportunities for interpersonal relationships that allow greater fulfillment and happiness. Appearance does count. Projecting the right visual clues can help a person along the road of life.

References

1. Gorney M, Martello J. Patient selection criteria. Medical-legal issues in plastic surgery. Clin Plast Surg. 1999;26:37.
2. Bulstrode NW, Waterhouse N, Forrester P. Male aesthetic patients to avoid, SLAP-SIMON. Plast Reconstr Surg. 2007;119:452.
3. Zebrowitz LA, Montepare JM. Social psychological face perception: why appearance matters. Soc Personal Psychol Compass. 2008;3(3):1497.
4. Eagly AH, Ashmore RD, Makhijani MG, Longo LC. What is beautiful is good, but: a meta-analytic review of research on the physical attractiveness stereotype. Psychol Bull. 1991;110(1):109–28.

Part I

Introduction

2 Social Media Marketing for the Male Aesthetic Practice

Ed Syring

Though many readers can still remember a time when marketing a medical practice was frowned upon, most of the physicians who remember when it was illegal have (hopefully) since retired. As the medical marketing world has evolved, there has been a consistent pattern of push back and approval. In a landscape fraught with regulation to protect against the vast minority of bad actors among medical professionals, it has been quite a journey for the more progressive and entrepreneurial physicians to successfully market themselves. Once marketing was even allowed, it remained frowned upon as established doctors felt that anyone who advertised did not have the skills, and therefore did not have the reputation or referral base, to be successful. Enterprising physicians persevered, however, and often became successful with great reputations despite their employment of more progressive marketing strategies.

With the advent of the internet, again it was the more enterprising physicians who created websites, much to the chagrin of many of their peers and the professional societies responsible for regulation. In hindsight, most doctors who waited to join the digital revolution wish they had been early adopters able to enjoy the more robust presence those with more mature websites now enjoy (as even the mere age of a website or URL is one of the many factors that Google weighs when ranking search results). Fast forward to the early 2000 s and it was becoming requisite for physicians, especially in the elective space, to have a website. Around the same time, the now most-popular social media platforms were just launching:

- 2003 saw the launch of LinkedIn
- 2004 saw the launch of Facebook, initially only aimed at college students
- 2005 saw the launch of YouTube, acquired by Google just a year later
- 2006 saw the launch of Twitter
- 2010 saw the launch of Instagram
- 2011 saw the launch of Snapchat
- 2016 saw the launch of TIKTOK.

Inevitably, surgeons slowly began posting their work, often drawing not only ire but formal complaint from societies like the American Society of Plastic Surgery. Just like traditional marketing decades earlier, the use of social media to promote a cosmetic practice was derided as unbecoming of the profession. The proliferation of social media led to physicians posting first on a personal level which naturally led to more professional posts from practices. Practices and physicians using social media professionally have crept into the majority, and even the societies

E. Syring (✉)
YellowTelescope, SEOversite, and iScreamSocialMedia, Miami, FL, USA
e-mail: ed@yellowtelescope.com

K. Jeffords et al. (eds.), *Aesthetic Surgery for Men*, https://doi.org/10.1007/978-3-032-03840-1_2

once castigating physicians for using the platforms now have their own feeds.

Social media has officially become a requisite part of a practice's holistic marketing strategy but it has not taken the place of more established forms of marketing, digital or otherwise. It is still paramount to have a beautiful website that converts visitors and to have a consistent, ongoing organic search engine optimization (SEO) strategy to continually improve (or, for those already well-ranked sites, maintain) rankings for terms prospective patients are searching. Content, in the form of written blogs and articles, photos, videos, patient testimonials, and more, needs to be continually added, refined, and optimized. Pay per click (PPC) marketing should be utilized to also appear at the top of a search engine page despite organic SEO rankings. Patient ratings and reviews on many platforms must be continuously added for practices to maintain a strong digital reputation in an ever more competitive cosmetic landscape. Marketing for the aesthetic practice has become the business of "*and*" not "*or.*" You can't consider having a website *or* performing SEO, *or* obtaining online reviews, *or* engaging in social media. You must have a strong website *and* perform SEO, *and* PPC, *and* obtain online reviews, *and*, once you have the digital foundation established with the aforementioned, you must engage in social media.

"Social media," however, is a blanket term with a definition that will continually evolve with the rapidly changing environment it embodies. For the purposes of this chapter, we will take a pragmatic approach to distilling the most practical, actionable information for the developing male aesthetic practice to monetize its social media presence. Indeed, an entire textbook could be written on the subject and would need to be updated at least semi-annually to keep up with the constantly shifting social media environment as platforms and consumers adapt to the developments of regulation, legislation, and economics of a lucrative and influential digital marketing industry. Indeed, this chapter was originally written in 2019, then essentially rewritten in time for publication due to Covid-related delays. Entire chapters could be devoted to the nuanced mechanics and minutiae regarding the algorithms of each social media platform, the implications of medical law through HIPAA and HITECH, ethical debate surrounding the effect glamorization of plastic surgery has on society's physical ideals, the neurological human response to prolonged exposure to aesthetic social media content, and more.

While we will briefly touch on some of these topics, in this single chapter we endeavor to outline the best, immediately usable practices to engage more male patients through social media marketing, written for the layperson, based on our combined decades of experience building aesthetic practices during what we surmise will be known as the Age of Social Media. We have divided the approach to successful social media marketing into two main categories: organic social media and paid social media. While associated, they are as related as swimming and diving—you need a pool for both, but you can't dive into the pool unless you can swim first, and each has fundamentally unique strategy, technique, and application. So, without further ado, let's wade into the shallow end to test the social media waters.

2.1 Organic Social Media

Just as a Google Ads campaign is moot without a superb website that is already ranking highly for organic Google search and converting organic leads, paying for posts or advertisements to appear at the top of a social media feed without a robust presence on a platform comprised of excellent content and engaged followers is imprudent. As we will describe, paid social media is growing faster and can be more directly monetized, but the need for a solid organic foundation remains. How do we make it worth doing? What constitutes engaging content, and how is it created or curated? How are followers amassed in a fashion that is accepted by platforms as authentic and transparent? How is engagement, and thus success, of an improving social media presence measured, and thus monetized? The answers are forthcoming, but let us begin with a brief description of the feeds in order of user engagement, beginning with the most engaging at the time of publishing (**bold** indicating a more prominent focus for medical social media marketing in this chapter):

- **Facebook**—the largest social media platform by far by almost every metric: 2.93 billion monthly active users (MAU).
- **Instagram**—owned by Facebook parent company, Meta Platforms, Instagram is the most inherently visual platform, and thus the most suited to aesthetic medicine. With more limited functionality than its parent platform, Instagram has also been the fastest growing platform in terms of users as of late, now up to 1.44 billion MAU.
- **Twitter**—known for its more limited post length and its focus on the most real-time posting, Twitter has lost share to other platforms and its growth has slowed despite its headlines for being a primary source of political communication. It currently has 450 million MAU.
- **LinkedIn**—the most "professional" platform, LinkedIn has developed into a primary source for business to business networking, recruiting, and content development. 310 million MAU.
- Snapchat—deserving of mention due to the 428 million MAU and its use by some notable physicians due to its relaxed content restrictions regarding nudity and intraoperative video. Snapchat has since lost tremendous share to other platforms in part due to the adoption of its original functionality (largely Facebook and Instagram creating the Stories function).
- **TIKTOK**—the newest social media platform to enter the fray, already has 1 billion MAU. Starting in China in 2016, the company focused on short-form content and has seen great success with that change.
- YouTube—needs to be mentioned due to the 1.9 billion MAU, but is a Google property more appropriately discussed as part of SEO, and only for the most devoted physician filmmakers.
- Podcasts—from Spotify to the Podcasts app, there are plenty of ways for people to listen to podcasts with 104 million Americans listening to podcasts regularly.

2.2 Branding and "Avatar"

Before content can be created or curated, let alone posted to any of the platforms mentioned above, the practice must first determine its identity. What defines the practice, authentically, that differentiates it personally and professionally from other practices offering identical treatments to male patients? If your brand was a person that accurately embodied yourself, your staff, the procedures you perform, and even your facility, what would that person be like, and how would they relate to the patients you would like to attract to your practice? Answer some simple questions about this "person":

- Do they identify as male, female, etc.?
- How old are they?
- What is their level of education?
- What kind of house do they live in?
- What kind of music do they like?
- What do they do for fun on evenings and weekends?
- What do they think is funny?
- What are their favorite colors?
- How much do they earn?
- Do they have pets? Kids? A significant other?
- Do they have an accent? What is their vernacular?
- Where did they grow up?
- Are they introverted and educational or extroverted and promotional? Occasionally both?
- And so on….

By having the questions answered, a clear identity of the avatar that embodies the presence will materialize and help dictate decisions on content, writing captions, and as we will see in the paid social media section, targeting the desired consumer demographic.

Here are two examples of determined brand identity:

- A Houston, TX, practice attracting a largely female clientele identifies a sassy but classy woman in her mid-30 s born and bred in town. She has elementary aged children, has a bachelor's degree, and works full time in a creative industry where boots and denim are encouraged in the dress code. Her husband has a demanding job as an oil industry executive. They have a four-bedroom house with a pool on a cul-de-sac in a master planned community. They have a golden retriever who isn't afraid to jump into the Gulf of Mexico when they take weekend family trips to Galveston. Rabid Houston Texan fans in the fall and Astros fans in the summer, they are frequent hosts to neighbors for barbecues that always involve a little rose for the ladies and whisky for the guys. She is fun loving but southern proper, not afraid to belt out a country tune if the lyrics aren't too gosh darned dirty.
- A NY, NY-based practice identifies as an early 40 s man that grew up in the mid-west but has lived in the city for 20 years. His wife and elementary age child share a three-bedroom apartment in a converted brownstone in Brooklyn's Boerum Hill. He works in a creative industry as a marketing executive with a passion for art and design, frequenting fine art and street art installations alike. He likes well-made clothing with a relaxed aesthetic and is comfortable aging gracefully but wouldn't mind some professional aesthetic help. His all-natural skin-care regimen has largely been pieced together from reading recommendations in Esquire and Men's Journal on his iPad, particularly in the summer weekends on Montauk. While he enjoys sports, he's equally happy listening to an NPR podcast from a City Bike in the cool fall weather.

Once you have a grasp on who you are and who you are appealing to, you can begin determining the appropriate content to create and curate. The keys to engaging organic social media content are variety and authenticity. Think of the new parent who only posts photos of the baby. Though you love kids, photo after photo of the kid can be as numbing as their repeated posts from every new restaurant they tried before becoming parents. The same goes for an aesthetic practice. The visual nature of social media naturally lends itself to showcasing patient results, but if the entire feed is before and after photos, followers become numb to the content and lose interest. Without the personality of the avatar reflected through a variety of authentic posts, the human element that differentiates the practice from others is lost. When considering content, remember the "and" principle. While the list of potential subjects is limitless, you will want to continuously amass:

- Before and after photos and videos
- Written and video patient testimonials
- Intraoperative photos and videos
- Videos of treatments being performed
- Candid photos and videos of the doctor and staff
- Photos and videos of the facilities
- Photos and videos of products sold in the office
- Links to blog posts or relevant articles
- Recordings of professional presentations
- Highlights of team meetings and social gatherings
- Celebrations of birthdays and anniversaries
- Personal photos of pets and families
- Features of the team enjoying local culture or on vacations
- Posts related to hobbies or interests
- Articles from the internet highlighting any of the above
- PR features and hits
- Highlights of training or working with colleagues
- And so much more…

While it is important to have a variety of subjects of posts, and to vary between photos, video, and linked content, the addition of logos, text, animations, and other design elements will also create more engagement with followers.

- Incorporate drawn or written elements on photos. Draw animated arrows or outline treated areas to draw more attention to results.
- Add logos to photos to brand them, which can also be much more aesthetically pleasing than a "watermark" to prevent unauthorized sharing without credit.
- Add music to videos.
- Add written text or captions to highlight key spoken phrases in a video.
- Have an animated logo created to "bookend" the beginning and end of a video.

It is paramount to adhere to the content standards set by each platform when it comes to realistic results and nudity. Many of the effects listed above can also be used to cover parts of the body that are not allowed to be displayed on most social feeds, a unique challenge to overcome when abiding by the "community standards" defined by each platform. These standards are more relaxed for male images than they are for female images, primarily in that male nipples do not need to be covered. Genitals can never be shown, making it all the more challenging to highlight any sort of male enhancement, though some surgeons redirect viewers to other feeds that allow, such as Snapchat.

Of course, successfully posting results also requires the applicable written consent from the patient. While it should be habitual to take photos of a patient prior to treatment, during follow-up to track progress and when final results have been achieved, it should be equally standard for the physician, practitioner, and office team to attempt to obtain consent to share these photos on social media. Willingness to provide consent will of course vary greatly from patient to patient, and depend on the nature of the treatment, but the effort to obtain consent should be consistent. We recommend the following word track to be ideally used by the doctor, personally asking each patient for consent:

> By the way, did you review my photos before you decided to proceed with me doing your surgery? Great. And did you find that process helpful in understanding who was right for you and what we could accomplish compared to our peers? Wonderful. One thing I'd love to ask is if you might be willing to 'pay it forward' and allow us to utilize your photos so other patients just like you can see our work and be helped just like other patients who gave consent helped you. I would love to be able to share your wonderful results on social media to help people hoping to achieve similar results. We can also simply keep them internally, meaning we will not use your images more publicly without your approval, but we can, for example, show your photos to patients in our photo book in the office or put them on our photo gallery on the website. If that'd be ok with you, I'll have our front desk get the quick permission and it would be a great help – of course no pressure at all as we want you comfortable.

More patients than you might think will be willing to share their results, but they almost never will unless you ask them. So, ask everyone. And if the patient initially declines, you can always offer more private options for sharing, like blocking out identifying features, if it makes them more comfortable.

When it comes to the nature of post creation, there are several elements to consider:

- Visual—though the visual nature of posts varies between platforms, given the visual nature of social media, and visual nature of aesthetic treatment, this should be the first consideration.
- Caption—once the visual is created, it must always be accompanied by a written caption that provides context and often a call to action (CTA) to drive engagement and create leads. This is also where the practice "voice" must be consistent and where the determined avatar particularly come into play.
- Hashtags—these are terms that are tracked within the platform and essentially link posts to each other within a catalog, allowing users to easily search for related posts.
- Hat tip—originally abbreviated "h/t" but has developed over time to simply mean the attribution of credit to the original source of content by listing the username, or "handle," of the account. It is also an opportunity to link to other accounts to increase exposure as accounts are alerted when others "tag" them in

their posts, increasing the chances of sharing with broader followers.

With your practice brand's avatar clearly defined and trove of locally sourced content amassed, it is important to create a written caption for each visual post. Think about what you are posting and why to provide context for what the viewer is looking at. This of course will differ greatly from post to post depending on the content, but as noted that variety will keep readers engaged and continuing to follow you. Writing in first person increases engagement even further. Too many aesthetic practices have someone in their office writing for them. Posts that are written about the doctor do not resonate with viewers like those that are written by the doctor, or someone who has the training and ability to write authentically as the doctor or practice. Post length limit is technically determined by the platform, as in Twitter's case you are limited to 280 characters. Facebook expanded their limit to 63,206 characters, Instagram limits to 2200 characters, and LinkedIn limits to 3000 characters. That also doesn't mean that you should write that much. Make your point and be succinct. For promotional posts announcing events or specials, or for posts highlighting great results, include a call to action (CTA) inviting the viewer to reach out through a direct message (DM), comment, call to the office, or visit to the link to your website.

Adding hashtags to a post can be crucial to optimization. All posts on a platform are indexed and tracked by every term that starts with a hash symbol (#). Note that hashtag terms cannot include spaces or punctuation ("#chicagogynecomastia" will work but "#chicago gynecomastia" will only index the first word attached to the hash mark, "Chicago"). While the number of hashtags does differ among platforms, the Goldilocks rule of thumb is 12 per post. Displaying as many as the allowed 30 on Instagram can make the post feel cluttered, but only using 1–6 on a post can limit the exposure of the post. When choosing hashtags, Goldilocks endures. It's a best practice to choose tags with high search volume but are more specialized to the location and procedure. You can research hashtag usage volume on Instagram, for example, by simply typing in the hashtag in the "tags" section of the search function.

- For example, at the time of writing this chapter, #gynecomastia yielded 84,600 posts. #gynecomastianewyork yielded 100+ posts.
- #maleplasticsurgery yielded 11,800 posts. #maleplasticsurgeryny yielded 500+ posts. #maleplasticsurgerynewyork yielded less than 100 posts.

Hat tips and tagging other handles is another best practice. If you are posting about any treatment, do some research to see if the manufacturer, or the treatment, or device itself has a social profile to which you can link. At an even more base level, it is important to credit other profiles if you are resharing their content.

Once you have your posts created with visuals, captions, hashtags, and hat tips, you can organize the posts into an editorial calendar for each platform you plan to post on. Some practices may elect to only post to Instagram or Facebook since they are the most popular, and they offer the option to mirror both feeds as they are connected under Meta's umbrella. At the other end of the spectrum, some practices will elect to post unique content to Facebook, Instagram, Twitter, and LinkedIn several times a week. Depending on resources and budgets, more is typically better but don't feel you have to do all or nothing. For the practice starting out, even posting 3 times per week can develop good habits and eventually lead to traction online. There are several tools available online like Hootsuite that also allow automated posting. While it's not quite "set it and forget it," and does require initial loading of content, these can be invaluable for efficient, automated posting to Instagram, Facebook, Twitter, and LinkedIn.

2.3 Increasing Followers, the Right Way

Posting fantastic, engaging content alone will not necessarily lead to more people seeing it appear on their feeds. As we will discuss in more detail in the forthcoming section on paid social media ads, organic reach from business feeds has waned dramatically in recent years due to algorithmic changes on platforms. Aside from strokes of luck with strong PR hits, appearing on a reality show, or being listed as one of Oprah's favorite things, there are no advisable shortcuts to increasing your followers without manually asking to follow users in the hopes they follow you back. While there are services that promise boosts in followers well into the thousands in a very short amount of time (days to weeks), these should not be utilized for any reason. Not only are these tempting short cuts ethically questionable, but they are often rife with fake accounts at worst, and unengaged accounts at best. Further, social platforms have started penalizing the performance of user feeds who have shown dramatic increases in follower counts in short time spans or evidence of fake follower accounts, particularly on Instagram and Twitter (Facebook business pages are not allowed to follow other personal accounts).

While there are limits on the number of accounts an Instagram or Twitter account can follow in a day, hours and hours every month must be invested in following other accounts related to your specialty. Some ideas, again non-exhaustively, include following all the followers of local gyms, fashion boutiques, restaurants, locally based companies, community organizations, cultural periodicals, other medial practices, and other similar feeds that might attract similar followers that you're after to form an engaged group of interested consumers. With consistency, it is reasonable to expect increases each month from dozens to hundreds of followers, which add up considerably over time, as will engagement.

2.4 Measuring Success and Engagement

As you consistently post and increase followers, it is important to be watchful for any engagement, which is what we are ultimately after. In essence, any like, comment, or DM is measurable engagement. Any comment or DM constitutes a lead and should be responded to as soon as possible with a thank you and an additional CTA directing them to the practice contact information to give yourself the best chance of turning engagement into procedures performed. We regularly see practices book procedures in the tens of thousands of dollars for patients who initially heard about them on social media, reached out to the practice via DM, and eventually come into the practice for consultation, thanks to diligent follow-up from a Patient Coordinator.

Even if this isn't happening regularly for you yet, you can still measure the success of your organic social media efforts with the following metrics, ideally monthly:

- Followers—the number of followers an account has is important, but more does not always equal better as we've mentioned above.
- Likes—again, positive sign of engagement but mostly good for the ego. More is better but tough to convert a like into a lead. Platform algorithms do recognize posts and feeds with more likes, as well as shares, in the sense there is virality of a post within the community.
- Comments and DM—more the better, and make sure your staff responded!
- Google analytics—you should also be logging into the Google analytics for your website, which specifically tracks visitors from social media sites. If your posts are consistently promoting visits to your website, this should increase over time, will help with your sites ranking, and any leads that convert from a social visitor are a social lead.

2.5 Practical Application

Everything discussed thus far can be executed in several ways largely depending on the nature of the practice ownership (and their proclivity for naturally posting several times a week on their own), the time they are willing to devote to this endeavor, and budget they are prepared to spend on improving their social media.

- Do it yourself—if you are the type of person that has a predisposition to post regularly for your own personal feeds, the time to devote several hours a week to creating content, writing captions, researching hashtags, editing photos and videos, let alone spending the time to follow hundreds of accounts to hopefully get them to follow you back, you might be able to do this yourself. Not only have we learned this is the vast minority of doctors, we also know that it still won't be as successful as if it were done by an expert who spends 40–100 hours a week on the art and science of social media.

- Hire an expert in house—many practices think that having someone in house will answer their social media prayers. Unfortunately, many also make the mistake of assuming that anyone born after 1990 and armed with a smartphone can provide the kind of leads they need to be successful. Actual social media experts earn between $35,000 and $70,000 per year, with many enterprise-level experts earning well into the six figures. If you have the budget for this person, it may still make more sense to outsource the content editing, automated posting, and metric tracking to an outside agency so you can devote the time of your local employee to helping you create excellent content in the office.
- Hire an outside expert—it is typically most prudent for a practice to find a partner who specializes in social media for their industry and subscribes to the best practices outlined in this chapter.

2.6 Paid Social Media

It is no secret that social media companies are in the business of advertising sales. Meta, the world's largest social media company (accounting for over 6 billion monthly active users across its properties Facebook, WhatsApp, Messenger, and Instagram), reported over $114 billion in ad revenue in 2021. Meta shows no signs of slowing down with a projected advertising revenue of over $200 billion by 2026. While the company does not disclose the specific ad revenue split between platforms, they did indicate that the most significant recent growth came from Instagram, and the vast majority of revenue comes from Facebook and Instagram, the two largest platforms that also offer the most robust advertising capabilities.

Part of the reason for the growth in ad revenue is because Facebook and other platforms have been changing their algorithms drastically reducing the reach of organic posts particularly from businesses. Depending on the type of patient, type of content, and quality of engagement with organic content, it's estimated that the average post from a business could be as low as 2%. Surely with rising users but a finite amount of real estate on a news feed, let alone a dropping consumer attention span, it is inevitable that a lower percentage of content produced will be seen. Economics of scale aside, Meta says it is intentionally burying more pubic content in the name of creating more "meaningful interactions." It also means that reducing the reach of a company's content to essentially zero, Meta expects businesses to pay for their content to be seen. This will only increase with time.

As nuanced and complex as the world of organic social media can be, it could be considered downright nebulous compared to paid social media advertising. From demographic selections to selecting the right budgets and A/B testing to track the success of a specific campaign, there are innumerable variables to consider. We will endeavor to simplify when it comes to what a practice should consider, and we will largely focus specifically on the largest, and therefore likely most effective, platform: Facebook. While all major platforms offer the opportunity to advertise, different platforms are going to offer different ways to achieve different goals. They also offer the ability to market to highly targeted demographics. For the aesthetic practice marketing to men, the ultimate goal is to increase lead generation—more prospective patients contacting the practice with questions or request for appointment. While we focus on Facebook, the best practices exemplified can be carried over to other platforms.

A recent Pew Research study determined social media usage across several platforms and

Table 2.1 Use of different online platforms by demographic groups

% of US adults who say they use...	YouTube	Facebook	Instagram	Pinterest	LinkedIn	Snapchat	Twitter	WhatsApp	TikTok
Total	81	69	40	31	28	25	23	23	21
Men	82	61	36	16	31	22	25	26	17
Women	80	77	44	46	26	28	22	21	24
White	79	67	35	34	29	23	22	16	18
Black	84	74	49	35	27	26	29	23	30
Hispanic	85	72	52	18	19	31	23	46	31
Ages 18–29	95	70	71	32	30	65	42	24	48
30–49	91	77	48	34	36	24	27	30	22
50–64	83	73	29	38	33	12	18	23	14
65+	49	50	13	18	11	2	7	10	4
<$30,000	75	70	35	21	12	25	12	23	22
$30,000–$49,999	83	76	45	33	21	27	29	20	29
$50,000–$74,999	79	61	39	29	21	29	22	19	20
$75,000+	90	70	47	40	50	28	34	29	20
High school or less	70	64	30	22	10	21	14	20	21
Some college	86	71	44	36	28	32	26	16	24
College+	89	73	49	37	51	23	33	33	19
Urban	84	70	45	30	40	28	27	28	24
Suburban	81	70	41	32	33	25	23	23	20
Rural	74	67	25	34	15	18	18	9	16

Note: White and Black adults include those who report being only one race and are not Hispanic. Hispanics are of any race. Not all numerical differences between groups shown are statistically significant (e.g., there are no statistically significant differences between the shares of White, Black, or Hispanic Americans who say the use Facebook). Respondents who did not give an answer are not shown

From: Auxier B, Anderson M. Social Media Use in 2021. Pew Research Center, April 7, 2021

demographics. Facebook was by far the most widely used across all platforms, with 69% of online Americans using it. Of those that use other platforms, an average of 90% also use Facebook. Further, it was used by 75% of online Americans earning over $75,000 a year, 73% of users with at least a college degree, 70% of online Americans age 18–29, 77% between the ages of 30–49, and 73% age 50–64. Most salient for our chapter, an estimated 61% of online American men use Facebook. Finally, 70% of total users access the platform every day. With Facebook reporting 1.93 billion daily users, estimating 10% of users are in the United States and 56.6% of users are male, the simple math means the national daily Facebook audience in the United States is just over 109 million men. With almost half of all men in the United States using Facebook every day, it is statistically one of the largest possible audiences for advertising male aesthetic treatment. With the capability to track a very specific male population, the efficacy and return on investment has the potential to be far greater than other platforms (Table 2.1).

We will describe the process to create and launch a paid ad campaign, the strategy to continually test the efficacy of a campaign, and review what results look like from actual iScreamSocialMedia client campaigns.

First, decide on the procedure you might want to advertise to men. While it can be appropriate to consider advertising for a wide array of treatments at different levels of pricing, from low-cost skin care to costly surgical body contouring, hair restoration, or facial rejuvenation, conversion rates may also differ. Inquiries for more expensive surgery with higher recovery/risk might not convert to treatment at a rate as high as lower cost treatments with lower recovery/risk. For the sake of illustration, let's assume we are advertising to attract more male prospects interested in CoolSculpting.

Make sure whomever is managing the campaign is an expert on the treatment you hope to promote. Each ad will be a combination of visual and written copy intended to solicit an emotional response from the viewer. To communicate the value of the treatment, the marketer must understand who the target audience is, what might peak their interest, what symptoms are being treated, how the treatment is performed, the nature of the recovery, what results might look like, and the costs. The marketer is, in essence, selling the procedure so should be as knowledgeable as Patient Concierge or Coordinator that might be responsible for converting the lead to a patient.

Visit www.facebook.com/business. Click "Create an ad." Prepare to be overwhelmed. We won't go into each and every variable that Facebook allows you to control. Tutorials abound online and Facebook elaborates on each variable within the Ads Manager. Variables should also be tested and tweaked over time to determine the most successful specific audience and budget. The more specific your audience, the lower the volume, though quality may be better, but marketing is always a balance between quantity and quality. Of course, a new patient referred by three previous patients and another physician is more likely to convert to a procedure than someone who hears about you for the first time from your Facebook ad. However, if our Facebook targeted audience directs the ad at men ages 30–50, with at least a college degree, a household income in at least the top 25%, who have children, and are interested in luxury goods, fitness, and men's clothing, our hope is to have more qualified leads likely interested in and able to afford CoolSculpting.

Determining budget is equally nuanced and requires testing. Facebook will help you estimate the volume of conversions you might expect from a campaign, but also think about the number you might need to at least break even on a monthly spend. First, let's define a few things related to tracking paid Facebook advertising:

- Impressions—the number of times a Facebook ad is actually displayed or appears on a users' feeds.
- Reach—the number of people in the selected audience who actually see an ad.
- Clicks—the number of times a user actually clicked on an ad.
- Landing page—a unique website that users are directed to once they click on an ad. This is a single page developed to be similar to your own practice website, but is specifically designed to convert visitors who have clicked link in a Facebook ad. If we are promoting CoolSculpting for men, all of the photos and written content will be devoted to that. There should not be any links to other pages or procedures, but there should be several opportunities to submit contact information to the practice. The entire page is a sales pitch and so should be professionally designed, include sharp photography, "trust builders" like the accolades of the doctor and practice (number of patients treated, board certifications, years in practice, training/certification/schools attended, etc.), details about the treatment, details about a special offer, and several calls to actions (CTA) directing the visitor to "request a consultation" or similar. This is often the final destination in the funnel and ultimately yields the "acquisition"—the lead.
- Lead Ad—a native contact form within a Facebook ad that auto-populates user contact information. An alternative or supplement to a landing page, Lead Ads direct the user to a pop-up within Facebook that fills in known information pulled from the user's Facebook profile, allowing the user to fill in any other info or edit it. Once the user submits that information, this is also considered an "acquisition."
- Cost per click (CPC)—the total cost divided by the number of clicks.
- Cost per acquisition (CPA)—the total cost divided by the number of leads actually submitted to the practice—what the practice pays per lead.

Now let's paint a few pictures to illustrate how these all come into play using metrics from actual iScreamSocialMedia campaigns with varying success (Table 2.2).

- Dr. One had a Facebook campaign advertising Orbera that ran from 10/01/21 through 12/31/21, spending $2924.37in that time. In that time, the ad appeared on Facebook feeds 24,580 times (impressions) and 11,712 Facebook users actually saw the ad (reach). Of those that saw the ad, 243 clicked the link (yielding a CPC of $12.03), and of those that clicked through to a landing page or Lead Ad, 24 submitted their information (acquisitions, leading to a CPA of $121.85). Let's assume an Orbera package price of $7000 that yields a profit to the practice of $6000 after disposables and other expenses totally $1000 (for simple math). That means they only need one sale to break even. If this is an average practice with a Patient Concierge handling all incoming leads and consultations who historically converts 10% of your digital leads, this practice should have converted 2 sales out of those 24 leads, leading to $12,000 in profit for the practice on a $3000 spend.
- Dr. Two had a Facebook campaign advertising Evolve/Evoke that ran from 10/01/21 through 12/31/21, spending $2776.49 in that time. In that time, the ad appeared on Facebook feeds 33,352 times (impressions) and 15,681 Facebook users actually saw the ad (reach). Of those that saw the ad, 338 clicked the link (yielding a CPC of $8.21), and of those that clicked through to a landing page or Lead Ad, 39 submitted their information (acquisitions, leading to a CPA of $71.19).
- Dr. Three had a Facebook campaign advertising Laser Treatments that ran from 10/01/21 through 12/31/21, spending $2985.52 in that time. In that time, the ad appeared on Facebook feeds 20,353 times (impressions) and 12,973 Facebook users actually saw the ad (reach). Of those that saw the ad, 219 clicked the link (yielding a CPC of $13.63), and of those that clicked through to a landing page or Lead Ad, 30 submitted their information (acquisitions, leading to a CPA of $99.52).

Facebook allows you to choose your bid strategy to help you spend the money efficiently. You are against all other companies targeting the same eyeballs in your audience, which is why costs can rise higher in more competitive markets. Facebook is essentially bidding on your behalf in ad auctions and gives you the choice how to manage the spend. There are several options to direct Facebook on how to manage your budget based on preference, but the metrics will allow you to know where you may need to make tweaks in the conversion funnel. The spend gets you impressions and reach. The design of the ad and landing page determine the conversion rate of people seeing it.

The ad is essentially built of two portions: the written and the visual:

- The written copy should succinctly outline the treatment being offered, why someone might want it, if there is a special offer, and a CTA. It might read "When diet and exercise fail to deliver the flat, toned midsection you have been looking for, CoolSculpt may be the best option. Click the link to schedule a consultation and save $250 today!"
- Develop the visual for the ad by finding images that will resonate with the viewer. Facebook offers many stock options which can make the ad look polished with professional photos. There are several types of ad format that also allow for a "carousel" of several images you can scroll through. If we are targeting men between 30 and 50 years of age who would like to slim down their midsection, we might select images that highlight the potential results with a photo of an athletic guy in that age range.
  - Be prepared to try alternate images over the course of a campaign to test photos or video that might resonate more with viewers and lead to better conversion. Also be prepared to try several prior to the ad even going live. Every ad is reviewed prior to being posted to make sure the content adheres to strict guidelines. When aesthetic practices often help people feel better naked, you have to be careful about the images you select.

Table 2.2 iScreamSocialMedia Campaigns

Campaign Name	Procedure	Leads	CPA	Link Clicks	CPC	Reach	Impressions	Amount spent (USD)	Reporting starts	Reporting ends
Dr. One	Orbera	24	$121.85	243	$12.03	11,712	24,580	$2924.37	10.01.2021	12.31.2021
Dr. Two	Evolve/Evoke	39	$71.19	338	$8.21	15,681	33,352	$2776.49	10.01.2021	12.31.2021
Dr. Three	Laser Treatment	30	$99.52	219	$13.63	12,973	20,353	$2985.52	10.01.2021	12.31.2021

CPA Cost per acquisition
CPC Cost per click

While their policies are listed https://www.facebook.com/policies/ads/, the approval process is almost completely subjective, and final approval, or rejection, is ultimately determined by artificial intelligence, or an algorithm. Pay particular attention to avoiding Adult Content ("implied nudity, excessive visible skin, and images focused on individual body parts" are non-compliant) and complying with Personal Health ("Ads must not contain 'before-and-after' images or images that contain unexpected or unlikely results. Ad content must not imply or attempt to generate negative self-perception in order to promote diet, weight loss, or other health related products"). We've had many frustrating rounds of re-submission for approval even though we thought the image would have easily passed based on previous ads.

Once the ad is created, the audience is targeted, and the budget is defined, it's time to go live. The Ads Manger dashboard within Facebook Business allows the marketer to monitor the performance in real time and adjust. With myriad variables, it's important to be patient and not make too many adjustments at once. Quality changes are more important than quantity. Too many changes can stall ad performance, as will making the wrong changes. To know what's working, be strategically patient and test few changes at a time. Once you've driven the CPA down, however, you can stick with what works and amplify your results with additional spend on that campaign.

2.7 Summary and Indications of What's on the Horizon

Though this non-exhaustive primer on the current best practices for building a strong male aesthetic social media presence will hopefully lead to the reader's success, there is much left unsaid. As noted at the beginning, an entire textbook would be needed to more fully address everything that can be done on every feed in a constantly changing landscape. Consumer behavior will continue to shift, particularly for men. While much progress has been made in the acceptance of male aesthetic treatment, more has to occur for male engagement to be as productive as possible. The idea of discussing cosmetic surgery was taboo mere years ago, but has become so mainstream that patients are openly discussing their procedures with strangers en masse on social media. The developing ideal of modern masculinity will see more acceptance of men treating their appearance, particularly as the population ages. The propensity for social media followers to select aesthetic providers based solely on social media exposure will increase.

As marketing technology continues to develop, so too will the techniques to maximize their usage. Video content is quickly replacing still photos and images due to newer formats like Tiktok, Reels, and streaming services replacing cable boxes in the recent wave of "cord cutting." With the added content platforms, those not charging subscription will respond to shareholders calls for higher revenues with more opportunities for advertising. Opportunities to pay for exposure will grow and ore feeds will become "pay to play" for businesses. With that will come increases in costs, but also increases in returns, particularly for the practices that have realized early enough that social media is no longer a trend. Those aesthetic practices that start with current best practices, patiently persist to see results, stay abreast of social media marketing developments, and plan to nimbly adapt as time goes on will be well served.

3 Designing a Practice for Men

Ali A. Qureshi and W. Grant Stevens

3.1 Introduction

Male plastic surgery continues to be a growing market within aesthetics. Men seek both nonsurgical and surgical procedures to improve and maintain their looks. The motivations behind these are often no different from those of women, but anecdotally, men will tell us they want to look as young as they feel and remain competitive in the workplace with the influx of younger male associates.

As societal norms and expectations change, plastic surgeons remain well suited from their training and aesthetic eye to meet the growing needs of male clientele. Additionally, as the millennial population increases their consumer power, their culture and willingness to spend on improving their appearance will also include a significant group of men whose aesthetic demands will need to be met.

For plastic surgeons and their practices to tailor their services to the needs of men, they must understand the market trends and popularity of services. According to the American Society for Aesthetic Plastic Surgery Cosmetic Data Bank, the top five most common plastic surgery procedures for men were liposuction, eyelid surgery, male breast reduction for gynecomastia, tummy tuck, and facelift [1]. For nonsurgical procedures in 2017, men accounted for about 9.2% of all injectables reported. The most common injection was with botulinum toxin, followed by poly-L-lactic acid, calcium hydroxyapatite, and lastly hyaluronic acid injectables. When it came to skin rejuvenation, men accounted for 6.3% of skin rejuvenation procedures, which was most commonly photorejuvenation with IPL followed by chemical peels. Interestingly, men accounted for almost 40% of all tattoo removal, 10.4% of all laser hair removal, and 13.0% of all nonsurgical fat reduction procedures [1].

In this chapter, we review our experience with male plastic surgery patients, including nonsurgical and surgical services and how to market to this growing clientele.

3.2 Nonsurgical Treatments and Marketing to Male Patients

Nonsurgical aesthetic services are a "disruptive technology" for many plastic surgeons because they happen outside of the familiar operating room. The reality is that these services are rapidly expanding, accounting for nearly $2 billion in 2017 according to the ASAPS Cosmetic Surgery Data Bank [1]. In 2007, a landmark study from the Cosmetic Medicine Task Force explored the disruption caused by non-core providers in

A. A. Qureshi (✉) · W. Grant Stevens
Aesthetic Surgery Fellow, Marina Plastic Surgery, Marina del Rey, CA, USA

K. Jeffords et al. (eds.), *Aesthetic Surgery for Men*, https://doi.org/10.1007/978-3-032-03840-1_3

aesthetics, the growth of nonsurgical procedures, and rise of medical grade spas. The most salient finding is known as the "747 effect." Surveyed patients were asked who they would choose to perform their cosmetic surgery—93% responded a plastic surgeon and 7% responded a dermatologist or non-core physician. When asked who they would ask to perform a minimally invasive procedure like laser or injectables, 42% chose a dermatologist, 33% non-core physician, and only 25% chose a plastic surgeon. A total of 46% of respondents that had a positive or good experience with non-invasive procedure with a non-plastic surgeon would stay with the non-plastic surgeon for cosmetic surgery [2].

We think about nonsurgical treatments in context of what we call the "Five Principles of Aesthetic Medicine" which are centered on patient care: acquisition, retention, optimization, education, and conversion [3]. This is how an individual becomes a "Patient for Life®" in a practice, including men. Nonsurgical services are on one end of a continuum whose other end is surgery. Successful plastic surgery practices offer the full range of nonsurgical services to their male clientele.

In Los Angeles, we noted that the addition of cryolipolysis in our office attracted more male patients and saw this actually impacted surgical volume. In 2017, nonsurgical fat reduction was one of the top 5 nonsurgical procedures; it is an ideal example of how a nonsurgical aesthetic service leads to patient acquisition. In 2013, Stevens et al. published a study in which 66% of the over 500 patients were new to the practice and specifically were seeking cryolipolysis with Coolsculpting ® (Allergan, Dublin, Ireland) [4]. Of these, 62% were "aesthetic neophytes" never before having had an aesthetic procedure. This created an opportunity to introduce patients to other aesthetic services in the practice. This included injectables, skin care, laser hair removal, and surgical procedures. Nearly 40% of these "aesthetic neophytes" actually came back to the practice for other aesthetic services. A total of 95% of patients never had an injectable treatment previously, and the practice found that the most commonly availed service by returning cryolipolysis patients was injectables [4].

The study noted that nonsurgical procedures expanded the male demographics of the practice. A targeted radio advertising and marketing campaign led to a dramatic increase in male cryolipolysis patients from 13% to 42% of all cryolipolysis clients being men over a 2 year period. The most popular treatments areas for men are flanks (55%), lower abdomen (35%), and upper abdomen (5%). Nonsurgical aesthetic services attract people into a surgical practice that they may have otherwise never considered. We believe this is a powerful tool for practices that seek to expand their male demographic and its financial implications have been studied elsewhere [5].

The nearly threefold increase in men coming to our office motivated us to launch a website targeted directly at men and the procedures they would be interested in. Additionally, what we have found is that men coming for cryolipolysis return for more nonsurgical fat reduction and other services. This includes skin care, hair transplantation, hair removal, treatment for hyperhidrosis, and other services. Men who never considered these services before are exposed to the wide range of aesthetic services our office offers during their cryolipolysis treatments, and we use this as an opportunity for patient education. At Marina Plastic Surgery Associated, men often opt for "dual-sculpting" where they have cryolipolysis and hair transplantation in the same visit (Fig. 3.1). Practices can become creative

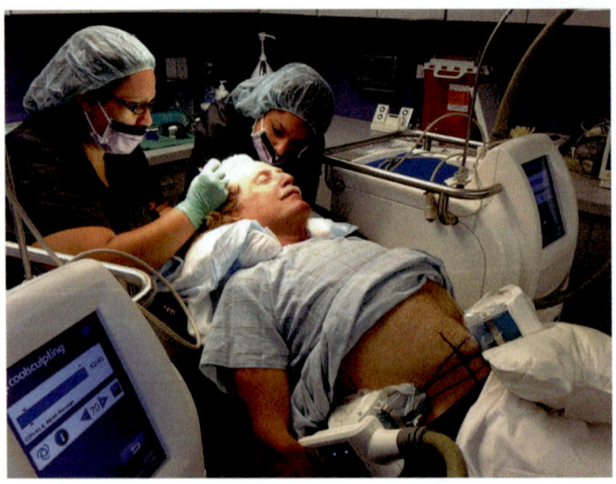

Fig. 3.1 Men undergoing nonsurgical procedures like cryolipolysis can undergo other nonsurgical procedures like hair transplantation at the same time. In our practice, this is referred to as "dual sculpting"

with combining nonsurgical procedures and offerings and increase their internal marketing. What is interesting is that the number of surgical patients who are men has also increased from 11% in 2012 to 18% in 2015 as a result of non-surgical service growth and targeted marketing campaigns.

3.3 Surgical Treatments and Marketing to Male Patients

While most patients want a "natural" result, men will emphasize this even more than women (Fig. 3.2). Generally, men do not want people, including friends, family, and partners, to know that they have had surgery. Scars are a stigma of any surgery and men can be incredibly sensitive to scar location, length, and final appearance. Unlike some women who may have had a C-section or breast biopsy or other surgery, many male patients have never had surgery before. This is true even for liposuction cases. Surgeons should consider being extra sensitive to incision placement and have a thorough discussion with male patients to ensure they are comfortable with the scar placement.

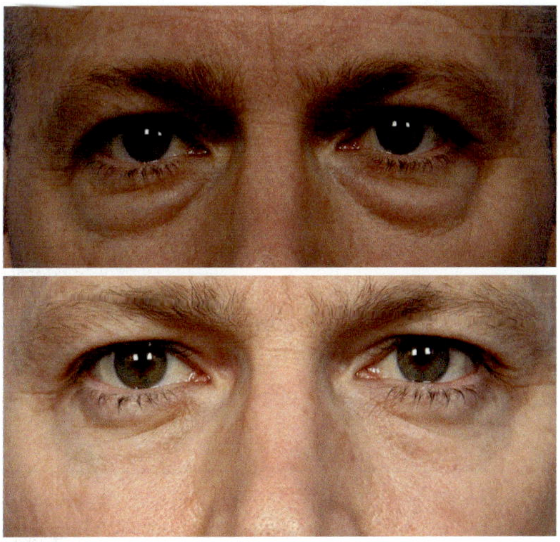

Fig. 3.2 This 43-year-old male came to the office reporting that his coworkers reported he always looked tired despite getting good sleep and rest. He underwent a lower blepharoplasty to remove bulging orbital fat. He wanted to maintain a natural look that would help him look as good as he felt

Male facelifts are on the rise, and one of the top five surgical procedures in 2017. Hairline and sideburn incisions are exceedingly important to men. As plastic surgeons, it is important to anticipate the questions and concerns that male patients will ask about. Pre-emptively discussing some of these concerns will reassure a patient who is considering surgery and increase the likelihood that they will schedule surgery. Offering hair transplantation is a great adjunct procedure for the postop facelift patient as well.

Men may perceive pain differently than women, and this may be because they have not had surgery before or given birth like their female counterparts. Setting expectations and managing concerns about pain at the preoperative consult is important. This is true of postoperative recovery and resumption of activities like working out or sexual activity. Men can tend to be quick to resume all their normal preoperative activities and this can lead to complications after surgery. Managing expectations preoperatively about when and what can be resumed postoperatively is imperative.

There are also opportunities to combine surgical and nonsurgical offerings to achieve optimal results in male patients. For example, all patients who have facelifts in our practice also have what is called "icing on the cake." Typically, 5–7 days after their procedure, patients begin a series of treatments to improve their skin quality and texture as well as have neurotoxin and soft tissue filler treatments. These nonsurgical treatments enhance the final surgical result and also allow the patient to develop an appreciation for what non-surgical services can do to maintain their surgical result. We have found that many male patients want to maintain the results they have achieved and return for nonsurgical maintenance.

3.4 Location, Location, Location

Creating an environment that men are comfortable in is imperative to the success of a plastic surgery practice that seeks to attract (and retain)

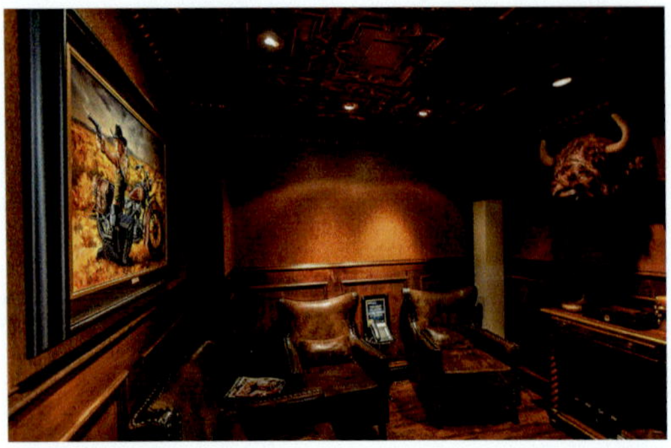

Fig. 3.3 The lounge in Marina ManLand caters specifically to the preferences of our male clientele. This includes leather chairs and a television among other amenities catering to men

a male clientele. Internal research that led to the creation of Marina ManLand® at Marina Plastic Surgery Associates revealed some interesting preferences that male patients have (Fig. 3.3). Men prefer leather chairs to sit separately versus a couch. They prefer a separate waiting room for their own privacy. They do not like to be kept waiting even when in a waiting room. They prefer a masculine décor with sports programs on the televisions and an attentive staff. The bathroom in ManLand even has a urinal. Smell is important to men too and creating an ambiance that appeals to all the senses enhances the experience for men in a plastic surgery office.

The reality is that men have different tastes than women, even when it comes to where and how they are seen in the office. Practices need to be sensitive to these subtle but powerful differences as they can impact how a man feels welcome or not welcome in a practice. Men are more likely to return to an office where they feel comfortable in their own skin.

3.5 Growing a Practice and Referral Patterns

A facelift patient once told us, "Men are just as vain as women. We just don't want anyone to know we are." Many plastic surgeons will attest to word of mouth referrals being a powerful marketing tool for practice growth, especially in women. However, men may hear about nonsurgical and surgical services from their spouses, partners, and media. But, not many men talk to other men about the services they have availed. In our experience, men are more willing to seek out information about aesthetic services once they are actually in the office. The challenge remains how to get men into the office, because once they are here, they are willing to learn and try things. Marketing efforts from practice may find it challenging to continue to try to attract new male clientele and not see the word of mouth referrals they see in their female clientele. This can be frustrating but is the nature of growing a male plastic surgery practice.

Another option to increase awareness of male services in a practice is to encourage clients to fill out online reviews. The internet remains a powerful tool in dissemination of information and patient experiences. With increasing reviews available online, we have found our male clientele to be more aware of what to expect in terms of recovery and downtime from both nonsurgical procedures like hair transplantation and surgical procedures like liposuction.

3.6 Conclusions

Demand for male aesthetic services is on the rise. Practices that seek to attract and retain male patients must be able to accommodate them with nonsurgical and surgical services. Many men are "aesthetic neophytes" never before having sought an aesthetic service like a facial but may be just as, if not more, concerned about their appearance than their female counterparts. Successful practices will be able to use their strengths to meet the growing and evolving needs of male patients.

References

1. Cosmetic Surgery National Data Bank Statistics. Aesthet Surg J. 2017;37(suppl 2):1–29.
2. D'Amico RA, Saltz R, Rohrich RJ, et al. Risks and opportunities for plastic surgeons in a widening cosmetic medicine market: future demand, consumer preferences, and trends in practitioners' services. Plast

Reconstr Surg. 2008;121(5):1787–92. https://doi.org/10.1097/PRS.0b013e31816c3c49.
3. Qureshi AA, Stevens WG. Why should young aesthetic plastic surgeons care about aesthetic medicine? Aesthet Surg J. 2018; https://doi.org/10.1093/asj/sjy273.
4. Stevens WG, Pietrzak LK, Spring MA. Broad overview of a clinical and commercial experience with CoolSculpting. Aesthet Surg J. 2013;33(6):835–46. https://doi.org/10.1177/1090820X13494757. Epub 2013 Jul 15.
5. Richards BG, Schleicher WF, D'Souza GF, Isakov R, Zins JE. The role of injectables in aesthetic surgery: financial implications. Aesthet Surg J. 2017;37(9):1039–43. https://doi.org/10.1093/asj/sjx136.

The HIV-Positive Male

4

Faisal Al-Mufarrej and Keith Jeffords

4.1 Introduction

Highly active antiretroviral therapy (HAART) has increased the life span of HIV infected patients by preventing the development of acquired immunodeficiency syndrome (AIDS). As people live longer, the long-term side effects of liporedistribution are more commonly recognized. While the treatment has greatly reduced mortality and also improved quality of life of patients, these long-term physical changes have secondary aesthetic sequelae with lingering psychological effects, including depression. These effects still negatively affect the well-being of patients and reduce their compliance with treatment [1, 2]. Addressing these sequelae can improve self esteem, mood, body image, quality of life, and compliance [3].

The physical liporedistribution seen in HIV patients is often referred to as HIV-associated lipodystrophy syndrome, but should be more appropriately called HAART-associated lipodystrophy. The majority of patients present with various degrees of both lipoatrophy and lipohypertrophy. Less commonly, patients present with only lipoatrophy, and rarely, patients present with only fat accumulation. Lipoatrophy typically affects the face, while fat accumulation is usually truncal. Truncal fat accumulation may be accompanied by visceral fat buildup. Lipohypertrophy of the neck may also be seen and is typically anterolateral with larger than normal amount of fat. Patients may also present with a cervicodorsal "buffalo hump" that causes disfigurement, pain, or difficulty sleeping.

Thymidine-based nucleoside analogue reverse transcriptase inhibitors, like zidovudine (AZT) and stavudine (d4T), are the usual cause of these aesthetic changes [4, 5]. Inhibition of mitochondrial DNA polymerase is thought to cause adipose cell dysfunction by depleting its mitochondrial DNA resources [6]. Newer non-thymidine reverse transcriptase inhibitors (tenofovir or abacavir) and protease inhibitors are associated with less lipoatrophy [7, 8]. Other risk factors of lipodystrophy include male gender, age > 40 years, white race, duration of HIV infection, low-density lipoprotein cholesterol, low CD4 counts (<100cells/mm3, especially if unchanged with treatment) [8], and weight loss on treatment [9].

It is important to note that pre-exposure prophylaxis (PrEP) in non-HIV patients using tenofovir/emtricitabine (Truvada) has been found to be extremely effective in preventing the transmission of HIV in high-risk individuals. High-risk

F. Al-Mufarrej (✉)
The Michael and Marian Ilitch Department of Surgery, Wayne State University School of Medicine, Detroit, MI, USA
e-mail: falmufar@wayne.med.edu

K. Jeffords
Private Practice, Paramount Plastic Surgery, Smyrna, GA, USA

K. Jeffords et al. (eds.), *Aesthetic Surgery for Men*, https://doi.org/10.1007/978-3-032-03840-1_4

non-HIV patients today are increasingly prescribed PrEP. Truvada has not been found to cause lipid dysregulation or lipodystrophy.

4.2 Evaluation

While aging is associated with soft tissue atrophy, it rarely is as severe as HAART-associated lipoatrophy [10]. Distinguishing the two is important. Unlike aging, rhytid formation and ptosis are less likely encountered with HAART. With HAART, atrophy can progress to almost complete loss of the subdermal facial fat loss with visibility of the underlying facial skeleton, giving an emaciated appearance. It mainly affects the cheeks, orbits, and temples [11]. In the cheeks, often a triangular area of depression is identified between the nasolabial fold, the malar arch, and the line connecting the two [12]. Injecting in this triangle provides improved cosmesis and patient satisfaction regardless of filler and technique.

In assessing the severity of facial lipoatrophy, the Carruthers Lipoatrophy Severity Scale [13] is useful. Grade 1 demonstrates mild and localized facial lipoatrophy, while with Grade 2, deeper, longer atrophy starts revealing the underlying facial muscles. In Grade 3, there is wider, deeper atrophy with the muscles clearly showing. Wide lipoatrophy extending up toward the orbital rims is seen in Grade 4, with skin directly on muscles and the bony skeleton clearly visible. The James Facial Lipoatrophy Scale is another similar scale that grades atrophy from mild to severe [14].

It is also important to note that salivary gland enlargement, particularly parotid, can occur in 1–10% HIV patients and may complicate the presentation. While it often occurs early on during HIV infection, it may occur with inadequate HAART treatment and confound one's assessment of facial aesthetics [15]. It can be bilateral and may or may not be associated with xerostomia. Parotid enlargement is often due to benign lymphoepithelial cysts.

HAART-associated lipodystrophy is often accompanied by metabolic lipid dysregulation [16]. A total of 44% have insulin resistance, 5% have diabetes, 38% hypertriglyceridemia, and 11% hypercholesterolemia. HAART can also increase the risk of developing hypertension, cardiovascular disease, and renal dysfunction [17]. Because of this, plastic surgeons must engage the patient's primary care physician to provide a multidisciplinary treatment strategy and preoperative optimization that includes blood testing, pharmacological intervention, dietary plan, and exercise regimen.

The Center for Disease Control has established that transmission of HIV is extremely rare in healthcare setting, and the risk is effectively nonexistent in patients with undetectable viral loads. However, proper sterilization procedures are still required. HIV, without AIDS, also does not affect surgical wound healing. While patients may present with aesthetic challenges, they are often healthy and safe to undergo surgery. Regardless, medical clearances, blood pressure, and glucose control, in addition to lab tests, HIV load, and T-cell counts, may be necessary.

4.3 Treatment

4.3.1 Medical Treatment, Exercise, and Therapy

A physically active lifestyle also has a protective effect on the development and recurrence of HAART-related lipodystrophy [17]. Intra- and extra-oral muscle contraction and stretching maneuvers can improve buccinator muscle volume and may be an option for patients with recurrent or persistent volume loss despite treatment or ones who cannot undergo other treatments. Such maneuvers are not helpful in augmenting zygomaticus and masseteric muscles [18].

Pharmacological strategies to prevent lipore-distribution have been generally ineffective. Cessation of thymidine-based nucleoside analogues can produce modest and very slow improvement of atrophy [6, 19–21]. Appetite stimulants such as megestrol acetate and dronabinol are options for rare patients with lipoatrophy and low caloric intake.

Human growth hormone naturally activates protein production in muscle cells and the release of energy from fats. The US Food and Drug Administration (FDA) approved recombinant growth hormone (rhGH), Serostim (somatotropin), in 1996 for the treatment of HAART-related fat redistribution. In one study [22], 5 mg subcutaneous treatments given daily for 6 months resulted in improvement in cheek soft tissue thickness by 19% in patients with moderate to severe facial lipoatrophy. The effect was sustained for at least 6 months after drug cessation. In randomized, placebo-controlled studies, rhGH significantly decreased abdominal fat, and improved both lean body mass and total body weight by approximately 3 kg each. In one meta-analysis, rhGH was found to have similar efficacy to anabolic steroids and testosterone in treating wasting, but rhGH was also associated with significant improvements in physical endurance, oxygen carrying capacity, and quality of life [23–25]. rhGH may also improve CD4 cell counts, a known risk factor for lipodystrophy, in patients on antiretroviral therapy. The treatment however does not appear to offer any survival advantage and is unlikely to help with limb atrophy. Reductions in "buffalo hump" and breast size have also been reported, although breast development in men has been noted as a side effect of rHGH [26]. Some self-limited side effects include diarrhea, arthralgia, myalgia, mastalgia, hyperglycemia, peripheral edema, and hand numbness. Side effects improve on stopping rhGH, but improvements may also reverse and are more likely among individuals with mild lipodystrophy.

4.3.2 Fillers

Many filler agents exist, and when the clinician decides on a treatment regimen, many factors should be considered. The degree and duration of improvement for each treatment option depend on the severity of lipoatrophy and the biophysical properties of each filler. Mild lipoatrophy requires few treatments and has more permanent correction. While fillers are generally safe, the volumes used with HIV patients are quite large placing them at higher risks of immediate and delayed complications. Studies comparing clinical efficacy are limited by injection technique heterogeneity as well as by the lack of valid lipoatrophy assessment tools. Studies often do not include patient ages and duration on HAART, which can confound the results. Studies also typically have 12–18 months, which is insufficient to demonstrate the long-term efficacy and safety, as filler agents may last longer. Natural fillers from autogenic, allogenic, and xenogenic sources are biodegradable and temporary, while synthetic fillers may be partially degradable or nondegradable.

4.3.2.1 Nonpermanent

Collagen, bovine or human, was one of the earliest products approved by the FDA for treatment of rhytids and the first studied for HIV lipoatrophy. It is no longer recommended for HIV lipoatrophy because it is extremely short-lasting (3-4 months) and requires pretreatment intradermal hypersensitivity screening (usually two tests four weeks apart) [27]. Hyaluronic acid, a naturally occurring polysaccharide, is less immunogenic and comes in various viscosities to improve stability and longevity when compared with collagen [28]. High-density hyaluronic is a safe option that provides immediate aesthetic improvement and soft tissue augmentation with high patient satisfaction and a sustained longevity of 12 months [29, 30]. Increased total skin thickness of >10 mm was noted on sonography in 60% patients at 1 year [31]. Midface injections can be performed using depot, fanning, and "smile-and-fill" techniques with a touch-up as needed in 2–4 weeks [11]. Depending on severity, 3–26 cc of hyaluronic acid may be necessary [11]. Injections may be repeated annually. Mild local redness, tenderness, and swelling are common early side effects.

4.3.2.2 Semipermanent

The only fillers specifically approved for HIV lipoatrophy by the FDA are two semipermanent fillers: [1] poly-L-lactic acid (PLLA, Sculptra, Dermik Laboratories, USA) and [2] calcium hydroxylapatite (CaHA, Radiesse, BioForm Medical Inc., USA).

PLLA was approved in August 2004 by the FDA as the first injectable treatment for facial lipoatrophy [14, 32, 33]. It had been already used as a cosmetic filler and filler for HIV atrophy in Europe under the name of New Fill. It is currently the most widely studied filler for HIV lipoatrophy with the most robust evidence (yet still only Grade B recommendation) [17, 34]. PLLA is a synthetic resorbable inert chemical that was previously used in orthopedic fixation devices and injectable drug delivery systems. PLLA causes an inflammatory reaction that leads to fibroblast accumulation, collagen deposition, and subsequent gradual increase in soft tissue volume [35, 36].

Data from the APEX002 and the Blue Pacific Study in the United States were used to get FDA approval [14, 37]. The studies included 97–99 patients who underwent PLLA injections (no more than 2 vials using a 3 cc dilution/vial) about 3–6 weeks apart until correction was obtained, up to 6 sessions. In both studies, patients demonstrated high satisfaction at the end of treatment, at 6 months, and at 12 months. Compared with baseline, when measured by calipers, patients at the end of their treatment demonstrated 65.1% increase in buccal skin thickness, increasing to 68.8% at 6 months and 73% at 12 months [14]. In the Blue Pacific Study, patients needed 3 treatment sessions at minimum (Grade 1), and 4–5 sessions for Grade 2–3 atrophy, with 6 sessions needed for the most severe cases. Two to five retreatments were needed 13 to 21.4 months after initial treatment [32]. More severe lipoatrophy was associated with shorter period to retreatment and greater number of retreatments (Fig. 4.1).

Calcium hydroxylapatite (CaHA, Radiesse, BioForm Medical Inc., USA) is safe, immediate, and long-lasting with high patient satisfaction [38]. CaHA is the most common mineral in bone. It was the second filler to be FDA-approved for HIV lipoatrophy. CaHA microspheres are delivered in a water-based gel that is slowly absorbed after injection, leaving behind a structure to support fibroblast growth [39]. In a prospective, open-label study of 100 subjects over three sites, all subjects noted improvement at 12 months, but 10% perceived return to baseline by 18 months. Most patients needed 3 injections over a 6-month period with an average volume of 8.4 cc (2.0–20.4 cc) [38].

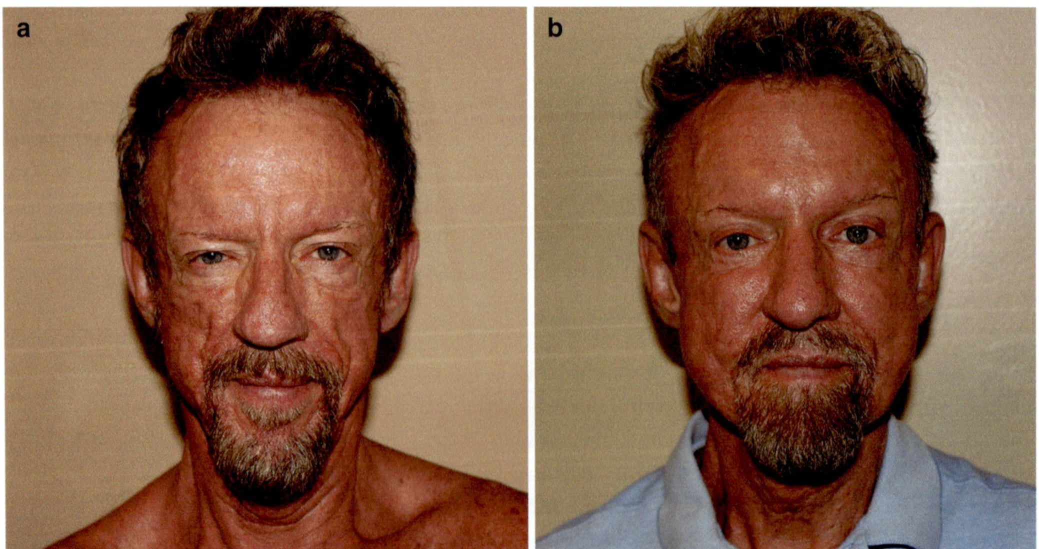

Fig. 4.1 Patient with HIV facial lipoatrophy and history of parotidectomy (**a**) treated with multiple filler injections (**b**)

4.3.2.3 Permanent

Polymethylmethacrylate (PMMA), while biocompatible and found in many medical devices, in its filler form (Bellafill, previously Atefill, Artes Medical Inc., USA), is suspended in bovine collagen that is immunogenic and requires pretesting [27]. As the collagen dissolves over 3 months, PMMA lays foundation for new collagen formation [35]. It is the only FDA-approved permanent filler. Increases in cheek thickness as seen on ultrasound are maintained for up to 5 years. Patients with severe lipoatrophy may still need repeat injections in 1–2 years, and delayed nodules may appear after 2–5 years [40].

Polyacrylamide hydrogel (Aquamid, PAAG) contains 2.5% cross-linked polymer made of biocompatible acrylamide and 97.5% water. After being injected, it stays in the tissues by forming a surrounding capsule. It can be safely removed by skin puncture or manual pressure [41]. Aquamid, while not FDA approved for use in the United States, can safely provide a significant increase in cheek soft tissue thickness with improved aesthetic result and patient satisfaction. Studies found it to be equally as effective as fat and PLLA at 2 years [42], but more so at 4 years [43]. It may be injected in multiple 1 cc monthly sessions until adequate correction is obtained [44]. Alternatively, attempts to correct the deformity in a single megafilling session (with further touch-ups) have been found to be quicker and safe [45]. On average, patients need 8-9 cc [34, 45]. Polyalkylimide hydrogel (Bio-Alcamid) is similar, but is made of 4% alkylimide amides, and on average requires 12-20 cc for adequate correction [46].

Although permanent products offer safe long-term solutions with lower overall cost, serious complications, when they do occur, are also long-lasting. Strict aseptic technique is crucial, and prophylactic antibiotics should be considered prior to dental procedures. While local infection, product migration, and foreign body reactions are extremely rare, small palpable permanent nonvisible nodules due to overfilling may be seen in one out of every 3–4 patients [47]. Rare, massive hemi-facial temporary edema has been reported after surgical removal of such nodules [48].

While the use of highly purified silicone oil has been described in treatment of HIV lipodystrophy [49], this is highly controversial and should not be attempted outside the context of a rigorous IRB-approved study.

4.3.3 Lipofilling

Lipofilling provides consistent long-term results, like permanent fillers, but without being immunogenic or generating a foreign body reaction. While volume and number of sessions are variable, lipofilling may offer better facial rehabilitation because surgeons can be more aggressive with fat and fill deeper than with permanent fillers [50] and it can be combined with a facelift (Figs. 4.2 and 4.3). Despite the need for anesthesia, it is often more cost-effective [51] and allows for global aesthetic improvement as it allows for other body contouring procedures to be performed at the same time (e.g., trunk liposuction) [50]. The Coleman technique is often used in preparing fat graft. Lipofilling is limited by the number of available donor sites. Also, in patients with HAART-related lipodystrophy, fat is often fibrous, of low quality, and is difficult to harvest. While fat is often harvested from abdomen, care has to be taken when harvesting from hypertrophied areas, as lipohypertrophy of grafted tissue has been reported when using hypertrophic donor sites [52]. In addition to subjective patient-reported improvement, studies demonstrated magnetic resonance imaging [53] and ultrasound [52] evidence of increased facial fat using the Coleman technique in HIV atrophy at 6 and 17.5 months by 10–10.5 mm and 5.5 +/−2.4 mm, respectively. Dermis-fat compound graft harvested from the inner arms or abdomen can also be transferred to the malar area through a transoral approach [54, 55]. Significant resorption within the first 3 years can occur in up to 25% of patients requiring multiple repeat attempts [54, 56].

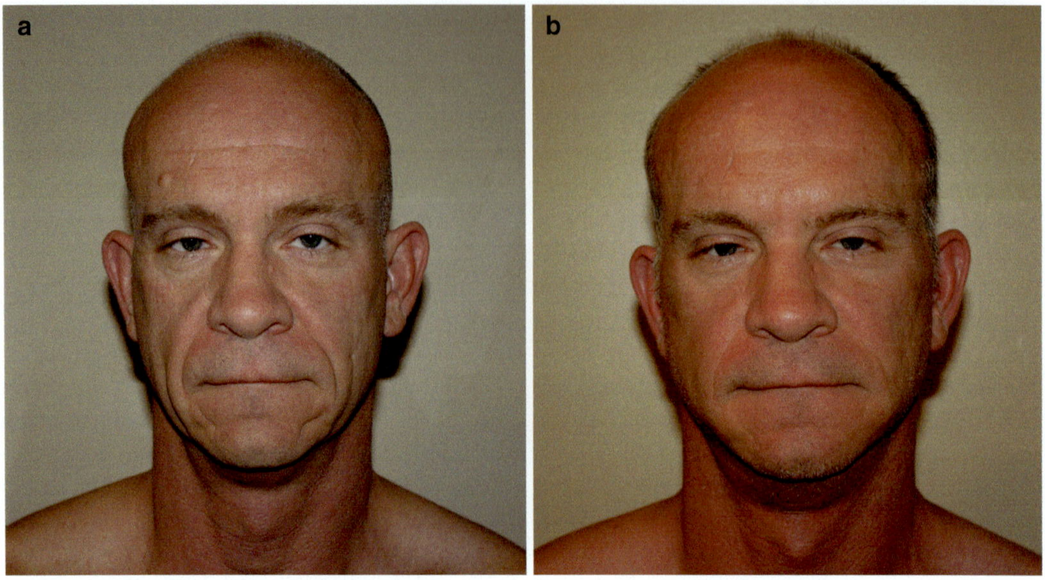

Fig. 4.2 Patient with HIV facial lipoatrophy (**a**) treated with facelift, submental liposuction, and facial fat grafting (**b**)

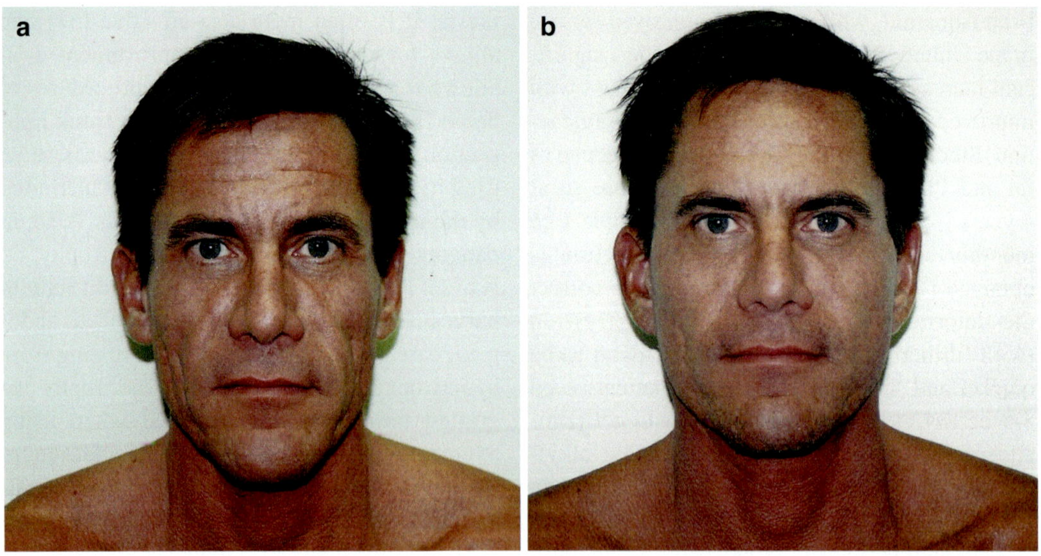

Fig. 4.3 Patient with HIV facial lipoatrophy (**a**) treated with facelift and fat grafting (**b**)

4.3.4 Implants

Submalar augmentation with alloplastic implants can offer permanent, and potentially reversible, correction with natural results [57, 58]. Implants include polymeric silicone, expanded polytetrafluoroethylene (e-PTFE), and porous polyethylene (Medpor) [59]. Implants are placed subperiosteally using a gingivobuccal incision. While the procedure is safe in HIV patients, implants are often costly and carry a risk of infection, displacement, extrusion, and capsular contracture. Infections are likely highest with silicone implants in HIV patients (7.8–9% infection rate) [60]. The procedure can be performed under local anesthesia and sedation, but often requires general anesthesia and is associated with postoperative downtime. With HAART, there is often thinning of the soft tissue envelope that is not adequately addressed with implants alone. Such implants are best reserved for patients interested in bony augmentation, giving them the appearance of higher cheekbones, and who already have an adequate soft tissue envelope. One must be careful not to use large implants in patients with severe lipoatrophy, as it may result in a more gaunt appearance unless treatment is augmented with fillers or fat too.

4.3.5 Truncal and Neck Surgery

Truncal lipodystrophy may present with asymmetric lipohypertrophy, lipoatrophy, and skin excess. This can involve the chest with varying degrees of gynecomastia. An individualized approach is necessary and may include lipectomy and/or liposuction (Fig. 4.4). As with any surgery, it is important to discuss goals and expectation preoperatively with the patients. It is important to educate patients on strategies to preventing fat recurrence or atrophy including dietary modification and exercise.

Treating the neck can be a very satisfying procedure for patients with HIV-related lipodystrophy. Liposuction is an effective treatment for cervicodorsal lipodystrophy [61]. Given the large amount of accumulated fat, the fibrous nature of the fat, and fat recurrence, excisional lipectomy is often necessary (Fig. 4.5) [62]. Cervical pre-platysmal and post-platysmal lipectomy/liposuction with platysmaplasty can be a great contouring technique for patients with anterolateral cervical lipohypertrophy [63[] Care must be taken to prevent seromas and hematomas, which may occur at higher rates in HIV patients than non-HIV patients [63]. Infection risks have not been found to be any higher and can be prevented with prophylactic preoperative antibiotic.

While lipoatrophy is often most distressing in the face, limb lipoatrophy can also occur, most notably in the gluteal area. Gluteal augmentation can be safely performed with intramuscular implants [64, 65] or subcutaneous lipofilling.

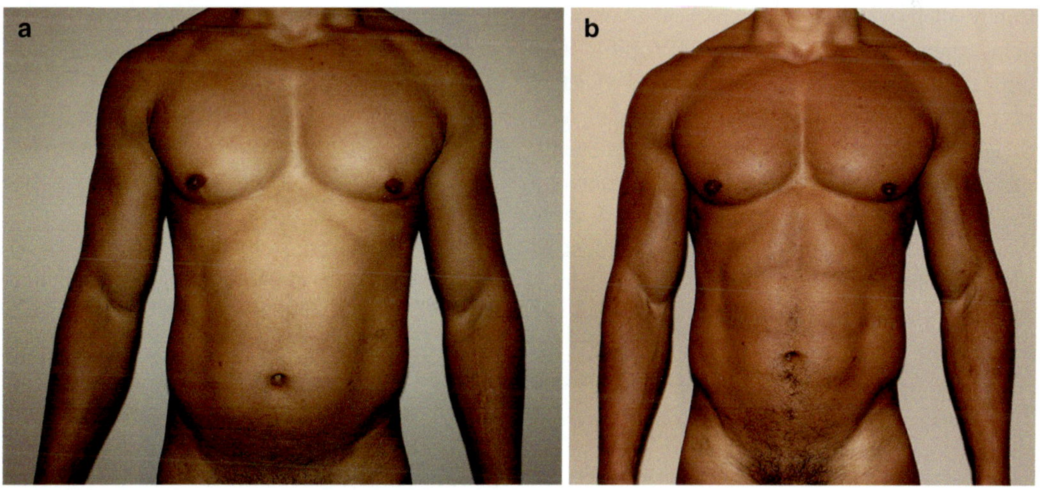

Fig. 4.4 HIV Patient with truncal lipohypertrophy (**a**) treated with liposuction (**b**)

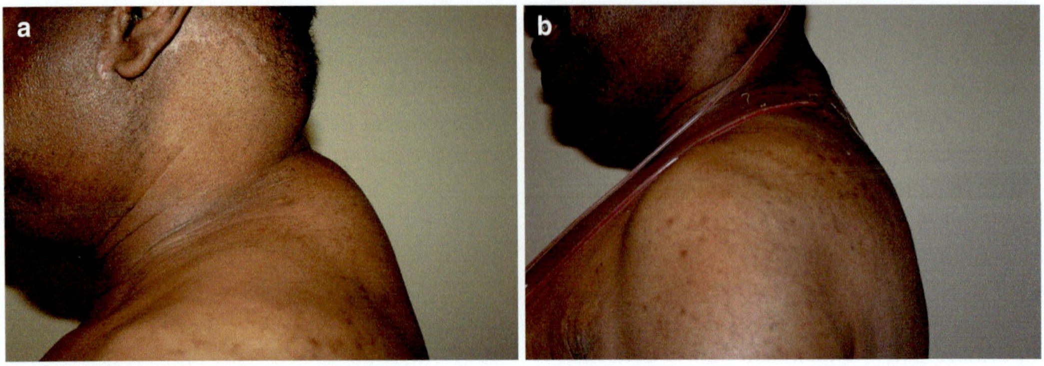

Fig. 4.5 HIV Patient with "buffalo hump" (**a**) treated with open lipectomy (**b**)

4.4 Conclusion

HAART can result in metabolic dysregulation and fat redistribution. The physical effects can adversely affect quality of life and compliance with HAART. Careful evaluation of the HIV patient presenting with liporedistribution is crucial. Treatment is important, often multimodal, and may include dietary modification, pharmacological intervention, surgery, percutaneous filler injections, therapy, and exercise. Since health insurance often does not typically cover treatment of HAART-associated lipodystrophy, such treatment may represent a considerable expense for patients with HIV [66]. It is critical that the surgeon understands and educates his or her patient on the risks and benefits of such treatments. Patients often must weigh the benefits of the treatment on their quality of life against its risks and costs before they can decide if they want to undergo treatment, which treatment to undergo, and if they should consider switching their HIV medications.

References

1. Blanch JRA, Martinez E, et al. Factors associated with severe impact of lipodystrophy on the quality of life of patients infected with HIV-1. Clin Infect Dis. 2004;38:1464–70.
2. Duran S, Saves M, Spire B, et al. Failure to maintain long-term adherence to HAART: the role of lipodystrophy. AIDS. 2001;15:2441–4.
3. Orlando G, Guaraldi G, De Fazio D, Rottino A, Grisotti A, Blini M, et al. Long-term psychometric outcomes of facial lipoatrophy therapy: forty-eight-week observational, nonrandomized study. AIDS Patient Care STDs. 2007;21(11):833–42.
4. Carr A, Workman C, Smith DE, Hoy J, Hudson J, Doong N, et al. Abacavir substitution for nucleoside analogs in patients with HIV lipoatrophy: a randomized trial. JAMA. 2002;288(2):207–15.
5. John M, McKinnon EJ, James IR, Nolan DA, Herrmann SE, Moore CB, et al. Randomized, controlled, 48-week study of switching stavudine and/or protease inhibitors to combivir/abacavir to prevent or reverse lipoatrophy in HIV-infected patients. J Acquir Immune Defic Syndr (1999). 2003;33(1):29–33.
6. Brinkman K, Smeitink JA, Romijn JA, Reiss P. Mitochondrial toxicity induced by nucleoside-analogue reverse-transcriptase inhibitors is a key factor in the pathogenesis of antiretroviral-therapy-related lipodystrophy. Lancet (London, England). 1999;354(9184):1112–5.
7. Gallant JE, Staszewski S, Pozniak AL, DeJesus E, Suleiman JM, Miller MD, et al. Efficacy and safety of tenofovir DF vs stavudine in combination therapy in antiretroviral-naive patients: a 3-year randomized trial. JAMA. 2004;292(2):191–201.
8. Price J, Hoy J, Ridley E, Nyulasi I, Paul E, Woolley I. Changes in the prevalence of lipodystrophy, metabolic syndrome and cardiovascular disease risk in HIV-infected men. Sex Health. 2015;12(3):240–8.
9. Huisin't Veld D, Balestre E, Buyze J, Menten J, Jaquet A, Cooper DA, et al. Determinants of weight evolution among HIV-positive patients initiating antiretroviral treatment in low-resource settings. J Acquir Immune Defic Syndr (1999). 2015;70(2):146–54.
10. Coleman S, Saboeiro A, Sengelmann R. A comparison of lipoatrophy and aging: volume deficits in the face. Aesth Plast Surg. 2009;33(1):14–21.
11. Ho D, Jagdeo J. Safety and efficacy of a volumizing hyaluronic acid filler for treatment of HIV-associated facial lipoatrophy. JAMA Dermatol. 2017;153(1):61–5.

12. Rauso R, Tartaro G, Freda N, Rusciani A, Curinga G. A facial marker in facial wasting rehabilitation. J Drugs Dermatol. 2012;11(2):202–8.
13. Jagdeo J, Ho D, Lo A, Carruthers A. A systematic review of filler agents for aesthetic treatment of HIV facial lipoatrophy (FLA). J Am Acad Dermatol. 2015;73(6):1040–54.e14.
14. Mest DR, Humble G. Safety and efficacy of poly-L-lactic acid injections in persons with HIV-associated lipoatrophy: the US experience. Dermatol Surg. 2006;32(11):1336–45.
15. Sekikawa Y, Hongo I. HIV-associated benign lymphoepithelial cysts of the parotid glands confirmed by HIV-1 p24 antigen immunostaining. BMJ Case Rep. 2017;2017.
16. Guaraldi G, Orlando G, Squillace N, De Santis G, Pedone A, Spaggiari A, et al. Multidisciplinary approach to the treatment of metabolic and morphologic alterations of HIV-related lipodystrophy. HIV Clin Trials. 2006;7(3):97–106.
17. Segatto AF, Freitas Junior IF, Santos VR, Alves KC, Barbosa DA, Portelinha Filho AM, et al. Lipodystrophy in HIV/AIDS patients with different levels of physical activity while on antiretroviral therapy. Rev Soc Bras Med Trop. 2011;44(4):420–4.
18. Gabana-Silveira JC, Mangilli LD, Sassi FC, Braga AF, Andrade CR. Adolescents with HIV and facial lipoatrophy: response to facial stimulation. Clinics (Sao Paulo, Brazil). 2014;69(8):574–8.
19. Carr A. HIV protease inhibitor-related lipodystrophy syndrome. Clin Infect Dis. 2000;30(Suppl 2):S135–42.
20. Carr A, Law M. An objective lipodystrophy severity grading scale derived from the lipodystrophy case definition score. J Acquir Immune Defic Syndr (1999). 2003;33(5):571–6.
21. Carey D, Liew S, Emery S. Restorative interventions for HIV facial lipoatrophy. AIDS Rev. 2008;10(2):116–24.
22. Honda M, Yogi A, Ishizuka N, Genka I, Gatanaga H, Teruya K, et al. Effectiveness of subcutaneous growth hormone in HIV-1 patients with moderate to severe facial lipoatrophy. Intern Med (Tokyo, Japan). 2007;46(7):359–62.
23. Moyle GJ, Schoelles K, Fahrbach K, Frame D, James K, Scheye R, et al. Efficacy of selected treatments of HIV wasting: a systematic review and meta-analysis. J Acquir Immune Defic Syndr (1999). 2004;37 Suppl 5:S262–76.
24. Esposito JG, Thomas SG, Kingdon L, Ezzat S. Growth hormone treatment improves peripheral muscle oxygen extraction-utilization during exercise in patients with human immunodeficiency virus-associated wasting: a randomized controlled trial. J Clin Endocrinol Metab. 2004;89(10):5124–31.
25. Evans WJ, Kotler DP, Staszewski S, Griffin GE, Isgaard J, Gertner JM, et al. Effect of recombinant human growth hormone on exercise capacity in patients with HIV-associated wasting on HAART. AIDS Read. 2005;15(6):301–3, 6–8, 10, 14.
26. Torres RA, Unger KW, Cadman JA, Kassous JY. Recombinant human growth hormone improves truncal adiposity and 'buffalo humps' in HIV-positive patients on HAART. AIDS. 1999;13(17):2479–81.
27. Elson ML. The role of skin testing in the use of collagen injectable materials. J Dermatol Surg Oncol. 1989;15(3):301–3.
28. Narins RS, Brandt F, Leyden J, Lorenc ZP, Rubin M, Smith S. A randomized, double-blind, multicenter comparison of the efficacy and tolerability of Restylane versus Zyplast for the correction of nasolabial folds. Dermatol Surg. 2003;29(6):588–95.
29. Pignatti M, Pedone A, Baccarani A, Guaraldi G, Orlando G, Lombardi M, et al. High-density hyaluronic acid for the treatment of HIV-related facial lipoatrophy. Aesth Plast Surg. 2012;36(1):180–5.
30. Bechara FG, Gambichler T, Brockmeyer NH, Sand M, Altmeyer P, Hoffmann K. Hyaluronic acid new formulation: experience in HIV-associated facial lipoatrophy. Dermatology (Basel, Switzerland). 2008;217(3):244–9.
31. Bugge H, Negaard A, Skeie L, Bergersen B. Hyaluronic acid treatment of facial fat atrophy in HIV-positive patients. HIV Med. 2007;8(8):475–82.
32. Mest DR, Humble GM. Retreatment with injectable poly-l-lactic acid for HIV-associated facial lipoatrophy: 24-month extension of the Blue Pacific study. Dermatol Surg. 2009;35(Suppl 1):350–9.
33. Mest DR, Humble GM. Duration of correction for human immunodeficiency virus-associated lipoatrophy after retreatment with injectable poly-L-lactic acid. Aesth Plast Surg. 2009;33(4):654–6.
34. Mansor S, Breiting VB, Dahlstrom K, Andersen AB, Andersen O, Christensen LH. Polyacrylamide gel treatment of antiretroviral therapy-induced facial lipoatrophy in HIV patients. Aesth Plast Surg. 2011;35(5):709–16.
35. Lemperle G, Morhenn V, Charrier U. Human histology and persistence of various injectable filler substances for soft tissue augmentation. Aesth Plast Surg. 2003;27(5):354–66; discussion 67.
36. Gogolewski S, Jovanovic M, Perren SM, Dillon JG, Hughes MK. Tissue response and in vivo degradation of selected polyhydroxyacids: polylactides (PLA), poly (3-hydroxybutyrate) (PHB), and poly (3-hydroxybutyrate-co-3-hydroxyvalerate) (PHB/VA). J Biomed Mater Res. 1993;27(9):1135–48.
37. Barton SE, Engelhard P, Conant M. Poly-L-lactic acid for treating HIV-associated facial lipoatrophy: a review of the clinical studies. Int J STD AIDS. 2006;17(7):429–35.
38. Silvers SL, Eviatar JA, Echavez MI, Pappas AL. Prospective, open-label, 18-month trial of calcium hydroxylapatite (Radiesse) for facial soft-tissue augmentation in patients with human immunodeficiency virus-associated lipoatrophy: one-year durability. Plast Reconstr Surg. 2006;118(3 Suppl):34s–45s.
39. Marmur ES, Phelps R, Goldberg DJ. Clinical, histologic and electron microscopic findings after injection

of a calcium hydroxylapatite filler. J Cosmet Laser Ther. 2004;6(4):223–6.
40. Cohen SR, Berner CF, Busso M, Gleason MC, Hamilton D, Holmes RE, et al. ArteFill: a long-lasting injectable wrinkle filler material--summary of the U.S. Food and Drug Administration trials and a progress report on 4- to 5-year outcomes. Plast Reconstr Surg. 2006;118(3 Suppl):64s–76s.
41. Nicolau PJ. Long-lasting and permanent fillers: biomaterial influence over host tissue response. Plast Reconstr Surg. 2007;119(7):2271–86.
42. Guaraldi G, Orlando G, De Fazio D, De Lorenzi I, Rottino A, De Santis G, et al. Comparison of three different interventions for the correction of HIV-associated facial lipoatrophy: a prospective study. Antivir Ther. 2005;10(6):753–9.
43. Negredo E, Higueras C, Adell X, Martinez JC, Martinez E, Puig J, et al. Reconstructive treatment for antiretroviral-associated facial lipoatrophy: a prospective study comparing autologous fat and synthetic substances. AIDS Patient Care STDs. 2006;20(12):829–37.
44. De Santis G, Pignatti M, Baccarani A, Pedone A, Spaggiari A, Orlando G, et al. Long-term efficacy and safety of polyacrylamide hydrogel injection in the treatment of human immunodeficiency virus-related facial lipoatrophy: a 5-year follow-up. Plast Reconstr Surg. 2012;129(1):101–9.
45. Rauso R, Gherardini G, Parlato V, Amore R, Tartaro G. Polyacrylamide gel for facial wasting rehabilitation: how many milliliters per session? Aesth Plast Surg. 2012;36(1):174–9.
46. Loutfy MR, Raboud JM, Antoniou T, Kovacs C, Shen S, Halpenny R, et al. Immediate versus delayed polyalkylimide gel injections to correct facial lipoatrophy in HIV-positive patients. AIDS. 2007;21(9):1147–55.
47. Rauso R. 5-year study of a polyacrylamide hydrogel-based filler for rehabilitation of HIV-related facial lipoatrophy. Aesthet Surg J. 2015;35(8):1021–9.
48. Zeltzer AA, Craggs B, Van Thielen J, Hendrickx B, Seidenstuecker K, Hamdi M. Massive hemi-facial Edema after permanent filler removal in an HIV-positive patient. Precautions and patient information. Aesth Plast Surg. 2015;39(3):425–7.
49. Jones DH, Carruthers A, Orentreich D, Brody HJ, Lai MY, Azen S, et al. Highly purified 1000-cSt silicone oil for treatment of human immunodeficiency virus-associated facial lipoatrophy: an open pilot trial. Dermatol Surg. 2004;30(10):1279–86.
50. Rauso R, Curinga G, Santillo V, Corvo G, Tartaro G. Comparison between lipofilling and a non-absorbable filler for facial wasting rehabilitation in HIV-positive patients. J Craniofac Surg. 2011;22(5):1684–8.
51. Vallejo A, Garcia-Ruano AA, Pinilla C, Castellano M, Deleyto E, Perez-Cano R. Comparing efficacy and costs of four facial fillers in human immunodeficiency virus-associated lipodystrophy: a clinical trial. Plast Reconstr Surg. 2018;141(3):613–23.
52. Guaraldi G, De Fazio D, Orlando G, Murri R, Wu A, Guaraldi P, et al. Facial lipohypertrophy in HIV-infected subjects who underwent autologous fat tissue transplantation. Clin Infect Dis. 2005;40(2):e13–5.
53. Levan P, Nguyen TH, Lallemand F, Mazetier L, Mimoun M, Rozenbaum W, et al. Correction of facial lipoatrophy in HIV-infected patients on highly active antiretroviral therapy by injection of autologous fatty tissue. AIDS. 2002;16(14):1985–7.
54. Martins de Carvalho F, Casal D, Bexiga J, Sousa J, Martins J, Teofilo E, et al. HIV-associated facial lipodystrophy: experience of a tertiary referral Center with fat and dermis-fat compound graft transfer. Eplasty. 2016;16:e31.
55. Strauch B, Baum T, Robbins N. Treatment of human immunodeficiency virus-associated lipodystrophy with dermafat graft transfer to the malar area. Plast Reconstr Surg 2004;113 (1):363–70; discussion 71–2.
56. Domergue S, Psomas C, Yachouh J, Lesnik A, Reynes J, Goudot P, et al. Fat microinfiltration autografting for facial restructuring in HIV patients. J Cranio-Maxillo-Facial Surg. 2006;34(8):484–8.
57. Claude O, Domergue Than Trong E, Blanc R, Ascher B, Bagot M, Meningaud JP, et al. Treatment of HIV facial lipoatrophy with a submalar porous polyethylene implant (Medpor). Annales de chirurgie plastique et esthetique. 2009;54(1):21–8.
58. Burres S. Midface volume replacement with a transmaxillary implant. Aesth Plast Surg. 2005;29(1):1–4; discussion 5.
59. Romo T 3rd, Baskin JZ, Sclafani AP. Augmentation of the cheeks, chin and pre-jowl sulcus, and nasolabial folds. Facial plastic surgery : FPS. 2001;17(1):67–78.
60. Binder WJ, Kamer FM, Parkes ML. Mentoplasty--a clinical analysis of alloplastic implants. Laryngoscope. 1981;91(3):383–91.
61. Onesti MG, Fioramonti P, Carella S, Spinelli G, Scuderi N. Nd:YAG laser-assisted liposuction for an HIV patient. Aesth Plast Surg. 2010;34(4):528–30.
62. Warren AG, Borud LJ. Excisional lipectomy for HIV-associated cervicodorsal lipodystrophy. Aesthet Surg J. 2008;28(2):147–52.
63. Ion L, Raveendran SS. Open neck lipectomy for patients with HIV-related cervical lipohypertrophy. Aesth Plast Surg. 2011;35(6):953–9.
64. Andrade GA, Coltro PS, Barros ME, Muller Neto BF, Lima RV, Farina JA Jr. Gluteal augmentation with intramuscular implants in patients with human immunodeficiency virus with lipoatrophy related to the use of antiretroviral therapy. Ann Plast Surg. 2017;79(5):426–9.
65. Benito-Ruiz J, Fontdevila J, Manzano M, Serra-Renom JM. Hip and buttock implants to enhance the feminine contour for patients with HIV. Aesth Plast Surg. 2006;30(1):98–103.
66. Hornberger J, Rajagopalan R, Shewade A, Loutfy MR. Cost consequences of HIV-associated lipoatrophy. AIDS Care. 2009;21(5):664–71.

Asian Male Aesthetic Ideals

5

Walter J. Joseph and Clyde Ishii

5.1 Introduction

The US population is predicted to increase by 50% between the years 1995 and 2050, with 90% of this growth projected to occur within the ethnic demographic, including Asian communities [1]. Asian Americans represent the second fastest growing ethnic group within the USA, behind the Hispanic population. In turn, it has been estimated that the percentage of Asian Americans requesting cosmetic procedures has increased by greater than 200% in recent years and is only projected to increase further over time. The proportion of Asian males seeking treatment has increased in conjunction with these trends, from 12% in 2005–2009 to 19% in 2010–2014 [2]. As such, it is of great importance for the plastic surgeon to garner a thorough understanding of the history of Asian aesthetics, the aging Asian male face, and Asian aesthetic ideals in order to deliver successful and optimal outcomes to our Asian male patients

W. J. Joseph (✉)
Private Practice, Beverly Hills, CA, USA
e-mail: drjoseph@leifrogersmd.com

C. Ishii
Department of Surgery, University of Hawaii John A. Burns School of Medicine, Honolulu, HI, USA
e-mail: cishii@ishiiplasticsurgery.com

5.2 History

Interestingly, much of Asia's history was predominated by isolation from the West. It was not until 1853—after nearly 250 years of isolation during the Tokugawa Period—that Japan reopened its ports at Tokyo Bay to American influence, led by the ships of Commodore Matthew Perry. The societal role of Asian women prior to this time was largely limited to that of the housewife. However, with this Westernization in the 1850s, women began leaving their homes to work in industry, schools, and hospitals [3].

This public exposure began to empower Asian women, who typically were subservient to their male counterparts, allowing things like beauty and aesthetics to come to the forefront of female interest. M. Mikamo, a Japanese surgeon, capitalized on this new focus on physical attractiveness, and, in 1896, published the first case of Asian double-eyelid surgery [3]. Contrary to popular belief, Mikamo's medical journals do not emphasize a "Westernization" of the Asian eyelid; rather, he describes an effect to enhance the Japanese aesthetic [3, 4]. Needless to say, with a greater Asian female interest in aesthetic surgery, Asian men, too, began to pursue surgical aesthetic enhancement across the continent, including both Korea and China. However, it was not until the twentieth century that Asian aesthetic surgery shifted from enhancing the Asian

K. Jeffords et al. (eds.), *Aesthetic Surgery for Men*, https://doi.org/10.1007/978-3-032-03840-1_5

aesthetic toward the goal of creating features inspired by Caucasian ideals [5].

5.3 Skin

As plastic surgeons, the skin is our canvas. In order to deliver superb cosmetic outcomes to the Asian male patient, one must have a strong foundation of understanding regarding Asian skin and its unique properties. In general, Asian skin ranges in Fitzpatrick skin types III–V. Eastern Asians tend to be slightly fairer skinned (III–IV), whereas South Asians (Indian, Pakistani) can be type V. Histologically, despite Asian skin being a darker complexion than Caucasian skin, the number of melanocytes is nearly the same across ethnicities. Rather, it is the greater number of melanosomes and therefore greater production of melanin from melanocytes that confers the skin pigment [6]. In addition, photoprotection is a result of the more densely present melanin found in Asian skin. It has also been shown that Asian skin has a thicker dermis than Caucasian skin as well as a greater abundance of collagen. A consequence of greater collagen density is the tendency for Asian skin to mount a more vigorous fibroblastic response during wound healing, which may result in hypertrophic scarring and prolonged redness during scar maturation, seen across the spectrum of Asian skin types [6–8].

It is thought that because of the thickness and complexion of Asian skin, ablative modalities for skin treatments—such as CO_2 laser resurfacing, medium to deep chemical peeling, and dermabrasion—have been wrought with undesirable side effects leading to a prolonged recovery [7]. These effects include either hyper- or hypopigmentation, erythema, and scarring. However, that is not to say that these treatments are never indicated in Asian skin. Rather, ablative therapies in Asian skin should be performed more conservatively and to localized areas of concern, after having obtained a thorough informed consent.

More common and successful in Asian skin are nonablative skin treatments, which target particular chromophores in the skin rather than entirely effacing the epidermis. In particular, Q-switched lasers (Nd:YAG and KTP) have demonstrated good success in evening pigmentation in Asian skin, with shorter down times than those seen with CO_2 lasering. Intense pulsed light (IPL) has also been shown to be successful among the Asian population; however, IPL may require more treatment sessions than targeted Q-switched lasering to demonstrate the same benefit. Lastly, lighter chemical peels (15 to 35% TCA, Jessner's solution, or glycolic acid) can be used in combination or separately from nonablative therapy for maximal improvement in cutaneous dyschromias and finer wrinkles.

5.4 Facial Aging

It has been well documented in the literature that those with a higher grade (III-V) Fitzpatrick skin type tend to have a later onset of aging than those with a lower grade (I–II). This paradigm particularly holds true when juxtaposing Asian and Caucasian skin types. The naturally darker pigment seen in Asian skin, along with a greater dermal thickness as described above, seems to thwart the aging process [9]. This is particularly evident when men were asked to rate various features of their aging faces. On average, the onset of facial rhytids occurred 10–20 years earlier for Caucasian men than Asian men. This included forehead lines, nasolabial folds, crow's feet, glabellar lines, and oral commissures [10].

Despite the later *onset* of aging in the Asian male, the *velocity and severity* of aging AFTER onset appear to also vary between Asian and Caucasian males [11]. In general, the Asian male upper face tends to age more slowly, especially when compared to Caucasian counterparts. Interestingly, one area of exception appears to be the forehead. Although transverse rhytids in Asian men have a much later onset than Caucasian men (see above), this facial feature tends to be more pronounced and severe than Caucasian men of similar age [5]. In contrast, the vertical rhytids of the glabella region in Asian males are less pronounced than Caucasians. As for the lower face, the aging process tends to be comparable between Asian and Caucasian men, with somewhat more severe evidence of aging in Asians when examining the nasolabial folds and the marionette lines.

As described above, naturally darker complexion in Asians renders the face less susceptible to the damaging effects of UV rays. As such, the fine rhytids associated with aging Caucasian skin are less of an issue with Asian men. The darker Asian pigmentation also provides for a more homogeneous complexion, less visible vascularity, and less visible and smaller pores as compared to Caucasians. Asians—and Asian men in particular—are instead more affected by superficial dyschromias, including solar lentigines, melanocytic nevi, ephelides (freckles), nevi of Ota, and melasma.

Table 5.1 Facial skeletal features within the Asian race and correlated soft tissue appearance

Skeletal features in Asians	Related physical appearance in Asians
Increased bitemporal width	Wide forehead
Increased bizygomatic width	Wide midface
Increased intergonial angle	Wide lower face
Retruded forehead	Flat, backward slanted forehead
Retruded orbital rims	Puffy, heavy eyelids
Low nasal bridge with deficient anterior nasal spine	Flat, short nose with retruded collumella
Retruded medial maxilla	Under-eye darkness, central midface concavity, broad nasal width

5.5 Facial Skeleton

The Asian facial skeleton is characterized by a mesocephalic or "medium head" with a wider, shorter vertical height than the Caucasian head which is longer and narrower [1, 5]. The wider appearance to the Asian face is often due to prominent malar eminences and pronounced definition of the zygomaticomaxillary complex. This prominence, in association with a relative deficiency of the maxillary and infraorbital regions, results in shallowness of the mid-facial area [13]. A wide gonial angle combined with prominence of the mandibular angles is often noted in the Asian face—especially in Koreans. These characteristics contribute to a square, flat appearance of the face (Table 5.1).

Despite the "Westernization" of the Asian eyelid with double eyelid blepharoplasty, the opposite trend in terms of the ideal facial shape appears to hold true in the Asian population. More specifically, while Caucasians seek to achieve a "sculpted" and "defined" facial structure with high, defined malar eminences and a sharp jawline, Asians tend to view their natural skeletal structure as "masculine" and seek to soften or smooth their facial contours. This cultural paradox tends to hold truer for Asian females than Asian males. However, with the recent surge in the "KPop" phenomenon in Korea and across much of Asia, male Asian pop-stars are depicted in the media with smoother, more effeminate facial contours, influencing some Asian men to seek skeletal reduction surgery, including malar reduction and mandibular reduction surgeries [9]. Although this particular "ideal" certainly encompasses a cultural subset of Asian men, this does not apply to all men across the Asian ethnicity. Therefore, it is of paramount importance to clearly elicit the goals of the Asian male patient in terms of facial contouring surgery and the application of non-surgical facial contouring treatments. Some Asian men may seek reductive surgeries for a less-chiseled appearance while others may wish to augment their angular contours for a masculinizing effect [9].

5.6 Eyes

See Chap. 13 on Asian blepharoplasty.

5.7 Nose

The Asian nose is characterized by a low radix, low dorsum, weak lower lateral cartilage complexes, columellar retraction, and thick sebaceous skin [12, 14]. In contrast, the Caucasian nose is classically noted to have a more defined and projected tip, a higher dorsum, more defined lower lateral cartilage complexes, a longer columella, and thinner overlying skin. Similar to Asian blepharoplasty, rhinoplasty remains one of the most common aesthetic procedures among Asians and in particular among Asian men, with the overall goal of augmenting the nasal framework to create a more defined and projected nasal dorsum and tip. However, the combination of a weak cartilaginous framework, along with abundance of fibrofatty tissue seen in Asian noses, makes Asian rhinoplasty particularly challenging. Furthermore, although it might be assumed that goals of an Asian rhinoplasty are indicative of a "Westernization" of the nose, it should be noted that in Asian cultures, a high, narrow nasal bridge is desirable and has been described as an aesthetic ideal. Nonetheless, rhinoplasty remains one of the most controversial aesthetic procedures among this particularly ethnic population.

References

1. Sturm-O'Brien AK, Brissett AEA, Brissett AE. Ethnic trends in facial plastic surgery. Facial Plast Surg. 2010;26(2):69–74.
2. Liew S, Wu WT, Chan HH, Ho WW, Kim HJ, Goodman GJ, et al. Consensus on changing trends, attitudes, and concepts of Asian beauty. Aesth Plast Surg. 2016;40(2):193–201.
3. Mikamo M. Mikamo's double-eyelid operation: the advent of Japanese aesthetic surgery. 1896. Plast Reconstr Surg. 1997;99(3):664; discussion -9.
4. Cheng J, Xu FZ. Anatomic microstructure of the upper eyelid in the oriental double eyelid. Plast Reconstr Surg. 2001;107(7):1665–8.
5. Rhee SC. Differences between Caucasian and Asian attractive faces. Skin Res Technol. 2018;24(1):73–9.
6. Chan IL, Cohen S, da Cunha MG, Maluf LC. Characteristics and management of Asian skin. Int J Dermatol. 2019;58(2):131–43.
7. Chao YYY, Chhabra C, Corduff N, Fabi SG, Kerscher M, Lam SCK, et al. PAN-ASIAN CONSENSUS-key recommendations for adapting the world congress of dermatology Consensus on combination treatment with injectable fillers, toxins, and ultrasound devices in Asian patients. J Clin Aesthet Dermatol. 2017;10(8):16–27.
8. Zhu YQ, Xie YH, Liu FH, Guo Q, Shen PP, Tian Y. Systemic analysis on risk factors for breast cancer related lymphedema. Asian Pac J Cancer Prevent. 2014;15(16):6535–41.
9. Flament F, Amar D, Feltin C, Bazin R. Evaluating age-related changes of some facial signs among men of four different ethnic groups. Int J Cosmet Sci. 2018;40(5):502–15.
10. Lam SM. A new paradigm for the aging face. Facial Plast Surg Clin North Am. 2010;18(1):1–6.
11. Rossi AM, Eviatar J, Green JB, Anolik R, Eidelman M, Keaney TC, et al. Signs of facial aging in men in a diverse, multinational study: timing and preventive behaviors. Dermatol Surg. 2017;43(Suppl 2):S210–S20.
12. McCurdy JA, Lam SM. Cosmetic surgery of the Asian face. 2nd ed. New York: Thieme Medical Publishers; 2006.
13. Ira D, Papel M. Facial plastic and reconstructive surgery. 3rd ed. New York: Thieme Medical Publishers; 2009.
14. Li Z, Unger JG, Roostaeian J, Constantine F, Rohrich RJ. Individualized Asian rhinoplasty: a systematic approach to facial balance. Plast Reconstr Surg. 2014;134(1):24e–32e.

Hispanic Aesthetic Ideals

6

Christian L. Stallworth and Jaime R. Garza

6.1 Hispanics in North America

According to the US Census Bureau, the Hispanic population reached 58.9 million people in 2017. Currently, Hispanics comprise 18% of the US population constituting the largest racial or ethnic minority group. And these numbers are only projected to grow with estimates of 111 million people in the USA by 2060 [1]. While people of Hispanic origin were once predominantly living in southern US border states and in historically culturally diverse major metropolitan cities like New York and Miami, population growth and dispersion find their numbers increasing throughout the entire USA. So too will their numbers increase in our practices. More than ever before, surgeons must understand the Hispanic patient and how their ideals, and treatment plan may be the same or unique to other patient populations.

In order to understand the traits that comprise the aesthetic ideal in Hispanic patients, we should first consider the history of the Hispanic people. With Spanish conquest of the north, central, and south Americas in the fifteenth and sixteenth centuries came a co-mingling of races between western European and Native American Indian populations. Further still, the addition of African slaves in the eighteenth century provided further genetic diversity to this population. Thus, while the term "Hispanic" classically refers to descendants of Spanish-speaking countries, the ethnic diversity of these peoples can be argued to be better described as *Mestizo*, or mixed, owing the mergers of the African, Indian, and European populations [2].

Today, Hispanic populations remain extremely heterogeneous and have great variation in their individual racial identification. When compared to all other racial groups, Hispanics demonstrate a greater tendency (2–19%) to identify with more than one racial group [1]. These can draw from numerous individual and combinations of global populations from Mexico, Central and South America, Native American populations, Western European, Caribbean, and Southeast Asian. These identifications are intertwined with an individual's social and economic status, overlap in cultural beliefs and practices, and can also influence aesthetic norms within individual subgroups that identify as Hispanic.

C. L. Stallworth (✉)
Department of Otolaryngology—Head & Neck Surgery, Division of Facial Plastic and Reconstructive Surgery, Long School of Medicine, University of Texas Health Science Cente, San Antonio, TX, USA
e-mail: Stallworth@uthscsa.edu

J. R. Garza
Plastic and Reconstructive Surgery—Medical Arts & Research Center—MARC, San Antonio, TX, USA

K. Jeffords et al. (eds.), *Aesthetic Surgery for Men*, https://doi.org/10.1007/978-3-032-03840-1_6

6.2 Facial Aesthetics in the Hispanic Male

A review of the literature finds sparse and sporadic descriptions of the aesthetic ideals in the Hispanic patient, especially in men. This is likely due to relatively fewer male patients in aesthetic practices, and the historically overwhelming emphasis on Caucasian norms above other races. But it may also stem from the difficulty in defining a singular description for such a diverse population. Mestizo characteristics certainly vary from other ethnic groups, but even demonstrate variability from within the Latino population as well. Here, we highlight a number of traits inherent to the Mestizo population and describe what of these is found to be most attractive in the male patient.

As is true of all human faces, the Mestizo aesthetic ideal is similarly rooted in harmony among facial subunits and proportions. Balance between horizontal facial thirds and vertical fifths remain. However, Mestizo patients tend to exhibit a broader face with more prominent eminences. Owing to their generally thicker skin and underlying bone structure, distinctive frontal, malar, and mandibular prominences are more common and found to be aesthetically pleasing. For the male patient, maintenance and even accentuation of these traits not only help to preserve their ethnicity, but also enhance their masculinity [3]. While the term "machismo"[1] can carry a negative connotation, it actually stems from Spanish and Portuguese cultural pride for self-reliance, strength, honor, and the concept of a man's ability to provide for and protect the well-being of his family. These are important personal and cultural attributes for the Hispanic male [2, 3]. Altering these inherent physical traits or failing to enhance them when deficient can be detrimental to the patient that desires to exhibit these qualities.

Mestizo skin types deserve considerable attention when looking for an aesthetic ideal in male patients. Latino patients have inherently thicker, heavier, and relatively more oily skin than Caucasian patients. The consequence is a soft tissue envelope that is weightier and more difficult to surgically lift and drape. Hispanics are also not bound to a discreet Fitzpatrick skin type. Based on an individual's ancestry, Mestizo skin types can range from lighter Fitzpatrick types 2 and 3 to Fitzpatrick type 5. In general, though, many individuals fall within Fitzpatrick types 3 or 4. Of these, men with lighter skins tones have traditionally been recognized as more attractive. By virtue of having darker skin types, Hispanic patients are more prone to development of post-inflammatory hyperpigmentation (PIH) too. This can arise from any inflammatory instigator including eczema, acne, local trauma, or surgical wounds. And even though some Hispanics may have fairer skin tones, they remain more prone to these pigmentary changes than their Fitzpatrick counterparts from other European ancestry. And like Latino women, Hispanic men are equally susceptible to the development of melasma over time. These pigmentary changes can be isolated to the epidermis, the dermis, or a combination of these layers and treatment should be based on appropriate diagnosis of which case exists. Finally, people with darker skin tones have been known to consider their risk of skin cancer to be less than that of fairer skinned individuals. However, they, too, are equally susceptible to skin malignancies that arise from ultraviolet light exposure. The use of sunscreen should be similarly emphasized in Hispanic men—not only for protection from malignancy but to also protect from the aging effects of UV light. Taken as a whole, maintenance of a uniform, lighter skin complexion without hypo- or hyper-pigmentation is idyllic for Latino males.

There are distinct periocular aesthetics for the Latino male as well. In general, Hispanic men tend to have fuller, darker brows. Together, the

[1] Machismo: (/məˈtʃiːzmoʊ, mɑː-, –ˈtʃɪz–/; Spanish: [maˈtʃismo]; Portuguese: [maˈʃiʒmu]; from Spanish macho "male," and -ismo) [1] is the sense of being "manly" and self-reliant, a concept associated with "a strong sense of masculine pride: an exaggerated masculinity." [2] Machismo is a term originating in the early 1930s and 1940s best defined as having pride in one's masculinity. It is associated with "a man's responsibility to provide for, protect, and defend his family." [3] https://en.m.wikipedia.org/wiki/Machismo

underlying bone structure and heightened skin thickness lend to a full brow and upper lid complex. Eyelid hooding can then result, creating an almond-shaped, more Asian-appearing aperture of the eye [2]. Similar to all individuals, maintenance of native upper lid architecture free of skin laxity and excess skin creates a more rested, youthful appearance. However, caution should be heeded in addressing the upper lid and brow to avoid skeletonization of the orbit. Doing so can yield a more gaunt, feminized appearance that is not optimal for the Hispanic male. The lower lid should also maintain a shortened vertical height with a smooth lid-cheek junction that is supported by upper cheek and malar volume.

Normative measures of lip architecture exist for the Caucasian patient but do not adequately translate to that of the Mestizo patient. While there is relatively little objective data, there is some evidence that, in general, Hispanics have and prefer slightly larger lips. In a study comparing upper and lower lip measures between Mexican-Americans and European-Americans, Mexican-American upper and lower lips were found to respectively protrude 3 mm and 0.6–2.4 mm more than their European-American counterparts. This was thought due not only to variance in skin and soft tissue volume but also due to dental and facial skeletal factors as well. These differences were consistent for both female and male patients [4]. In addition to inherent physical differences in lip size, a study by Heidekrueger [5] demonstrated a preference by Latin-American laypersons and surgeons alike to find larger lips more attractive than any other nationality

One aspect of the Hispanic face that has garnered considerable attention and study is the Mestizo nose [6]. Latin noses can be relatively smaller in comparison to the facial whole. They tend to have shorter nasal bones and a smaller nasal vault, together creating a lower radix and obtuse nasofrontal angle. The upper lateral cartilages tend to be longer and, with the septum, create a predominate cartilaginous dorsal convexity. Tip cartilages are typically thin and weak and burdened beneath a heavy soft tissue envelope. Together with a weaker and more retrused caudal septum, Mestizos tend to have less tip support and a more acute, deeper nasolabial angle. Despite these native attributes, ideal nasal aesthetics in Hispanic males share common objectives held for other male noses—a straight nasal complex that has a narrow pyramid, along with a less prominent nasal hump on profile [7]. Patients and surgeons equally desire a harmonious nose that balances other facial attributes including frontal and mental projection on profile. Even so, maintaining a slightly higher dorsum and wider tip-defining points and base width can ensure Hispanic males continue to reflect their ethnic origins. More than any other facial trait, a thorough understanding of the patient's perception of their own aesthetic ideal in relation to their gender and ethnicity is paramount.

6.3 Conclusion

As with any patient, consultation with the Hispanic male patient is tantamount for a successful treatment outcome. Understanding their concerns, motivations, and aesthetic ideals will only come from a frank discussion of these factors. And while some ideals will hold true across gender and ethnic lines, the surgeon must consider the Hispanic patient's own perceived aesthetic ideals, their goals, and priorities for correction or augmentation, together with their ancestry. These will often be influenced not only by the patient's perceptions and preferences for attractiveness but also by exerted influence of their family and social structure as well. Facial symmetry and a youthful, homogeneous skin complexion will be desired along with a stronger jaw line and wider cheek bones that provide some angulation yet without harshness. A lower, dark, full trichion with slight temporal recession is also preferable. Eyebrow and upper eyelid volume should be maintained, along with an almond-shape eye that is supported by adequate malar volume. And finally, nasal lines should remain smooth, yet define a slightly higher nasal dorsum. The nasal base width should be at or slightly beyond the intercanthal distance and without alar flare. In concert, these attributes will work to create an archetypical beauty in the Hispanic male while preserving masculinity and ethnicity.

References

1. https://www.census.gov/newsroom/facts-for-features/2018/hispanic-heritage-month.html
2. Cobo R. Facial aesthetic surgery with emphasis on rhinoplasty in the Hispanic patient. Curr Opin Otolaryngol Head Neck Surg. 2008;16:369–75.
3. Cobo R, Garcia CA. Aesthetic surgery for the Mestizo/Hispanic patient: special considerations. Facial Plast Surg. 2010;26(2):164–73.
4. Kollipara R, Walker B, Sturgeon A. Lip measurements and preferences in Asians and Hispanics: a brief review. J Clin Aesthet Dermatol. 2017;10(11):19–21.
5. Heidekrueger PI, Szpalski C, Weichman K, et al. Lip attractiveness: a cross-cultural analysis. Aesthet Surg J. 2017;37(7):828–36.
6. Patel AD, Kridel RH. Hispanic-American rhinoplasty. Facial Plast Surg. 2010;26(2):142–53.
7. Cobo R. Nuances with the mestizo tip. Facial Plast Surg. 2012;28:202–12.

Part II

Face

7 African American Male Aesthetic Ideals

Lisa B. Bootstaylor and Sumayah Taliaferro

7.1 Introduction

Historically consistent across different cultures and regions of the world, the concept of a "physically powerful" masculine ideal permeates ancient paintings and sculptures and is evident in our contemporary icons and maverick athletic figs [1, 2]. With social media, easy Internet access, and direct consumer marketing, paired with seductive marketing phrases such as "Brotox," men consumed close to 10% of all cosmetic treatments delivered in the United States [3, 4]. Over 15.6 million surgical and minimally invasive cosmetic procedures were performed in the United States in 2020, and the African American population is the fastest-growing ethnic population receiving cosmetic procedures [5, 6]. African American men with more disposable income and exposure to plastic surgery procedures, like women of color, are increasingly seeking aesthetic procedures and surgery [7, 8]. Men have similar motivating factors as women and seek to restore a more youthful appearance and physique [9, 10]. With a paucity of clinical data on African American men in the aesthetic literature, the importance of managing skin of color (SOC) for an optimized aesthetic outcome is essential. In fact, in a recent survey, 47% of dermatology residents reported that their medical training was inadequate in training them on skin conditions in blacks [11]. These findings highlight the urgent need to expose and train both clinicians and surgeons on a more diverse patient population, especially as the demographic of our country shifts over the upcoming decades. The fundamental principles of aesthetic surgery can create successful outcomes in populations of color. However, the global patient experience must be based on rigorous vetted principles which evolved from ethnic and cultural nuances. With nuanced and culturally sensitive knowledge, the surgeon can develop confidence in managing common issues in skin of color and their unique subset of aesthetic surgery concerns and aesthetic ideals.

Ideal care for skin of color requires the integration of how the basic science of darker skin types impacts the global care and treatment plan for this population. There are myriad morphologic and physiologic differences between Fitzpatrick system 1 and 6 skin types. However, pigmentary distribution difference, an increased number and size of melanocytes, and fibroblast activity and morphology dominate most studies.

Assessing skin color type can be challenging because of variations in skin tone, hue, and pigment [12]. The Fitzpatrick Classification scale, established for photosensitivity measures, is also used by clinicians for skin type classification and

L. B. Bootstaylor (✉)
Dr. Lissa Plastic Surgery, Atlanta, GA, USA

S. Taliaferro
Private Practice, Atlanta, GA, USA

K. Jeffords et al. (eds.), *Aesthetic Surgery for Men*, https://doi.org/10.1007/978-3-032-03840-1_7

the basis of aesthetic treatment plans. The African American population generally ranges from Type IV through Type VI. Type IV often refers to a beige/olive tone; Type V, a brown tone; and Type VI, a very dark brown tone. The Fitzpatrick classification limited to six skin type choices may not be ideal for the more analytical surgeon searching for a way to more accurately stratify patients to obtain predictable and seamless aesthetic results [13]. The Roberts skin classification system is a 4-part serial profile based on a combination of a quantitative and qualitative assessment such as (a) a review of ancestral and clinical history, (b) visual examination, (c) test site reactions, and (d) physical examination of the patient's skin. The Roberts skin classification system is increasingly being used by dermatologists. With the Roberts classification and skin color charts such as the Felix von Luschan chart, surgeons can acquire more relevant clinical data points [14]. Key assessment principles and technique modifications can be incorporated to provide strategies that are specific to the African American male client and help ameliorate the impact of dyschromia, other pathologic entities, and suboptimal scarring [15].

It is well established that the number of melanocytes in different skin types remains relatively constant and is defined by the epidermal melanin unit. Skin pigmentation is dictated by the quantity and distribution of melanin. Melanin exists in two isoforms: dark-brown eumelanin and light pheomelanin, which remains constant between dark and lightly pigmented skin types. Skin complexion and photosensitivity are predominantly determined by the levels of eumelanin in the epidermis [16]. Characteristics of the melanocyte's phenotypic expression of pigment are confounded by the genetic polymorphism of select pigmentation genes [17, 18], and predicting a patient's skin response to procedures based on the patient's skin color can be fraught with disappointment. Despite skin phenotype, early intervention of post-procedure pigmentary irregularities and scarring is the best opportunity to minimize unaesthetic sequelae of procedures. The author's decision-making tree is based on biological data and the author's experience which may help clarify and optimize the management of the African American male patient who seeks aesthetic procedures (Table 7.1).

Table 7.1 African American male rejuvenation timetable

Age	Problem	Treatment (Consider)
20–30 years	Dyschromia Pseudofolliculitis barbae (PBF) Aesthetic concern Hairline protection	Chemical peels Laser hair removal and PBF Rx Gynecomastia and prominent ear surgery Topical agents

30–40 years	Dyschromia
	Maintain assets
	  Jawline
	  Cheeks
	  Aesthetic concern
	  Hairline protection
		Chemical peels
		Fillers
		Gynecomastia
		Liposuction
		Nonsurgical or surgical

40–50 years	Wrinkle reduction Volume loss nasolabial fold, tear trough Skin elasticity Dsychromia (dark circles) Lower lid puffiness Aesthetic concern Hairline protection	Neuromodulators Stimulatory fillers Non-invasive skin tightening Cosmeceuticals Eyelid surgery (transconjunctival) Body contouring surgery Surgical or nonsurgical
50–60 years (midface/temple)	Volume deficient Event wrinkle reduction Aging eyes	All of the above Skin tightening Eyelid surgery
70–80 years	Volume maintenance	All of the above Facial surgery

7.2 The Aging Process

The aging process in men of color varies significantly within ethnicity and significantly compared to age-matched Caucasian men, given the skin pigmentary and cellular difference of the skin [19, 20]. There is at least a decade delay in the visual signs of aging in men of color, which consist of middle and lower face volume deficiency, dyschromia, and hair loss (Table 7.2). A study of self-reported signs of aging in multiple ethnic groups demonstrated reduced signs of aging in African American men compared with other racial ethnic groups, including Asians, Hispanics, and Caucasians [21, 22]. Again, nuances include a later onset of photoaging, a greater focus on uneven pigmentation and volume loss, and a concern for hair loss. African American hair has flat elliptical-shaped hair shafts with curved hair follicles with few elastic bands anchoring hair follicles to the dermis, and thus, hair fragility and sensitivity must be addressed with combination therapy. The thicker, more compact dermis and stratum corneum with more cornified layers create a unique opportunity to use non-invasive rejuvenation techniques to achieve the prolonged youthful appearance desired by African American men [23]. Depending on the age of presentation, monotherapy and/or a combination approach with energy-based devices, neurotoxins, fillers, and cosmeceutical formulations can produce profound results which can be maintained annually by this often-loyal customer base (Table 7.1).

Table 7.2 Optimizing aesthetic outcome in men of color: recognizing different biological baselines

Biological differences	Clinical manifestations
Increased melanin and pigment gene polymorphism	Hyperpigmentation, hypopigmentation
Compact and thicker dermis	Wrinkle resistance
Enhanced fibroblast activity	Hypertrophic scar, keloid formation, hair fragility/sensitivity

7.3 Non-surgical Facial Rejuvenation: Neuromodulation, Fillers, and Lasers

7.3.1 Pre-op Assessment

The common primary request from these patients is to obtain a natural look and a more rested appearance. This population usually leaves it up to the physician to decide on a treatment plan, and they are loyal to the practice and tend to return 1–2 times per year for touch-ups. Patient behavior is influenced by socioeconomic status and/or the level of education. Patient procedure interest and the experience and knowledge of the clinician will influence therapy and treatment selection. Recognizing pre-op procedure dyschromia and aberrant scarring should impact the treatment plan.

7.3.2 Treatment Plan

Treatment strategies for African American men will be influenced by scientific data which suggest that stimulatory fillers such as calcium hydroxyapatite (CaHa) (i.e., Radiesse; Merz Aesthetics, Raleigh, NC) and poly-L-lactic acid (PLLA)) (i.e., Galderma, Fort Worth, TX) injected as supportive and foundational products may last longer and require fewer treatments than their white counterparts [23]. Ideal areas of injection should include the malar eminence, jawline, temporal area, and the tear trough (Fig. 7.1). When injecting fillers in the cheek, attention must be paid to careful placement in order to avoid feminizing the face [24] (Fig. 7.2). Botulinum toxin-A is used for dynamic rhytids (furrows and frowns arising from smiling, laughing, or frowning). Increased doses of neurotoxin are required for thicker procerus and corrugator muscles, and treatment of the frontalis is needed to maintain a preferred flattened brow [25]. As initial treatments, radiofrequency devices with or with microneedling or non-ablative fractional laser resurfacing are often employed because the delivered thermal energy is chromophore inde-

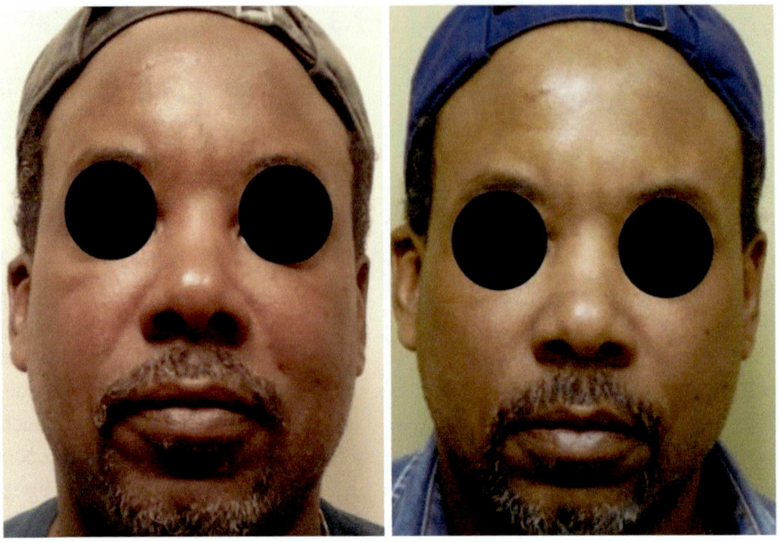

Fig. 7.1 Frontal views of a 48-year-old African American male with descent of the malar eminence and dyschromia who underwent combination therapy over 3 months which consisted of cosmeceuticals, full face radiofrequency, and a semi-permanent filler, Radiesse. Post-procedure results noted at 3 months. Advantage: Non-invasive and avoidance of post-inflammatory hyperpigmentation (PIH). Hyperpigmentation avoidance with linear threading technique

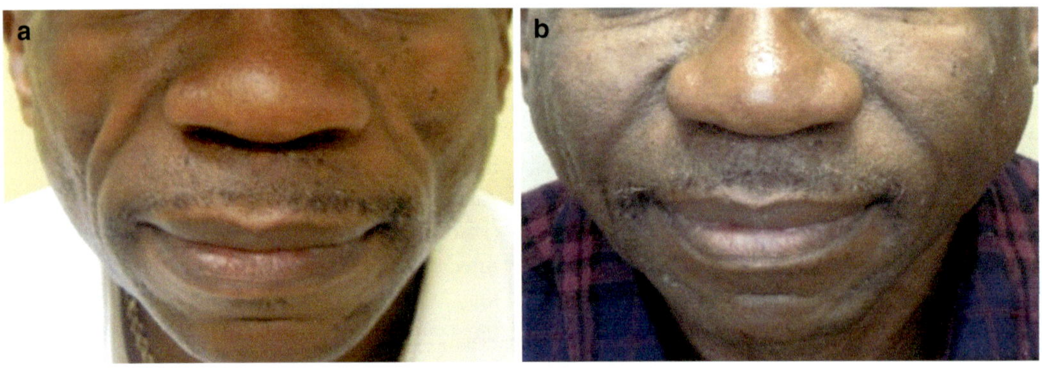

Fig. 7.2 (**a**) Frontal views of a 68-year-old African American male with lipodystrophy who underwent 5 poly-L-lactic acid filler sessions for cheek and lower face restoration. (**b**) Post-procedure results noted at 6 months. Advantage: Stimulatory filler with dermal thickening. Disadvantage: Patient and provider patience over the course of treatment

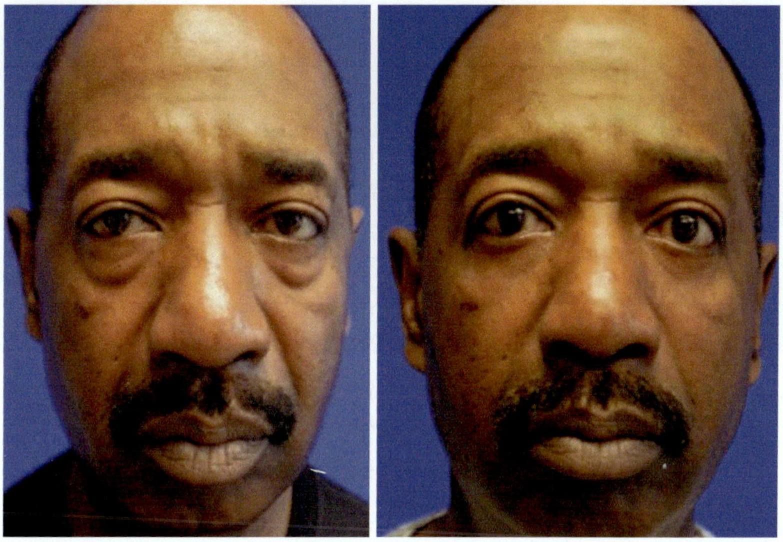

Fig. 7.3 Frontal views of a 65-year-old African American male who underwent a bilateral lower lid blepharoplasty with lateral canthopexy. His lateral cantal position is maintained, and he exhibits improved blending of his lower lid-cheek junction. Post-procedure results are noted at 7 months. Advantage: Subciliary incision tolerated well if required. Disadvantage: Suture removal post-op. Dyschromia avoided by running 6.0 Prolene intracuticular suture used with loops tied at each end for easy removal. (Courtesy: Wright Jones, MD Atlanta, GA)

pendent, and these devices provide excellent safety for use in ethnic skin with little downtime. Post-inflammatory hyperpigmentation (PHI) can be avoided with a slow injection rate and the linear threading techniques [26].

7.4 Body Contouring

7.4.1 Pre-op Assessment

Body contouring rejuvenation is grounded in traditional techniques and treatments tailored to the African American male that are focused on select modifications, which are influenced by cultural differences, geography, and individual aesthetic ideals [27–29]. Although there are a paucity of studies specifically focused on African American men in cosmetic surgery, studies on achieving an attractive aesthetic physique and non-invasive rejuvenating procedures dominate the literature [30, 31]. Popular surgical procedures sought are comparable to the general population in the following order: non-invasive procedures, body contouring surgery, and facial surgery [5, 6] (Fig. 7.3).

7.4.2 Treatment Plan

Liposuction and gynecomastia surgery, both invasive and non-invasive, are the most common procedures sought by African American men. Having similar goals and expectations for body contouring, satisfaction with the results of body contouring is common and associated with a speedy recovery and compliance. Discretion and privacy are paramount in this population when seeking any aesthetic procedure, and well-concealed, small, and muted scars are desired (Figs. 7.4 and 7.5). During the perioperative period, explicit instructions to care providers, early optimized pain management, length of time for garment utilization, and physician extender surveillance are needed to deliver and re-enforce concrete post-op instructions to meet both provider and patient expectations (Fig. 7.6). Tumescent analgesia liposuction with minimum

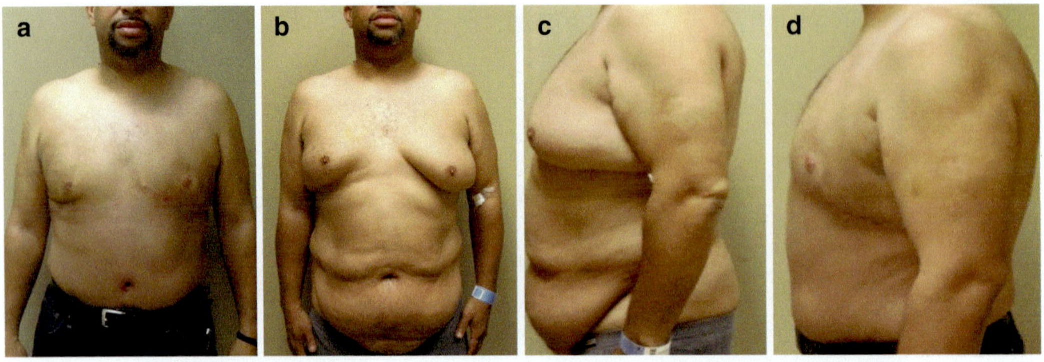

Fig. 7.4 (**a**, **b**) Frontal and lateral views of a 42-year-old male with gynecomastia and panniculitis with a body mass index of 33.5 kg/m^2 who underwent a full lipoabdominoplasty, right breast liposuction, and left breast crescent excision with a free nipple graft under general anesthesia. Pannus weight 4688 grams, and total liposuction aspirate was 3675 cc. (**c**, **d**) Postoperative results are noted at 3 months. Author's Insight: Rely heavily on the thick dermis to decrease the scar burden by substituting liposculpture for optimum results. High tension areas use additional sutures or maneuvers to offset tension to prevent wide and thick scar; intermittent buried vertical mattress 2-0 or 3-0 (Polydioxanone (PDS)) was used. The right breast was treated with liposuction alone

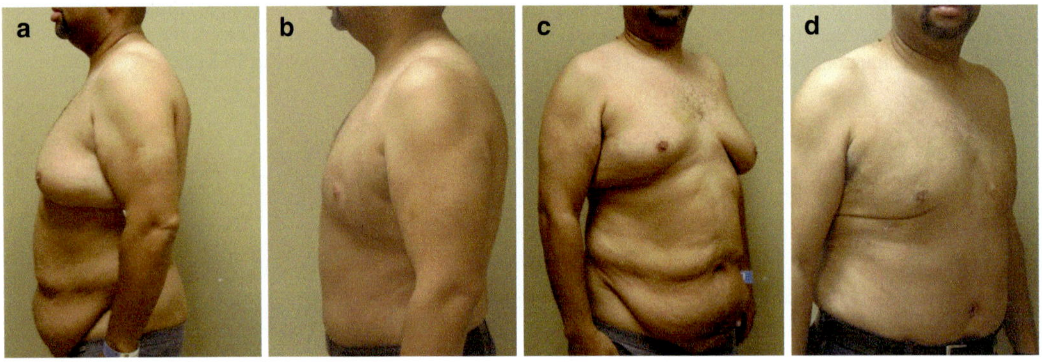

Fig. 7.5 (**a**, **b**) Frontal and right oblique views of a 42-year-old male with gynecomastia and panniculitis with a body mass index of 33.5 kg/m2 who underwent a full lipoabdominoplasty, right breast liposuction, and left breast crescent excision with a free nipple graft. (**c**, **d**) Postoperative results are noted at 3 months. Pre-op notes with multiple surgical options are ideal to reduce the scar burden for the patient

sedation has gained popularity because this technique reduces the intraoperative and postoperative complications associated with general anesthesia. Tumescent analgesia liposuction, also called "awake liposuction" or "twilight liposuction," has other advantages such as increase affordability, patient preference, a higher BMI treatment range and an easier cognitive rebound from sedatives [32, 33]. With careful patient selection, physiologically monitored awake liposuction patients can achieve comparable results to liposuction performed under general anesthesia (Fig. 7.7). Patient self-positioning during the procedure allows for optimum liposculpture of the desired area [34]. Surgeon's satisfaction with this technique requires careful patient selection, identifying and treating the contouring deformity, as well as carefully integrating abdominal etching and skin tightening intraoperative modalities to optimize the overall aesthetic physique of the male (Fig. 7.8). As an additive technique to the liposuction process, abdominal etching requires absolute patient compliance because protracted custom garment use is required. The author's liposuction device of choice is the pulse-assisted microaire device for debulking, followed

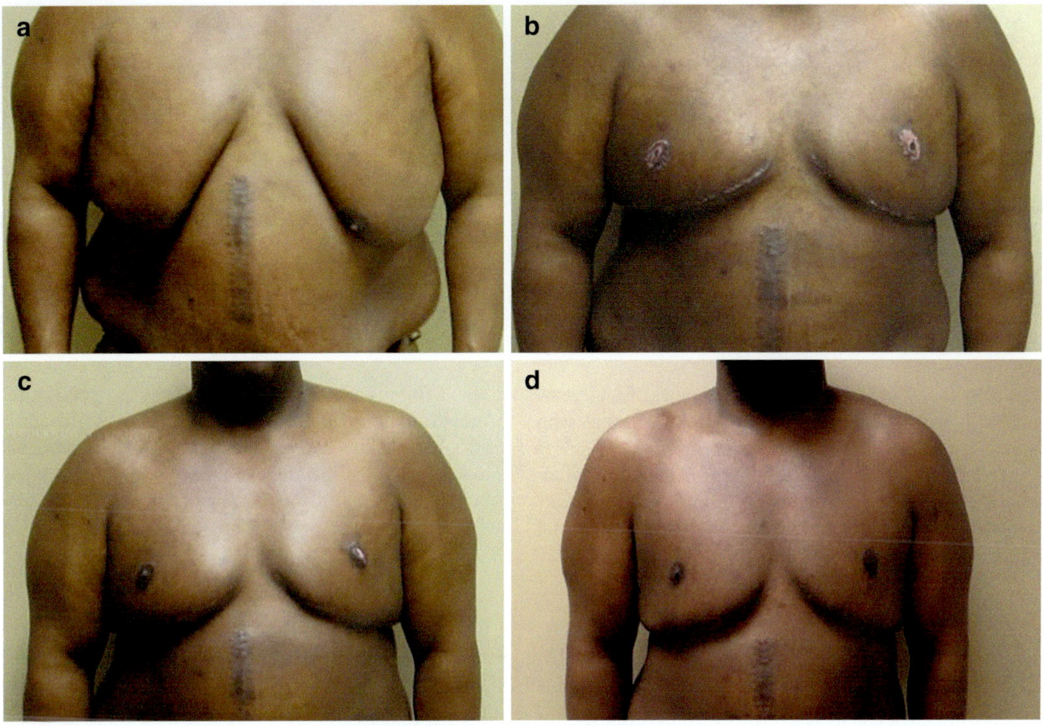

Fig. 7.6 Frontal views of a 38-year-old male with a body mass index of 41. kg/m2, who underwent bariatric surgery and lost 150 lbs., and developed symptomatic gynecomastia-Stage 4. He underwent an en bloc resection of excessive skin and breast tissue using a crescentic transverse incision placed in the inframammary crease. Bilateral free nipple grafts and liposuction of the chest, bra roll, and upper abdomen was also performed. Postoperative results are noted: (1) Pre-op, (2) Post-op: 2 months, (3) at 6 months, and (4) 3 years. Author's Insight: Hypopigmentation of the nipple areolar complex generally resolved within 2 years. Skin retraction of the bilateral breast and chest amenable to an additional 100 pound weight loss

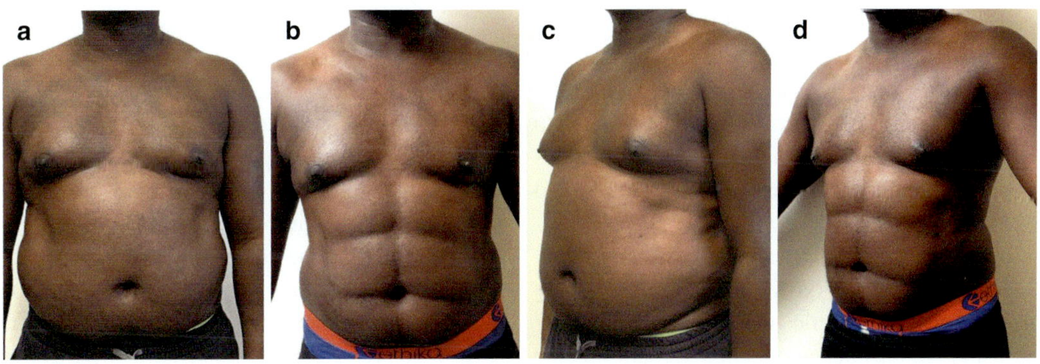

Fig. 7.7 (**a**, **c**) Frontal and left oblique views of a 45-year-old male with a body mass index of 34.1 kg/m2 who underwent chest and trunk liposuction with abdominal etching under local anesthesia using power-assisted liposuction. Total aspirated fat was 4800 ml. (**b**, **d**) Post-procedure results are noted after 3 months of follow-up. Author's Insight: Liposuction alone chosen based on excellent skin quality despite patient's age. Intradermal low-dose Kenalog injections and skin protectors are used to avoid post-inflammatory hyperpigmentation which is more noticeable in skin of color

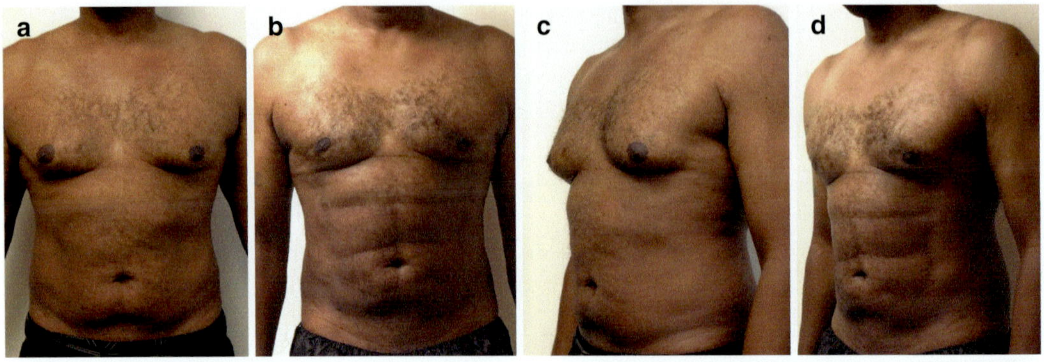

Fig. 7.8 (**a**, **c**) Frontal and left oblique views of a 44-year-old male with a body mass index of 31.2 kg/m2 who underwent chest and flank liposuction with excisional gynecomastia under local anesthesia using ultrasound-assisted liposuction at 70% power followed by power-assisted liposuction and abdominal etching. Total aspirated fat: 1400 ml and breast tissue average weight 21 grams. (**b**, **d**) Postoperative results are noted after 6 months of follow-up. Author's Insight: Skin protectors conceal liposuction entry sites extremely well. Intradermal dermal injection of 2.5 mg of Kenalog per cc; helps mask entry sites. Dermal thickness must be assessed carefully before Kenalog use

by brief laser-assisted liposuction and radiofrequency devices to improve the collagen-tightening process of the skin. Skin protectors are used at all sites to avoid protracted PHI and scar deformities.

7.5 Considerations of Pigmentation

Skin of African descent has been demonstrated to have fibroblasts which are larger, often multinucleated, with closely packed smaller collagen fibers running parallel to the epidermis. These fibroblasts can demonstrate hyperactivity and decreased collagenase enzyme activity thought to produce keloid formation [35] and a higher incidence of keloid formation in this population and skin of color [36, 37].

As the African American male aesthetic population continues to grow, surgeons must stay abreast of the aesthetic interests of this population and the prevalence of skin disorders specific to this racial group. Moreover, the phenotypical presentation of the aesthetic client may not correlate with the pigmentary traits expressed in the post-procedure period. Treatment approaches should take into account basic molecular biological differences which may impact the result. PHI and the unique scarring patterns of the population should be addressed pre-procedure and post-procedure.

7.5.1 Post-Inflammatory Hyperpigmentation (PIH)

Addressing aesthetics in men of color often requires the careful consideration of hyperpigmentation. Thus, this section discusses causes of hyperpigmentation that are relevant in a common evaluation of the male cosmetic patient. Hyperpigmentation is one of the most common concerns among patients of color who visit a skin specialist [38]. Halder et al. reported post-inflammatory hyperpigmentation to be among the top three diagnoses among African Americans in a dermatology clinic [39, 40]. Inevitably, similar concerns will be raised when men of color present to plastic surgeons. Hyperpigmentation commonly accompanies postsurgical scars (Fig. 7.9). Also, a recent report cited PIH as one of the most common complications of laser treatments [41].

Post-inflammatory hyperpigmentation (PIH), a darkening of the skin beyond its normal color, is a common occurrence, particularly among persons with dark skin. It is a manifestation of cuta-

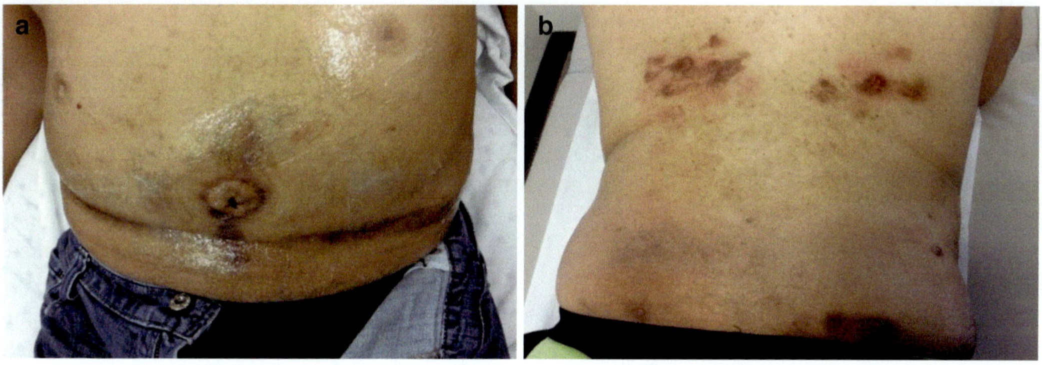

Fig. 7.9 (**a**) Frontal and (**b**) posterior view of post-inflammatory hyperpigmentation after a liposuction procedure. Treatment: Fraxel and custom-compounded cosmeceuticals

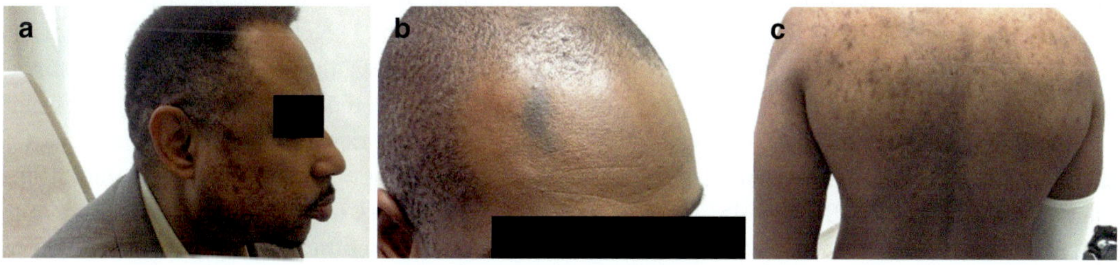

Fig. 7.10 (**a**–**c**) Examples of post-inflammatory hyperpigmentation in African American Men on the Face, forehead, and back

neous inflammation and injury. PIH is a frequent sequela of skin disease as well as cosmetic procedures. While it is overall benign, PIH causes significant psychological distress in many patients (Fig. 7.10).

The pathogenesis of PIH involves inflammatory processes which stimulate melanocyte activity. Cytokines and inflammatory mediators cause hyperpigmentation by their direct stimulation of melanocytes. An increase in melanogenesis occurs, and melanin is transferred through dendrites to adjacent keratinocytes. Most often, this results in epidermal hyperpigmentation. If the basal layer is damaged or disrupted by inflammation, melanin is absorbed by macrophages through phagocytosis and forms melanophages. This results in dermal hyperpigmentation, which is more resistant to treatment. A clinical sign of epidermal pigmentation is a brown discoloration on the skin. A clinical indicator of dermal pigmentation is a grayish or bluish hue [41] (Fig. 7.10).

Many of the treatments used for melasma are also used to treat post-inflammatory hyperpigmentation. The gold standard treatment for hyperpigmentation in the United States is topical hydroquinone. Hydroquinone inhibits melanin synthesis by acting as a substrate for tyrosinase, the enzyme required for melanin synthesis, causing a decrease in melanin production. In recent years, the use of hydroquinone has been under greater scrutiny. Questions of potential carcinogenicity have been raised but not substantiated (for typical clinical applications), and its use remains controversial. While hydroquinone 4% is the most common strength, various concentrations are used in the therapeutic treatment of hyperpigmentation. Combination treatments are frequently used, particularly triple combination creams. A triple combination cream (fluocinolone acetonide 0.01%, hydroquinone 4%, tretinoin 0.05%), while FDA-approved for melasma, is very effective in the treatment of PIH. Combining hydroquinone with other ingredients enhances its efficacy but may also increase its cutaneous absorption and potential for adverse effects. Potential adverse effects include irritation and allergy, exogenous ochronosis, loss of elasticity of skin, and impaired wound healing [42].

7.5.2 Retinoids

Retinoids interfere with melanogenesis by increasing cellular turnover. This decreases the transfer of melanosomes. The three main types of retinoids used to treat hyperpigmentation are retinoic acid (tretinoin), adapalene, and tazarotene. Studies demonstrate the efficacy of tretinoin cream 0.1% for the treatment of PIH [43]. However, in clinical practice, other strengths (e.g., 0.025–0.05%) are generally better tolerated. All three retinoids have demonstrated efficacy in the treatment of PIH [44, 45].

Numerous other agents aid in the treatment of hyperpigmentation. The list of products to address hyperpigmentation increased in recent years as research expanded on alternatives of hydroquinone [46–49] (see Table 7.3).

7.5.3 Chemical Peels

Chemical peels are mainstays of treatment for hyperpigmentation and photorejuvenation. While chemical peels are most often utilized in lighter skin for an anti-aging benefit and to improve actinic damage, they are more frequently used in darker skin for the treatment of hyperpigmentation, acne, pseudofolliculitis barbae, and scars. Superficial and low-to medium-depth chemical peels are generally best tolerated in darker skin types (Fitzpatrick IV—VI). Glycolic acid (30–70%), salicylic acid (20–30%), and trichloroacetic acid (TCA: 10–25%) peels are among the most common peels used, but other combination peels are frequently used.

Table 7.3 Therapies for hyperpigmentation

Aleosin	Mulberry extract
Arbutin	N-acetylglucosamine
Azelaic acid	Niacinamide (B3)
Glutathione	Other antioxidants
Glycolic acid	Polyodium
Kojic Acid	*leucotomos*
Licorice (glabridin)	Salicylic acid
Lignin peroxidase	Soy
Magnesium ascorbyl	Topical retinoids
phosphate	Tranexamic acid
Mequinol	Vitamin C

Before treating patients of color with a chemical peel, it is important to know whether the peel has proven safety in darker skin tones. A conservative approach is recommended. With new patients, it is best to start with lower concentrations first. With certain chemical peels, such as TCA, the peeling solution is often left on the skin until it produces the appearance of "frosting." However, as noted by Roberts [50], "frosting" may not be a desired effect, as it indicates a deeper penetration of the peeling solution and increases the risk of post-inflammatory hyperpigmentation. A neutralizing agent, such as bicarbonate solution, should be used after glycolic acid peels to avoid continuous keratolytic activity and potential adverse effects. In skin of color, caution should be used when performing many types of chemical peels. For example, the Jessner's peel, a popular combination originated by Dr. Max Jessner, which is composed of resorcinol (14 g), salicylic acid (14 g), and lactic acid (85%) in ethanol, is used successfully in many patients of color, but can cause hyperpigmentation in some patients of Fitzpatrick skin types V and VI [50].

Taking a detailed medical history is important before proceeding with a chemical peel. Written consent and photographs should be obtained. Patients should be asked about their ancestry to assess ethnicity and nuances for predicting skin reactions (see Table 7.4) [14, 51–54], systemic and topical medications, and all products used on the affected skin areas. Retinoids and any products containing exfoliating ingredients should be discontinued at least one week before commencing a chemical peel. Patients should be asked specifically about agents that increase photosensitivity (e.g., tetracycline antibiotics, contraceptives, antidepressants, vitamin supple-

Table 7.4 Skin classification scales

1. Fitzpatrick Skin Phototype Classification System	A classification of human skin color based on melanin content and cutaneous response to ultraviolet light. It predicts the skin's ability to tan and likelihood of burning. Developed by Dr. Thomas Fitzpatrick in 1975, it was originally developed to help select appropriate treatment levels for phototherapy, but continues to be a tool of skin color classification for dermatologic research. Type I always burns, never tans Type II usually burns, tans minimally Type III sometimes mild burn, tans uniformly Type IV burns minimally, always tans well (moderate brown) Type V very rarely burns, tans very easily (dark brown) Type VI never burns (deeply pigmented dark brown to darkest brown)
2. Roberts Skin Type Classification System	A more comprehensive skin categorization tool to help predict cutaneous response to treatment. Useful in planning cosmetic procedures and preventing complications. Based on evaluation of 4 components: Phototype, hyperpigmentation, photoaging, and scarring. Takes into account ancestral history, visual and physical examination of the skin, and test site reactions
3. Lancer Ethnicity Scale	Identifies skin type by combining knowledge of ancestry with Fitzpatrick skin classification. Assists in treatment selection and assessment of healing times from cosmetic procedures such as lasers and chemical peels
4. Taylor Hyperpigmentation Scale	A visual scale composed of laminated cards of 10–15 skin colors and 100 gradations of these hues. Designed to be a quick tool for categorization of skin color
5. Felix von Luschan Skin Color Chart	An early skin classification scale developed to establish racial identity. Skin color is ranked from 1 to 3, used primarily in studies during the first half of the twentieth century

ments). Patients should be asked about the history of herpes simplex virus (HSV). If a positive history of HSV is noted, antiviral prophylaxis treatment should be administered. Skin classification scales include: (1) Fitzpatrick Skin Phototype Classification System, (2) Roberts Skin Type Classification System, (3) Lancer Ethnicity Scale, (4) Taylor Hyperpigmentation Scale, and (5) Felix von Luschan Skin Color Chart (Table 7.4).

In all patients, but particularly in patients of color, patient education and after-care are of paramount importance. Proper timing of chemical peels should also be discussed beforehand. Avoidance of the sun is important before and after treatments and should be emphasized. It is important to manage patient expectations prior to a chemical peel. Patients should understand that treatments generally require a series of sessions. One of the most common adverse effects is hyperpigmentation. The combined effect of poor post-treatment skin care and sun exposure can lead to devastating post-inflammatory hyperpigmentation that may last for years. In patients of color, consistency is important as well. Even small variations (technique in application, number of layers applied, and post-peel activities) may affect the outcome of chemical peels.

7.5.4 Microneedling

Various resurfacing modalities are more limited for ethnic skin types. Fortunately, microneedling has successful outcomes among patients of color and is emerging as a reliable alternative to laser resurfacing. Microneedling has gained popularity for the treatment of numerous skin conditions, including the treatment of facial rejuvenation, scars, hair loss, acne, and hyperpigmentation [55]. While considered safe, risks of complications may be higher in skin of color patients, and include post-inflammatory hyperpigmentation, hypertrophic scarring, and infection. Thus, a more conservative approach to microneedling depth is recommended in darker skin types. Pre- and post-treatment with topical hydroquinone and/or other skin correcting agents is recommended.

Microneedling has also grown in popularity for its potential for transdermal delivery of therapeutics. For example, there are various protocols

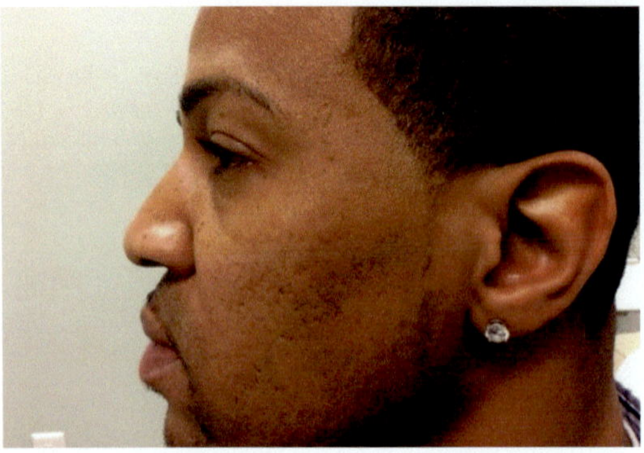

Fig. 7.11 Lateral view of an ideal candidate for treatment of scars with radiofrequency and microneedling

of microneedling combining growth factors and platelet-rich plasma (PRP) in skin rejuvenation, microneedling with the infusion of hair growth factors for the treatment of alopecia, and microneedling with the infusion of pigment correcting agents in the treatment of melasma. Additionally, the introduction of radiofrequency with microneedling (such as Intracel) has enhanced the treatment of skin rejuvenation, surgical scars, acne scars, and pore size for patients with darker skin (Fig. 7.11).

7.5.5 Laser Treatments

Lasers may enhance the treatment of PIH and are often useful adjunctive therapies. The Fraxel laser has demonstrated efficacy in the treatment of PIH [56, 57]. The 1064 Nd:YAG lasers, such as Laser Genesis and, more recently, the Neo Aerolase 650 microsecond laser, are popular lasers in the treatment of hyperpigmentation [58]. With delayed photo-aging of darker skin types and increased propensity for scarring, it is important to consider non-invasive modalities for men of color presenting with mild to moderate skin laxity. These patients often desire a "non-surgical lift" for skin tightening and slight adipose reduction. Laser-assisted lipolysis may be helpful combined with options such as fractionated laser (Fraxel), radiofrequency microneedling (e.g., Intracel), and fractional bipolar radiofrequency devices (Fractora/Morpheus8)—each showing a good safety profile with minimal downtime [59, 60].

7.6 Scar Management

Hypertrophic scarring and keloids are more common among skin of color patients. Hypertrophic scars display elevated skin at the wound site, while keloids involve scar tissue extending beyond the wound site. There is a greater propensity for hypertrophic scars and keloids to develop on earlobes, the central chest, shoulders, and upper back. The pathogenesis is complicated and may involve aberrant cytokine activity. There are three main phases of wound healing: (1) Inflammatory phase, (2) proliferation phase, and (3) maturation phase [61]. Some have proposed that hypertrophic scars and keloids may result from a prolonged or overly intense inflammatory stage during the steps of wound healing.

7.6.1 Prevention

A common adage states that it is easier to prevent scars than to treat them. Thus, a few steps taken preoperatively, intraoperatively, and immediately postoperatively may be of great benefit in the long run. For example, postoperatively, early use of topical silicone may reduce scar thickness and improve color. Silicone sheets facilitate healing and should be applied 12–24 hours a day for up to 2 months. Silicone gel applied twice daily may be used. Silicone treatments are more beneficial for new, fresh scars [62].

7.6.2 Treatment

While there are numerous treatments available for the treatment of scars, very few treatments are used as widely as intralesional corticosteroids. Intralesional triamcinolone (Kenalog) is a first-line treatment for keloids and a second-line treatment for hypertrophic scars [63]. Side effects of intralesional triamcinolone include hypopigmentation, skin atrophy, telangiectasia, comedone and cyst formation, folliculitis, and pain and sensitivity. Patients should be informed about possible side effects before beginning treatments.

In clinical practice, a combination of treatments is used to obtain optimal results for scar treatment. For example, classic "chicken pox" scars or atrophic scars can be improved by scar revision followed by microneedling or fractionated laser treatments. While there are various fractionated lasers, Fraxel is preferred for skin of color patients. To prevent hyperpigmentation, it is often effective to treat the affected areas with hydroquinone 1–2 weeks after treatment. In patients particularly vulnerable to hyperpigmentation, pretreatment (1–2 weeks prior) with hydroquinone should be considered. Successful treatment of acne scarring may occur with a set of microneedling treatments alternating with the Fraxel laser. Treatments may begin with 2 consecutive Fraxel treatments (spaced 1 month apart), followed by 2 sessions of microneedling (also spaced 1 month apart). Afterwards, the clinician and patient can consider treatment with a radiofrequency microneedling laser (favored for scars with significant atrophy). Injection of Belotero or other hyaluronic acid fillers to larger atrophic scars also works well in combination with the above treatments.

For the treatment of mild hypertrophic surgical scars, the author recommends a series of Fraxel treatments, along with a course of topical hydroquinone, and sometimes sessions of a low dose of intralesional triamcinolone (3–5 mg) to improve hyperpigmentation. A series of radiofrequency with microneedling laser treatments (e.g., Intracel) also works well. These devices are preferred over microneedling for hyperpigmented scars, as texture often improves, but hyperpigmentation may worsen with microneedling alone. The 1064 Nd:YAG Neo Aerolase nanometer laser has patented 650 microsecond technology which makes it a useful adjunct in the treatment of scars that consist of marked hyperpigmentation.

7.6.3 Keloids

The treatment of keloids remains challenging. Few clinical trials have been performed on scar treatments, particularly in pigmented skin. Multimodal therapy is the best approach to hypertrophic and keloid scars and ultimately leads to the lowest recurrence rate. The treatment must be at least a combination of pressure and massage which progresses to intralesional injection therapy with cryotherapy [63, 64]. Cryotherapy is not a good option in patients of color due to the risk of permanent hypopigmentation. Excision followed by radiation therapy has proved to be the most effective with recurrence rates of nearly 20%. Surgical excision, followed by multiple radiotherapy sessions (over 24–72 hours of excision) and post-procedure intralesional steroid injection, yields the best treatment to date [65]. For the co-author, intralesional Kenalog injections (10—40 mg) remain the initial gold-standard treatment. The co-author has achieved success in treating hypertrophic scars and keloids with a series of intralesional injections in combination with flurandrenolide (Cordran) tape. For 2–4 weeks before and after injections, patients are instructed to cut strips of Cordran tape and apply it to the scars to leave on for 10 to 12 hours daily. For patients reluctant to undergo injections, flurandrenolide tape may be used alone or along with silicone adhesives. The Fraxel laser is helpful after the former treatments to blend the scars with the surrounding skin to improve cosmetic appearance. Care should be used to avoid blistering of atrophic skin surrounding the scar or keloid that may have developed from intralesional cortisone injections. With conservative settings and a gentle touch, this is not usually a problem, and the atrophy itself improves with the fractionated laser treatments. Again, the Fraxel laser is preferred. Fraxel may aid in the delivery of topical treatments into scar tissue. Lasers reported in the literature for the treatment of scars, such as CO2, Er:YAG, pulsed dye laser (PDL), and IPL, often have limited use in skin of color (SOC).

7.7 Pseudofolliculitis Barbae

The issue of folliculitis is frequently raised when evaluating men of color for cosmetic procedures. Often, before mentioning concerns about wrinkles and aging skin, men often express a desire for skin that is smooth and even in color on the face, particularly the beard area. Thus, when evaluating the male aesthetic patient, it may be important to address the common concern of pseudofolliculitis barbae and consider it in the overall treatment plan.

Pseudofolliculitis barbae (PFB), also known colloquially as "ingrown hairs" or "razor bumps," is an inflammatory skin disorder characterized by erythematous follicular and perifollicular papules, often with concomitant hyperpigmentation in areas of hair growth after shaving. Hypertrophic scars and keloid formation are common sequelae in the affected areas. Secondary infection may develop and complicate the condition. Itching and pain also commonly occur (Fig. 7.12).

PFB may affect persons of any race, but high rates are found in African American men. PFB is also prevalent among persons of Hispanic and Middle Eastern ancestry. The incidence among African American men is reported to be between 45 and 83% [66]. While the morphology of the curled hair pattern is felt to be responsible for the predisposition to develop PFB, a genetic risk factor has been identified. A recent study linked a mutation in the 1A alpha helical segment of keratin 75 ((K6hf) to an associated higher risk for PFB [67].

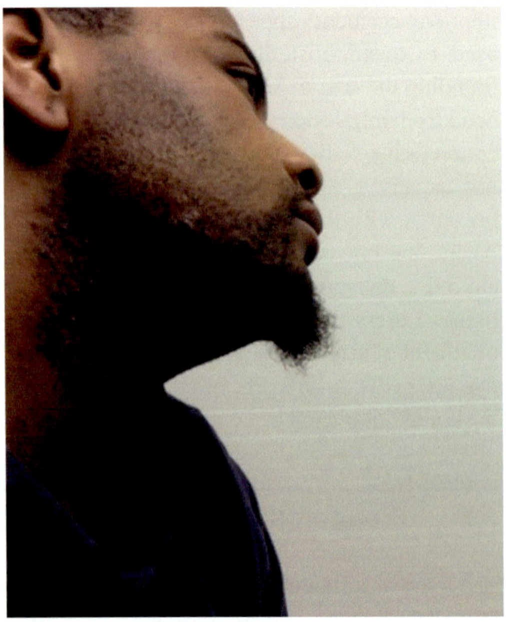

Fig. 7.12 Pseudofolliculitis barbae. Ideal candidate for treatment

The pathogenesis of PFB involves the creation of a sharp and curly hair from a razor which increases the risk of penetration of the hair into areas of adjacent skin. Reentry of hairs into the surrounding skin leads to an inflammatory reaction, and the hallmark papules ("razor bumps") ensue. The inflammatory process can progress to lead to pustules or abscesses. On close inspection, one may observe loops of hair re-entering the skin or buried under overlying skin. The reentry ignites a foreign body immune reaction. Indeed, histology of areas of PFB typically displays a foreign-body-like reaction to the hairs.

Treatment of PFB involves a combination of medical and pharmacologic therapies, modification of shaving practices, and the use of procedural modalities. Overall, various treatments may mitigate disease, but are often not curative. The goal of treatment is to improve the appearance and prevent complications of hyperpigmentation, keloids, hypertrophic scarring, and infection. Some experts have advocated the use of pre-shave and post-shave regimens (68,69). Generally, it is recommended that men begin shaving by washing the area with warm water to soften the hairs using a gentle cleanser. Exfoliating with scrubs, a brush, or a washcloth moved in a circular motion (physical exfoliation) assists in dislodging ingrown hairs and in prepping the area. Consistent use of a clean, sharp razor is important.

The use of electrical razors often significantly improves PFB. Electrical razors cut hairs while maintaining a length of 0.5 mm to 1 mm, which helps to prevent early reentry of hairs into the skin and lessens buried hairs. Similarly, many patients find that switching from razors to the use of clippers assists in decreasing follicular reentry and entrapment of hairs by maintaining a length of 1 mm to 3 mm [68, 69].

Topical steroids remain a mainstay of treatment for PFB. Very short-term use (1–2 weeks) of moderate to high potency steroids may be used as rescue therapy to clear patients rapidly, but use of low potency steroids is frequently used for maintenance, with frequencies of 1–3 times per week. For example, a common approach would begin with a short course of treatment with topical fluocinonide 0.05% followed by maintenance with topical desonide three times a week. Moreover, intralesional steroids (triamcinolone in a range of concentrations from 3 to 5 mg injected into the papules) are generally very effective. It is important to warn of possible hypopigmentation and take steps to avoid this potential side effect. Injecting slowly decreases the tendency for peripheral spread of the solution into the surrounding skin which can lead to peripheral hypopigmentation.

Retinoids (tretinoin, adapalene, and tazarotene) are now considered first-line treatments as well. Adapalene is often a safe first choice as many patients find it less irritating than other retinoids. Trifarotene, a new fourth-generation retinoid recently approved for the treatment of acne vulgaris, might also demonstrate similar benefits in the future [70]. Chemical exfoliation is very helpful in minimizing PFB. Washes and topical products containing glycolic acid, salicylic acid, and lactic acid are often therapeutic. In addition, studies and reports have indicated the effectiveness of oral and topical antibiotics [71, 72], topical eflornithine, chemical depilatories, and electrolysis.

Addressing the hyperpigmentation that often accompanies PFB is an essential part of treatment, as often patients are more bothered by the hyperpigmentation than the papules (or "bumps") of PFB. Hydroquinone is the gold standard of the topical treatments used to improve hyperpigmentation. Other products containing ingredients that correct pigmentation, such as azelaic acid, kojic acid, arbutin, and licorice extract, are useful adjuncts.

While PFB is extremely common, it often remains a therapeutic challenge. Most experts claim no cure for the condition but agree that more definitive treatments include growing a beard or having the hair permanently removed. Growing out the beard has, in fact, been reported to completely clear PFB in many patients. However, this may not be acceptable for some patients. Fortunately, treatment of PFB is often successful with laser hair removal. The long-pulse Nd: YAG (1064 nm) laser is the gold standard, remaining the laser of choice for patients of color. The diode (810 nm) laser has gained popularity for its safe use among patients with darker skin types as well [73, 74]. Studies have demonstrated that destruction of hairs and follicular miniaturization leads to a decrease in the number of papules. While hair regrowth is common, a series of multiple laser hair removal sessions when performed over 4–6 consecutive months generally yields a significant long-term reduction in hairs. Male patients, in particular, must be warned of possible regrowth. Many hairs may grow back, as men are genetically wired to grow hair in certain areas, but generally after a series of treatments, the hair grows back thinner than the hair prior to treatment. Dramatic improvement in PFB is often noted after laser hair removal treatments. One study showed that up to 80% reduction in bumps and hairs was still observed after 6 months of final treatment [73].

Since more conservative measures are used for hair removal in darker skin, it is important to inform patients that in order to attain the best state of consistent hair reduction, they will require multiple sessions. They should also be encouraged to plan for maintenance sessions, which may be performed quarterly or every 3 months.

Pseudofolliculitis barbae affects self-esteem for many patients, leading to challenges socially and professionally. Physicians in a position to offer treatments to improve the condition can make a huge impact on quality of life. Properly addressing PFB can greatly improve satisfaction among male aesthetic patients.

7.8 Laser Hair Removal

When treating patients with lasers for hair removal, it is important to discuss the risks of the procedure, ask about all products used on the affected skin, and provide very clear pre- and post-care instructions. This is critical for patients of color to avoid complications. Patients should discontinue topical treatments one week before laser procedures and switch to a basic regimen consisting of only a mild cleanser and sunscreen. After laser treatments in some patients, it is helpful to advise the use of a topical antibiotic (e.g., benzoyl peroxide/clindamycin cream) and a mild topical steroid for three days afterwards. Antiviral prophylaxis is recommended. Acyclovir 800 mg or valacyclovir 1 g dosed daily is commonly used three days before and after treatments. In skin of color patients, lower fluences and longer pulse durations are recommended for laser treatments. The Nd: YAG (1064 nm) and diode (810 nm) lasers are considered the safest for this population (Fitzpatrick IV–VI). Cooling the skin (using cool compresses, chilled lubricant) before and after treatments is helpful to reduce adverse effects [74].

7.9 Conclusion

Cosmetic procedures in the African American male can produce aesthetic ideals which are culturally based and nuanced. The pursuit of these aesthetic ideals will be increasingly desired, and aesthetic surgeons catering to this population must be sensitive not only to male anatomy but also to unique skin challenges of this population. Aesthetic ideal physiques and facial profiles can be safely delivered by both invasive and noninvasive treatment options. The Aesthetic African American male ideal reflects optimum surgical outcomes without pigmentary or aberrant scarring consequences.

References

1. Burn SM, Ward AZ. Men's conformity to traditional masculinity and relationship satisfaction. Psychol Men Masc. 2005;6:254–63.
2. DeBruine LM, Jones BC. Correlated preferences for facial masculinity and ideal or actual partner's masculinity. Proceeding of the Royal Society B. Published 28 February 2006. Accessed 25 Mar 2022.
3. Lazar CC, Deneuve S. Patients' perceptions of cosmetic surgery at a time of globalization, medical consumerism, and mass media culture: a French experience. Aesth Surg. 2013;33(6):878–85.
4. Available from: https://www.plasticsurgery.org/news/plastic-surgery-statistics. Accessed 25 Mar 2019.
5. American Society for Aesthetic Plastic Surgery. 2020 cosmetic surgery national data bank statistics. Available from :https://cdn.theaestheticsociety.org/media/statistics/aestheticplasticsurgerynationaldatabank-2020stats.pdf. Accessed 1 May 2022.
6. American Society of Plastic Surgery. 15.6 million cosmetic procedures performed 2020. Available at: https://www.plasticsurgery.org/documents/News/Statistics/2020/plastic-surgery-statistics-full-report-2020.pdf
7. American Society of Plastic Surgery. 2017 Cosmetic demographics. Available at: https://www.plasticsurgery.org/documents/News/Statistics/2017/plastic-surgery-statistics-full-report-2017.pdf.
8. Wimalawansa S, McKnight A, Bullocks J. Socioeconomic impact of ethnic cosmetic surgery: trends and Potential Financial impact the African American, Asian American, Latin American and Middle Eastern Communities have on cosmetic surgery. Sem Plast Surg. 2009;23(3):159–62.
9. Frederick DA, Lever J, Peplau LA. Interest in cosmetic surgery and body image: views of men and women across the lifespan. Plast Reconstr Surg. 2007;120:1407–15.
10. Sobanko JF, Taglienti AJ, et al. Motivations for seeking minimally invasive cosmetic procedures in an academic outpatient setting. 2015;35(8):1014–20.
11. Buster KJ, Yang L, Elmets CA. Are dermatologist confident in treating skin disease in African Americans? J Invest Dermatol. Meeting Abstracts. 2011;abstract 235 (61–65).
12. Treesirichod A, Chansakulporn S, Wattanapan P. Correlation between skin color evaluation by skin color scale chart and narrowband reflectance spectrophotometer. Indian J Dermatol. 2014;59(4):339–42.
13. He SY, et al. Self-reported pigmentary phenotypes and race are significant but incomplete predictors of Fitzpatrick skin phototype in an ethnically diverse population. J Am Acad Dermatol. 2014;71:731–7.
14. Roberts WE. The Roberts skin type Classification system. J Drugs Dermatol. 2008;7:452–6.
15. Burgess CM. Special considerations in African American skin. In: Alam M, Bhatia A, Kundu R, et al., editors. Cosmetic dermatology for skin of color. McGraw-Hill Companies; 2008. p. 163–7.
16. Vincensi MR, d'Ischia M, Napolitano A, et al. Phaeomelanin versus eumelanin as a chemical indicator of ultraviolet sensitivity in fair skinned subjects at high risk from melanoma: a pilot study. Melanoma Res. 1998;8(1):53–8.
17. Visser M, Palstra RJ, Kayser M. Human skin color is influenced by an intergenic DNA polymorphism regulating transcription of the nearby BNC2 pigmentation gene. Hum Mol Genet 2014;23(21):5750–5762. -1DOWU.
18. Sturm RA, Duffy DL. Human pigmentation genes under environmental selection. Genome Biol. 2012;13(9):248 –IDOWU.

19. Szabo G, Gerald AB, Patnak MA, et al. Racial differences in the fate of melanosomes in human epidermis. Nature. 1969;222(5198):1081–2.
20. Motangna W, Carlisle K. The architecture of black and white skin. J Am Acad Dermatol. 1991;24:929–37.
21. Brissett AE, Naylor MC. The aging African American face. Facial Plast Surg. 2010;26(2):154–63-IDOWU.
22. Vashi NA, de Castro Maymone MB, Kundu RV. Aging differences in ethnic skin. J Clin Aesthet Dermatol. 2011;9(1):31–8.
23. Harris MO. The aging face in patients of color: minimally invasive surgical facial rejuvenation a targeted approach. Dermatol Ther. 2004;17:2006–11.
24. De Maio M. Ethnic and gender considerations in the use of facial injectables: male patients. Plast Reconstr Surg. 2015;136(5S):40S–3S.
25. Green JB, Keaney TC. Aesthetic treatment with botulinum toxin: approaches specific to men. Dermatol Surg. 2017;43(11S):S153–6.
26. Henry M. Cosmetic concerns among ethnic men. Dermatol Clin. 2018;36:11–6.
27. Singh D. Female judgement of male attractiveness and desirability for relationships: role of waist to hip ratio and financial status. J Pers Soc Psychol. 1995;69(6):1089–101.
28. Granberg EM, Simmons LG, Simmons RL. The role of body size in mate selection among African American young adults. Sex Roles. 2015;73(7–8).340–54. Epub 2015.
29. Thakerar JN, Iwawaki S. Cross-cultural comparison in interpersonal attraction of females toward males. J Soc Psychol. 1979;108:121–2.
30. Singh B, Keaney T, Rossi AM. Male body contouring. J Drugs Dermatol. 2015;14(9):1052–9.
31. Vagianos A. What the "ideal man's body looks like in 19 countries. Women section Huffington Post 2/18/2016.
32. Seify H. Awake plastic surgery procedures: the use of a sufentanil tablet to improve patient experience. Aesthet Surg J Open Forum. 2022;4:ojab056.
33. Gutowski KA. Tumescent analgesia in plastic surgery. Plast Reconstr Surg. 2014;134(4s-2)50S–57S.
34. Chai CT, Theodorou SJ. 1000 consecutive cases of laser-assisted liposuction and suction-assisted lipectomy managed with local anesthesia. Aesth Plast Surg. 2012;36(4):795–802.
35. Taylor SC. Skin of color: biology, structure, function, and implications for dermatologic disease. J Am Acad Dermatol. 2002;46:S41–62.
36. Burgess GM. Special considerations in African American skin. In: Alam M, Bhatia A, Kundu R, et al., editors. Cosmetic dermatology for color. McGraw-Hill Companies; 2008. p. 163–7.
37. http://www.surgery.org/sites/default/files/2014-Stats.pdf
38. Alexis AF, Sergay AB, Taylor SC. Common dermatologic disorders in skin of color: a comparative practice survey. Cutis. 2007;80:387–94.
39. Halder RM, Grimes PE, McLaurin CI, Kress MA, Kenney JA Jr. Incidence of common dermatoses in predominantly black dermatology practice. Cutis. 1983;32:388–90.
40. Halder RM, Nootheti PK. Ethnic skin disorders overview. J Am Acad Dermatol. 2003;48:S143–8.
41. Silpa-archa N, Kohli I, Chaowattanapanit S, Lim HW, Hamzavi I. Post inflammatory hyperpigmentation: a comprehensive overview: epidemiology, pathogenesis, clinical presentation, and noninvasive assessment technique. J Am Acad Dermatol. 2017;77:591–605.
42. Taylor S, Grimes P, Lim J, Im S, Lu H. Postinflammatory hyperpigmentation. J Cut Med Surg. 2009;13:183–91.
43. Bulengo-Ransby SM, Griffiths CEM, Kimbrough-Green CK, et al. Topical tretinoin (retinoic acid) therapy for hyperpigmented lesions caused by inflammation of the skin in black patients. N Engl J Med. 1993;328:1438–43.
44. Grimes P, Callender V. Tazarotene cream for postinflammatory hyperpigmentation and acne vulgaris in darker skin: a double-blind, randomized, vehicle-controlled study. Cutis. 2006;77:45–50.
45. Jacyk WK, Mpofu P. Adapalene gel 0.1% for topical treatment of acne vulgaris in African patients. Cutis. 2001;68(suppl):48–54.
46. Rossi AM, Perez MI. Treatment of hyperpigmentation. Facial Plast Surg Clin N Am. 2011;19:313–24.
47. Chaowattanapanit S. Postinflammatory hyperpigmentation: a comprehensive overview: treatment options and prevention. J Am Acad Dermatol. 2017;77:607–21.
48. Davis EC, Callender VD. Postinflammatory hyperpigmentation: a review of the epidemiology, clinical features, and treatment options in skin of color. J Clin Aesthet Dermatol. 2010;3:20–31.
49. Nestor M, Bucay V, Callender V, Cohen JL, Sadick N, Waldorf H. Polypodium leucotomos as an adjunct treatment of pigmentary disorders. J Clin Aesthet Dermatol. 2014;7(3):13–7.
50. Roberts WE. Chemical peeling in ethnic/dark skin. Dermatol Ther. 2004;17:196–205.
51. He SY, McCulloch CE, Boscardin WJ, Chren M-M, Linos E, Aaron ST. Self-reported pigmentary phenotypes and race are significant but incomplete predictors of Fitzpatrick skin phototype in an ethnically diverse population. J Am Acad Dermatol. 2014;71:731–7.
52. Lancer HA. Lancer ethnicity scale (LES). Lasers Surg Med. 1998;22:9.
53. Taylor SC, Arsonnaud S, Czernielewski J. Hyperpigmentation Scale Study Group. The Taylor hyperpigmentation scale: a new visual assessment tool for the evaluation of skin color and pigmentation. Cutis. 2005;76:270–4.
54. Treesirichod A, Chansakulporn S, Wattanapan P. Correlation between skin color evaluation by skin color scale chart and narrowband reflectance spectrophotometer. Indian J Dermatol. 2014;59:339–42.
55. Cohen BE, Elbuluk N. Microneedling in skin of color: a review of uses and efficacy. J Am Acad Dermatol. 2016;74:348–55.

56. Ghannam S, Al Otabi FK, Frank K, Cotofana S. Efficacy of low-fluence Nd:YAG 1064nm laser for the treatment of post-inflammatory hyperpigmentation in the axillary area. J Drugs Dermatol. 2017;16:1118–23.
57. Woolery-Lloyd H, Viera MH, Valins W. Laser therapy in black skin. Facial Plast Surg Clin North Am. 2011;19:405–16.
58. Roberts WE, Henry M, Burgss C, Saedi N, Chilukuri S, Campbell-Chambers A. Laser treatment of skin of color for medical and aesthetic uses with a new 650-microsecond Nd:YAG 1064 nm laser. J Drugs Dermatol. 2019;18(4):s135–7.
59. Dayan E, Rovatti P, Aston S, Chia CT, Rohrich R, Theodorou S. Multimodal radiofrequency application for lower face and neck laxity. Plast Reconstr Surg Glob Open. 2020;8(8):e2862.
60. Alexiades M, Munavalli GS. Single treatment protocol with microneedle fractional radiofrequency for treatment of body skin laxity and fat deposits. Lasers Surg Med. 2021;53(8):1026–31. https://doi.org/10.1002/lsm.23397.
61. Lee HJ, Jang YJ. Recent understandings of biology, prophylaxis and treatment strategies for hypertrophic scars and keloids. Int J Mol Sci. 2018;19:711.
62. Perez JL, Rohrich RJ. Optimizing post-surgical scars: a systematic review of best practices in preventative scar management. Plast Reconstr Surg. 2017;140:782e–92e.
63. Andrews JP, Marttala J, Macarak E, Rosenbloom J, Uitto J. Keloids: the paradigm of skin fibrosis-pathomechanisms and treatment. Matrix Biol. 2016;51:37–46.
64. Arna AI, Gauglitz GG, Barret JP, Jeschke MG. Up-to-date approach to manage keloids and hypertrophic scars: a useful guide. Burns. 2014;40:1255–66.
65. Jones MJ, Hardy C, Ridgway J. Keloid Management; A retrospective case review on a new approach using surgical excision, platelet-rich plasma, and In-office superficial photon x-ray radiation therapy. 2016;29(7):303–7.
66. McMichael AJ. Hair and scalp disorders in ethnic populations. Dermatol Clin. 2003;21:629–44.
67. Winter H, Schissel D, Parry DAD, Smith TA, et al. An unusual A1q2Thr polymorphism in the 1A alpha-helical segment of the companion layer-specific keratin K6hf: evidence for a risk factor in the etiology of the common hair disorder pseudofolliculitis barbae. J Invest Dermatol. 2004;122:652–7.
68. Alexis A, Heath CR, Halder RM. Folliculitis keloidalis nuchae and pseudofolliculitis barbae: are prevention and effective treatment within reach. Dermatol Clin. 32:183–91.
69. Perry PK, Cook-Bolden FE, Rahman Z, Jones E, Taylor SC. Defining pseudofolliculitis barbae in 2001: a review of the literature and current trends. J Am Acad Dermatol. 2002;2014(46):S113–9.
70. Cosio T, Di Prete M, Gaziano R, et al. Trifarotene: a current review and perspectives in dermatology. Biomedicine. 2021;9(3):237.
71. Bridgeman-Shah S. The medical and surgical therapy of pseudofolliculitis barbae. Dermatol Ther. 2004;17:158–63.
72. Cook-Bolden FE, Barba A, Halder R, Taylor S. Twice-daily applications of benzoyl peroxide 5%/clindamycin1% gel versus vehicle in the treatment of pseudofolliculitis barbae. Cutis. 2004;73(Suppl 6):18–24.
73. Ross VE, Cooke LM, Overstreet KA, Buttollph GD, Blair MA. Treatment of pseudofolliculitis barbae in very dark skin with a long pulse Nd:YAG laser. J Nat Med Assoc. 2002;94:888–93.
74. Battle EF, Hobbs LM. Laser-assisted hair removal for darker skin types. Dermatol Ther. 2004;17:177–83.

Pretragal Facelift

8

David Mattos and William G. Austen, Jr.

8.1 Introduction

The male facelift population, as discussed in Chap. 9, is a unique patient population that has increased in number over the years and often requires a different approach than the female facelift. There are differences in the patients' anatomy and goals. Anatomical differences include facial hair, different hairlines, shorter hairstyles, wider lower-third facial proportions, thicker skin, more prominent nasolabial folds, and increased facial skin vascularity [1]. The goals of the male patients are also different, as the patients have a desire to preserve a masculine look and an increased reluctance of undergoing surgery due to common surgical stigmata. While facelift surgery dates back to the early twentieth century, only in the last few decades has the stigma of surgery for men diminished enough to see a significant increase in male facelifts [2]. Additional challenges for this patient population include a significantly higher risk of developing a hematoma, increased prevalence of hypertension, and a reluctance to wear makeup to conceal their healing incisions and bruising. For these reasons, patient selection and education are both critical to patient satisfaction.

D. Mattos
Massachusetts General Hospital, Boston, MA, USA
e-mail: dmattos@alumni.harvard.edu

W. G. Austen, Jr. (✉)
Division of Plastic and Reconstructive Surgery,
Massachusetts General Hospital, Boston, MA, USA
e-mail: wausten@mgh.harvard.edu

Prevention of hematoma formation must be stressed in men, as they occur in approximately 4.2–12.9% of the time [3–9]. In one institution, the incidence of postoperative hematomas decreased from 8.7% to 3.9% over a 30-year period with the institution of normotensive anesthesia. In contrast, the overall hematoma rate when considering women is only 1.9% [9]. As such, it is important to assess risk factors for bleeding preoperatively, including history of hypertension and postoperative nausea, personal or family history of a bleeding diathesis, and medications that may contribute to bleeding. In terms of medications, it is worthwhile to ask patients to continue taking their antihypertensives, except for diuretics, before surgery. Patients should stop NSAIDs, aspirin, or anticoagulant medications for at least a week before surgery. Patients should also stop supplements, including ginkgo biloba, St. John's wort, and other supplements with unknown effects. Finally, given the significantly increased risk of complications with smoking, including a 12-fold increased risk of skin slough after facelifts, patients must stop smoking for at least 4 weeks prior to surgery [10]. If the patient is not able to stop smoking, a procedure with more limited dissection and undermining can sometimes be considered.

In preparing patients for surgery, one has to have frank discussions with the patients about

K. Jeffords et al. (eds.), *Aesthetic Surgery for Men*, https://doi.org/10.1007/978-3-032-03840-1_8

realistic expectations to make sure they understand and would be happy with the expected outcome. It is not unusual for high-profile patients or people in high-visibility jobs to consider facelifts, and for these patients, clarity of the expectations is especially important [3]. The preoperative supine test is utilized to give each patient a sense of what his postoperative result may look like [11]. If the patient's desired outcome is realistic, he is encouraged to proceed with surgery. There are also risk factors for dissatisfaction with surgery that one should consider before offering surgery, which include young age, unrealistic expectations, minimal deformities, familial problems, and patients with frequent history of surgery, among other factors [12]. Finally, given how hesitant some men are of showing any signs of surgery, they should be counseled that most patients can get back to light work at 1–2 weeks, but bruising may persist, and they need to be prepared for that possibility.

In the senior author's practice (W.G.A.), the preferred male facelift technique utilizes a pretragal incision. In men, this incision preserves the distribution of facial hair and avoids redraping hair-bearing skin over the tragus, which can be difficult to shave, is abnormal, and unattractive [3]. Previously, some surgeons advocated leaving the strip of hairless skin in the pretragal region intact by making the incision at the anterior portion of hairless skin, but this needlessly narrows the sideburns and can lead to a more visible scar. The loss of the hairless skin, however, is less noticeable if the sideburn width can be preserved, and the incision can be camouflaged well. The senior author normally follows a skin crease in the preauricular region that is simple to identify and is ideal for healing and camouflaging.

8.2 Technique

8.2.1 Preoperative Course

In their consultation visit, patients are photographed with the standard views and are given preoperative instructions, including which medications to avoid or continue. They are instructed to take all of their antihypertensive medications the morning of surgery. We also allow them to shave before surgery, as the follicles are usually still easy to see. On arrival to the preoperative area, the patient's blood pressure is measured, and if greater than 120 mmHg, a 0.1 mg/24 hours clonidine patch is applied to improve control. Jewelry is removed.

8.2.2 Intraoperative Course

8.2.2.1 Anesthesia and Positioning

Pneumatic compression boots are placed on both legs. An endotracheal tube is inserted and secured with tape to the chin, avoiding significant lateral extensions into the area that is going to be undermined, and avoiding the submental region. Corneal shields are placed in each eye with lubricant. The operating room table is turned counterclockwise approximately 120 degrees, and the arms are tucked in for access from both sides of the table. Nauseogenic and paralytic anesthetic agents are avoided. The face is prepped with saline, and sterile straight extension tubing is added to the endotracheal tube to maximize mobility of the tubing and allow easy access to the submental incision. The head is wrapped with sterile towels, but the marking and incision line into the posterior hairline must still be visible.

8.2.2.2 Incision Markings

Markings are done before infiltrating the wetting solution to prevent distorting the anatomy. The preauricular skin is evaluated carefully for natural skin creases. The skin crease closest to, but anterior to, the tragus is chosen. For bald men, the incision markings begin in the temporal region, at or below the most superior aspect of the crus helicis. It is extended inferiorly, gently curving along the preauricular sulcus until it reaches the tragus, where it follows the chosen skin crease in the pretragal region. This should be in the most posterior aspect of the hairless skin between the tragus and the facial hair, to preserve the width of the sideburn and facial hair preauricularly. For men with hair, the superior aspect of the incision is extended anteriorly along the hairline, and care should be taken to avoid significantly altering the width of skin from lateral orbital rim and eyebrow to the temporal hair, as it can create an unnatural look. The anterior extension of this incision follows the chosen hairline of the patient. If horizontal, the course is horizontal, and if oblique, the course is oblique. More importantly, a W-plasty incision is used along the anterior extent of the hairline, as in short-scar facelift described by Tonnard [13–15]. An example of the markings is seen in Fig. 8.1. It is also marked a few millimeters into the hairline, so that after beveling the eventual incision perpendicular to the hair follicles, some hair will grow from the deep flap of tissue that remains inferior to the scar line and camouflage it [16]. The inferior extent of the incision then curves around the earlobe in the natural crease. The incision then transitions again into a W-plasty above the postauricular sulcus to prevent the scar from migrating down into the neck. The W-plasty incision along the sideburn and posteriorly increases the length of the recipient side of the incision, so that any redundant skin from the skin flap raised can be spread out and the dog ear can be minimized. At the point where the posterior hairline comes underneath or closest to the helix of the ear, the marking travels posteriorly into the hairline. If minimal skin excess is present, the incision can be carried horizontally into the hairline, as it can be better concealed. However, when using this approach, one must be careful to avoid an occipital notch in the hairline. If significant amount of skin laxity is expected, the markings can follow the posterior hairline, though this approach is less often needed. Finally, a submental incision is marked, which should be 3–4 cm, and hidden along a skin crease. Consideration of the expected amount of skin resection must be taken again, as an incision drawn too anteriorly in a patient with severe skin laxity could end up on the anterior, visible portion of the chin after undermining is done.

8.2.2.3 Fat Grafting

Fat grafting is rare during a male facelift in the senior author's practice. While there is some volume loss as we age, fat grafting can be overdone and lead to an unnatural appearance postoperatively, and can also be somewhat unpredictable in

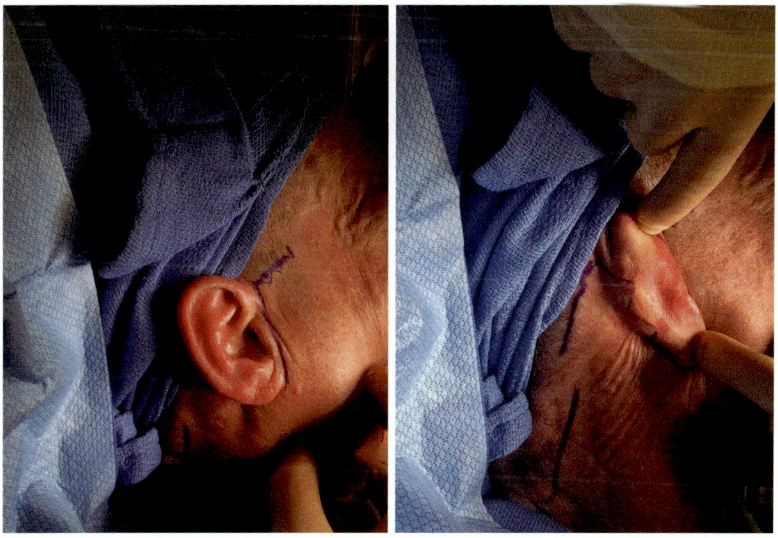

Fig. 8.1 Incision markings, patient 1: The preauricular, pretragal incision is seen on the left. The extension of the pretragal incision through the hairline zig-zags to be able to distribute some of the excess skin during inset of the facelift skin flap. Similarly, the posterior incision on the right goes up onto the conchal cartilage and zig-zags as well for skin distribution and to minimize the extension of that scar lower into the neck, where it becomes more visible

terms of survival. Most of the time, not doing any fat grafting allows the face to look younger yet remain in harmony with the patient's preoperative appearance. In severe cases, fat grafting will be done to the nasolabial fold. However, if the patient has very deep nasolabial folds, a spatulated 3 mm cannula can be used to break up the adhesions along the nasolabial fold to smoothen it out. There is controversy in the literature as to whether it should be done up front or after the dissection. A 3 mm cannula can also be used without suction to remove a small amount of fat from the fold.

8.2.2.4 Local and Tumescence

Local anesthesia is injected along the pretragal and submental incisions with epinephrine before moving onto tumescence. A wetting solution made with 125 mg of lidocaine, 2.5 mEq of sodium bicarbonate, and 1 mg of epinephrine in 1000 mL of Lactated Ringer's is infiltrated into the subcutaneous plane throughout the areas to be dissected. The infiltration is done with a 12-gauge cannula and a power injector at 250 cc/minute. Both sides of the face are infiltrated with approximately 400–500 cc per side. Tumescent technique can also be done more slowly in the awake patient. There is a 15-minute pause before proceeding to allow the vasoconstrictive effect to take hold. The incision is then made perpendicular to the hair follicles in areas with hair. As previously mentioned, this approach allows hair follicles to survive on both sides of the incision and conceals the scar more effectively [16],

8.2.2.5 Flap Elevation

Curved iris scissors are used with double hooks to sharply and carefully elevate the preauricular skin, as it is more difficult to define the subcutaneous layer in this region. The curved iris scissors afford more precision and avoid cautery burns of the hair follicles. Dissecting at the appropriate level is particularly critical in men, as great care must be taken to leave the hair follicles up with the skin to prevent alopecia in this region postoperatively, which would have a feminizing effect. The hair follicles should be visible on the undersurface of the flap. Once the appropriate layer is established, facelift scissors are used under direct vision with transillumination to define the plane. The scissors are beveled up to minimize risk of nerve injury, especially around the border of the mandible and the anterior edge of the parotid. If there is appreciable jowling, the mandibulocutaneous ligament must be released. The submental incision is made, and any further dissection necessary can be done. Using first double hooks and then a small lighted retractor, the pre-platysmal plane is developed sharply with scissors, avoiding the external jugular vein. The submental region plane of dissection is connected with the facial skin plane of dissection, and care is taken to ensure there is an even thickness of skin and fat on the elevated flap. This typically requires leaving down a bit of fat over the platysma in the central neck, which can be removed with a 6 mm spatula to even it out.

8.2.2.6 Platysma

Attention is then turned to the platysma, where its redundancy and subplastysmal fat layer are assessed. Any redundancy in the midline can be removed with cautery, and any prominent region of subplatysmal fat resected directly, albeit carefully. Liposuction is not typically done for the subplatysmal fat but is often done for the preplatysmal fat. In patients with a thicker layer, a spatulated cannula is used to carry out suction lipolysis of the neck and jawline for better definition. If there is significant platysmal banding, the platysma is cut at the cervicomental angle for a few cm, allowing the platysma to drape more sharply after the partial transection of each side. The platysma is then plicated with two layers of 3-0 vicryl running sutures. A platysmal suspension suture is not used, though some authors prefer to use it when they don't think they're able to get enough definition of the jawline with other techniques [1].

8.2.2.7 SMAS Plication

A distinct difference in men and women is the importance of the wide, prominent lower third of the face for men compared to the importance of malar prominence with a narrow lower third of the face for women. Therefore, in women, the goal is malar augmentation as well as pulling up of the superficial musculoaponeurotic system (SMAS), whereas in men, defining the mandibular angle and jawline is more critical, and malar over-augmentation should be avoided. The vector of pull may be more posterior with a male plication. Typically, in the senior author's practice, SMAS is plicated instead of resected or elevated as a flap. There is a diminished risk of nerve injury, less surface area that may bleed, and the technique is effective. When setting the tension, a line is drawn from the junction of the zygoma and arch to the mandibular angle, approximately parallel to the nasolabial fold, creating a perpendicular vector of pull that can efface it more effectively. The vector is tested and adjusted as needed. The ellipse is plicated, starting at the angle and traveling to the zygoma to create fullness. Developing a dog ear at the superior end of the plication is helpful with malar augmentation, but the dog ear at the inferior end should be flattened out with buried vicryl sutures. To accentuate the cervicomental angle, the plication should be carried into the neck. Some authors prefer to resect the SMAS before suturing it to get fresh fascial edges [17]. The senior author only resects tissue if the patient has significant SMAS excess, such as after massive weight loss. The tension of the SMAS is set to smoothen out the jowls without undue tension or an unnatural appearance. Some authors, such as Rohrich, believe their own results are improved by also elevating a lateral platysmal window that is suspended to better define the angle of the mandible [1]. This window can often be sutured to the mastoid. Similarly, other authors, such as Marten, prefer to raise an SMAS flap for male facelifts [18]. For his SMAS flap, he believes that raising it above the zygomatic arch is advantageous, as he feels that allows him to better elevate and rejuvenate the periorbital region and midface more effectively than SMAS flap elevated below the zygomatic arch. Despite the variations in technique, no technique has been proven to be statistically better than another technique in direct comparison studies, which suggests that the most important is the ability to execute one's preferred technique well [19]. Before moving on to the skin redraping, symmetry on both sides of the face should be confirmed. A 7 French round drain is brought out posteriorly above the most superior aspect of the incision, and hidden in the hair on either side before beginning the skin closure.

8.2.2.8 Skin Redraping

The skin edges are clamped with Allis clamps, and redraped conservatively to avoid an operated-on look. The vector of pull for setting the tension of the skin can differ from the one used to set the SMAS tension, which primarily determines the longevity of the facelift outcome. The skin should be redraped to maximally define the angle of the mandible and the jawline, yet minimally impacts the facial hair pattern and hairline. Typically, this balance requires a vector perpendicular to the nasolabial fold. Minimal skin resection should be done around the earlobe and tragus, to prevent a pixie ear deformity and an unnatural eversion of the tragus. There should be no tension at these two points. Instead, the tension should be set in the superior corners of the incision preauricularly and postauricularly. Posteriorly, the posterior end of the flap should be pulled superiorly and anteriorly to set the hairline in a natural location and avoid the stigmata of notching. Additionally, the cuts in the skin are straight or curved, as opposed to zigzags as were done in the initial incisions, as the skin flap always has some redundancy, and therefore can be spread out more evenly throughout the zigzagging segments of the opposing side of the incision, which distributes the extra skin while avoiding a dog ear. The skin acts to redrape over the face, but should not be thought of as a support layer. If it is drawn too tight, ischemia will ensue, which can cause delayed healing, poor scarring, scar hypertrophy, and alopecia.

8.2.2.9 Skin Closure

The first sutures set are the tension-setting sutures in the anterior and posterior corners. After, the incision in the hair posteriorly is stapled together, and the remainder of the incision is closed meticulously. Posteriorly, the flap skin is tied with deep dermals to the exposed conchal cartilage, which allows for a strong suture bite and minimizes descent of the incision over time. Some more deep dermals are placed anteriorly as well for support. The W or zigzagging segments of the incision are sutured evenly to spread out the redundancy, insetting with interrupted nylon sutures at each corner of the zigzag. 3-0 monocryls are used to set the tension, and 5-0 nylon sutures are used for external sutures. Anteriorly, a nylon suture is run from the tragus and up to the sideburn, before again continuing with interrupted sutures in the zigzag segment. The submental incision is closed with deep dermals and a running nylon also.

8.2.2.10 Dressing and Wake-Up

If any hair is present, it is washed with shampoo. Bacitracin and xeroform are placed along the incisions, and a headwrap is placed with iced gauze underneath. The patient is woken up in a deep state by the anesthesiologist to minimize the risk of coughing from the endotracheal tube stimulation. Pneumatic compression boots are kept on.

8.2.3 Postoperative Course

The patient is admitted to the hospital overnight for blood pressure monitoring. This is especially important for men, given their increased risk for hematomas. The blood pressure is monitored closely all night, and if the clonidine patch that was placed preoperatively is not maintaining systolic blood pressure < 130 mmHg, IV hydralazine is given for blood pressure control. No antibiotics are used postoperatively. The head of the bed is elevated at all times overnight to minimize swelling, and the headwrap is loosened slightly for comfort during the postoperative check.

On postoperative day 1, the headwrap is changed to a fresh gauze bandage roll headwrap, and the drains are removed if the output is appropriate. The transdermal clonidine patch and the pneumatic compression boots are removed before discharge. Patients are allowed to take off their gauze bandage roll headwrap when they get home, but should sleep with 2–3 pillows to minimize swelling. They may wash their hair 3 days after surgery. At the one-week follow-up visit, the submental and preauricular sutures are removed. The postauricular sutures and staples are removed at the two-week follow-up visit. Patients should continue applying bacitracin to their incisions for 2 weeks after their sutures are removed. Lifting anything over 10 lbs. should be avoided until 4 weeks after surgery.

8.2.4 Advantages

The benefits of this technique are multiple. It is safe, reproducible, accentuates masculinity, and preserves the patient's facial hair distribution. Figures 8.2, 8.3, and 8.4 are representative comparisons of preoperative with 3-month postoperative photos of the expected result. Figure 8.5 shows a 6-month postoperative comparison. Lastly, Figs. 8.6 and 8.7 compare preoperative photos with a 7-year follow-up photo. The advantages mentioned throughout the text include reproducibility, by avoiding unnecessary steps that the senior author does not think are necessary in his hands, such as elevating a lateral platysmal window or a high SMAS flap. The same techniques also allow the procedure to remain safe, by avoiding going under the SMAS or the platysma, where patients are more at risk for nerve injury that, although rare, can be devastating and leave visible stigmata of surgery. By remaining conservative with the amount of patients that are fat grafted, one avoids potentially overfilling the face and creates a more natural appearance. A focus on the jawline definition helps accentuate the patient's masculinity. Finally, the pretragal approach allows the preservation of the patient's facial hair distribution, and the zigzag scars eliminate the need for extending incisions by allowing for better distribution of the redundancy in the skin flap that is inset.

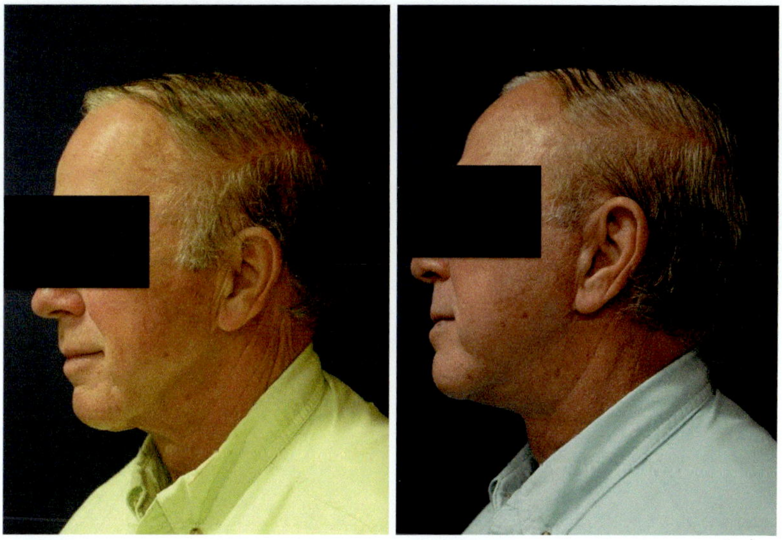

Fig. 8.2 Lateral view comparison, patient 2: Left preoperative photo with mild jowling and decreased definition of the cervicomental angle, with resolution in the 3-month postoperative photo on the right. The hairline is preserved and the incision is concealed

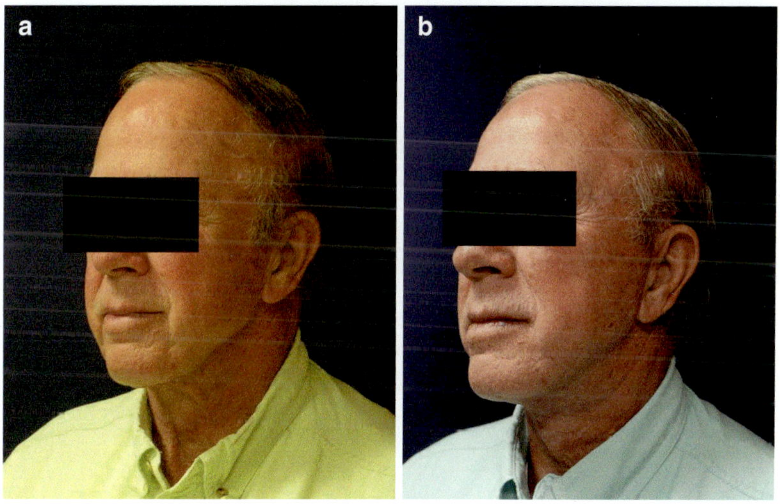

Fig. 8.3 Oblique view comparison, patient 2: Left preoperative photo and right 3-month postoperative photo showing an improvement in the mandibular definition, jowls, and platysmal banding

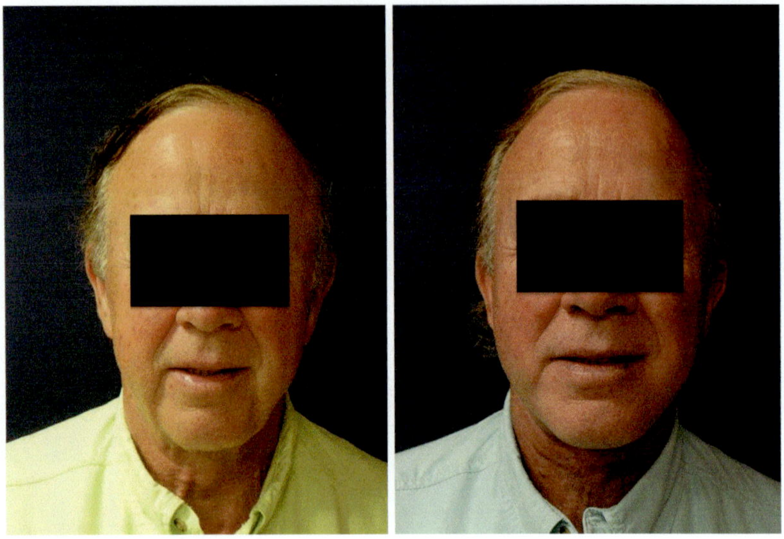

Fig. 8.4 Frontal view comparison, patient 2: The left preoperative photo shows moderate jowling, decreased mandibular definition, and platysmal banding. The right 3-month postoperative photo shows improvement of those three components

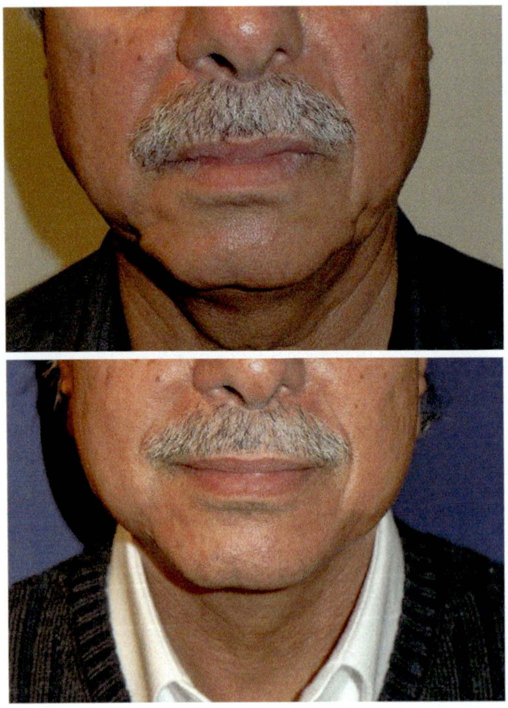

Fig. 8.5 Frontal view comparison, patient 3: The top preoperative photo shows moderate jowling, decreased mandibular definition, and neck skin laxity banding. The right 6-month postoperative photo shows improvement of those three components

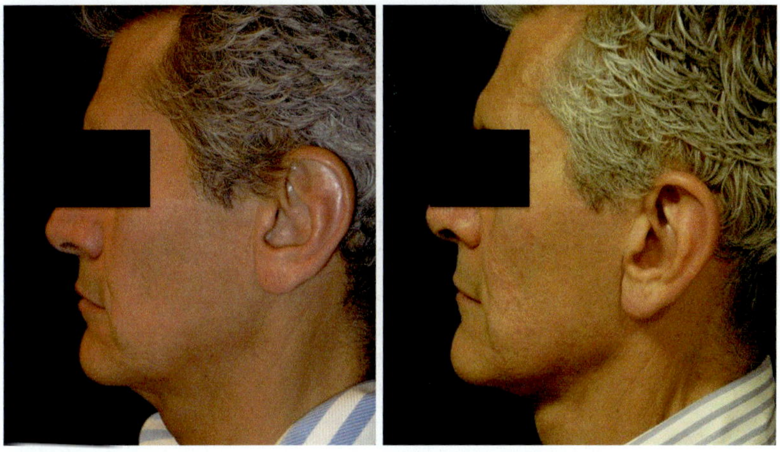

Fig. 8.6 Lateral view comparison, patient 4: Left preoperative photo with some jowling and again decreased mandibular definition with an obtuse cervicomental angle. The right 7-year postoperative photo shows a natural result with improvement in all components, which continues to look better than the preoperative photo 7 years later

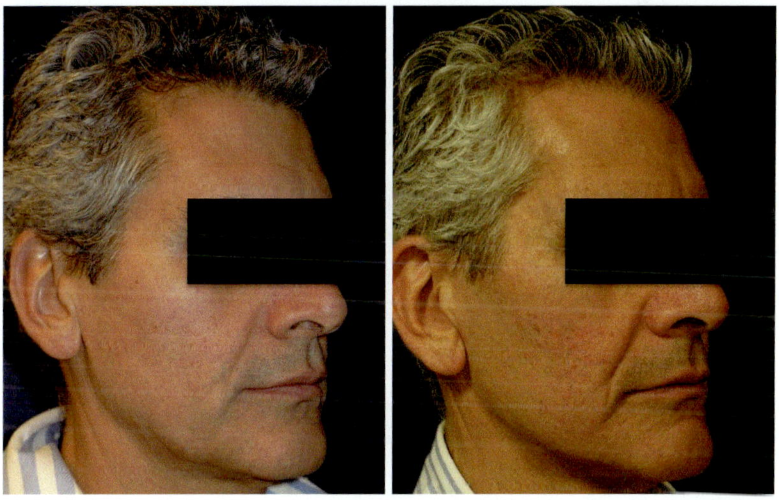

Fig. 8.7 Oblique view comparison, patient 4: Left preoperative photo and right 7-year postoperative photo with improved mandibular definition and jowling

References

1. Rohrich RJ, Stuzin JM, Ramanadham S, Costa C, Dauwe PB. The modern male rhytidectomy: lessons learned. Plast Reconstr Surg. 2017;139(2):295–307.
2. Joseph J. Hangewangenplastik. Dtsch Med Wochenschr. 1921;47:287.
3. Baker DC, Aston SJ, Guy CL, Rees TD. The male rhytidectomy. Plast Reconstr Surg. 1977;60(4):514–22.
4. Ramanadham SR, Costa CR, Narasimhan K, Coleman JE, Rohrich RJ. Refining the anesthesia management of the face-lift patient: lessons learned from 1089 consecutive face lifts. Plast Reconstr Surg. 2015;135(3):723–30.
5. Pitanguy I, Ramos H, Garcia LC. Filosofia, tecnica e complicacoes das ritidectomias atraves de observacao e analise de 2600 casos pessoais consecutivos. Rev Brasil Cir. 1972;62:277.
6. Lawson W, Naidu RK. The male facelift. An analysis of 115 cases. Arch Otolaryngol Head Neck Surg 1993;119(5):535–9; discussion 40–1.
7. Grover R, Jones BM, Waterhouse N. The prevention of haematoma following rhytidectomy: a review of 1078 consecutive facelifts. Br J Plast Surg. 2001;54(6):481–6.
8. Abboushi N, Yezhelyev M, Symbas J, Nahai F. Facelift complications and the risk of venous thromboembolism: a single center's experience. Aesthet Surg J. 2012;32(4):413–20.

9. Baker DC, Stefani WA, Chiu ES. Reducing the incidence of hematoma requiring surgical evacuation following male rhytidectomy: a 30-year review of 985 cases. Plast Reconstr Surg. 2005;116(7):1973–85. discussion 86-7.
10. Rees TD, Liverett DM, Guy CL. The effect of cigarette smoking on skin-flap survival in the face lift patient. Plast Reconstr Surg. 1984;73(6):911–5.
11. Hsu C, Gruber RP, Dosanjh A. Prediction of face-lift outcomes using the preoperative supine test. Aesth Plast Surg. 2009;33(6):828–31.
12. Herruer JM, Prins JB, van Heerbeek N, Verhage-Damen GW, Ingels KJ. Negative predictors for satisfaction in patients seeking facial cosmetic surgery: a systematic review. Plast Reconstr Surg. 2015;135(6):1596–605.
13. Tonnard PL, Verpaele A, Gaia S. Optimising results from minimal access cranial suspension lifting (MACS-lift). Aesth Plast Surg. 2005;29(4):213–20. discussion 21
14. Tonnard P, Verpaele A. The MACS-lift short scar rhytidectomy. Aesthet Surg J. 2007;27(2):188–98.
15. Baker DC, Nahai F, Massiha H, Tonnard P. Short scar face lift. Aesthet Surg J. 2005;25(6):607–17.
16. Camirand A, Doucet J. A comparison between parallel hairline incisions and perpendicular incisions when performing a face lift. Plast Reconstr Surg. 1997;99(1):10–5.
17. Imber G, Silich RC. Limited-incision face lift technique. Aesthet Surg J. 2001;21(3):216–26.
18. Marten TJ, Elyassnia D. Chapter 6.9 Facelift: Male Facelift. In: Neligan PC, editor. Plastic Surgery, 4th ed. 2018.
19. Mustoe TA, Park E. Evidence-based medicine: face lift. Plast Reconstr Surg. 2014;133(5):1206–13.

9 Facial Rejuvenation in the Male Patient

Richard J. Greco

Men are living longer, working longer, and are having multiple relationships. Men were fortunate because as they aged they were thought to become "more distinguished" as we aged, but since we are living longer—men eventually just starting to look old too. This has led to a huge increase in interest in facial rejuvenation in our male patient population.

Men have different interests from women. They are LESS tolerant of having any obvious sequela or appearance of having had cosmetic surgery performed. Patients are interested in non-invasive procedures to help with wrinkles and folds, but the most common complaints are the extra skin and puffiness of their eyes and the loose skin of their necks.

The goals of this chapter are to discuss my approach to the male rejuvenation patient. I will discuss how to decide the best options within the limitations of what the patient will allow you to perform. Men are where women were 30 years ago—they want to look younger—but don't want anyone to know they are having it done. Their recovery time is longer (return to work without looking obvious about their procedure), as they don't like wearing makeup and have less ability to explain the swelling and bruising.

R. J. Greco (✉)
The Georgia Institute For Plastic Surgery, Savannah, GA, USA

9.1 Patient Evaluation

I meet all new patients in my office. We sit down and discuss their areas of concerns about which they would like my opinion and suggestions. One of my goals is trying to have the patient explain the changes in their personal or work life that have stimulated them to come visit with me. We will discuss their overall health history and whether they are an acceptable health risk to operate on.

We then take standard photographs of the patient from multiple angles, including the entire area of concern, and then close-ups of specific areas that may require assistance. These are digital photos that are immediately uploaded. I then perform an examination of the patient and discuss my findings immediately while I am doing the exam with the patient:

- Hair—density, color, quality, with specific discussions of hair loss patterns. I also note the pattern of the patient's sideburns and post-auricular hairline.
- Skin textures—discussion of deep pitting, wrinkles, actinic changes, and color changes.
- Brow—position and ptosis, forehead, and glabellar wrinkle pattern.
- Upper eyelids—laxity of skin, excess fat, eyelid ptosis.

K. Jeffords et al. (eds.), *Aesthetic Surgery for Men*, https://doi.org/10.1007/978-3-032-03840-1_9

- Lower lids—entropion, ectropion, lower lid laxity, excess skin and fat—and in which compartments, festoons.
- Jowls—laxity and actual sag.
- Neck—this is usually the biggest concern. Loose skin, platysma bands, excessive submental fat, ptotic submandibular glands.
- Nasal labial folds—how deep and the degree of cheek sag.
- Oral commissure lines—depth and degree of laxity.
- Loss of volume—as we age, many individuals lose volume in the face, causing facial sag. An evaluation of tissue sag versus volume loss helps determine the correct way to treat the change in appearance.

Additional areas of concern that I look at—but do not comment on unless the patient discusses—are the shape and size of the patient's ears and nose.

We now look at the photographs together to see which areas of concerns bother the patient enough to discuss. Once we know which areas are their primary concern, we can offer noninvasive, minimally invasive, and surgical options to obtain the improvements they desire. We discuss the degrees of improvement versus the recovery and risks of each technique. We then discuss what combination of techniques can be utilized to reach their goals.

I like to use morphing technology to simulate some of the improvements that we perceive that we can obtain for the patient. It is not a guarantee of result, and we try to under promise the result—but allows the patient and significant other a preview of what is possible. We provide technology that allows the patient to look at these photographs and altered images at home. Using the same program, we review many before and after photographs of some of my previous patients that had similar problems, how we treated them, and their short-term and long-term results. We demonstrate each of the procedures they are considering.

The goal is to educate the patient as to their options, likely improvements, risks and complications, and length of recovery so they can make an informed decision with us as to their best course of action. Many times, this could involve doing the procedures in multiple smaller steps—but the majority choose to do as many as possible at one time to reduce their overall recovery times.

We always offer the least invasive and quickest recovery procedure possible to solve the problem. Noninvasive procedures including toxin treatment for forehead, glabella, and lateral periorbital regions and fillers to the nasal labial and oral commissure regions are extremely well received. They will be discussed by others in this book.

Our focus will be on our approach to the neck and face.

9.2 The Neck

We will see men of all ages with an imperfect neck. This could be from extra fat, loose skin, muscle bands, inadequate chin, or a combination of the above. Younger individuals usually have fullness from too much fat and can be treated with noninvasive fat dissolving methods or liposuction. If the patient has significant fullness, my preference is liposuction.

9.2.1 Liposuction of the Neck

In the correct patient with submental fullness due to extra fat, we perform liposuction under local or local and light sedation. We typically make three small puncture wounds—one under the chin and one behind each earlobe. We start by creating a small skin wheal with a 30-gauge needle and infiltration of 1% lidocaine with 1: 100,000 epinephrine. Next, we will either use our facelift infiltration technique utilizing with 60 cc syringes and 22 G spinal needles utilizing ½ % Lidocaine with 1:400,000 epi or infiltrate with a liposuction infiltrating needle (mix 50 cc of 1% lidocaine in 1 liter NSS and 2 cc of epinephrine).

Liposuction is performed with a 3 mm cannula with all ports aiming down from the skin surface. You want to avoid suctioning directly on the undersurface of the skin flap to help avoid adhe-

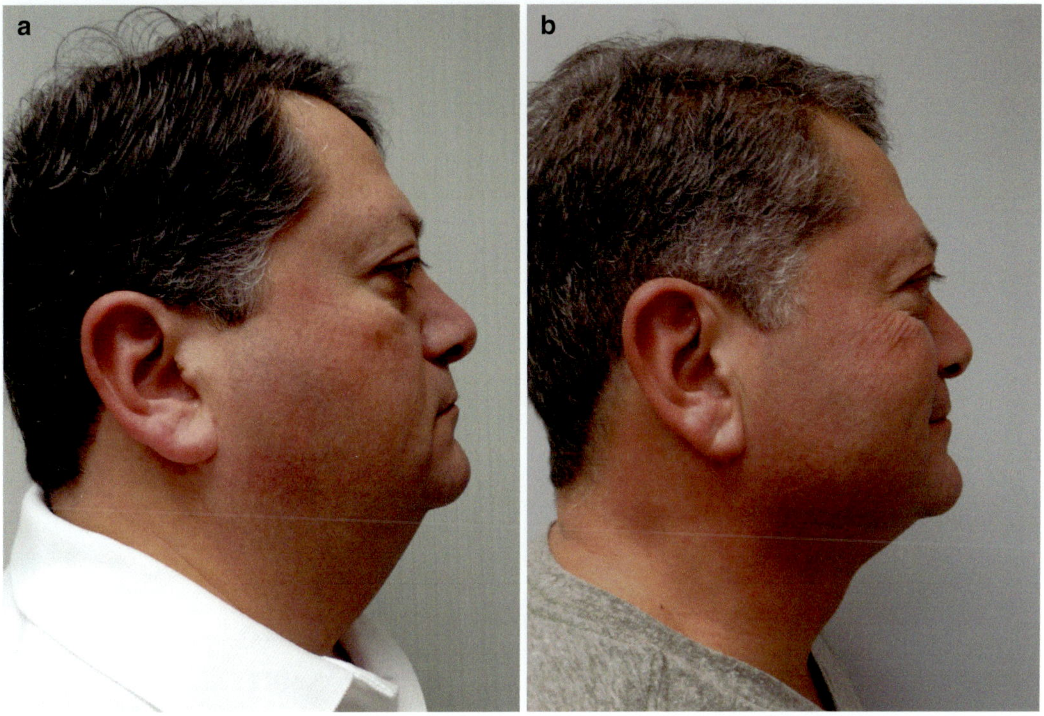

Fig. 9.1 (**a**) Liposuction of neck preoperative; (**b**) Liposuction of neck postoperative

sions or puckers from direct connections between the dermis and the underlying musculature. The amount of fat aspirated is always underwhelming. But the disruption of the fat, injury, and scar formation leads to excellent results (Fig. 9.1).

9.2.2 Direct Excision of Neck

Many men come in with different degrees of aging, but there is only one area of concern—the extra skin of their neck. It flops around and hangs over their collar. They often will state, "I don't care about getting older and looking it, but I hate this neck (while grabbing the loose skin of their neck)". After careful examination of the patient – some will accept the concept that a neck lift or a facelift will do a better job of improving the neck without any visible scars on the neck, others are not willing to accept the cost or downtime associated with bigger procedures and are willing to accept the scar to get an improvement of the neck silhouette. The results can be very rewarding, and the scars usually become imperceptible with years (Figs. 9.2 and 9.3).

9.2.3 Neck Lift

Thorough evaluation of the patient shows occasional laxity of the neck, no jowl formation, and a relatively youthful face. This is the perfect patient for a post-auricular neck lift. It avoids the visible scars of the anterior neck and allows for the creation of an improved neck. Many of these patients can benefit from a submental liposuction at the same time as the neck lift, for example, removal of some of the fullness associated with extra submental fat. We routinely improve the shape and lines of the neck by tightening or advancing the platysma muscle posteriorly on each side.

Neck lifts are performed under intravenous sedation and local infiltration. After the hair is combed and secured with small rubber bands, incision lines are drawn in the postauricular sul-

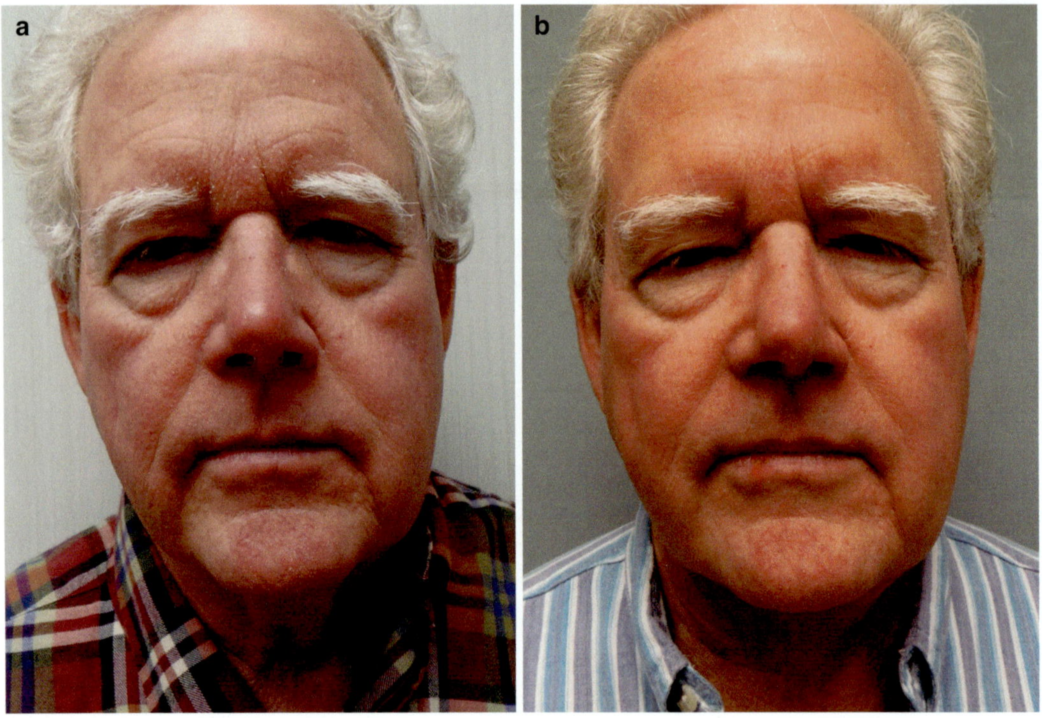

Fig. 9.2 (**a**) Preop direct neck excision front; (**b**) Postop direct neck excision front

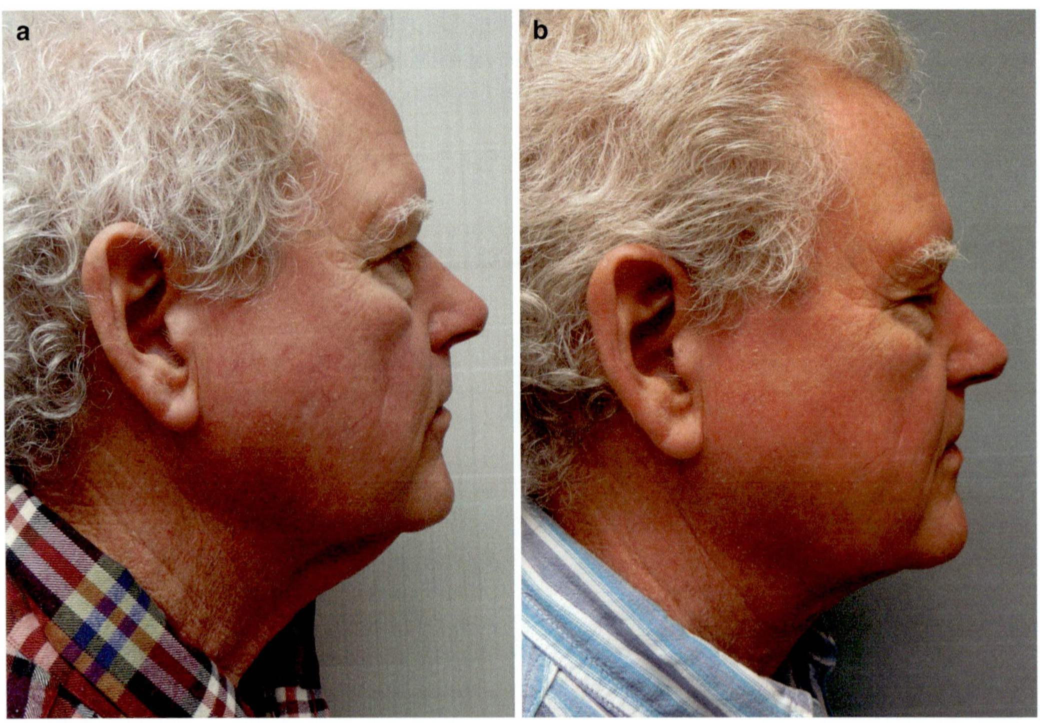

Fig. 9.3 (**a**) Preop direct neck excision side; (**b**) Postop direct neck excision side

cus and then arched and brought back into the postauricular scalp. Infiltration of the incisions is performed with a 30-gauge needle with 1% lidocaine with 1:100,000 epinephrine. Next, we will use our facelift infiltration technique utilizing 60-cc syringes and 22-G spinal needles utilizing ½% lidocaine with 1:400,000 epinephrine throughout the neck region.

After 10 minutes for the local anesthetic to take effect, we will make the incision from the bottom of the ear, along the post-auricular sulcus, in an arched fashion above a line straight back from the tragus. Into the scalp for about 3 cm on the line straight back from the tragus. We will now elevate the skin flap at a level beneath the dermis and a small amount of fat and blood supply—but above the fascial plane of the platysma, mastoid fascia, and sternocleidomastoid muscle. The lateral border of the platysma is found and opened along its edge. Care is taken to avoid the greater auricular sensory nerve.

The platysma edge is then advanced posteriorly, and we trim a segment of it away, depending on the degree of laxity Figure of eight sutures of 3(0) PDS are used to secure the lateral edge of platysma to the Mastoid fascia and then the lateral neck fascia. Care to avoid the external and internal jugular veins and greater auricular nerve is important. Once the right side is secured, the excess skin is elevated and removed to hide the scars in the sulcus and in the scalp posteriorly. A suction drain for two days and close the defect with 4(0) PDS post-auricular and 3(0) PDS in the scalp followed by staples. The skin behind the ear is closed with 4(0) PDS subcutaneoulsy and then a 3(0) Prolene running dermal suture with 2 or three external loops to help with the ease of removal at 2 weeks. A similar procedure is performed on the opposite side.

9.3 Facelift

Men interested in facial rejuvenation are often very different from my female patient population. They usually come in at a later stage of aging, often at the recommendation of their significant other, and are very concerned about the appearance of having had something done. In addition, they often have very heavy and advanced jowling and loose skin on their neck. Their expectations are also "less" perfect and would prefer an improvement that gets rid of all of this loose skin—usually grasping the skin of their neck and sometimes jowls—with the least surgery as possible. Performing a neck lift alone allows us to only redistribute their excess neck skin in an anterior/posterior vector, whereas if they have a facelift, we can redistribute their laxity in a blend of vertical and posterior vectors leading to the best resolution. They may not want a browlift or eyelid surgery at the same time, but they get a lot of improvement and satisfaction from a facelift alone.

I meet all new patients in my office. We sit down and discuss their areas of concerns, about which they would like my opinion and suggestions. One of my goals is having the patient explain what the changes are in his personal or work life that have stimulated them to come visit with me. We will discuss their overall health history and whether they are an acceptable health risk to operate on.

The patient is then taken to an exam room where we do a very thorough evaluation of the head and neck region, starting with the hair density, patterns of balding, hairlines, and degree of brow ptosis. As we work our way down, we note the degree of skin excess of the upper and lower lids and the amount and locations of lid fat pocket prominence. A snap test of the lower lid is performed. As we examined the cheeks and neck, we note the degrees of skin laxity, locations of such, and the influences of facial fat atrophy or excess. When considering the possible facial rejuvenation incisions, it is important to note how much skin laxity the patient has, where the patient's hair pattern is presently, and how your planned incisions may ultimately result in a change in the hair pattern and visibility of the subsequent scars.

The artistic nature of plastic surgery is to meticulously plan to leave as little evidence as possible that we have been involved in the patient's rejuvenation. Our goals will include leaving the sideburn at a height not higher than the top of the ear, to not increase the width from the lateral canthus to the temporal hairline greater than 4 cm, to avoid a step off in the postauricular hairline, to have a natural junction between the earlobe and the facial skin, the for the postauricular scar to fall in the natural crease, and for the preauricular scar and color transition to be as hidden as possible.

I believe in taking standard photographs of the patient, putting them on the computer screen, and reviewing with the patient what they see and what concerns them. Most patients have never actually sat and looked at what others see when they look at them. We review before and after photographs of many patients who have had similar procedures and what I consider to be a good result. It allows the patient to get an idea of what your artistic direction is. We then morph the patient's photographs using Mirror software to begin the discussion about what is and is not possible. We are careful not to over correct the simulated result so that the patient does not have unrealistic expectations. If a patient has expectations that are not what I can safely and reliably provide, I would rather not operate on the patient. In addition, I explain to the patient that is my job to give them a thorough evaluation of everything that I see that we can improve, it is their job to tell me what bothers them, or feel is worth addressing. I do not want them to tell me afterwards—why didn't you tell me that we could have addressed that while I was there.

A thorough health history and physical is performed. Most of these procedures are done under deep intravenous sedation and can last as long as six hours, depending on what they have decided to address. If there are health concerns, a medical clearance is obtained.

9.3.1 Decisions

There are a series of decisions that we will make after discussions with the patient. Some are more dependent on our personal experience with previous patients, while others will be made by the patient.

9.3.2 Operative Procedure

Once the patient has decide that a "facelift" is the best choice, we will consider the following three options: skin-only facelift, Dual Plane, Deep Plane (SMAS) facelift , and the "Deep Plane" facelift. My experience is that male patients want a very natural look and as little downtime as possible. This limits my personal choice in most patients to a Dual Plane Deep Plane SMAS operation.

Skin-only facelifts are the simplest and low-risk procedures, but there are two major drawbacks to this technique: the results last only for a short time and a significant number of patients will have an "overdone" or windswept appearance. Men cannot tolerate this potential consequence—so the only patients that I use this procedure in are Acne Patients and young patients with minimal to moderate facial aging that want a refreshed look and short downtime.

"Deep Plane" facelifts often are performed with deeper anesthesia, more operative time, and a much longer recovery due to the prolonged postoperative swelling depending on the amount of anterior dissection performed. The majority of my male patients are not willing to be out in public until they do not appear to if they had "something done." I find that the results of elevating the SMAS in the Deep Plane separately from the overlying skin allows for the perfect elevation of the deep structures—securing a natural base to redrape the skin in the best directions to remove as much of the appearance of aging without tension or a "pulled look". This allows for the most Natural Result with the quickest recovery for me.

My preferred technique is a compendium of thoughts, concepts, and techniques that I learned from my professors at the University of Pittsburgh, modified from my experience at the Manhattan Eye and Ear, and refined through 32 years of experience, reflection, and modifications. Facial rejuvenation is artistic, and each surgeon has a different vision of what a good result is. This is important to share with your patient through pre- and postoperative photographs to demonstrate your vision and results. In addition, using "morphing" programs to demonstrate what they might appear like after surgery can help discuss what they are hoping for and whether it is actually possible to meet their needs. My opinion is that patients do not want a "done" result. They want to be as young as possible, while looking natural.

Details such as placement of scars, preservation of hairlines, tension of rejuvenation forces on the deeper structures in order to leave the skin lift and incisions without tension, and replacement of soft tissue volume when necessary are important to obtain the ideal results. The choices change based on the patient's degree of skin laxity and facial volume atrophy, location of hairlines, and the skin coloration on the face, ear, and pretragal regions. We will review how we make these decisions preoperatively and intraoperatively.

9.3.3 Scar—Preauricular Versus Posttragal

We evaluate each patient in the following areas to help us make up our minds on the best option to recommend to the patient—the decision is ultimately theirs to make after discussing our thoughts on the best option.

Preoperative wrinkle/folds in the preauricular area. If the patient is already used to significant folds in the preauricular area and the scar will fall in this line, the patient is less likely to notice or object to the scar. It falls into the previous fold's position (Fig. 9.4).

1. Coloration of the tragus and the location of the advanced skin. If there is a distinct difference in the coloration or ruddiness in the coloration of the skin, it would lead more to a post-tragal incision.
2. Length and density of sideburn in conjunction to the width of preauricular non-hair-bearing skin in comparison to the amount of skin laxity. We do not want significant hair density directly in the preauricular space and on the tragus. If we feel that it is likely to "crowd" the area, leaving a small area of non-hair bearing preauricular skin is preferable.
3. Definition of preoperative tragus. The postoperative appearance of a typical posttragal incision allows for the lack of a preauricular scar at the expense of a blunted preauricular /tragal junction. The less defined the tragal/preauricular skin juncture is, the less noticeable the lack of definition of the postoperative posttragal incision will be.

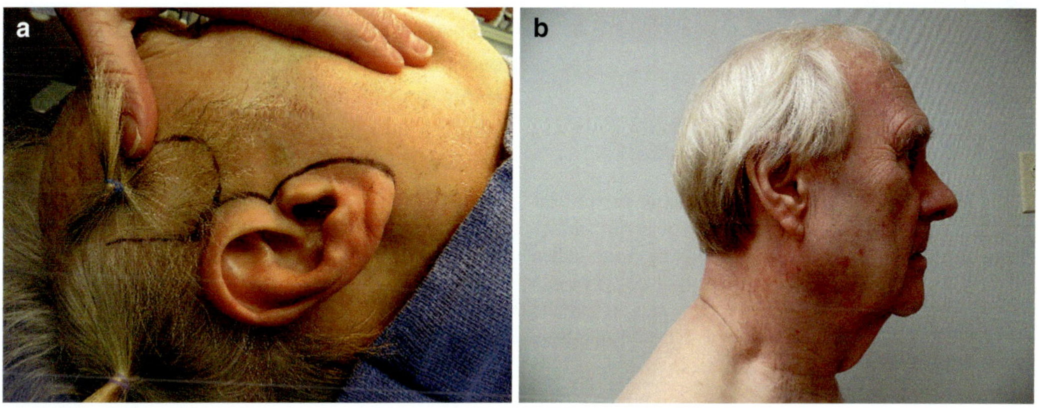

Fig. 9.4 (**a**) Well-defined tragus with even coloration and preexisting preauricular folds; (**b**) Demonstration of the option of hairline or a super auricular temporal incision

9.3.4 Post Auricular Scar

We discuss with patients that they will have to shave more posteriorly and behind their ears because of the advancement of hair-bearing cheek and neck skin. Our goal is to hide the scar, but not allow for hair-bearing skin on the posterior aspect of the ear. The incision is planned to either go posteriorly into the scalp at the level of the tragus or along the hairline (Fig. 9.5).

I do not prefer the incision along the hairline because it is visible, especially in men with short hair styles or if they wear their hair back in a ponytail (maybe you should offer them a stylist for advice). The only reason that I make an incision along the hairline is if they have had a previous incision there, or if there is so much laxity, we will create a significant step off in the posterior hairline. We can try to work the hairline forward and still prefer this to the scar. We also try not to have a straight line back from the ear to the scalp and try to take the scar up a bit higher postauricular in the non-hair-bearing skin to break up the scar and hide it higher behind the ear.

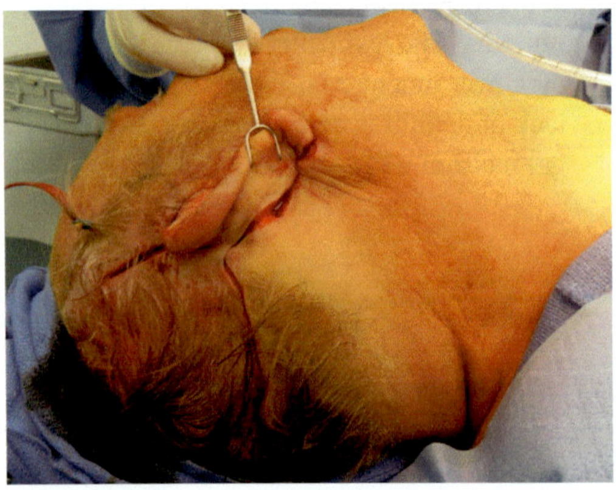

Fig. 9.5 The postauricular scar falls just in the postauricular groove. Care not to go up on the posterior surface of the ear to prevent hair-bearing skin from being pulled on the posterior aspect of the ear. The incision goes into the posterior scalp at the level of tragus, and we avoid a straight-line scar by elevating the scar in the non-hair-bearing area as well

9.3.5 Temple Scar

All decisions tend to be made based on what is the likelihood that we will make the person look "done" or "post-surgical." Every individual has a different degree of space between their lateral orbit and their hairline, a different degree of skin laxity, a different position and inferior placement of their sideburn, and a different degree of hair density. One must imagine if you make a temporal incision, how far up you will take their sideburn, and how far back their hairline will go based on their laxity and your planned procedure. Even though I generally prefer the super-auricular temporal incision, one should not allow the sideburn to go higher than the top of the ear and bring the temporal hairline too far posteriorly, or you will both feminize and make the patient look "operated" on.

9.3.6 SMAS Elevation

After the skin has been opened and the dissections performed, it is important to elevate the SMAS and suspend the actual facial enhancement on these deeper structures. In men, I start the incision at the inferior border of the zygomatic arch and anterior to the ear by 1 cm (Fig. 9.6) and continue down (Fig. 9.7) to the confluence of the lateral platysmal border (Fig. 9.8). Elevation continues over the anterior edge of the parotid and until the elevation allows for improvement of the jowls and the upper half of the nasal labial fold (Fig. 9.9). If the patient needs further cheek definition, we fold over the SMAS and suture it into place (Fig. 9.10). If this would feminize the patient, we excise it and suture it into position with buried figure-of-eight sutures of 4(0) PDS.

We then excise the excess anterior to the ear and create a pendant of SMAS to attach postauricularly to the mastoid fascia (Fig. 9.11) or just pull the lateral border of the platysma posteriorly to suture to the mastoid fascia and SCM fascia with buried figure-of-eight sutures of 3(0) PDS (Fig. 9.12). We

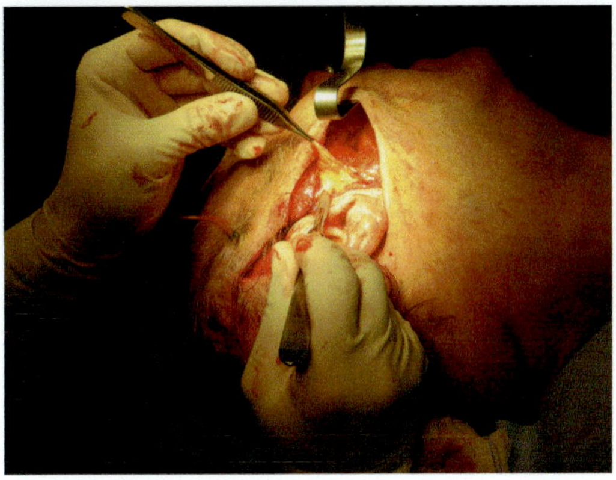

Fig. 9.6 Beginning of the SMAS dissection at the level of the bottom of the zygomatic arch

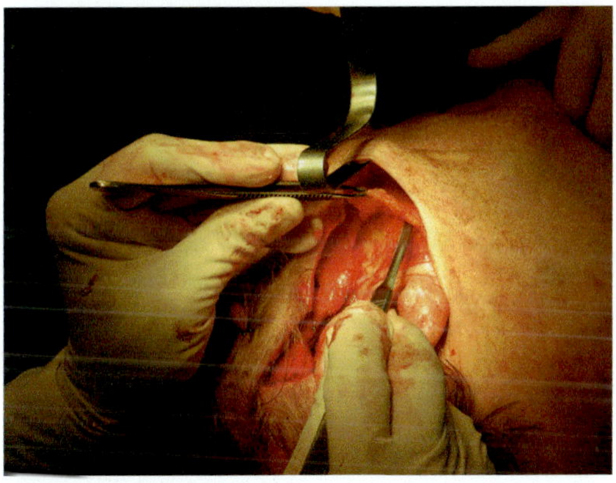

Fig. 9.7 Sharp dissection for the first 1.5 to 2 cm, then facelift scissor dissection

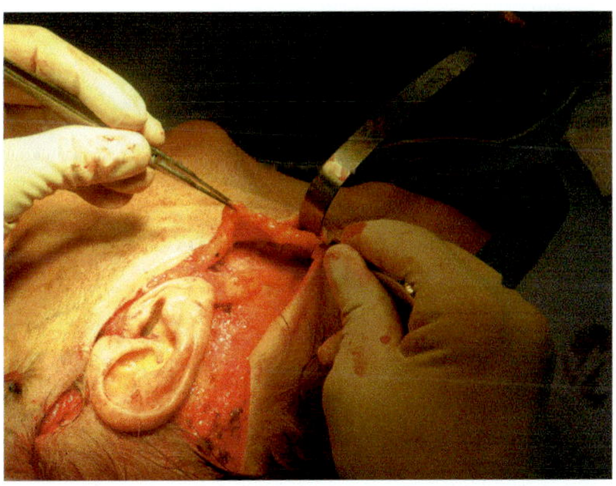

Fig. 9.8 Elevation of the confluence of the SMAS and the lateral platysmal border

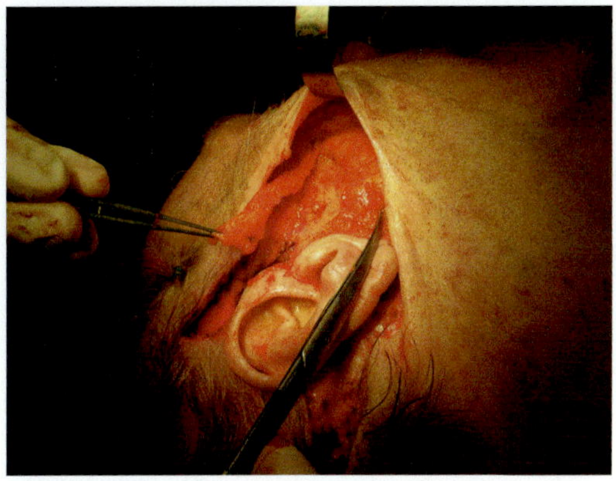

Fig. 9.9 After elevating to the best superior tension, excision of excess SMAS

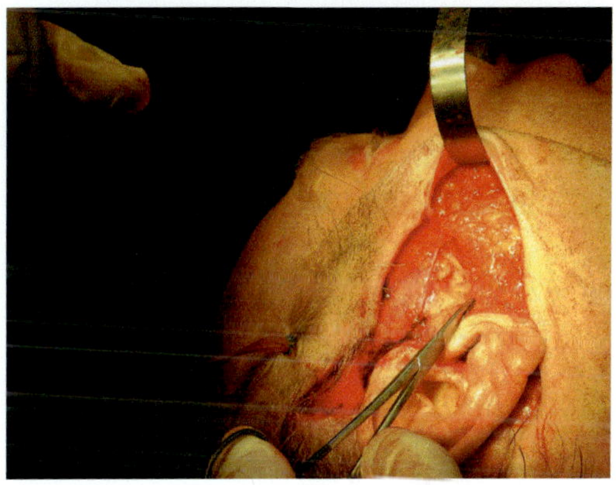

Fig. 9.10 Securing SMAS elevation with buried 4(0) PDS figure of eights

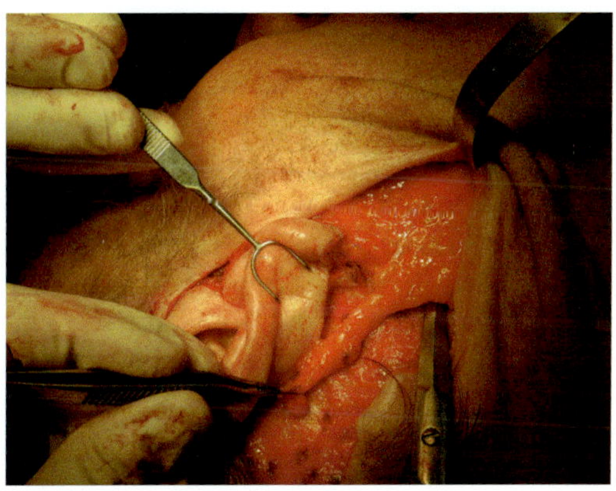

Fig. 9.11 Creation of a SMAS pendant used to secure the pull at the neck margin in a posterior and superior vector

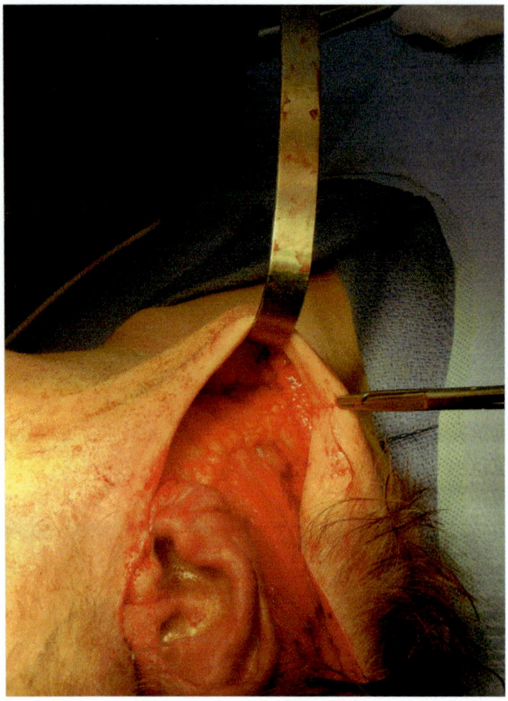

Fig. 9.12 The closure of the lateral platysma border to the posterior neck fascia

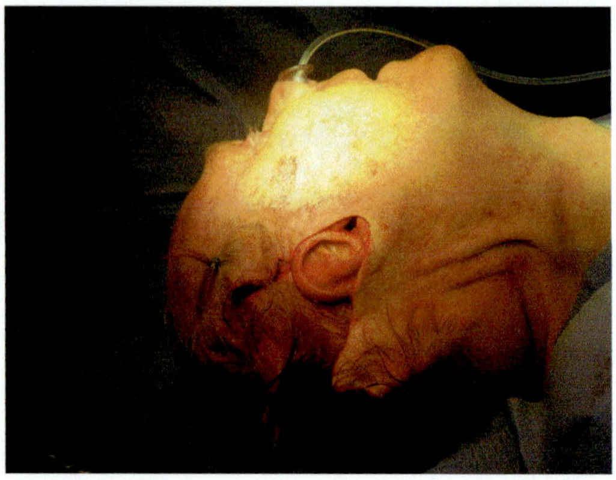

Fig. 9.13 Redraping of skin laxity with all tension on SMAS closure—none on skin

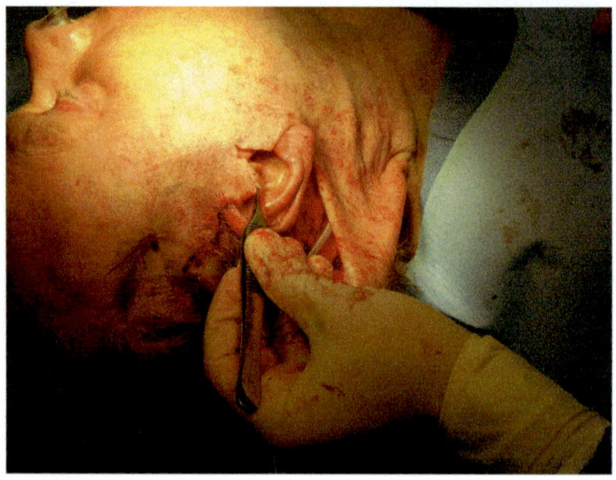

Fig. 9.14 Setting the posterior resection with a vertical vector as well

suture down 4 or 5 centimeters until an adequate lateral pull has been performed without creating a bulge or "dog ear" of the fascia.

9.3.7 Closure of Facelift

After SMAS elevation, repositioning, excision of excess SMAS, and securing of the closure, we now start the closure of the skin without tension (Fig. 9.13). Two TLS drains are placed—one in the temple down along the cheek and one posterior down into the neck. The first suture is either at the top of the ear and set the sideburn at its maximal vertical elevation—or if it is not an issue—it is peak of the posterior resection (Fig. 9.14), at the peak of the pre tragal incision with a 5 (0) PDS. We then set the temporal resection and excise the excess skin superior to the ear and close with 3(0) PDS and staples (Fig. 9.15). One can trim the excess skin in the superior aspect of the preauricular area and close with 5(0) PDS.

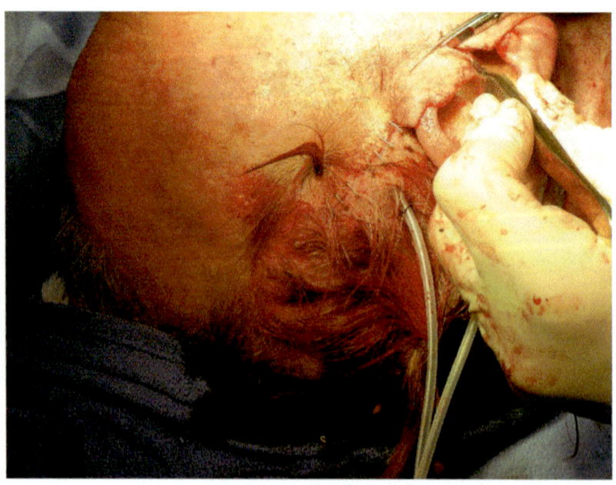

Fig. 9.15 The temporal area has been secured with 3(0) PDS and staples. Trimming preauricular excess

The next step is to set the postauricular closure with close attention to the hairline step off. We often set the point right behind the ear and then move the hairline closure forward (Fig. 9.16). This reduces the step off, but it cannot compromise the posterior/ vertical vector of pull on the neck. The postauricular skin is secured with 4(0) PDS and the scalp with 3(0) PDS and staples (Fig. 9.17). The inferior ear is then fitted for closure with careful resection of skin excess. It is important not to create pixie ears by cutting too much tissue at the earlobe closure. It is better to have the skin tucked up into this area with no tension (Fig. 9.18).

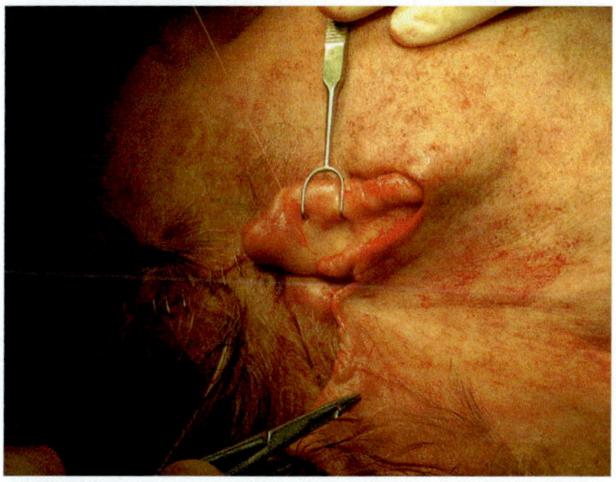

Fig. 9.16 Excess has been measured and incised. The peak of postauricular elevation is secured with 5(0) PDS

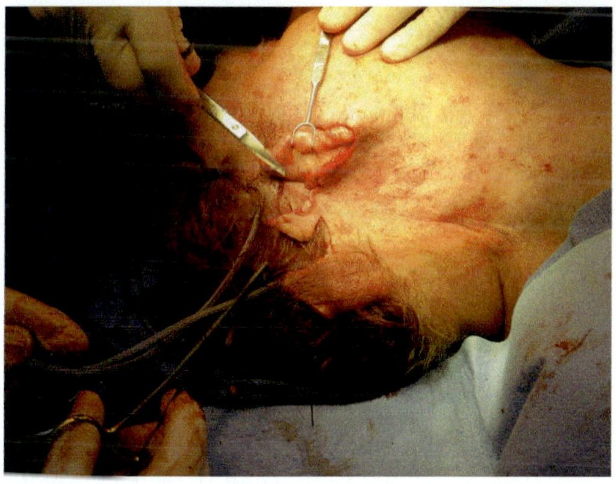

Fig. 9.17 Posterior hairline is re-established and excess trimmed. Closed with 3 (0) PDS and staples

The anterior region is closed with buried 5(0) PDS and running 6(0) Nylon sutures (Fig. 9.19). Postauricularly, we use a 4(0) PDS dermal closure and then a running 3(0) subcuticular Prolene suture with a few external loops for ease of remaoval (Fig. 9.20).

9.3.8 Open Submental Incision

The majority of the patients do not need a submental incision. Most patients have lax skin and

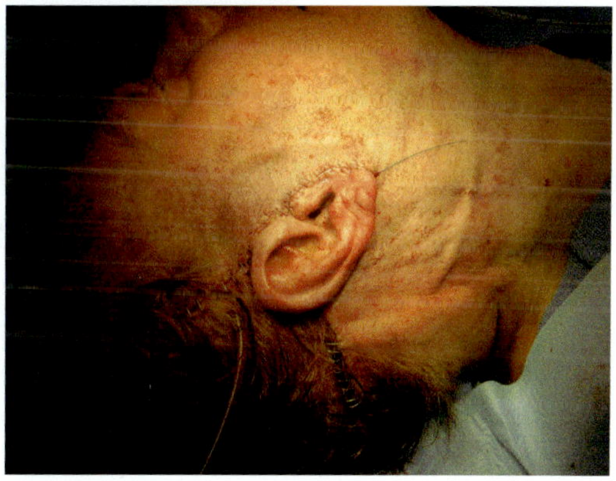

Fig. 9.19 Final closure with interupted subdermal 5(0) PDS sutures followed by a running 6 (0) Nylon suture anteriorly followed by 4(0) interrupted subdermal PDS sutures and a running subcuticular 3(0) Prolene with pull out loops

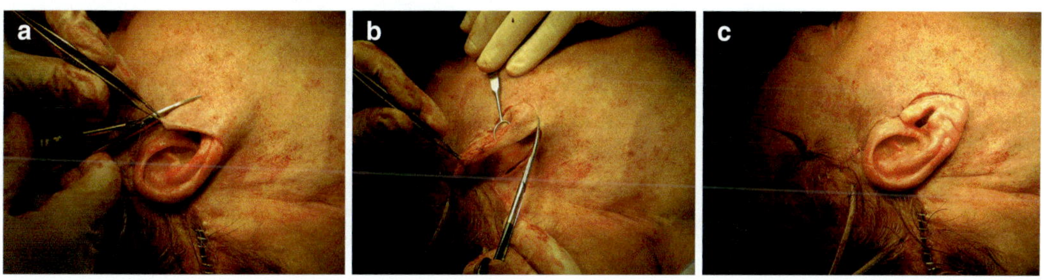

Fig. 9.18 Trimming of the excess facial skin (**a**) anteriorly and (**b**) posteriorly; (**c**) Leaving laxity at the base of the ears to avoid pixie ears

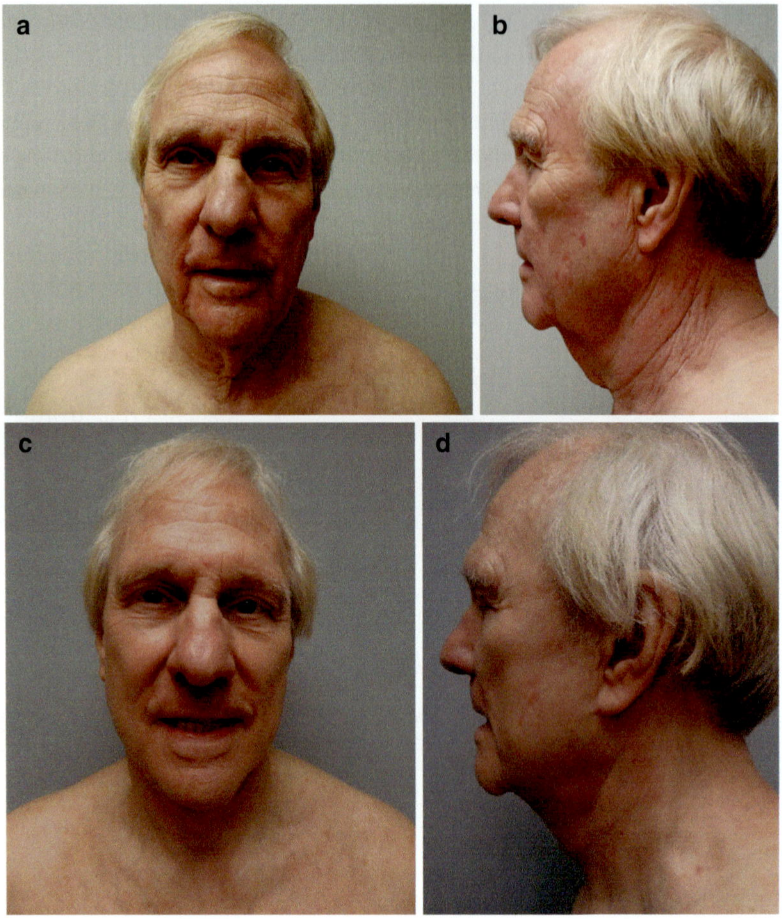

Fig. 9.20 (**a**) Facelift preop front; (**b**) facelift preop side; (**c**) facelift postop; 20 (**d**) facelift postop side

some extra fatty fullness that can be handled with liposuction. In my hands, the indications to open the neck are to approximate the medial edges of the platysma. We ask the patient to bite down and look at the anterior neck to see if there are definable bands. These bands will reappear in a few years if one only pulls the platysma posteriorly. By creating a platysma sling anteriorly and then tightening it posteriorly as well, the neck is nicely recontoured and the bands are less likely to recur. If necessary to improve the bands after the midline platsymal repair, we divide the platysma distally beyond the mid-thyroid cartilage region until they have dissipated. The submental incision is closed last with 5(0) PDS and 6 (0) Nylon.

9.3.9 Fat Grafting

There have been many advancements in the understanding and treatment of facial aging. For many decades, facial rejuvenation procedures have focused on the repositioning of skin and the underlying soft tissues. It is only recently that we have begun to understand that facial aging is caused by not just skin and soft tissue laxity but also volume loss that comes from fat atrophy. This has led to the concept of enhancing the rejuvenation result by restoring volume with small fat grafts. These have been useful to reduce lip lines or wrinkles, as an adjunct to soften the nasal labial and oral commissure folds, soften glabella and forehead wrinkles, and to fill in cheek hollows.

9.4 Conclusion

Men are living longer, working longer, and having multiple relationships at an older age. Men used to become "distinguished" and now they just become old. Although men are interested in looking younger, they do not tolerate the appearance of being "done." There are many decisions to be made based on the individual's specific anatomical features to design an operation that has the most potential to improve their appearance with the least risk of leaving signs of surgery.

Direct Neck Lift: Cervical Wave-Plasty

10

Fereydoun D. Parsa, Nicholas Yim, and Natalie N. Parsa

10.1 Introduction

A youthful neck is characterized by a distinct inferior mandibular border, visible subhyoid depression, visible thyroid cartilage bulge, anterior sternocleidomastoid line at a 90-degree angle with the submental line, and cervical angle of 105 to 120 degrees. However, as people age, the neck loses its natural shape and contour due to loss of elasticity that is often combined with fat accumulation in the submental and anterior neck region [1–8].

Neck rejuvenation is achievable through several different surgical options. A full face and neck lift results in the best improvement and has well concealed pre-auricular scars. However, an increasing number of patients, in particular aging men, are only interested in improving their neck contour and prefer a shorter, less extensive, and less costly procedure or are not suitable for longer operations due to medical reasons.

There is a wide array of procedures for neck rejuvenation through direct skin excision [1–7]. The major approaches are summarized in Fig. 10.1. These procedures may include fat removal and platysma plication. A major problem with these approaches is the relatively subjective nature of skin markings prior to surgery [1–7]. Lacking full satisfaction with these methods, we designed the present approach that is simple, easily teachable, and reproducible with precise preoperative markings.

This technique incorporates curved incisions, resulting in a final wave-like scar that we refer to as cervical "wave-plasty." Curved incisions are known to result in better healing and are less likely to result in hypertrophic or keloid scars [7].

F. D. Parsa (✉) · N. Yim
Department of Surgery, Division of Plastic Surgery, University of Hawai'i, John A. Burns School of Medicine, Honolulu, HI, USA
e-mail: nyim2022@hawaii.edu

N. N. Parsa
University of Hawai'i, John A. Burns School of Medicine, Honolulu, HI, USA
e-mail: parsa@hawaii.edu

K. Jeffords et al. (eds.), *Aesthetic Surgery for Men*, https://doi.org/10.1007/978-3-032-03840-1_10

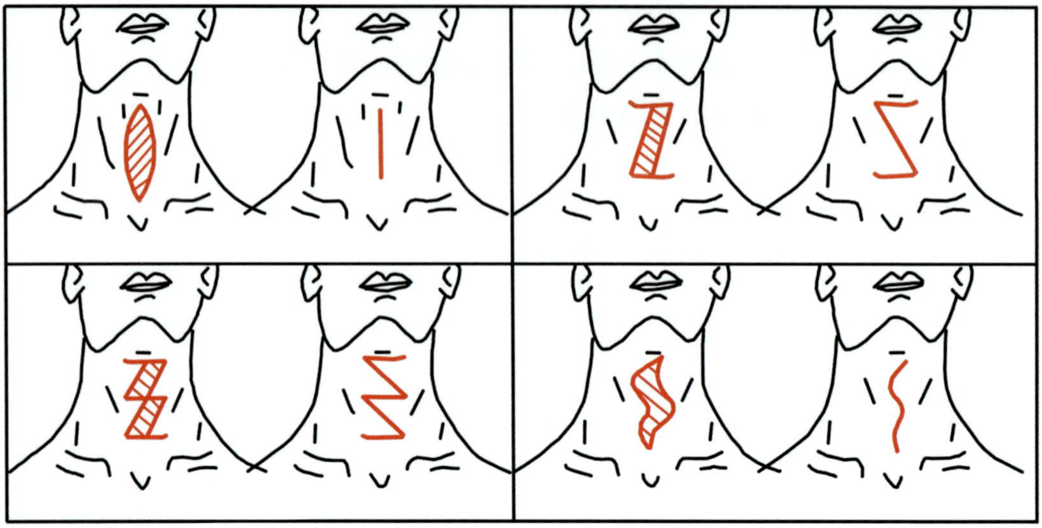

Fig. 10.1 Different excisional techniques. Top left figure shows lentiform excision that was described in 1903 with simple vertical closure. Top right is based on Z-incisions (1964, Marino) with a Z-plasty closure. Bottom left figure shows multi-Z-incisions (1971, Cronin and Biggs) with multi-Z-plasties. Bottom right figure is the current waveplasty technique with wave-like incisions

10.2 Patient Selection

Patient selection is paramount to patient satisfaction since not all patients with redundancy of cervical skin are candidates for this procedure primarily because of the resulting visible scars. It is advisable that patients be clearly informed preoperatively that there will be a visible permanent scar as a trade-off for improved neck contour. Since patients in general have poor understanding of pathologic scars, we recommend that photographs of hypertrophic scars be shown to them prior to surgery.

10.3 Markings

The anterior neck is marked while the patient is sitting or standing. A horizontal submental line is drawn within the submental crease and point X is marked on the left lateral side of this line (Fig. 10.2). A vertical midline is drawn from the mid aspect of the horizontal line down to the sternal notch and Point Y is marked. The vertical line is divided into four equal parts (Fig. 10.3). Excess cervical skin is pinched at each division marking to determine points A, B, C, D, E, and F (Fig. 10.2). These points are connected to result in two curves: X-A-C-E-Y and X-B-D-F-Y (Fig. 10.3). The latter curve is drawn after the skin is pinched gently several times with forceps to assure that the entire length of the incisions will be closed under no tension.

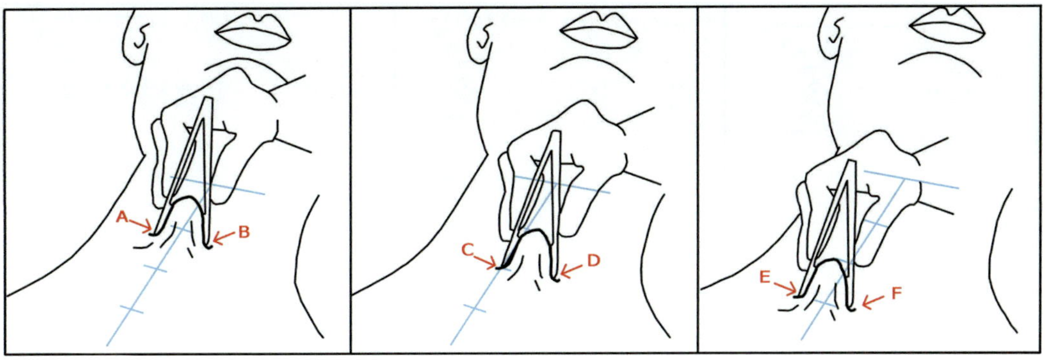

Fig. 10.2 Skin markings are done with patient either sitting or standing. The margins of skin are pinched with minimal force to allow for a tension-free skin closure

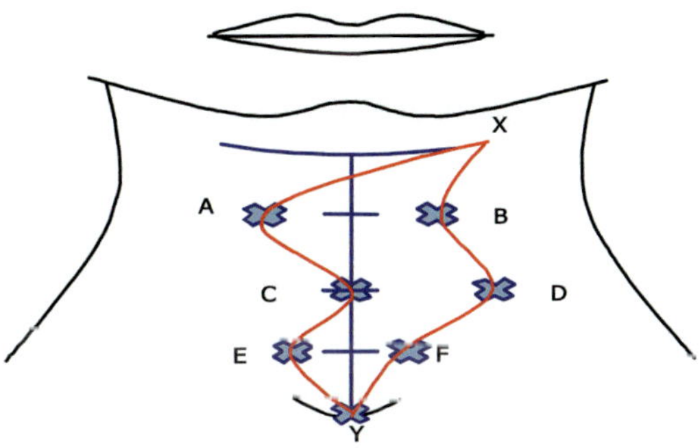

Fig. 10.3 Points X to point Y are joined with two wave-like curves

10.4 Surgical Technique

The operation may be performed under local anesthesia supplemented if necessary with light intravenous sedation. We recommend the presence of an anesthesiologist during the operation to monitor patient's vital signs.

Incisions are made along the two wave-like curves joining point X to point Y (Fig. 10.3). Redundant skin is excised and platysmal muscles are plicated in the midline when indicated with interrupted buried 4-0 absorbable monofilament sutures. Flap elevation by undermining the skin and separating the skin from platysma is rarely required and therefore vascularity to skin margins is minimally compromised and the risks of hematoma, skin necrosis, and hypertrophic scarring are reduced. Lipectomy is performed if there are excess subcutaneous, submental, and/or subplatysmal fatty deposits.

Based on the extent of redundant skin and skin laxity, three types of final wound closures may be performed as shown in Fig. 10.4. Type I closure is the most common (Fig. 10.4, left, and Fig. 10.5). In type II closure, any resulting dog ear is excised within the submental area (Fig. 10.4, center). In type III closure, excess skin is removed horizontally or obliquely (Fig. 10.4, right). For final wound closure, we prefer the use of interrupted intradermal 4-0 monofilament absorbable sutures and simple interrupted 5-0 nylon skin sutures (Fig. 10.5).

Wounds are covered with 1- or 1/2-inch micropore paper tape and patients are instructed to continue paper tape application for 6 months at least while at home and during sleep [19, 20]. External sutures are removed 7 to 10 days after surgery.

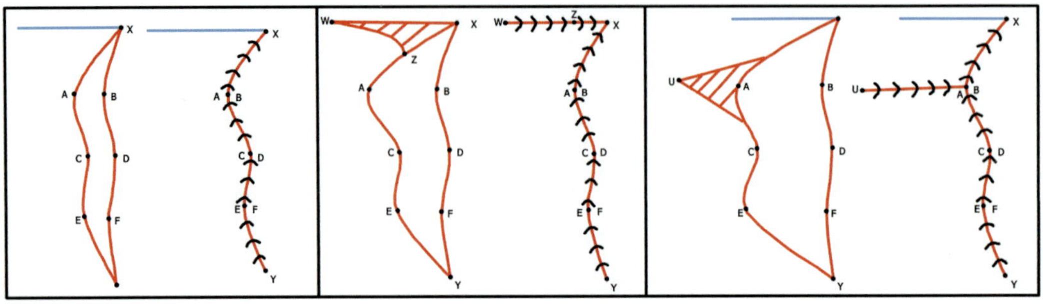

Fig. 10.4 The three types of wound closures are based on the extent of skin laxity and the amount of skin redundancy. Type 1 closure is shown on the left and is the most common type (Fig. 10.5). Type 2 is shown in the center and requires excision of a dog ear in the submental region. Type 3 wound closure (on the right) is indicated in patients with great skin redundancy and least skin elasticity. This type of closure was done in a 75-year-old patient shown in figs. 11 through 15

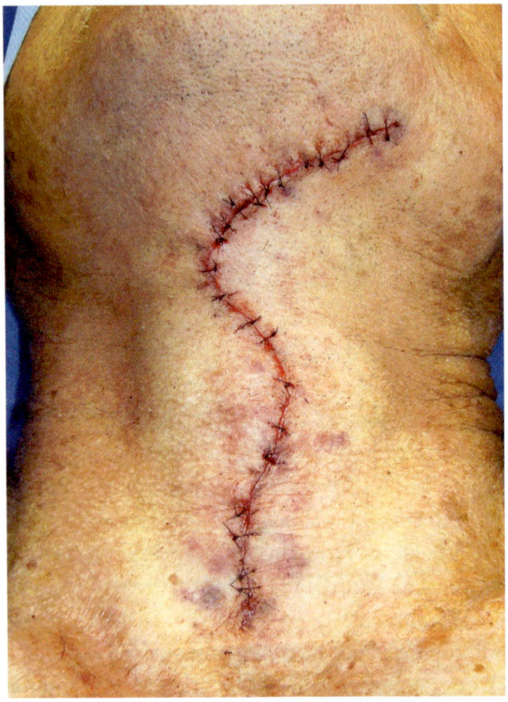

Fig. 10.5 Type 1 wound closure in a 69-year-old male who is shown in Figs. 10.6, 10.7, 10.8, 10.9, and 10.10

10.5 Results and Complications

Before and after photographs of patients that underwent cervical wave-plasty are shown in Figs. 10.6, 10.7, 10.8, 10.9, 10.10, 10.11, 10.12, 10.13, 10.14, and 10.15.

Limited wound dehiscence and scar hypertrophy may occur if incisions are closed under tension as seen in one of the earlier patients in our experience who underwent wave-plasty. This patient was a 75-year-old male smoker who required type 3 wound closure (Figs. 10.11, 10.12, 10.13, 10.14, and 10.15). He developed a 1 × 1 cm wound separation at the T-junction of wave-plasty and dog ear excision. This wound healed uneventfully by secondary intention with conservative management. Figures 10.13 and 10.14 show the scars at 3 months and Fig. 10.15 shows the same scars at 12 months after surgery with the neck extended to better present the entire scars. Wound dehiscence as well as hypertrophic scarring may be minimized significantly with tension-free wound closure and avoidance of sig-

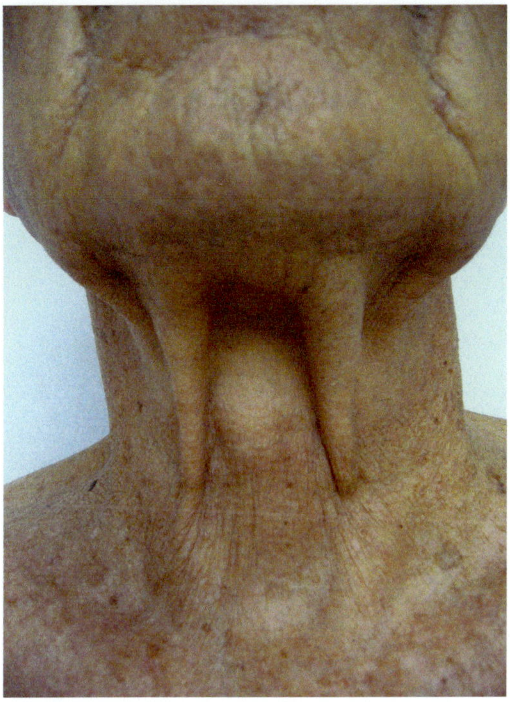

Fig. 10.6 Views of a 69-year-old male before cervical wave-plasty with type 1 skin closure

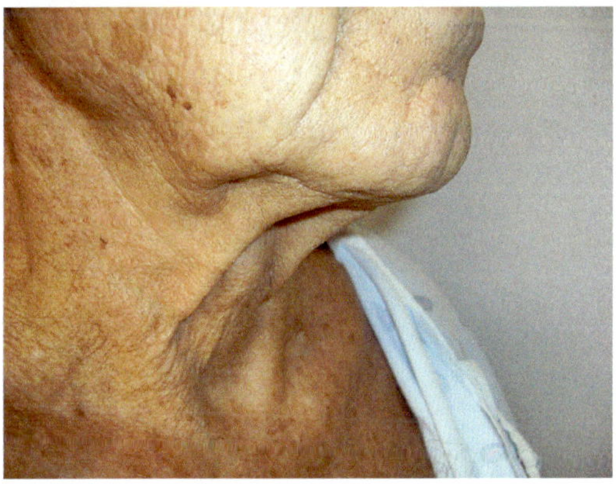

Fig. 10.7 Views of a 69-year-old male before cervical wave-plasty with type 1 skin closure

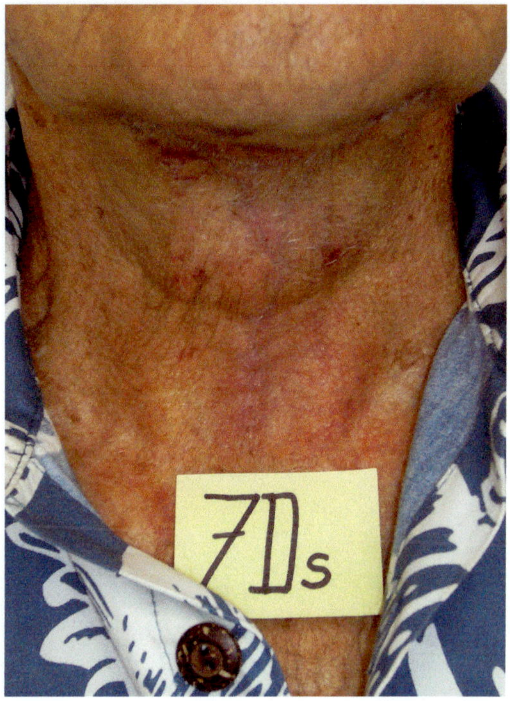

Fig. 10.8 Same patient as in Figs. 10.6 and 10.7 on the seventh postoperative day immediately after suture removal

nificant undermining. Wound infection and hematoma may occur as with any other operation and are very rare [11]. Preoperative oral administration of gabapentin and celecoxib has been shown [8–10] to significantly reduce postoperative pain and are recommended in doses of 600 mg and 400 mg respectively about 30 minutes before surgery. With this regimen we have found that the majority of patients do not require any analgesics other than acetaminophen and are able to return to limited routine daily activities the day after surgery

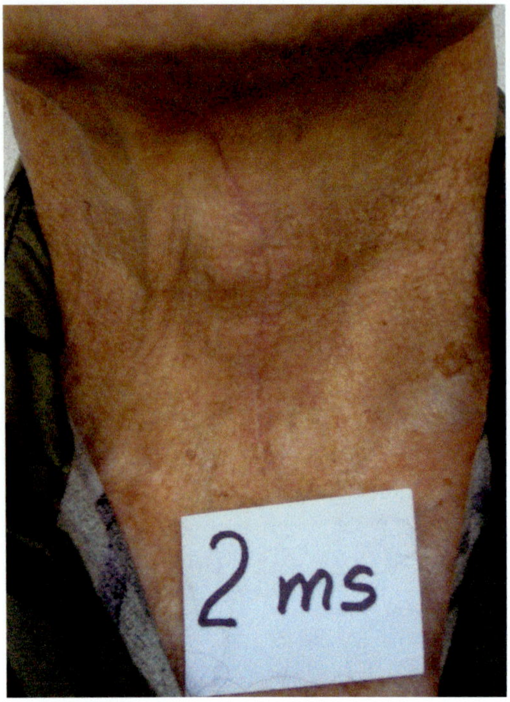

Fig. 10.9 Same patient as in Figs. 10.6 and 10.7 is shown 2 months after surgery

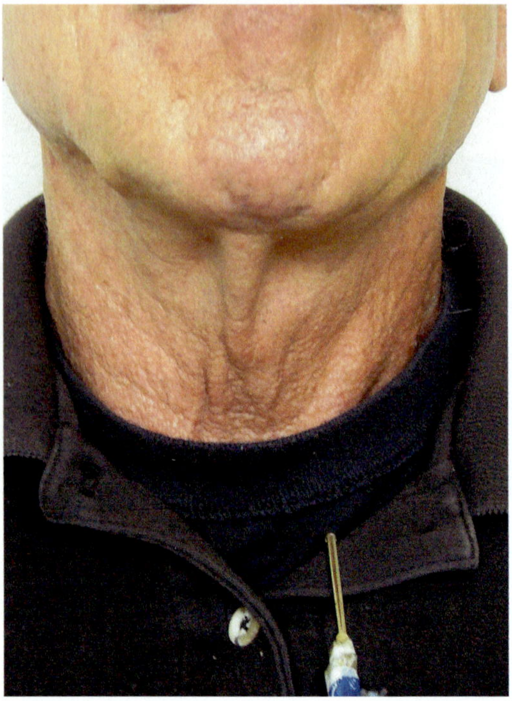

Fig. 10.11 A 75-year-old male smoker before cervical wave-plasty that required type 3 skin closure

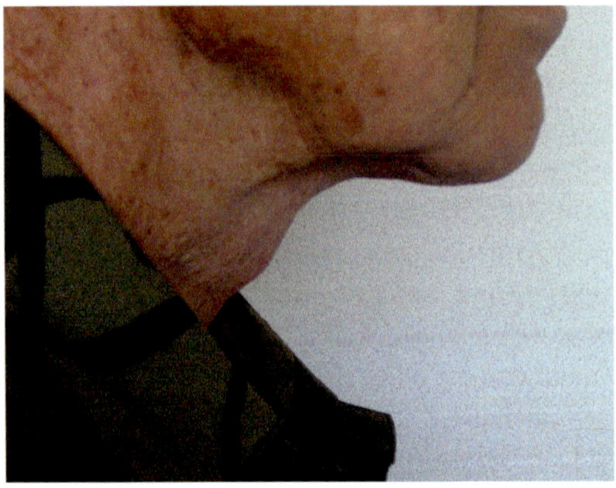

Fig. 10.10 Same patient as in Figs. 10.6 and 10.7 is shown 2 months after surgery

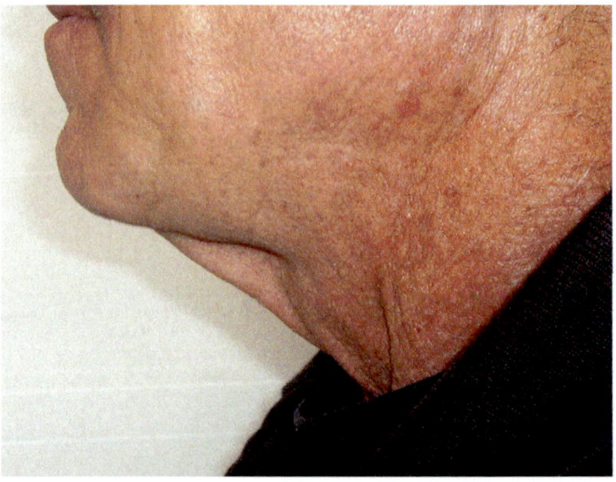

Fig. 10.12 A 75-year-old male smoker before cervical wave-plasty that required type 3 skin closure

10.6 Discussion

Although women constitute over 90% of patients who seek aesthetic face and neck rejuvenation procedures [11–13], over 50% of patients in our practice that undergo direct neck lift (cervical wave-plasty) are men. We believe this discrepancy is due to the fact that men accept more readily a visible scar on their anterior neck than women do. However, it is important that patients clearly understand that scars are permanent and noticeable hypertrophy may occur (Fig. 10.13). Review of photographs that show hypertrophic scars is most helpful in preoperative patient education since very few patients are familiar with these conditions. Previous studies of standard face and neck lift have reported an incidence of hypertrophic scarring from less than 2% to as high as 18% [14, 21–23]. Smokers, including former smokers, have been reported to carry a significantly higher risk of postoperative wound complications such as delayed healing, dehiscence, hematoma, and infection [15, 16].

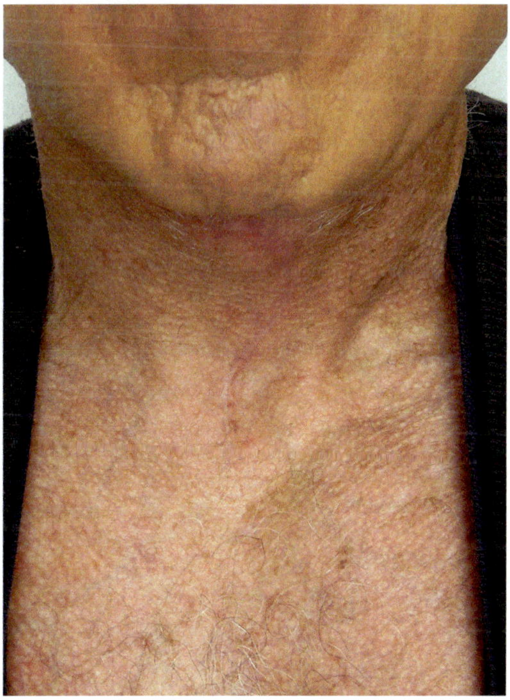

Fig. 10.13 Postoperative views of patient in Figs. 10.11 and 10.12 at 3 months after surgery. Note scar hypertrophy

Despite the fact that age, obesity, diabetes, hypertension, and smoking are among important comorbid factors in wound healing [16], we encountered only one case of limited wound dehiscence in a 75-year-old smoker with type 3 wound closure. The wound separation measured about 1 by 1 centimeter and occurred at the T-junction of wound closure. It healed by secondary intention and did not require revision. Figures 10.13 and 10.14 show this patient at 3 months and Fig. 10.15 is a photograph taken at one year after surgery. Hypertension that is not well controlled is another important comorbidity because of the potential for postoperative hematoma [17].

We have found that curve-like incisions with no significant undermining of skin, and tension-free skin closure are essential in minimizing wound complications and hypertrophic scarring. Platysma muscle plication is likely helpful in both reducing tension on wound margins and in improving neck contour. The use of micropore paper tape over the incisions for 6 months is also helpful in improving the long-term appearance of the scars [18–20].

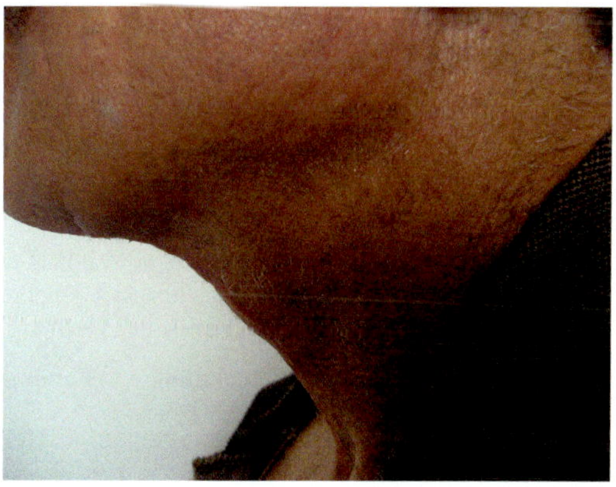

Fig. 10.14 Postoperative views of patient in Figs. 10.11 and 10.12 at 3 months after surgery. Note scar hypertrophy

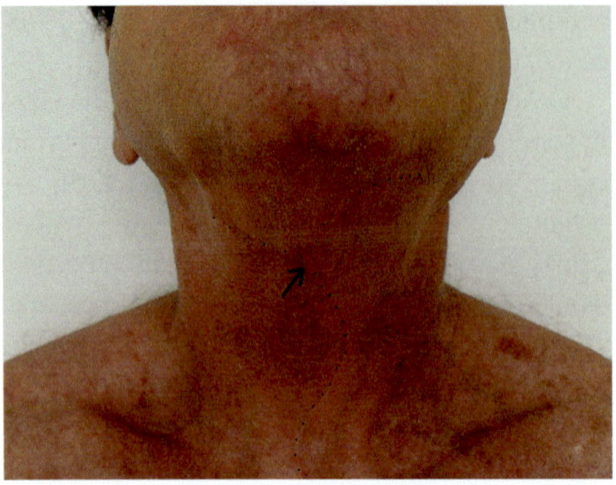

Fig. 10.15 Frontal view of patient in Figs. 10.11, 10.12, 10.13, and 10.14 with neck extended to better show the appearance of the scars with type 3 wound closure at 12 months after surgery. As one of our earlier patients who underwent wave-plasty, the incisions of this 75-year-old patient had been closed under tension that we believe resulted in wound dehiscence of about 1 × 1 cm at the T-junction between wave-plasty and dog ear excision shown with an arrow

10.7 Conclusion

Neck rejuvenation in men with wave-like incisions (wave-plasty) is simple, reproducible, and easily teachable. It allows for accurate preoperative planning and skin markings, results in a pleasing wave-like scar and allows for quick return to daily activities with minimal or no need for postoperative analgesics. This procedure has resulted in great satisfaction in men who understand and accept the resulting visible scars as a trade-off for improved neck contour.

Conflict of Interest The authors report no conflicts of interest, including, but not limited to, financial support, connections to pharmaceutical companies, and patents.

Financial Disclosure (Including Funding Sources) None.

References

1. Rohrich RJ, Rios JL, Smith PD, Gutowski KA. Neck rejuvenation revisited. Plast Reconstr Surg. 2006;118(5):1251–63.
2. Ramirez OM. Cervicoplasty: nonexcisional anterior approach. A 10-year follow-up. Plast Reconstr Surg. 2003;111(3):1342–5.
3. Miller TA. Excision of redundant neck tissue in men with platysma plication and Z-plasty closure. Plast Reconstr Surg. 2005;115(1):304–13.
4. Chaput B, Grolleau JL, De Bonnecaze G, Eburdery H, Chavoin JP, Garrido I. Anterior medial cervicoplasty. Ann Chir Plast Esthet. 2012;57(6):612–7.
5. Bitner JB, Friedman O, Farrior RT, Cook TA. Direct submentoplasty for neck rejuvenation. Arch Facial Plast Surg. 2007;9(3):194–200.
6. Bruneau S, Nguyen P, Foletti JM, Bellot V, Casanova D, Bardot J. Neck rejuvenation by anterior cervicoplasty: an original technical modification. J Plast Reconstr Aesthet Surg. 2013;6(11):1627–8.
7. Jordan JR, Yellin S. Direct cervicoplasty. Facial Plast Surg. 2014;30(4):451–61.
8. Sugai DY, Deptula PL, Parsa AA, Parsa FD. The importance of communication in the management of postoperative pain. Hawaii Med J. 2013;72(6):180–4.
9. Parsa AA, Sprouse-Blum AS, Jackowe DJ, Lee M, Oyama J, Parsa FD. Combined pre-operative use of celecoxib and gabapentin in the management of postoperative pain. Aesth Plast Surg. 2009;33(1):98–103.
10. Parsa AA, Soon CWM, Parsa FD. The use of preoperative celecoxib in reduction of postoperative pain after subpectoral breast augmentation. Aesth Plast Surg. 2005;29(6):441–4.
11. Parsa FD, Castel N, Parsa N. A modified, direct neck lift technique: the Cervical Wave-plasty. Arch Plast Surg. 2016;43:181–8.
12. Conway H. The surgical face lift - rhytidectomy. Plast Reconstr Surg. 1970;45(2):124–30.
13. Kamer FM, Frankel AW. Isolated submentoplasty: a limited approach to the aging neck. Arch Otolaryngol Head Neck Surg. 1997;123(1):66–70.
14. Friel MR, Shaw RE, Trovato MJ, Owsley JQ. The measure of face-lift patient satisfaction: the Owsley facelift satisfaction survey with a long-term follow-up study. Plast Reconstr Surg. 2010;126(1):245–57.
15. Riefkohl R, Wolfe J, Cox E, McCarty K. Association between cutaneous occlusive vascular disease, ciga-

rette smoking, and skin slough after rhytidectomy. Plast Reconstr Surg. 1986;77(4):592–6.
16. Parsa AA, Nakasone GK, Soon CW, Hsu A, Brickman M, Parsa FD. Smoking and breast reduction. Plast Reconstr Surg. 2006;117(7):2506–7.
17. Baker D, Stefani W, Chiu E. Reducing the incidence of hematoma requiring surgical evacuation following male rhytidectomy: a 30-year review of cases. Plast Reconstr Surg. 2005;116(7):1973–85.
18. Parsa FD, Parsa NN, Murarui D. Surgical correction of the frowning mouth. Plast Reconstr Surg. 2010;125(2):667–76.
19. Reiffe RS. Prevention of hypertrophic scars by long-term paper tape application. Plastic Reconstr Surg. 1995;96(7):1715–8.
20. Atkinson JA, McKenna KT, Barnett AG, McGrath DJ, Rudd M. A randomized, controlled trial to determine the efficacy of paper tape in preventing hypertrophic scar formation in surgical incisions that traverse Langer's skin tension lines. Plast Reconstr Surg. 2005;116(6):1648–56.
21. Henderson J, O'Neill T, Logan A. Direct anterior neck skin excision for cervicomental laxity. Aesth Plast Surg. 2010;34(3):299–305.
22. Matarasso A, Elkwood A, Rankin M, Elkowitz M. National plastic surgery survey: face lift techniques and complications. Plast Reconstr Surg. 2000;106(5):1185–95.
23. Thompson D, Ashley FL. Face-lift complications: a study of 922 cases performed in a 6-year period. Plast Reconstr Surg. 1978;61(1):40–9.

Blepharoplasty in the Male

11

Dennis Hurwitz

Blepharoplasty is an invasive procedure that improves the appearance of the eyelids, which may include operations on both brow and mid-cheek. Functional blepharoplasties that relieve visual obstruction, correct eyelid malposition, or reconstruct after trauma or tumor resection are not presented. According the 2018 Cosmetic Surgery Data Bank, eyelid surgery was the third most popular operation (17,593 cases) in males, after liposuction and gynecomastia correction [1].

From the senior author's experience, there are a dozen distinctive features of male blepharoplasty (Table 11.1). Working men desire blepharoplasty to ameliorate worn, tired, and old appearance. These attributes place males competing with younger executives at a disadvantage. Accompanying facelift, the seventh ranked procedure in men, is uncommon (1). Large fat bags and sagging tissues are more likely an issue than wrinkled skin. Heavier tissues are considered in the resection and support. Minimal and flat eyebrow elevation through a pexy is appropriate. Avoid feminizing by creating high arch brows, deep set eyes, and upward horizontal axis. Gaunt upper midcheek hypoplasia is common.

Periorbital aesthetics considers the forehead shape and brow position. Handsome men look even more rugged with prominent, overhanging brows. So flat eyebrow arches and drooping to the superior orbital rim are acceptable. A lower position than that, and a brow lift or pexy, is considered. When the patient requests a browlift, then a short hairline scar or endoscopic lift is offered. Without fixation of the lateral brow, the lateral canthal extension of the supratarsal skin excision may slightly lower it and, thereby, unattractively shorten the width from lateral brow to eye lashes. Adequate skin fullness between the brow and eyelid margin is more aesthetic. However, loose skin overlapping the superior

Table 11.1 Distinctive male features

1.	Successful in business
2.	Isolated procedure for rejuvenation
3.	Skin wrinkling rarely a concern
4.	Large lower eyelid bags
5.	Always removal of upper lid orbicularis to better define the supratarsal fold
6.	Conservative supra tarsal skin resection to avoid overly deep sulcus
7.	Extra lower lid lateral canthal support needed
8.	Avoid resection of thick brow skin between the eyelid skin and eyebrow
9.	Amenable to a limited eyebrow elevation from a suture Browpexy
10.	Shape a flat brow with suture fixation lateral to angle of the brow
11.	Avoid horizontal axis upward tilt
12.	Midcheek hypoplasia amenable to adipose fascia flap advancement

D. Hurwitz (✉)
University of Pittsburgh Medical Center, Department of Plastic Surgery, Pittsburgh, PA, USA

K. Jeffords et al. (eds.), *Aesthetic Surgery for Men*, https://doi.org/10.1007/978-3-032-03840-1_11

eyelid margin is rejected and may interfere with superior gaze. Bags of eyelid fat are also not acceptable. While flat cheeks are masculine features often seen in youth, exposed infraorbital rims and lower eyelid bags are objectionable.

11.1 Preoperative

The patient must describe his eyelid deformity, its impact, and expectation of results. Be alert to excessive narcissism, aggressive behavior, exaggeration of deformity and its impact on life, as well as unrealistic expectations. These patients are difficult at best. There must be an acceptance of imperfect result and possible need and costs for revision surgery. The aesthetic impact of eyebrow ptosis and/or midcheek hypoplasia with the negative aesthetic consequences of ignoring them as well as the technical options to correct is presented. Excessive skin laxity needs to be excised and deep crow's feet wrinkles are ideal to hide lateral canthal extension to the lid closures. A preoperative history and physical is obtained looking for evidence of medical, anesthetic, or psychiatric risks. A complaint of restriction of superior visual field is collaborated by an ophthalmologist examination of visual fields and thereby make the patient eligible for some insurance compensation.

Examine the patient with documentation of visual acuity, dermatochalasis, blepharochlasis, skin elasticity with a pinch and snapback test, festoons, pseudoherniation of fat from the lower three compartments, degree of scleral show, presence of tear trough deformity, and negative midface vector and eyebrow ptosis. A history of dry eye, photophobia, excess scleral show, or epiphora prompts a Schirmer test and perhaps an ophthalmology consult. A simple visual acuity exam is recommended. Preoperative frontal photographs of open lids, closed lids, and upward gaze should be taken and available in the operating room. If there is a history of hypertension, then review and be sure of optimal management. Poorly controlled hypertension or any other medical problem necessitates the operation be performed under general anesthesia. Otherwise we routinely perform blepharoplasty under local anesthesia supplemented with appropriate does of Xanax and Clonidine with continuous monitoring of pulse oximeter and vital signs.

11.2 Technique

Summaries of operative blepharoplasty is followed by a single complex case report with a detailed operative note that combines blepharoplasty with browpexy and adipose fascial flap advancement to the cheek. A decade ago, the senior surgeon mastered the technique of both facelift and blepharoplasty under local anesthesia, and because of its simplicity, cost effectiveness, and facilitation of the surgery, it has become the preferred approach. Even Browpexy and advancement of adipose fascial flap to the midcheek can be comfortably performed under local anesthesia. A brief presentation of radiofrequency blepharoplasty completes the chapter.

11.2.1 Upper Blepharoplasty

11.2.1.1 Marking

The excess skin of the upper eyelids produces redundancy even to overhang of the lash margin and is the source of restricted superior vision. Pulling this excess skin superior, draw the inferior incision line millimeters inferior to the tarsal fold. Drawing the superior incision, which determines the width of skin excision, requires judgment to adequately remove excess skin. Once drawn, following the infusion of local anesthetic, the surgeon is committed to its removal. The only adjustment can be the removal of an additional strip of skin. So, this decision on width of resection needs to be accurate and perhaps conservative. I scrutinize all the wrinkled thin skin between the supratarsal fold and the brow and included most of it for the transverse resection. The superior incision, including this crepey skin, tapers at each end to the lower incision to form of a crescent extending from nearly the medial canthus to just beyond the lateral canthus. Later, the exact width of resection can be confirmed by gentle forceps pinching of the skin prior to injecting the local anesthetic. If significant redundant tissue is present, the lateral incision is extended through the Crow's feet, with the patient aware of this visible scar that should fall into a natural wrinkle. When concerned about over resection of the width make the upper incision within the inked marking and if preliminary approximation leaves redundancy, simple trim out the inked skin with scissors.

Check the patient for symmetry and then mark the opposite upper eyelid accordingly.

11.2.1.2 Operation

While commonly recommended, the senior author does not use eye shields because they distort the lid and can stress the awake patient. Carefully prep and drape eyelids to ensure no disruption of markings or antiseptic enters the conjunctiva. 1% lidocaine with 1/100,000 epinephrine is slowly infiltrated subdermally painlessly along the excision site with a 1.5 inch 25-gauge needle.

With the assistant pulling medial canthal skin nasally, a #15 blade scalpel is used to make a 2 millimeter stairstep perimeter incision through skin and less widely through the gritty orbicularis muscle. Lateral to medial resection of both skin and muscle over the orbital septum are cut with a scalpel. Direct needle tip electrocautery stops bleeding. Spreading scissors are used to open the medial orbital compartment to expose fat. Easily teased-out fat is amputated through direct electrocautery. Additional fat and bleeding vessels may be directly cauterized. When the upper orbit would be too depressed following this composite resection, then only the eyelid skin is removed.

Mild pressure is placed on the upper eyelid wound by the assistant as the opposite upper eyelid is similarly treated. Upon returning to the original eyelid, a final search for hemostasis through needle point electrocautery is made. Starting from lateral to medial, the right upper eyelid is closed with an over and over full thickness skin suture above the lateral canthus and then switching to intracuticular horizontal bites across the supratarsal fold. Troublesome eyelid milia are minimized by this intracuticular closure. Then the opposite lid is treated similarly. A slight eversion of eyelashes is the desired effect. A steri-strip secures the long medial end of the suture to the glabella.

11.2.2 Lower Blepharoplasty

Lower eyelids are reached through either a subciliary or transconjunctival incision. If excess skin needs to be resected or an orbicularis flap neeeds to be sutured to across the lateral canthus, then a cutaneous approach is chosen. To minimize postoperative inferior malposition, the shortest possible trans orbicularis opening is made. If only orbital fat is excised, then a transconjunctival approach is preferred.

11.2.3 Subciliary Approach

11.2.3.1 Marking

A sub-eyelash incision is marked 1.5 millimeters below the lashes from lateral to the lower punctum to the lateral commissure and turned inferiorly at a 45 degree angle over the malar eminence.

11.2.3.2 Operation

Lower lid is infiltrated between the dermis and orbicularis muscle with about 1 cc of 1% lidocaine with 1:100,000 epinephrine. For the least pain, skin is penetrated at the termination of the lateral canthal extension and anesthetic is injected along the mid-lower eyelid, along the lower eyelid, the eyelid cheek junction, and lastly along the subciliary margin. With downward distracting the eyelid with the helping hand finger, a 15 blade precisely incises along the subciliary markings followed by several millimeters of scalpel undermining. A wide double hook retractor distracts the thin skin as forceps push down the orbicularis muscle to allow for a paint brush–like sweep of the muscle from the dermis. After undermining skin from 5 to 7 millimeters toward the infraorbital rim, the muscle is entered centrally through spreading scissors. With inferior traction on the cheek skin to tent the orbicularis muscle over the orbital septum, it is then incised along the central half of the orbit.

Prominent fat is teased free for direct electrocautery excision. Gentle pressure on the globe delivers the remaining excess fat for removal from each of the three fat pockets. Alternatively, through an incision through the arcus marginalis, the orbital fat pad can be dissected off the floor and released to be advanced over the rim and sutured to the periorbital. When this extensive surgery to cover the boney orbit and fill the infraorbital hollow is done, then a supported canthopexy is essential and may be supplemented with trans lid Frost sutures. The skin is redraped over the subciliary incision and a conservative tangential skin excision of 2 to 4 millimeters is made. The lateral orbicularis is usually suspended to the lateral orbit soft tissue with an interrupted 5-0 Maxon placed under the lateral canthal tendon. A wedge resection of skin is removed from the lateral canthal extension.

Lateral canthal region skin closure is by running 6-0 Prolene. The subciliary closure is then performed with interrupted 6-0 fast absorbing gut. Cold compresses are placed over the eyelids intermittently for the next 36 hours and then as desired with the advent of safe and even compression of the eyelids with the skin goggle we now using that aid.

11.2.4 Transconjunctival Operation

Topical anesthesia of the conjunctiva is followed by placement of corneal shields. The one-centimeter transverse conjunctival sulcus incision is sighted 4 millimeters up from the cul-de-sac prior to injection of local anesthetic. Frost-type sutures are placed to tautly retract the eyelids. The transverse conjunctival incision in scored followed by electrosurgical incision. Spreading dissection is carried through the lid retractors until the orbital septum is penetrated with identification of the medial, central, and lateral fat pads.

Forceps carefully tease out the excess fat which is amputated by electrosurgical coagulation. Direct coagulation of fat by the needle may be needed. The inferior oblique muscle is usually identified and preserved. Close the incision with several rapidly absorbing catgut sutures.

Adjunctive procedure can now be performed including facial fat grafting, fillers, neurotoxin, chemical peel, laser resurfacing, bipolar radiofrequency microneedling, microdermabrasion, or skin-pinch excision. The same procedure is then carried out symmetrically on the contralateral lower eyelid. The corneal shields are removed, and the eyes irrigated with balance ophthalmic saline, followed by application of ophthalmic ointment to the incisions. Cold compresses are placed for 36 hours.

11.3 Postoperative Care

Before discharge, the patients' vision and extraocular muscle movements and incisions should be checked. Strict blood pressure control, head of bed elevation at 30—45 degrees, and cold compresses should be continued at home. Wound care consists of ocular lubrication. The patient may shower in 24 hours; however, physical activity should be limited for two weeks.

At follow-up, patient should be carefully examined. Possible postoperative complications include the following: asymmetry, retrobulbar hematoma, ectropion and lid malposition, lagophthalmos, asymmetry, eyelash loss, corneal injury, chemosis, dry eyes, epiphora, and extraocular muscle injury.

11.4 Demonstrative Case

Operative note of four-lid blepharoplasty with Browpexy and adipose fascial advancement flap under local anesthesia (Figs. 11.1, 11.2, 11.3, and 11.4):

- *Diagnosis*: excess skin and fat of the upper and lower eyelids, brow ptosis, midcheek atrophy
- *Operation*: bilateral lateral suture browpexy, bilateral upper blepharoplasty, and lower blepharoplasty, with lower eyelid adipose

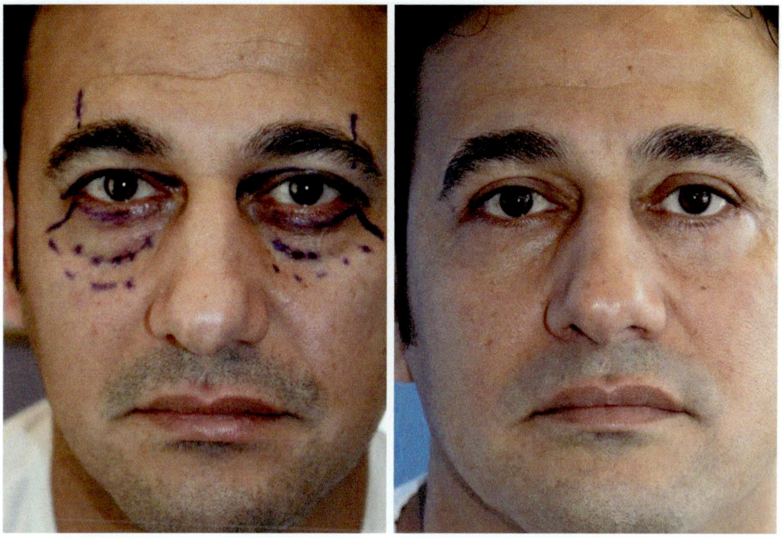

Fig. 11.1 Preoperative with operative marking and postoperative frontal views with eyelids open. (Left) Low lying flat eyebrow with lateral vertical brow markings indicating point of 4–0 Prolene browpexy. Several deep horizontal central forehead wrinkles. Excess upper lid skin rolling to nearly the lash margin, encircled with excision plan. Bulging medial and central fat bags dominate the lower eyelids. Prominent infraorbital rim leads to a depressed central midcheek. (Right) Brow tail is slightly raised. Eyelid margin is free of overhanging skin. Appropriately wide space between lateral lashes and brow. Forehead wrinkles are diminished. Lower eyelid bulges absent. Smooth transition over orbital rim to filled midcheek. Lower eyelid scar with canthal extension not seen

Fig. 11.2 Preoperative and postoperative frontal views with eyelids closed. (left) Excess eyelid skin is better seen as well abnormal contours. (Right) Faint scars, excellent contours, and no loose skin

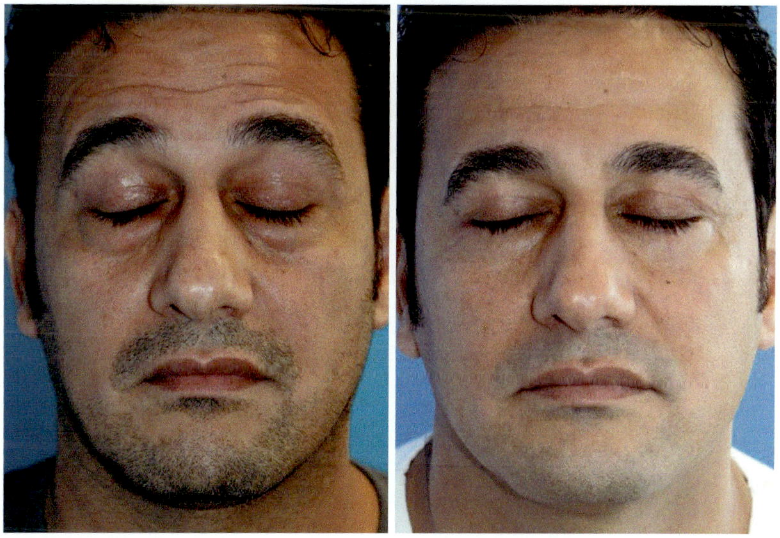

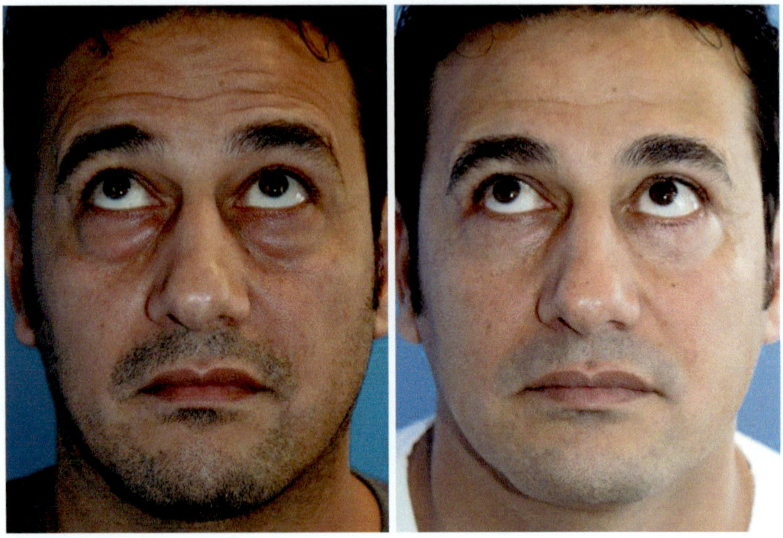

Fig. 11.3 Preoperative and postoperative frontal views with eyelids looking up. (Left) Furrowed forehead in animation. Severely bulging lower orbital fat bags. (Right) Faint forehead lines and blepharoplasty scars. There are no lower eyelid bags

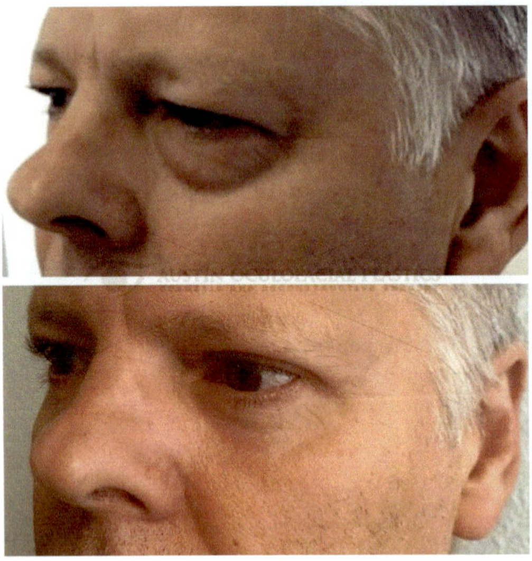

Fig. 11.4 (Top) Pre- and (bottom) postoperative frontal views for Accutite and Morpheus8 radiofrequency tightening of the lower eyelids and lateral upper eyelid

fascial flap advancement to the midcheek and lateral canthopexy with transcanthal suspension of lower orbicularis muscle

- *Anesthesia*: preop: xanax 2 mg oral sedation followed by 20 cc's 1% xylocaine with epinephrine mixed with 20 cc's ½% marcaine and 2 cc's sodium bicarbonate
- *EBL*: 5 cc's

The patient has moderately wrinkled, hyperactive forehead with symmetrical lateral brow ptosis and overhanging excess upper eyelid skin. He has prominent lower eyelid fat bags with defined infraorbital rim and deep nasojugal sulcus, worse on the right. The infraorbital cheek moderate soft tissue atrophy is also worse on the right. He desires removal of excess skin and fat bags from the lower eyelids. He accepted that the upper eyelid transverse skin excision should be conservative to avoid too deep a sulcus. He liked that the lateral brow pexies will be elevated and better shape his eyebrow as well as maintain if not slightly elongate the distance between his lateral eyelashes and the tail of the brow. Along with the lid excisions, the brow pexies should reduce frontalis hyperactivity leading to less animated and static wrinkles. He also accepted that his lower lid adipose hypertrophy and hernia should be mobilized as an adipose fascial flap and advanced across the infraorbital rim, which will correct his midcheek and nasojugal hollowness and midcheek fat atrophy. He understood that the high risk for lower eyelid malposition would be reduced by lateral canthopexies and transposition of the orbicularis muscle to the inner aspect of the superior orbital rim just above the lateral canthus. His lower eyelid subciliary scar as well and the upper supratarsal scar should be difficult to see, but the lateral canthal extensions if easily seen would appear like a wrinkle. Should lower lid malposition occur, vigorous massage and taping would be necessary over months, and if not relieved, then lower lid corrective surgery may be necessary. Failure to understand and accept the risk of symptomatic ectropion would eliminate the option of adipose fascial flap advancement.

He was marked and then explained the operation while looking into a mirror; he was assured once again that all could be accomplished comfortably under local anesthesia. Short vertical lines indicate the point of eyebrow pexy that elevates just lateral to the angle of the brow (Fig. 11.1). While slightly lifting his lateral brow as expected from the pexy, and sighting his superior tarsal fold, an inverted crescent excision of skin position over the fold was drawn from his medial to just beyond the lateral canthus. The width of excision included redundant thin inelastic eyelid but no thick brow skin. For access to the lower orbital fat, a subciliary line 1.5 millimeters from the lashes was drawn ending in a right angle lateral canthal extension.

After photographs were taken, the relaxed patient was transferred from the exam room to a quiet, minimally lit operating room with music of his choice. Talking is kept to essentials or to comfort the patient. Local anesthesia from a 10-cc syringe with a 1 ½-inch 25 gauge needle starts with one cc. supraorbital, infraorbital and zygomaticorbital direct puncture preperiosteal nerve blocks. Starting near the lateral canthus, anesthetic is slowly balloon injected along the marked upper eyelid excision infiltrated into the eyelid. From the malar bone subdermal injection tracts slowly between the cheek and lower eyelid. A fanlike infusion over the maxilla is made, followed by injection along the lower ciliary margin. The opposite periorbita are similarly anesthetized.

One set of eyelids and brow is operated before starting the other. The preop upper eyelid perimeter incisions are made. The skin and underlying central strip of orbicularis muscle are resected off the orbital septum. Alternatively, separate resection of the skin and then the muscle is bloodier and takes longer. As the preoperative exam suggested medial fat pad bulge, local anesthetic was infiltrated and allowed to sit. One centimeter of either side of the lateral marked brow verticals supra periosteal dissection frees the lateral brow. A horizontally place 4–0 Prolene suture places a secure bite through the retained periorbita. Then, it is passed through infra eyebrow tissue up to the dermis. Tie down raises the lateral brow to the desired height, or the suture is redone. The medial fat compartment is opened by spreading to expose the fat pad. Excess fat is teased out and removed through direct electrosurgery. Closure of the upper eyelid excision must wait for lower orbicularis muscle/lateral canthal suspension.

As the lower eyelid is pulled down, the subciliary incision site is reinjected with local anesthetic to provide a stable anesthetized platform for incision through the skin 1.5 mm from the lash margin, completed by a short right angle canthal extension. An incision 0.5 mm along the margin may damage the hair follicles, whereas an incision 2 millimeters or more away will leave visible scar. A lower eyelid skin flap is sharply elevated with the 15 blade from the orbicularis muscle for about 6 millimeter or slightly longer than the width of anticipated transverse skin resection. Bleeding is controlled with needle point electrocautery.

With the assistant both firmly retracting the dissected skin flap with a wide double hook and inferiorly distracting the midcheek, the suborbicularis space is entered by spreading sharp pointed scissors. The taunt orbital fascia is easily identified for scissor dissection over that plane, leading to the infraorbital rim and beyond. Sweeping spreading scissors and electrocautery cautery dissection proceeds through the SOOF (suborbicularis oculi fascia) fibrofascia to the extent that the depressed midcheek space is unroofed. With a double hook distracting the lower eyelid, a 15 blade widely detaches the bloodless orbital floor Arcus Marginalis origin to expose the infraorbital fat pad. A teasing and nipping of fascia supra periosteal dissection releases the fat pad for as much advancement over the rim and on to the upper maxilla as desired. Look for the inferior oblique extraocular muscle and protect it. The fibroadipose flap is suture advanced with 5–0 horizontal Maxon on a small, tapered needle sutures to the retained SOOF and maxillary periosteum. First the medial adipose fascial flap spans the nasojugal depression. The lateral portion of the flap is then suture advanced towards the malar eminence. Finally, the central flap is advance superior to the infraorbital nerve foramen. After tying each advancement suture, the lower eyelid margin is distracted toward the brow to ensure that it is not tethered inferiorly.

Next, the lateral canthal support and lateral orbicularis muscle advancement are started through the exposed left upper eyelid. The interior of the superior lateral orbit is exposed. Supra periosteal dissection proceeds bluntly under the lateral canthus. After placing a 5–0 Maxon suture into the superiolateral inner periorbita, the needle end is passed under the lateral canthus. After a substantial bite of lateral orbicularis muscle is taken, the needle is passed back under the lateral canthal tendon. Upon tying the lower orbiculars muscle to the superiolateral orbital rim, the lower eyelid was observed to have adequate suspension.

After careful electrocautery hemostasis. The upper eye wound is closed with a running skin closure above the lateral canthus which is transition from a 6–0 Prolene over and over running laterally to an intracuticular along the supra tarsal fold. Light eversion of the lash line is ideal tension. A wedge of skin along the lateral canthal extension was excised. Then the lower eyelid skin is draped over the lid allowing the excess width 4 millimeters to be excised. 6–0 Prolene-interrupted sutures close the lateral canthal extension. 6–0 rapid absorbing cat gut interrupted sutures close along the ciliary margin.

A similar procedure is performed on the opposite eyelids. Patient experienced an uncomplicated course. The results 18 months later demonstrate that aesthetic goals were achieved.

11.5 Minimally Invasive Treatment of Lower Lid Wrinkling, Minimal Deformity, Malar Bags, Festoons

The removal of adequate skin to treat lower lid wrinkling hazards lid malposition. Similarly, blepharoplasty to treat minimal deformity seems too risky. Malar bags and festoons either primary or secondary to lymphatic obstruction may simply be aggravated by traditional blepharoplasty. Likewise, direct excisions may not solve and even accentuate the deformity.

Radiofrequency microneedling and subdermal bipolar probe treatments appear ideally suited for what used to be nearly insoluble problems. The recent application of the combination of topical Morphous8 with Accutite Bipolar probe has routinely obtained satisfactory improvement (Fig. 11.4).

Reference

1. 2018 Cosmetic (Aesthetic) Surgery National Data Bank Statistics. https://www.surgery.org/sites/default/files/ASAPS-Stats2018.pdf. Accessed 26 July 2019.

12 Asian Blepharoplasty

Lawrence Tong and Clyde H. Ishi

12.1 Introduction

The term Asian Blepharoplasty refers to a constellation of aesthetic procedures performed on the Asian upper lid, which typically has supratarsal crease formation as a central objective. Although Asian blepharoplasty is one of the most widely performed aesthetic procedures worldwide [1], Asian blepharoplasty is less well-understood in countries outside of Asia. With the continued growth (both in numbers and affluence) of the Asian population worldwide, increasing demand is expected to continue for the foreseeable future. Management of this patient population requires a thorough understanding of the needs, expectations, and unique surgical techniques intrinsic to this demographic.

The natural occurrence of a supratarsal crease in Asians is approximately 50% [2]. There is a broad spectrum of crease presentation, ranging from absent, to low placement, to high placement on the lid. The character of the crease also varies among individuals from well defined, to poorly defined, to sometimes intermittently present or absent. The surgery to create the crease is also commonly called *double-fold surgery*, or *double lid surgery*. Beyond the creation of the supratarsal crease, other procedures are commonly incorporated to improve upper lid aesthetics. These include skin excision, medial epicanthoplasty, ptosis correction, and lateral canthoplasty.

Blepharoplasty is the most commonly performed aesthetic surgery in Asia. Female patients seek Asian blepharoplasty more frequently than males, comprising an estimated 85–90% of patients. Although females comprise 85–90% of the Asian blepharoplasty population, males do undergo this procedure, and their numbers are likely to increase and parallel the growth of male aesthetic surgery in general. The procedure skews to a younger patient demographic when compared to Caucasian blepharoplasty, with the majority of patients under 30 years of age. This chapter will discuss the anatomy, patient evaluation, surgical indications, and surgical techniques important to the management of patients seeking Asian blepharoplasty.

12.2 Motivation to Seek Asian Blepharoplasty

At its core, patients undergo Asian blepharoplasty to make the eyes look more attractive. Creation of a supratarsal crease creates the illusion of a larger palpebral fissure and makes the eye look more expressive. Large, expressive eyes are identified as being more attractive than small, inexpressive eyes across all cultures. Aside from

L. Tong · C. H. Ishi (✉)
Division of Plastic and Reconstructive Surgery, Yorkville Institute of Plastic Surgery, University of Toronto, Toronto, ON, Canada
e-mail: cishii@ishiiplasticsurgery.com

K. Jeffords et al. (eds.), *Aesthetic Surgery for Men*, https://doi.org/10.1007/978-3-032-03840-1_12

supratarsal crease formation, removal of excess skin can make a patient look younger, while modification of the epicanthal fold and correction pseudoptosis/ptosis further enhances aesthetics and aperture size.

The presence of a supratarsal crease is termed a double lid (or double fold), whereas an absence of the crease is termed a monolid (or monofold). The translated Chinese term describing an eyelid with a crease is literally 'double eyelid skin', referring to the two segments of skin (upper and lower) divided by the supratarsal crease.

The natural occurrence of a double lid/fold in Asians is approximately 50% [2]. In Asian culture, a double lid is deemed to be more attractive than a monolid. This viewpoint may be attributed to several factors: (a) the decreased apparent expressiveness of the eyes with monolids, (b) the perceived decrease in eye (aperture) size with monolids, and (c) the preference for an aesthetic influenced by Western ideals of beauty.

12.2.1 Expressiveness

The presence of an upper lid crease is generally thought to be a more attractive trait in Asian culture because it conveys a warmer, more expressive, or even welcoming look. An upper lid without a crease is variously described as appearing 'sleepy eyed', lacking expressiveness, or having an inscrutable look.

12.2.2 Eye (Palpebral Fissure) Size

Larger eyes are identified as being more attractive. Certain anatomic features of the Asian lid predispose the eyes to appear smaller. The lack of a supratarsal crease makes an eye appear smaller compared to one with a crease, even if the actual aperture size is no different. Double fold surgery produces a crease that creates the illusion of a larger palpebral fissure. Pseudoptosis orientalis is the term given when an Asian patient has skin that hangs below the upper lid margin, giving the appearance of ptosis and a smaller palpebral fissure. Correction of pseudoptosis occurs in patients undergoing Asian blepharoplasty, and a real increase in aperture size is achieved. The presence of an epicanthal fold will decrease the aperture width by concealing part of the medial canthal region. Epicanthoplasty enlarges the palpebral fissure in a horizontal direction by eliminating excess skin that covers the medial canthus.

12.2.3 The Influence of Western Culture and Beauty Ideals

Double fold surgery has been popular for decades in Asia. Globalization and rapid modernization in Asia since the 1980s have led to Asian culture adopting many aspects of Western society. This includes ideas of beauty and an appreciation for Caucasian eyelid aesthetics. In South Korea, which has the highest worldwide per capita rate of Asian blepharoplasties performed, cosmetic surgery is heavily influenced by an aesthetic amalgamation of Asian and Western beauty. Despite this, the specific viewpoint of Asian beauty is still distinct from Western beauty. Many surgeons (and patients) assert that patients who seek double fold surgery are motivated to emulate other Asians who naturally possess double folds, not Caucasians. It is vitally important to understand that westernization is not the goal in this patient demographic [3]. There is still a strong desire to appear Asian, but with some attributes customarily seen in Caucasians. In fact, most patients will be unhappy if the creases are made 'too high' or the eyes made to look 'too Westernized'.

12.3 Anatomic Considerations for Asian Eyelids

12.3.1 Surface Anatomy of the Supratarsal Crease

The surface anatomy of the upper lid has relevant landmarks to the discussion of Asian blepharoplasty. A clear distinction should be made between the terms supratarsal crease, supratarsal

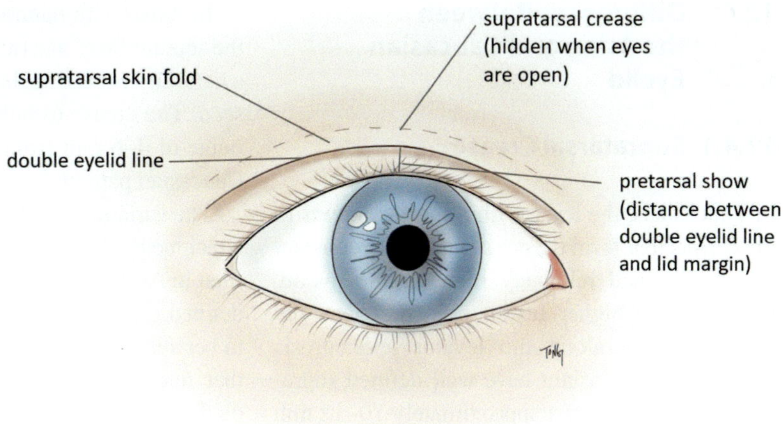

Fig. 12.1 Surface anatomy relevant to Asian blepharoplasty

fold, double eyelid line, and pretarsal show. They are sometimes referred to interchangeably, and although closely related, they are *not* synonymous. The *supratarsal crease* (also called the upper eyelid crease) is the horizontal line along which the skin folds when the eye opens (Fig. 12.1). The skin that overhangs the crease (with the eye open) is known as the *supratarsal fold* (also called the superior palpebral fold, and upper lid fold) (Fig. 12.1). Creation of a crease will obligatorily result in the creation of a fold. When observing the open eye from a frontal view, the inferior border of the supratarsal fold forms a line. This line is known as the *double eyelid line*. The distance between the double eyelid line and the lid margin (with the eye open) is called the *pretarsal show* or pretarsal skin exposure (Fig. 12.1).

A patient usually identifies the result of double lid surgery in terms of the amount of pretarsal show, and they usually refer to the pretarsal show as the 'crease height'. Although understandable, this is technically *incorrect*. From a surgeon's perspective, crease height is not the pretarsal show. Crease height is the distance between the lid margin and the supratarsal crease. If a patient states that they desire a crease height of 2 mm, they are usually indicating that they desire 2 mm of pretarsal show, the surgeon should keep this discrepancy in mind when discussing goals and formulating a surgical plan.

The height of the supratarsal crease is measured when the patient has their eyes *closed*, at the mid pupil. The pretarsal show is measured with the eyes *open looking straight ahead*. The pretarsal show *changes as a patient looks upward or downward*, hence standardization of the measurement is important.

12.3.2 Internal Anatomy of the Supratarsal Crease

A supratarsal crease is believed to be formed by anatomical fibrous attachments from the levator aponeurosis to the dermis [4] (Fig. 12.2). These attachments originate from the distal levator aponeurosis, travel through the orbicularis muscle, and attach to the dermis along a horizontal line on the upper lid skin. These attachments originate at (and inferior to) the fusion line of the orbital septum and levator aponeurosis [5]. In non-Asians, the fusion line is 2–5 mm above the superior tarsal border. In Asians, the orbital septum often fuses between the eyelid margin and the superior border of the tarsus [5]. The level of the fusion line between the septum and aponeurosis is thought to be a critical factor in explaining the principal differences between Asian and Caucasian upper lids.

12.4 Differences Between the Asian and Caucasian Eyelid

12.4.1 Supratarsal Crease

In Caucasians, the levator fibrous attachments to the dermis that form the crease are fairly constant and are located relatively high on the eyelid, reflecting the higher fusion point between the orbital septum along the levator aponeurosis (Fig. 12.2). Caucasians have well-defined supratarsal creases that start approximately 10–12 mm above the lid margin. The crease is almost universally present, and it runs roughly parallel with the lid margin along its entire width.

In Asians, the fibrous attachments can vary considerably in presence, location, and robustness among individuals. The variability stems from the fact that the distal septum can extend much lower in Asians than in non-Asians, before it fuses with the aponeurosis. A lower septum fusion point affects where the dermal levator fibers originate. The location of the fibers will start much lower on the lid and can be much less robust. This results in a low-lying crease or absent crease [5].

In Asian with naturally occurring double lids, the septum fuses at a more cephalad location, and a naturally occurring defined supratarsal crease is seen. The crease usually sits much lower (in the range of 4–6 mm from the lid margin) than in a Caucasian patient.

The variability in the nature and location of the attachments leads to the wide degree of diversity seen in Asian eyelids, ranging from a wide, well-defined crease, to no crease, to any combination in between. Patients may present with double lids that intermittently become monolids depending on the state of edema of the upper lids. These eyelids are believed to have dermal crease attachments that are either flimsy or fewer in quantity.

12.4.2 Shape

In most Asians with a supratarsal crease, the crease usually tapers toward (and commonly merges) with the lid margin as it moves medially (Fig. 12.3). This type of lid is referred to as a 'tapered crease' or 'inside crease'. This tapering of the crease is due to the presence of the epicanthal folds. In contrast, when the fold runs parallel with the lid margin all the way to its termination,

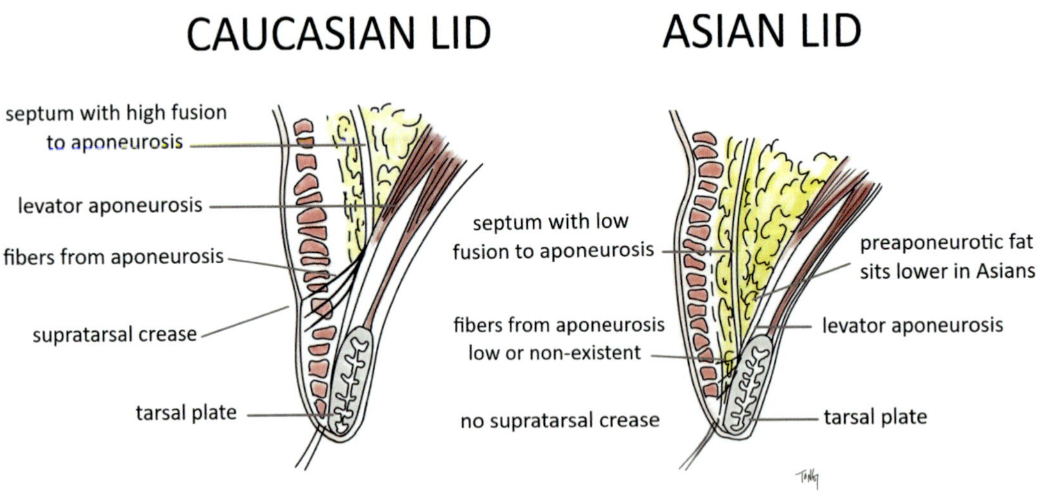

Fig. 12.2 Difference between Caucasian and Asian upper lid. In Caucasians, the orbital septum fuses above the tarsal plate, and aponeurotic fibers originate and extend to the dermis. This results in a well-defined, high supratarsal crease. In Asians, the septum fuses low, frequently below the upper edge of the septum. This allows the preaponeurotic fat to sit lower, giving the lid a puffy appearance. In addition, aponeurotic fibers to the dermis sit much lower (or are non-existent), producing a very low or non-existent supratarsal crease

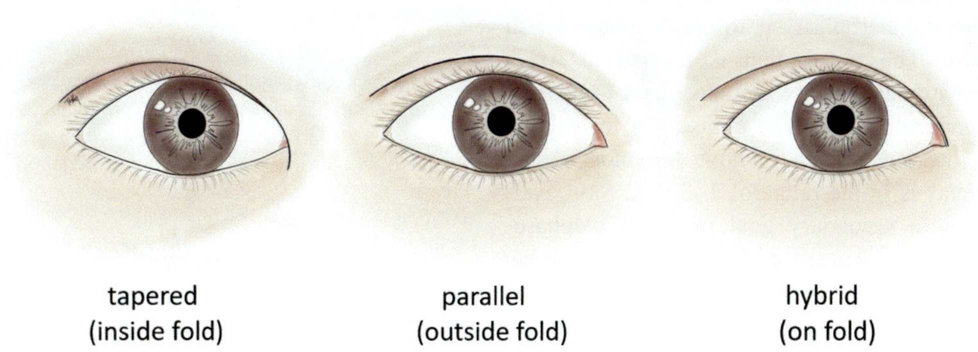

Fig. 12.3 Examples of tapered, parallel, and hybrid fold configurations. Right eye depicted

the lid is referred to as having a 'parallel crease', or 'outside crease' (Fig. 12.3). Almost all Caucasians possess a parallel crease because epicanthal folds are rare. Asians may also have a supratarsal crease with a parallel configuration, although it is the least common presentation. For many Asians, this configuration is also one of the most admired when it occurs naturally, possibly because of its relative infrequency.

12.4.3 Epicanthal Folds

Epicanthal folds are almost unique to Asians. The fold represents a band of skin that spans over the medial canthus, starting from approximately the medial third of the upper eyelid, traversing the medial canthus, and ending variably at the medial portion of the lower lid. The epicanthal fold can take on differing degrees of severity. Increasing severity manifests with the lacrimal caruncle progressively hidden from view, and the medial canthus appearing increasingly rounded. In the most severe forms, the eyes may take on an appearance of strabismus (pseudostrabismus) due to the horizontal shortening of the medial triangle with the accompanying illusion of esotropia. Aside from altering the medial canthus appearance, the epicanthal fold affects the supratarsal fold as the fold traverses medially. The epicanthal fold represents a band of tight skin, and a supratarsal fold will tend to taper toward it or merge with this line of greater skin tension. This affects the shape as previously discussed. When it joins the epicanthal fold or lid margin, it creates a '*tapered crease*' or 'inside fold'. When the supratarsal fold remains distinct from the lid margin, it is termed a '*parallel crease*' or 'outside fold'. A third possible configuration, referred to as an 'on fold', is seen when the fold joins the lid margin but only at its most medial aspect (Fig. 12.3). Later in this chapter, epicanthoplasty will be discussed as a means to minimize the appearance of the epicanthal fold.

12.4.4 Preaponeurotic Fat

Preaponeurotic fat in the Asian lid usually extends more caudally toward the lid margin than in the Caucasian lid (Fig. 12.2). This is due to the fact that the septum extends much lower on the levator than in Caucasian patients [5]. The result is an upper lid that may look full or puffy. Double fold surgery corrects the puffy appearance as fat is typically cleared away in the area of the planned crease. Aside from the new crease line, removal of preaponeurotic fat in more cephalad areas of the lid is performed conservatively in select patients.

12.5 Goals for Asian Blepharoplasty Versus Caucasian Blepharoplasty

The goals of Asian blepharoplasty are different from Caucasian blepharoplasty. These are two distinct patient populations seeking lid surgery for different concerns. The primary goal in Asian blepharoplasty is to create a supratarsal crease. The crease that is formed in Asian blepharoplasty is not the same as a Caucasian supratarsal crease. The crease sits lower, and the desired pretarsal show for most Asian patients is in the range of 1–3 mm. Skin excision is a secondary goal in Asian blepharoplasty. The degree of skin excision in Asian blepharoplasty is typically small because the patient population skews younger. In contrast, Caucasian blepharoplasty is focused primarily on the elimination of excess skin due to aging. Finally, little if any preaponeurotic fat is removed in Asian blepharoplasty. Fat is seldom removed and usually done conservatively, except where it lies in the area of the new crease. Aggressive removal of fat in double lid surgery may cause the appearance of multiple folds postoperatively. Contemporary Caucasian blepharoplasty involves much less fat removal than in the past, but it is still considered to be an important component of the procedure.

12.6 Differences Between Male and Female Asian Blepharoplasty

There is more demand from female Asian patients than male as with most cosmetic surgeries. Culturally, it is considered much more important for females to have double lids as compared to male Asian patients. When performing male Asian blepharoplasty, the principles of evaluation and surgery will be the same for male and female patients alike. The main difference is that male patients generally seek less pretarsal show when compared to females. The typical range for males should be 1–2 mm. Greater degrees of pretarsal show may come across as feminizing for some male patients (Table 12.1).

Table 12.1 Differences between Asian and Caucasian blepharoplasty

	Asian blepharoplasty	Caucasian blepharoplasty
Age of patient	Typically young (20's and up)	Typically middle age and up
Supratarsal crease creation	Primary goal	Rarely required
Typical degree of pretarsal show after surgery	Average: 1–3 mm	Average: 5–8 mm
Skin excision	Usually a minor amount, but depends on age	A primary goal
Fat removal	Minor degree, usually only at the level of the crease	Preaponeurotic fat excision is common compared to Asian blepharoplasty

12.7 Indications for Surgery

The surgery is performed for dissatisfaction with the appearance of Asian upper eyelids. The specific causes of dissatisfaction vary. Each indication is listed below and is discussed in detail in the section pertaining to formulating the surgical plan.

- Absent crease
- Low crease
- Ill-defined creases or intermittent loss of crease
- Crease Asymmetry
- Excess skin
- Epicanthal folds
- Ptosis

12.8 Consultation/Evaluation

Ideally, the consultation should be conducted without makeup, false lashes, or eyelid tape/glue. The presence of these items may obscure the true anatomy and/or mask asymmetries. The evaluation comprises three components:

1. Eliciting the patient's desired outcome
2. Examination of the patient's anatomy
3. Formulating a surgical plan to achieve the desired outcome based on the patient's existing anatomy

12.9 Patient's Desired Outcome

Patients usually have a general idea regarding what they would like to achieve. An important goal of the consultation is to attain enough information to understand the patient's wishes and formulate a surgical plan to achieve them. The following specific items should be elicited during the consultation:

- Patient concerns about the eyelids
  - Desires a crease? Height of pretarsal show desired?
  - Concerns about asymmetry?
  - Concerns about excess skin?
  - Concerns about lid puffiness/fullness?
- Specific details about the crease
  - Height: Specific crease height (expressed descriptively by the patient, and/or in sample photos, and/or simulating a fold using a bent paperclip, wire, or forceps)
  - Shape: Desired crease shape medially (tapered, parallel, or a hybrid of tapered and parallel)? Desired lateral shape (flared, or following the lid margin)?
  - Epicanthal folds: Does patient desire alteration of the epicanthal fold?

12.9.1 Crease Height

The patient will usually request a certain 'crease height'. This specifies the desired amount of pretarsal show they wish to achieve. Patients may have difficulty describing the degree of pretarsal show they desire. Even with an adequate description, it is not a precise value that can be used to perform the surgery. The patient should explicitly show/demonstrate what they would like to achieve to the surgeon. This can be demonstrated by using a curved paperclip to simulate a crease on the lid, or having the patient show the surgeon photographs of eyelids they desire. If a patient uses eyelid tape or glue, they may show a photo of themselves with the tape/glue in place with the preferred result.

12.9.2 Medial Crease Shape (Tapered /Inside Versus Parallel/ Outside)

The surgeon should ascertain the patient's preference for the medial fold appearance. Patients sometimes refer to the appearance of the medial crease as an *'inside fold'* (tapered crease), *'outside fold'* (parallel crease), or *'on fold'* (crease merges with the lid at the end of the medial canthus) (Fig. 12.3). If a patient is unfamiliar with these terms, the surgeon should show the patient examples of each. It should be noted that the patient's request may not always be possible or aesthetically desirable. For example, a high pretarsal show should not be combined with an inside/tapered medial crease as the transition from central to medial would be steep and unnatural. The anatomy may affect the medial crease shape as well. When simulating the crease with a curved paperclip (or other implement), the medial fold will naturally establish itself. A naturally occurring parallel fold indicates that a parallel or tapered fold (based on the patient's preference) may be created without adding epicanthoplasty. If the medial fold is naturally tapered, epicanthoplasty should be considered if the patient desires parallel folds. While the crease is simulated with a paperclip, the appearance of epicanthoplasty can be simulated by pulling the medial canthal skin slightly nasal. This maneuver is also useful to show the patient how epicanthoplasty can convert a tapered crease to a parallel.

12.9.3 Lateral Crease Shape

Finally, the patient may comment on how they would prefer the lateral portion of the fold. It may continue to follow the general shape of the lid margin, or follow a more horizontal path, creating a slightly flared appearance. A slightly flared appearance balances out the natural sagging of tissues laterally that occurs with aging.

12.10 Examination

Examination of the lids should start with the patient looking straight ahead. The following directed assessment points should be noted as part of a more comprehensive periorbital examination.

- Overall symmetry of the eyes, lids, and brows
- Presence or absence of a supratarsal crease.
- Measurements of any existing crease (from lid margin to crease with eyes closed with slight traction)
- Symmetry existing of creases
- Presence and severity of epicanthal folds
- Presence of brow ptosis
- Evidence of frontalis compensation for brow or lid ptosis
- Presence of ptosis or pseudoptosis

12.11 Formation of the Surgical Plan

12.11.1 Indications for Incisional Versus Non-incisional Techniques

An incisional (open) technique is mandatory when skin excision or adipose removal is required as non-incisional (closed) double fold techniques do not allow for skin or fat removal. Likewise, if ptosis correction is planned, the open method is utilized. Otherwise, the choice is up to the patient. The main differences between open and closed double fold surgery will be discussed.

- Incisions made
  - The incision for the open method spans most of the lid and is similar to Caucasian blepharoplasty, while the closed method requires three short stab incisions medially, laterally, and centrally, along the intended crease
- Skin removal/fat removal
  - Skin and/or fat removal can only be accomplished with the open technique
- Ptosis correction
  - Ptosis corrections can only be accomplished with the open technique
- Permanence
  - The open technique is permanent, while the closed technique is not. The creases will eventually disappear with the closed method as the sutures gradually cut through the tissues over time. The average duration is 3–5 years.
  - The closed method is usually reversible by removing the suture, while the open method is difficult to fully reverse.
- Healing time
  - The healing time is shorter for the closed method, and patients may be socially presentable in as little as 3 days. The average time for the open method is in the range of 5–10 days.

12.11.2 Absent Crease

The most common reason for Asian blepharoplasty is absent supratarsal creases or low-lying creases that are too low to be visible. The appropriate surgical plan is double fold blepharoplasty with supratarsal crease formation at the desired height.

12.11.3 Crease Height Planning

After the consultation, the surgeon should have a clear understanding of the patient's desired pretarsal show. The pretarsal show is determined by the location of the supratarsal crease AND the amount of skin that drapes over the supratarsal crease (i.e., the quantity of skin of the superior palpebral fold). Setting a higher supratarsal crease increases the amount pretarsal show (and vice versa), as does the removal of skin. An open technique allows for the manipulation of both variables.

When performing an open technique, the general concept is to achieve the desired result by affecting the two variables responsible for determining pretarsal show: the height of the supratarsal crease (i.e., the location of the incision), and the extent of supratarsal fold skin (i.e., the amount of skin that drapes over the crease). In order to make results more easily reproducible, the technique employs varying the height of the supratarsal crease while removing supratarsal skin in a manner to 'standardize' the extent of skin draping that occurs after surgery. The skin of the supratarsal fold is therefore made to be a constant, while the incision height is the variable. The advantage of this approach is that a given incision location will create a consistent pretarsal show for any patient, regardless of skin quantity. With this method, a 'low' crease is set at 4–5 mm above the lid margin, a 'medium' crease at 6–7 mm above the lid margin, and 'high' crease at 8–9 mm. The actual distances will vary from surgeon to surgeon as there can be differences in how the markings are made and the surgery is performed but should be constant for a given individual surgeon.

When performing a closed suture technique, the amount of skin is not altered. The amount of excess skin can vary from patient to patient; therefore, placing the sutures at a given distance from the lid margin does not produce a consistent pretarsal show. For these cases, the desired appearance is first simulated with the aid of a paperclip or other instrument pressing into the skin. The suture locations are then marked, based on the locations of where the instrument was 'pressed' into the skin. If the closed technique is limited to be used in patients with minimal degrees of skin excess, placing sutures at a given suture distance from the lid margin will provide a consistent pretarsal show.

12.11.4 Crease Asymmetry

Patients may present with creases that are asymmetric in height. Symmetry may be achieved by elevating *both* creases to a new level. As an alternative approach, the lower crease may be elevated to match the higher crease. In this circumstance, *both* lids should undergo double lid surgery. Even though only the lower crease would be elevated, the 'normal' level crease would be re-anchored at the same height. The rationale for operating on both lids is to achieve more predictable symmetry. When only one lid is altered, the crease levels may be made symmetric, but the definition of the new crease may differ from the native crease. Operating on both lids provides the best likelihood of symmetry in most cases. Lowering of an elevated crease is more difficult as the result is not as predictable. The general method of lowering a crease is discussed in the section in this chapter dealing with post-operative asymmetry.

12.11.5 Ill-Defined Creases or Intermittent Loss of Crease

Patients may complain that their creases lack definition (ill-defined creases) or are intermittent (the creases occasionally revert to monolid appearance). Intermittent creases seem to be affected by factors that affect swelling of the lid (such as crying, rubbing the eyes, lack of sleep, dehydration, dietary salt load, time since waking in the morning). More swelling appears to be associated with loss of a visible fold in these patients. These changes may be reflective of dermal attachments that are 'flimsy', resulting in supratarsal creases that are easily influenced by edema. These cases are treated by re-anchoring both side at the desired (same or new) level.

12.11.6 Excess Skin

Patients may present with excess skin in addition to a lack of a satisfactory crease. In these patients, an open approach is employed, and skin excision is incorporated into the double fold surgery.

Occasionally, a (typically) older patient may present with naturally occurring double folds requesting skin excision. They are satisfied with the appearance of the crease but complain that the upper lid excess skin has 'become droopy' and has narrowed the appearance of the pretarsal show. These cases are treated in a similar manner to Caucasian blepharoplasty and do not require double fold creation or alteration.

Pseudoptosis orientalis is a form of excess skin. In patients without a crease, excess skin can hang over the edge of the lid margin, giving the appearance of ptosis. In reality, there is no ptosis, but only the illusion that the lid margin is sitting too low. In the course of double fold surgery, the excess skin is corrected. More significant pseudoptosis requires the open approach. With the open technique, the excess skin is removed as dictated by the marking process. With the closed approach, *minor* degrees of pseudoptosis orientalis are also able to be corrected. Although no skin is excised, the creation of the crease can effectively stabilize the caudal skin, preventing it from hanging below the lid margin.

12.11.7 Brow Ptosis

If a patient has brow ptosis, the descent of the forehead tissues shifts the skin of the brow/upper lid transition area into the upper lid region. The result of double fold surgery may give the appearance of a puffy or rounded appearance to the supratarsal fold, especially if the brow ptosis is significant. Asians with brow ptosis commonly present with a significant degree of lateral hooding as well, giving the lateral lid area a downward slanted look. This effect is even seen in fairly young Asians whose brow ptosis appears mild. Lateral hooding can be somewhat mitigated by extending the lateral extent of the skin excision during open double fold surgery, but the results are typically suboptimal. The effect of brow ptosis on the central lid is diminished by removing more supratarsal skin during double fold surgery. There are limits to this approach as the supratarsal fold starts to appear bulky when the thicker skin from the superior upper lid is shifted inferiorly. Additionally, the brow position may descend even further with this approach. The management of brow ptosis is analogous to Caucasian patients; when lid surgery may not be sufficient to attain the patient's desired outcome, brow lift surgery should be offered. As a valuable educational tool, patients should be shown similar examples of past patients who have undergone double lid surgery with and without a brow lift. If a brow lift is planned, it should occur before the lid procedure, similar to combined browlift and blepharoplasty in non-Asians.

12.11.8 Epicanthal Folds

If epicanthal folds are present, they may be modified through epicanthoplasty. The decision to modify the epicanthal folds is based on the patient's wishes. Many patients may not even be aware of epicanthal folds or that epicanthoplasty exists. Depending on the practice and how the surgeon approaches the issue, epicanthoplasty may be rarely performed or frequently included with double lid surgery. The most common indications for epicanthoplasty are:

- To minimize the appearance of the epicanthal folds to achieve a sharper, less rounded appearance at the medial canthus.

- To correct severe epicanthal folds that create the appearance of pseudostrabismus.
- To create parallel folds in the presence of prominent epicanthal folds. Prominent epicanthal folds will create a strong tendency for the supratarsal fold to merge with the epicanthal fold medially, thus creating a tapered medial fold. Epicanthoplasty usually eliminates this effect so that a parallel fold can be created.
- To improve aesthetics in a patient with prominent epicanthal folds who wants a wide pretarsal show. The combination of wide pretarsal show in the presence of a strong epicanthal fold will result in a tapered medial crease and suboptimal aesthetics. The result will look unnatural due to the steep angle of descent the high crease follows as it merges into the epicanthal fold. The epicanthoplasty allows for a parallel crease to be created so it can follow a 'flatter' trajectory as it travels medially.

12.11.9 Preaponeurotic Fat Removal

Oftentimes, Asian patients will complain that their upper lids look full or puffy. It is important to discern the area of concern. Preaponeurotic fat sits low on the lid due to the caudal extension of the septum along the levator aponeurosis. Double-fold creation involves the removal of adipose tissue in the area and is generally sufficient to correct the 'puffy' appearance in the inferior lid. If the patient is concerned about preaponeurotic fat more cephalad in the lid, some fat may also be removed in a conservative manner. Aggressive fat resection in the upper lid is not recommended as it may lead to aesthetic complications such as an aged appearance or unwanted multiple creases ('triple fold') being formed. Retro orbicularis oculi fat (ROOF) may be more prominent in Asian patients, causing upper lid bulkiness. ROOF may be excised judiciously to decrease the appearance of bulkiness.

12.11.10 Ptosis

Correction of small degrees of ptosis is generally not indicated, but it may be a cosmetic issue in double fold surgery, particularly when it is asymmetric (i.e., unilateral or bilateral but asymmetric). The discussion of ptosis in this chapter is focused on patients seeking Asian blepharoplasty who present with small degrees of ptosis that affect the aesthetic outcome. This narrows the scope of discussion to patients who have good levator function and mild or even subclinical forms of ptosis (usually 2 mm of difference between eyes or less). The appearance of ptosis should be differentiated from a form of pseudoptosis common in Asians. Pseudoptosis orientalis occurs when the skin in the upper lid hangs down *below* the lid margin, giving the appearance of ptosis when none in fact exists. This type of pseudoptosis is corrected when the excess skin is removed as part of the open double fold procedure. No additional procedures are required to correct pseudoptosis when excess skin is removed in the usual manner described later in this chapter. Correction is also achieved with the closed double fold technique if the lax skin near the margin is stabilized to prevent it from hanging.

If true ptosis is noted, the levator function is usually normal (>10 mm of excursion). Patients with unilateral ptosis should be assessed for latent ptosis of the contralateral lid. By slightly elevating the ptotic lid to simulate ptosis correction, the contralateral lid is observed for 30 seconds. If the contralateral eyelid droops, then a diagnosis of bilateral asymmetric ptosis is confirmed. Both lids should be corrected in this case. In this patient group, the most common presentation is ptosis with a difference of 1–2 mm between lid margin elevations. When this presentation of unilateral (or bilateral but asymmetric) ptosis is not corrected during double fold surgery, it will likely result in pretarsal show asymmetry. If double fold surgery is performed in the usual fashion, *the pretarsal show will be wider on the ptotic lid.*

Additionally, the asymmetry is almost always noted by the patient postoperatively. Ptosis should be pointed out to the patient during the consultation and management options discussed.

Small degrees of ptosis (<1 mm) can be left alone if the patient understands there will be some post-operative asymmetry. Alternatively, this ptosis can be managed without formal ptosis correction. In this situation, the incision line on the ptotic side would be marked lower on the ptotic lid by (approximately) the same amount as the degree of ptosis. For example, a patient with 1 mm of relative ptosis on the right side would have the incision line on the right side marked 1 mm lower than on the left. After the surgery is completed, the supratarsal crease location would be *asymmetric* between sides (the right crease would sit lower relative to the left (normal) side), but the pretarsal show would be *symmetric* because the ptotic lid margin would also sit lower, thus giving the same amount of pretarsal show as the normal side. For differences more than 1 mm, ptosis is better managed with levator advancement on the affected eye(s) during open double fold surgery. Simultaneous ptosis correction and double fold surgery is a much more difficult procedure to successfully accomplish as there are many dynamic aspects at play. Patients should be told about the possibility of revision surgery in these cases.

12.12 Operative Techniques

12.12.1 Open Incisional Method with Skin to Aponeurosis Anchoring

12.12.1.1 Concept

Given that the supratarsal crease is formed by a line of anatomical attachment between the levator aponeurosis and the dermis, the procedure aims to surgically create this attachment using sutures to connect the skin to the aponeurosis. The location of the new supratarsal crease coincides with the location of the incision. Skin excision is utilized to create a consistent amount of supratarsal fold (the skin above the incision line). This helps to ensure a predictable pretarsal show at a given incision height despite varying degrees of skin excess. Dissection along the incision is carried down to the level of the levator aponeurosis. The skin of the lower flap is attached to the aponeurosis with 4–5 evenly spaced anchoring sutures along the incision line.

12.12.1.2 Preoperative Markings

The surgery begins with the preoperative markings. This is facilitated with the patient on a stretcher, in the supine position with the head slightly elevated.

While the patient stares straight ahead, a vertical line signifying the mid-pupil location is marked on the upper lid. Next, a horizontal mark is made along this vertical line, at a distance from the lid margin corresponding to the (preoperatively chosen) crease height. The crease height is typically between 5 and 9 mm above the lid margin. For perspective, a crease height of 5 mm provides approximately 1 mm of pretarsal show ('small'), 7 mm crease height will give approximately 2–3 mm of a pretarsal show ('medium'), while 9 mm provides approximately 4 mm of pretarsal show ('large'). These stated numbers are approximate and are affected by the patient's anatomy, the way in which the surgeon makes the markings, and how the surgeon performs the surgery. This mark is made with the lid skin on slight upward traction with the surgeon's free hand. The amount of traction corresponds to the point at which the eyelashes are just beginning to move (into eversion). The traction serves multiple purposes. When placing the anchoring sutures, replicating the same degree of stretch verifies that the sutures are placed at the correct distance from the lid margin. Putting the skin on stretch during marking will eliminate any skin redundancy between the lid margin and the new crease postoperatively. Marking the skin with the slight traction also ensures that pseudoptosis is corrected. Finally, because patients present with varying degrees of lid skin redundancy and laxity, marking in this manner helps to establish an 'end point' to help achieve consistent results between each eyelid and between patients.

Once the initial mid-pupil horizontal mark is established, the remainder of the incision line is drawn laterally and medially, roughly following the contour of the lid margin. When a medially tapered (inside fold) crease is desired, the medial mark merges with the origin of the epicanthal fold (or runs inferior to it). If a parallel (outside fold) crease is desired, the line stays relatively horizontal, running superior and slightly medial to the origin of the epicanthal fold. The medial incision should not extend much beyond the punctum. Incisions beyond this point may venture into nasal skin, which is thicker and more prone to hypertrophic scarring. Creation of a parallel crease may not be successful in the presence of a prominent epicanthal fold, especially if the preoperative paperclip simulation demonstrates a tapered crease. In patients who express a strong desire to have a parallel crease, epicanthoplasty should be performed concomitantly. The lateral portion of the incision line parallels the lid margin, or it may continue relatively straight for a somewhat more flared crease laterally. This completed mark represents the line of skin anchoring and the eventual supratarsal crease.

Next, an upper line representing the extent of skin removal is marked. Varying degrees of excess skin occur from patient to patient. Removal of the excess skin allows for a consistent level of pretarsal show for a given incision height. For patients with minor skin excess, the surgeon gently lifts the brow/lid skin with the same upward traction as before. Under traction, a marking pen is held at mid-pupil, just over the marked incision line. The traction is relaxed as the pen is held stationary, and a mark is then made at mid-pupil on the relaxed skin. The distance from the marked incision line to this new mark signifies the degree of skin removal required. For young patients, it is typically minor (1–2 mm). In (older) patients with more skin excess, the excision marking may be made easier by using skin forceps at mid-pupil, starting at the marked line, to gather skin to initiate lash eversion as before. The upper limit of the grasped skin represents the upper limit of skin excision. The rest of this upper line is drawn in, tapering off laterally and medially to join the initial marked incision line. It is important to be conservative with skin excision medially, as lagophthalmos occurs more easily in double fold surgery due to the proximity of the incision to the lid margin. Additionally, accentuation of the epicanthal fold can occur with more medial skin removal.

An alternative method for determining skin excision in the older patient has been described by Zubriri [6]. The patient sits upright and looks in the mirror, and the surgeon uses a bent paperclip to simulate the crease at the desired crease height (e.g., 5 mm for a low crease). The amount of pretarsal show is noted. The surgeon's other hand then elevates the forehead (to simulate lid skin removal) to the level desired by the patient. The surgeon notes the pretarsal show difference between resting and elevation. This difference is multiplied by 2 to obtain the amount of skin that should be removed (×2 to account for the front and back surface of the fold). For example, if the resting pretarsal show is 1 mm and the desired pretarsal show 4 mm, the difference is 3 mm, and so the amount of skin excision should be 6 mm (3 mm × 2 = 6 mm).

Finally, vertical lines are added along the length of the incision to indicate the locations of the anchoring sutures. This typically consists of four or five evenly spaced lines, with the mid-pupil line considered as one of the anchoring points.

12.12.1.3 Incision

The surgery is performed in the supine position, under light sedation or local anesthesia. The choice of anesthesia depends on patient preference. The surgeon will confirm that the chosen anesthetic is appropriate for the patient at the consultation. Sedation is utilized more commonly.

Once the face is prepped and draped, the markings are re-checked with calipers to confirm measurements and symmetry. Lidocaine with epinephrine (0.5% with 1:200000 epi) is injected along the incision lines. Operating on both lids simultaneously helps to optimize symmetry between lids. After seven minutes has elapsed, the incision is made on the first lid, through the skin only (Fig. 12.4). The ellipse of skin is

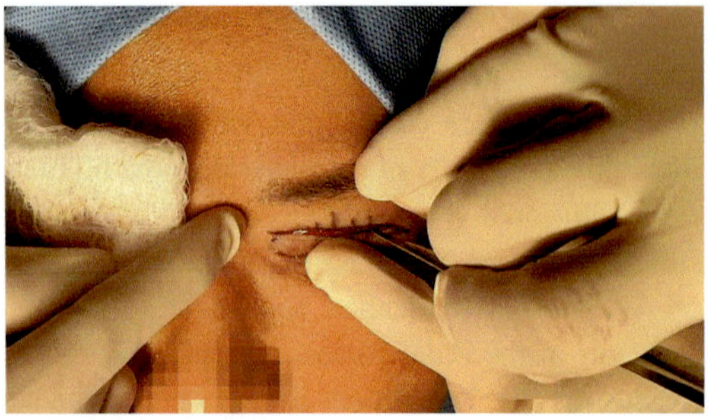

Fig. 12.4 Making the skin incision

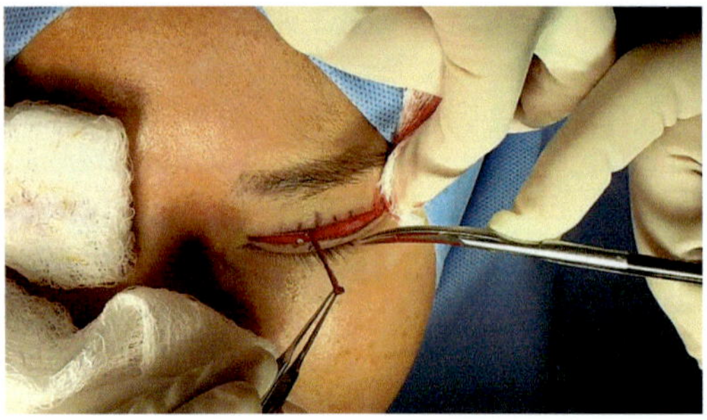

Fig. 12.5 Removing the strip of skin after initial incision

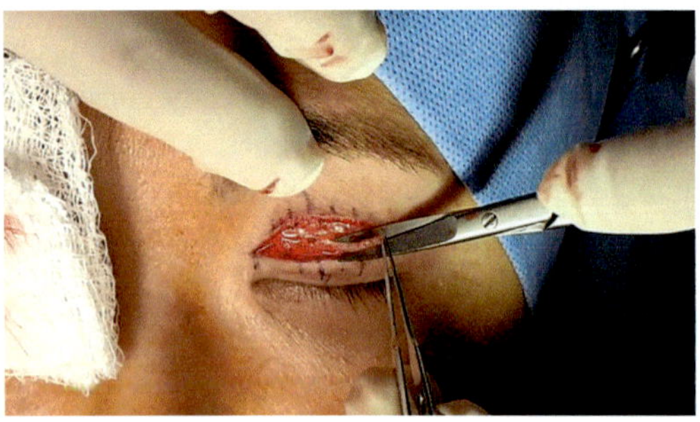

Fig. 12.6 Incremental removal of tissue along the edge of the lower flap, towards the levator aponeurosis

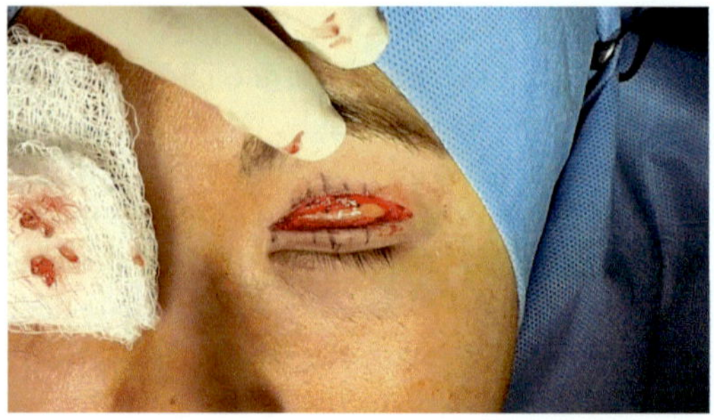

Fig. 12.7 Tissue sufficiently removed to depth of the levator aponeurosis

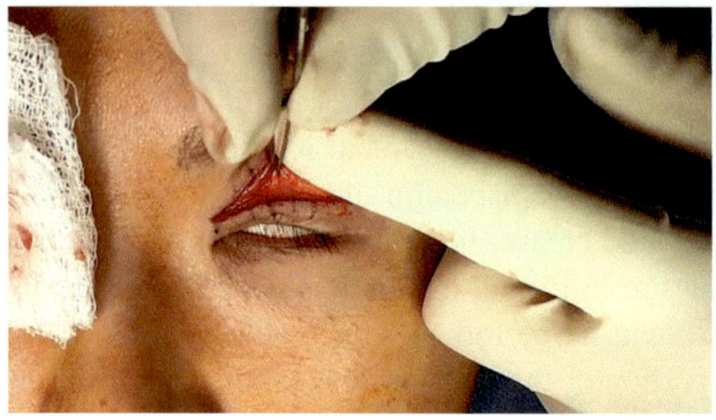

Fig. 12.8 Confirming the proper dissection depth for anchor suture placement with the distraction test. The base of the wound is grasped with fine forceps, and the lid is distracted upwards. If the lid margin moves in direct correspondence to the degree of distraction, the proper depth is achieved

removed using iris scissors (Fig. 12.5). Hemostasis is obtained using a needle tip cautery. The orbicularis and deeper tissues are then injected with local anesthetic. The skin is then removed on the contralateral lid in the same manner. Tissue excision along the incision line is started by progressively removing small strips of orbicularis and deeper tissues (Fig. 12.6) until the levator aponeurosis is encountered (Fig. 12.7). Prior to meeting the aponeurosis, the surgeon may encounter the distal portion of the orbital septum and preaponeurotic fat. This depends on the location of the incision and the patient's anatomy. The surgeon needs to recognize that there is significant variability of the anatomy here. The levator aponeurosis is shiny and white and may be difficult to identify, especially for the less experienced surgeon. The surgeon must be careful not the disinsert the levator aponeurosis by dissecting too deeply. A maneuver that is helpful to ascertain the correct level is termed the '*distraction test*'. The surgeon grasps the base of the incision with forceps and attempts to elevate the lid as if the lid were opening. If the lid margin moves in direct (1:1) fashion with the upward distraction, the proper depth is attained (this is a positive distraction test) (Fig. 12.8). If the lid margin moves upwards but somewhat indirectly with some 'slack' or 'give', dissection needs to continue deeper. Dissecting too deep beyond the aponeurosis (i.e., disinsertion of the aponeurosis) can also result in direct movement of the lid margin; therefore, tissue removal should proceed incrementally and stop once a positive distraction test is noted. The layer that provides a positive distraction test may not be the actual aponeurosis but instead represents superficially adherent tissue. This will still suffice provided that the anchoring sutures will be placed in the same tissues that are grasped by the forceps.

For the beginning surgeon, it may be helpful to initially identify the levator aponeurosis at a higher (more cephalad) level, which then can be followed back down towards the incision. This is done by finding and opening the orbital septum laterally and more cephalically. This area is safer to dissect as the levator aponeurosis is located much deeper than it is at the incision. Once the preaponeurotic fat is found, it is retracted upwards, and the levator aponeurosis should be visible directly underneath. The remainder of the anterior septum is carefully opened, and the aponeurosis can be followed inferiorly and preserved when excising other fat or soft tissues at the incision.

Adipose tissue is generally preserved in the upper lid except along the incision. The incision area should be relatively clear of fat to promote scar formation between the dermis and aponeurosis. In patients with significant excess, a conservative amount of upper lid fat can be removed. Aggressive removal of fat in the upper lid is not recommended as it may result in an aged appearance. Additionally, aggressive fat removal may result in the unsightly complication of triple or quadruple crease formation. This is believed to occur from the development of adhesions between the dermis and the levator at multiple levels in the absence of the interposed adipose tissue.

12.12.1.4 Placing Anchoring Sutures

After the contralateral lid has been dissected adequately, anchoring sutures are placed. The goal is to place a series of four to five sutures that will secure the edge of the inferior (caudal) incision to the levator aponeurosis at a distance corresponding to the desired crease height. A 6-0 nylon suture with a Castroviejo needle holder is used. The first anchoring suture is placed at mid-pupil. The initial bite of tissue is made at the subdermal level along the edge of the caudal flap. The next bite of tissue consists of the aponeurosis. A small portion of the aponeurosis next to the incision should be grasped with Bishops forceps, and the distraction test should be done to confirm that the suture bite will grasp aponeurosis. To eliminate the risk of corneal injury, the grasped tissue is slightly elevated, and the needle is then placed through the elevated tissue. The placement of the aponeurotic bite should set the lower flap tension to be similar as used in the marking process. The suture is then tied with ends cut close to the knot (Figs. 12.9, 12.10, 12.11, 12.12, 12.13, and 12.14). The superior (cephalic) skin flap is not incorporated in the anchoring suture. This helps to maintain optimal exposure of the aponeurosis while placing the anchoring sutures. After the ini-

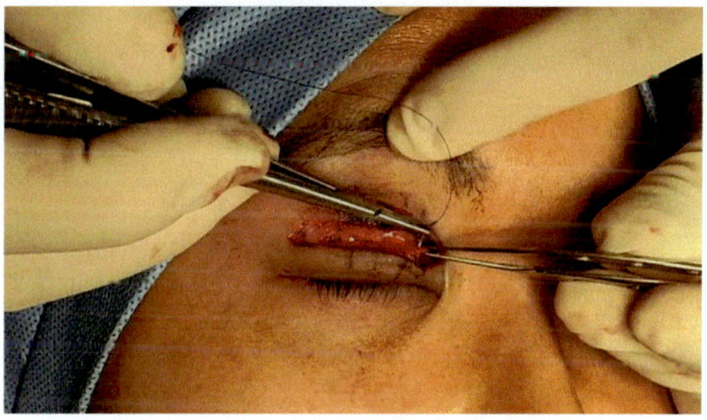

Fig. 12.9 A small bite of levator/peri-levator tissue is grasped with the forceps. The suture is placed through the grasped tissue. (The suture may be placed either in a backhand fashion initially through aponeurosis as shown, or forehand initially through dermis as described in the text)

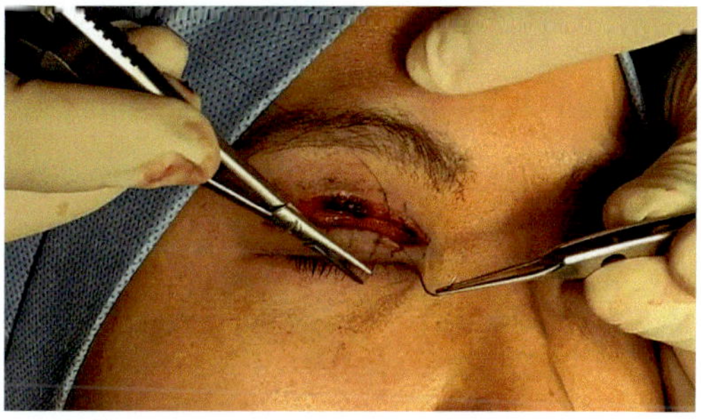

Fig. 12.10 The suture contines with a small bite of the dermis. (The suture may be placed either in a backhand fashion as shown, or forehand as described in the text)

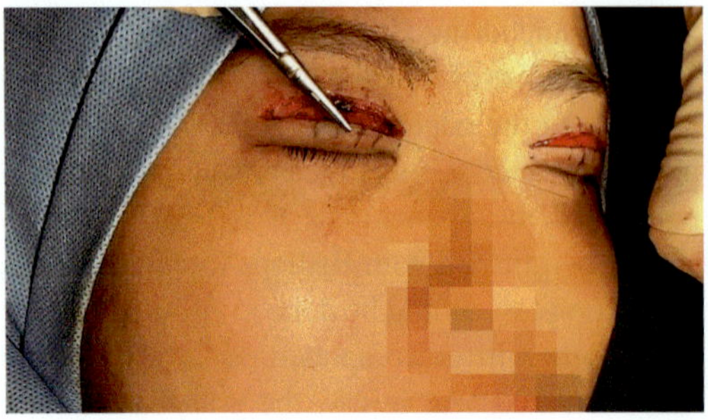

Fig. 12.11 The knot is tied down. To confirm proper placement, the surgeon should observe that the skin flap sits slightly taut, similar to the marking process. The series of anchoring sutures should create a smooth arc corresponding to the desired crease line

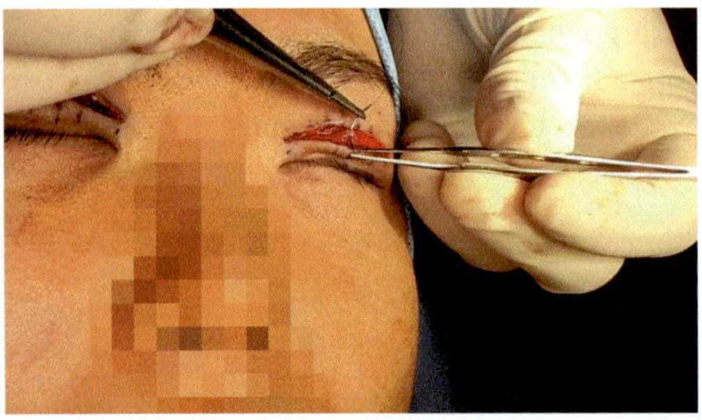

Fig. 12.12 Contralateral side anchoring suture through levator/peri-levator tissues. (The suture may be placed either in a backhand fashion as shown, or forehand as described in the text)

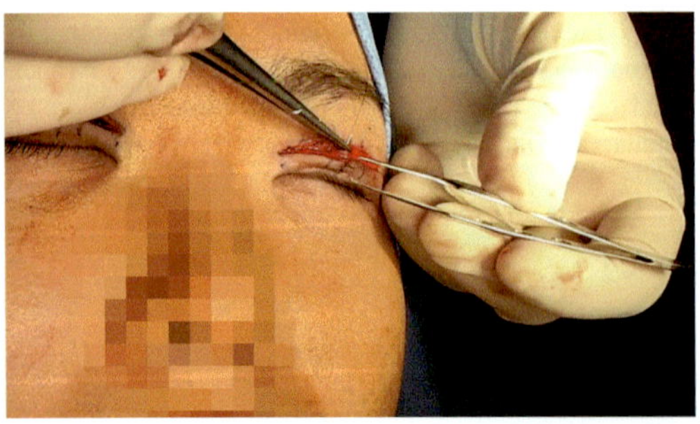

Fig. 12.13 Contralateral anchoring suture through levator/peri-levator tissue and dermis of skin flap. (The suture may be placed either in a backhand fashion as shown, or forehand as described in the text)

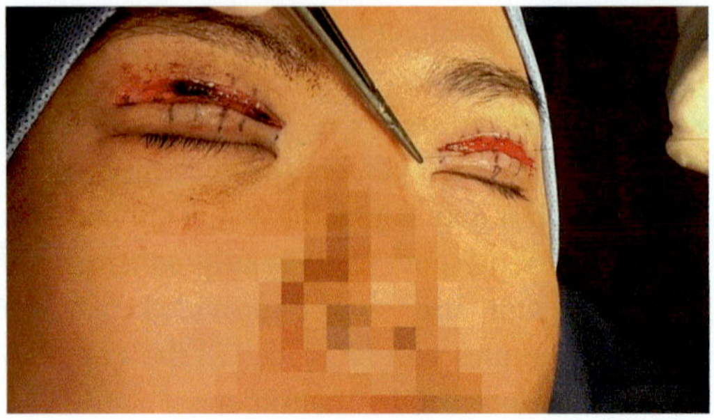

Fig. 12.14 Suture tied down with flap at proper level

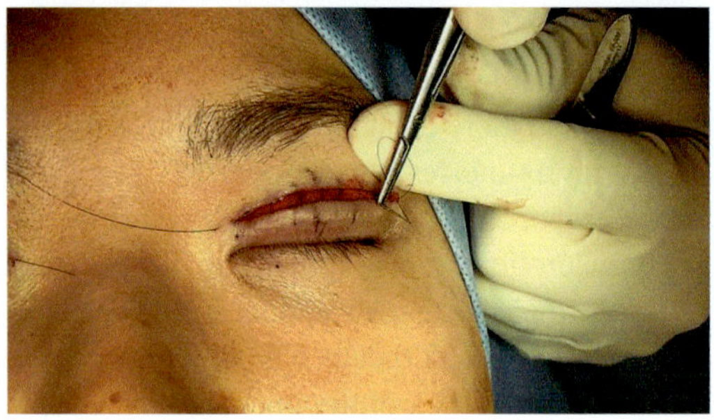

Fig. 12.15 Subcuticular closure of the incision

tial anchoring suture is placed, the same suture is placed on the contralateral lid. The next suture is placed on the first lid and then mirrored on the contralateral lid. The remaining anchoring sutures are placed in a back-and-forth fashion, until all anchoring sutures are completed.

12.12.1.5 Checking Symmetry and Closure

Once all anchoring sutures are placed, the patient is asked to open the eyes. The degree of sedation should allow for this. At this stage, it is normal for the amount of pretarsal show to look noticeably higher than what would be expected as the final result. Symmetry is checked. If asymmetry exists, the responsible anchoring suture(s) should be replaced and re-evaluated. The closure is performed with a running 6-0 subcuticular nylon suture with the ends left free (Fig. 12.15). A steristrip is placed over the incision.

12.12.2 Incisional Technique with Skin to Tarsal Plate Anchoring

This technique is very similar to the open technique described with anchoring of the dermis to the levator aponeurosis. The principal difference with this method is that the anchoring sutures are placed into the tarsal plate instead of the aponeurosis. The crease must be created within the height of the tarsal plate (which is almost always the case except in the highest placed incisions). The resultant crease is more static, as opposed to the dynamic nature of the aponeurotic anchoring. The crease tends to be visible even with the eyes closed. The procedure is somewhat easier to perform as the dissection does not need to be carried right down to the aponeurosis. Dissection only requires debulking of tissues until the sutures can be placed into the tarsal plate.

12.12.3 Non-incisional Suture Asian Blepharoplasty Technique (DST [Double Suture and Twist] Method)

Non-incisional (closed) methods utilize small stab incisions and rely on placing sutures to fix the anterior lamella to the posterior lamella along the intended supratarsal crease. There are multiple descriptions of suture methods for double-fold creation. One disadvantage commonly cited with non-incisional techniques is the lack of permanency. The double suture and twist method has gained popularity because of its relative simplicity and touted long-term results. The double suture and twist technique is summarized, as described by Kure and Minami [7].

12.12.3.1 Markings

The markings are performed with the patient in the sitting position. An open bent paper clip or other implement is used to simulate the crease on the patient's lid. Once the desired appearance is achieved, two or three small dots are marked along the midportion of the simulated crease line. A line is then drawn by connecting the dots, with the lateral and medial portions roughly equidistant from the lid margin. Excess skin is not removed with the closed approach. Therefore, to achieve a given pretarsal show, the height of the marked crease will vary depending on the amount of excess skin of the lid. The non-incision method should not be employed if the excess skin requires the crease to be more than 10 mm above the lid margin. The marked line should be rechecked with the paper clip for accuracy and symmetry with the contralateral side.

Once the lines have been confirmed, three spots are chosen along the line for the placement of stab incisions. The first should be at the center, and two others approximately 10 mm lateral and medial from the center.

12.12.3.2 Incisions

The surgery is performed under local anesthetic with or without light sedation. The external lids are anesthetized with 1% lidocaine with 1:100,000 epinephrine. Anesthetic eye drops are also placed. A corneal shield is inserted. The three horizontal stab incisions are made through the skin only, each approximately 3–5 mm in length. A Bishop's forceps is used to grasp the orbicularis muscle in each wound, and a small piece of muscle is removed. This will help the suture knots sit deeper to prevent postoperative visibility or palpability.

12.12.3.3 First Suture

A double- armed 6-0 prolene suture is used. The lid is everted, and the first needle pass starts on the conjunctival side, directly underneath the central stab incision. The needle is passed through the full thickness of the tarsal plate to exit the central stab incision. Next, the other end of the suture enters the same point on the conjunctival side but is directed laterally in the subconjunctival plane along the tarsal plate, towards the lateral stab incision. Here, the needle exits on the subconjunctival side and is passed through the same point, through the tarsal plate, to emerge through the lateral stab incision. This represents the first 'U-stitch' (Fig. 12.16).

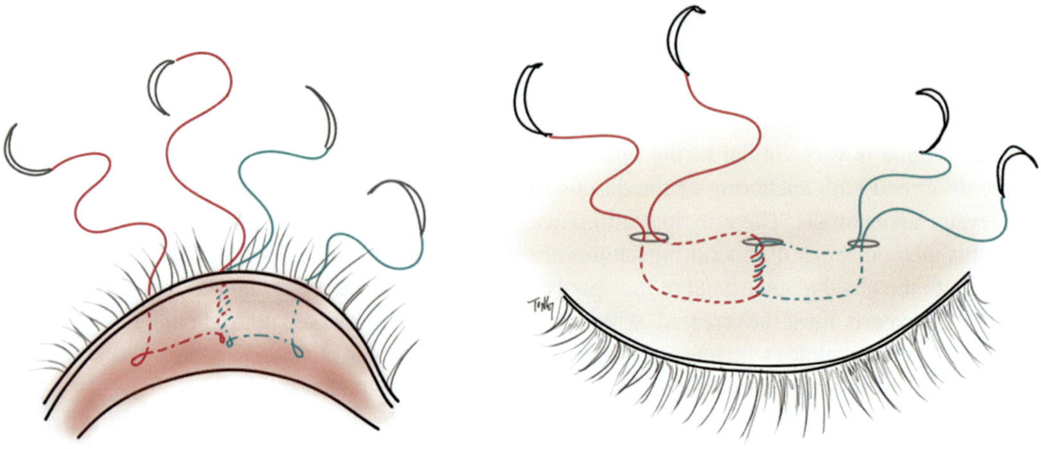

Fig. 12.16 Double suture and twist (DST) method: Two U-stitches are interlocked (twisted) after they emerge through the central stab incision (Conjunctival surface shown, right). The medial arms of the sutures are advanced subcutaneously and emerge through their respective medial or lateral stab incisions, joining with its other end (skin surface shown, left)

12.12.3.4 Second Suture

A second double-armed 6-0 prolene is utilized. This second suture is made in an analogous manner to the first one, except that the second end is directed to emerge through the medial stab incision. At this point, there are two U-stitches placed, with the two suture ends emerging from the central stab incision, as well as their respective lateral or medial stab incisions (Fig. 12.16).

12.12.3.5 Twisting the Sutures and Tying the Knots

The central needle ends are grasped and twisted together five times, keeping track of each suture with their respective U-stitch. The central needle of the lateral U-stitch is then passed into the central stab wound, along the subdermal plane, to exit the lateral stab incision. The central needle of the medial U-stitch is passed in a similar manner to exit the medial stab incision. At this point, the sutures have formed a loop back onto themselves and are interlocked at their central limbs (Fig. 12.16). The appearance of the creases should be checked by removing the corneal shields and having the patient open their eyes. If the aesthetics are unsatisfactory, the sutures are redone. Once a satisfactory result is verified, the sutures are tied at their respective lateral and medial stab incisions. The knots should not be over tightened as buckling of the skin or tarsal plate may occur. The knots are manipulated with forceps to allow them to sit deep from the skin's surface. Each stab incision is closed with a single simple suture or may be left as is, if well approximated on its own. Small steristrip pieces are applied over the stab incisions.

12.12.4 Epicanthoplasty Technique (Modified Root Z Epicanthoplasty)

12.12.4.1 Goals

The epicanthal fold can be thought of as a band of skin that originates in the region of the medial canthus, starting from the medial upper lid, spanning to the medial aspect of the lower lid. The fold presents with variable severity among individuals and shrouds the lacrimal lake to a variable extent. In the most severe instances, the epicanthal fold can make the medial canthus look rounded and create the appearance of pseudostrabismus. The presence of an epicanthal fold may prevent the formation of a parallel crease with double lid surgery. The goals of epicanthoplasty:

(a) Allow for the creation of a parallel crease when performed in combination with double fold blepharoplasty
(b) Correction of the appearance of a rounded medial canthus or pseudostrabismus
(c) Enlargement of the horizontal palpebral width

The design of the epicanthoplasty can be conceptualized as a transposition flap, with the epicanthal fold forming a triangular-shaped flap. The most inferior point of the epicanthal fold represents the tip of the triangle, and two other points: (i) the most medial point of the medial canthus, and (ii) the point on the epicanthal fold that directly overlaps (i), make up the other two vertices. When the skin is pulled medially, the base of the triangular flap is delineated by the two points (i) and (ii). This triangular flap is transposed from an axis that is predominantly inferior-medial to an axis that is roughly perpendicular to the original axis. This transposition relieves the line of skin tension along the original epicanthal fold to a more relaxed and horizontally oriented direction.

12.12.4.2 Markings

The description of this procedure is adapted from Park's technique of Modified Z-epicanthoplasty [8], using the same lettering arrangement. The first mark is located by following the epicanthal fold medially to its termination on the lower lid. A small dot is made here and represents the tip of the flap (point B). A second point is made by pulling the epicanthal fold medially to expose the canthus. A small dot is made at the most medial point of the medial canthus (point D). The third point (called point A) is made with the epicanthal fold relaxed, directly overlapping the medial canthus/second point (D). This third point (A) may be thought of as the 'pivot point'. Lines are drawn joining the tip (point B) to each of the other two points (A) and (D). Next, the location at which the tip will be inset is chosen. It is not an anatomical landmark as was the case for the points A, B, and D. This point (C) is made at a distance from point (A), equal to the flap's length (line AB), at roughly 45 degrees from horizontal. Making it 45 degrees from the horizontal will allow the flap to be inset roughly perpendicular to the original epicanthal fold, effectively releasing the original skin tension and exposing the lacrimal lake. This point C is (ideally) situated along the termination point of the double fold incision line, and its length may be modified to suit the aesthetic needs. A line is drawn from A to C. Finally, the last point (E) is chosen more medially on the double-fold incision line, at approximately the medial ⅓ junction. A line is drawn between E and A. The triangular skin flap AEC represents redundant skin that will be trimmed to allow proper fit when insetting Figs. 12.17 and 12.18 show the markings with the skin relaxed and pulled medially to expose the medial canthus.

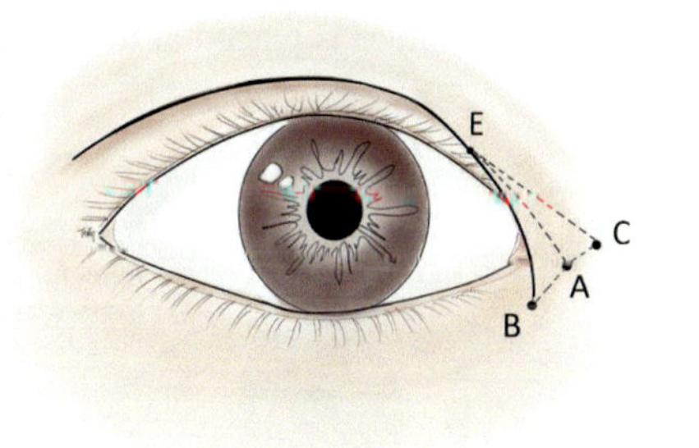

Fig. 12.17 Flap markings for modified Z epicanthoplasty

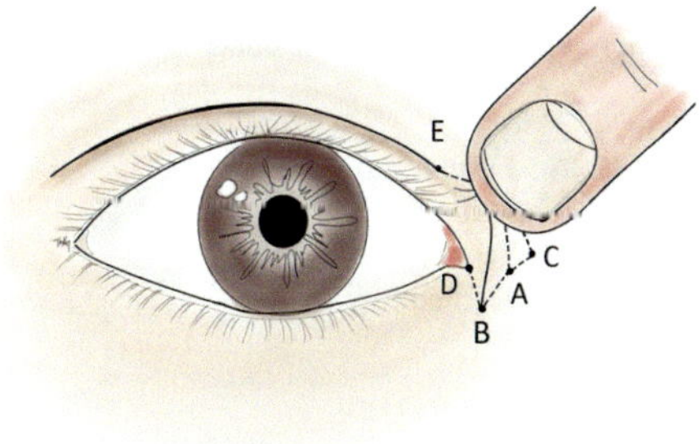

Fig. 12.18 Flap markings with epicanthal fold pulled medially. Point D is the medial canthus. Point A is the point on the epicanthal fold that directly overlaps point D (with skin relaxed). Point B is the termination of the epicanthal fold. DBA represents the tip of the flap. Point B will be rotated to point C. Triangle AEC will be excised to allow for proper fit during insetting

12.12.4.3 Creation of Flaps

The epicanthoplasty is performed first when combined with double fold surgery. After injection with lidocaine with epinephrine, the flap DBA is incised. With the epicanthal tissue pulled medially to expose the canthus, cut DB is made first. Next BA is incised. The area of skin, triangle AEC, is then incised and discarded. This discarded skin allows for a better fit of the flap (DBAE) once it is transposed. The flap DBAE is further mobilized with more undermining (particularly at DB) to free up the flap.

12.12.4.4 Rotation and Inset of Flaps

Assuming adequate release and proper design, point B should almost auto rotate into point C. A suture is placed to inset B to C. In addition, points D and A should come together without tension (as A corresponds to the same (overlapping) point as D). A suture is placed at the medial canthus where points A and D come together. A few more interrupted sutures are placed along the other suture lines as needed. Emphasis should be placed on tension-free closure (through adequate release) as a means to minimize scarring. The effect of the epicanthoplasty should be evident at this point with (i) the medial canthus no longer hidden by the fold, (ii) release of the skin tension along the medial upper lid with (iii) the elimination of any visible epicanthal fold (Figs. 12.19 and 12.20)

The rest of the double-fold procedure can then commence in the usual manner. By placing anchoring suture(s) at the desired position(s) along the medial incision, the medial crease shape and length can be further defined (now that the epicanthal fold is removed).

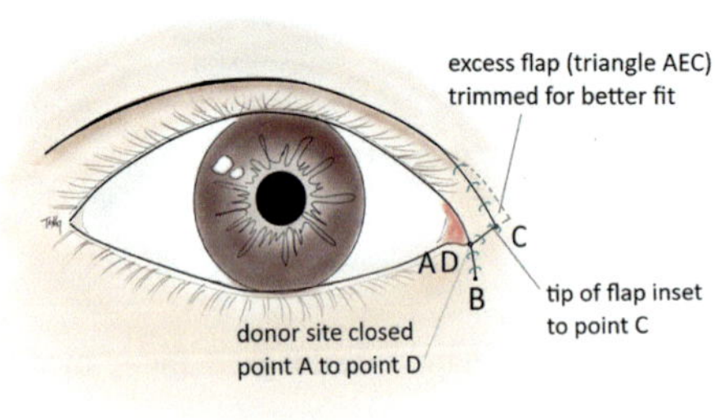

Fig. 12.19 Flap has been inset. Point A and D are brought together to close the donor site

12.12.5 Ptosis Repair (Levator Advancement)

Ptosis repair is usually performed as an adjunct procedure in conjunction with double-fold surgery. The focus of this discussion is on small degrees of ptosis that occur with younger patients. Most cases considered for ptosis repair in Asian blepharoplasty are due to asymmetry. The decision to perform repair should be reserved for patients with 1 mm or more difference in lid margin position. Performing surgery for less difference may not be worthwhile as the variability of the result may be greater than the preoperative difference. Ptosis repair results are generally

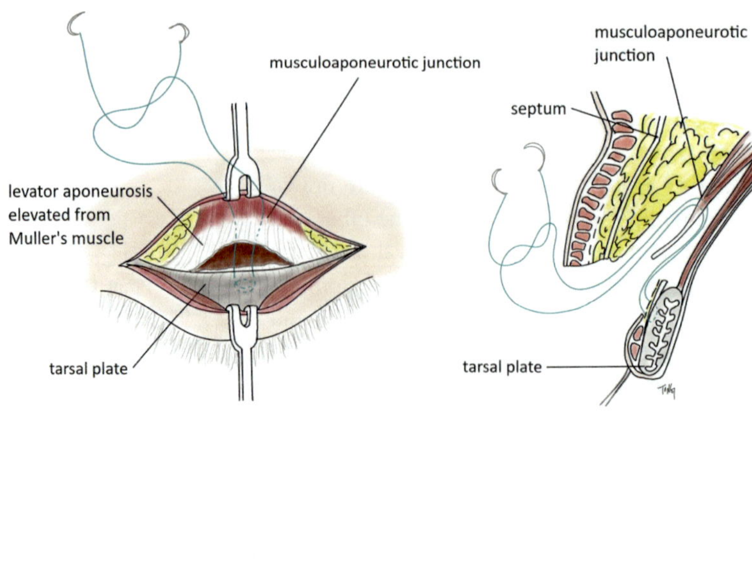

Fig. 12.20 Frontal and cross-section views depicting the concept of levator advancement

more difficult to control due to intrinsic difficulties with intraoperative adjustments and postoperative stretching of the tissues. Patients should be told that asymmetries may still exist post-surgery.

12.12.5.1 Markings

The markings for ptosis repair are made in conjunction with the open double-fold surgery. A vertical mid-pupil marking line is drawn for reference, indicating where the advancement suture will be placed.

12.12.5.2 Dissection

Open double-fold surgery is performed in the usual manner until the point at which the anchoring sutures would be placed. Beginning at the mid-pupil line, along the edge of the lower flap, the levator aponeurosis was gently lifted with forceps and dissected from the tarsal plate with scissors. Gentle inferior traction is placed on the inferior flap using a small double-pronged skin hook for countertraction. The plane between the levator aponeurosis and Muller's muscle is carefully dissected cephalically as the levator aponeurosis is lifted. Once dissection has reached the musculoaponeurotic junction, the levator advancement suture may be placed.

12.12.5.3 Advancement

A double-armed 6-0 silk suture is used. The surgeon elevates the tarsal plate (to protect the globe) and grasps a suture bite of the tarsal plate a few millimeters below the upper border, at the mid pupil. A second bite at the same location is made to establish firm fixation to the tarsus. Both needle ends are passed under the dissected aponeurosis to emerge centrally at the level of the musculoaponeurotic junction. The suture is tightened on a looped end of the suture. This allows the knot to be released if needed by pulling the end of the suture with the loop. The operating table is then adjusted to put the patient in the sitting position, and the patient is asked to open their eyes. The corrected lid should sit 1–2 mm higher than the normal lid. Slight overcorrection is performed to compensate for postoperative stretching and account for the epinephrine effect acting on Muller's muscle. The suture is re-adjusted as needed before finally securing the knot once the proper tension has been achieved.

Excess aponeurosis distal to the tarsal suture may be trimmed. A cuff of levator should be kept and used to anchor the crease. The double-fold surgery may be performed in the usual manner. Symmetry will be more difficult to judge as the ptotic lid will now be overcorrected.

12.13 Post-op Care of Asian Blepharoplasty

During the first week, patients should sleep with their head elevated to minimize swelling and bruising. Bruising fades between 5 and 10 days postoperatively. Discomfort is typically minimal, and patients seldom need more than one or two doses of light narcotic following surgery. Sutures are removed at approximately day 5 after surgery. At the initial postoperative visit, the appearance of the lids will invariably be higher than the final outcome due to edema. Asymmetry of the lids is also not unusual at this time. Patients should be counselled preoperatively about these expectations and anticipate the pretarsal show to settle to the desired outcome within a few weeks to several months after surgery. The closed non-incisional approach usually has a much faster recovery period, as there tends to be less edema and bruising compared to the open approach. The patient is instructed to refrain from any strenuous activity for 4 weeks beyond surgery.

With the open approach, the scar may become slightly pink and slightly raised over the initial few months. The scars will mature to become flat, and the color will fade to match the surrounding skin at approximately 6 months to one year after surgery. The immature scar is generally not visible unless the eyes are closed and is easily covered with makeup during this time.

Scars from epicanthoplasty may be slightly thicker than the crease scars. This is likely due to the increased tension on the incision lines of the epicanthoplasty, and the fact that the skin in this area may be thicker. Fortunately, this area also fades and flattens, albeit in a slower manner.

If a patient has had ptosis repair, the result may be slightly overcorrected at the first visit. With time, the lid is expected to stretch to look more natural and symmetric. If the lid looks significantly overcorrected, the lid can be stretched out manually. The patient is instructed to grasp the upper lid lashes while looking upwards. This is maneuver performed for 5–10 minutes per day

Follow-up visits are scheduled several weeks and a few months afterward to ensure that the final outcome meets the expectations of the surgeon and patient.

12.14 Complications of Asian Blepharoplasty

Most of the complications arising from Asian blepharoplasty are non-acute, with the vast majority of complications being observed several weeks post-surgery. Early complications such as hematoma and infection are rare.

12.14.1 Asymmetry

Asymmetry is the most common complication of double lid surgery. It is usually due to factors such as failure to identify asymmetry preoperatively, improper marking, and suboptimal surgical execution. As these factors are within the control of the surgeon, the best way to avoid asymmetry is prevention. This is accomplished with proper diagnosis and surgical design, precise preoperative markings, and impeccable execution. Beyond prevention, asymmetry is best managed after the result has been allowed to heal and settle.

Asymmetries are common immediately post-surgery due to edema and tissue inflammation. These early asymmetries are managed with patient reassurance and monitoring only. One should assume that a symmetrical result will eventually manifest if symmetry was checked and confirmed during surgery. Early surgical management should not be entertained unless there is gross asymmetry, such as the failure to create a fold on one side. Should asymmetry still be present months after surgery, the likelihood of revision increases. The surgeon should judge whether or not the edema and scar tissue have subsided sufficiently to deem the result as being final. In general, waiting 6 months before committing to revision of an incisional double fold surgery is reasonable. If the double-fold surgery was performed with a non-incisional technique, a revision may be performed much earlier, as scar tissue is less of an issue.

12.14.2 Correction of Asymmetry from the Non-incisional Technique

Correction of complications arising from non-incisional techniques can usually be remedied by removing the sutures. Very little scar tissue is created with these techniques, and removal will usually result in the lids reverting back to their original appearance. The non-incision double fold surgery can then be redone in the desired manner.

12.14.3 Correction of Asymmetry from the Incisional Technique

With the incisional technique, the two variables responsible for the degree of the pretarsal show are i) the crease height and ii) amount of skin above the crease. These two variables may be altered to correct postoperative pretarsal asymmetry.

If the crease height is symmetric but the pretarsal show is asymmetric, the problem is likely to be excess supratarsal skin on the side with less pretarsal show. This assumes ptosis is not a contributing factor to the asymmetry. Correction is a matter of supratarsal skin excision, in a similar fashion to upper lid blepharoplasty. This strategy may also be employed even if the height of the creases is (mildly) asymmetric. Removal of skin in this situation can achieve pretarsal show symmetry, but the crease heights will remain asymmetric.

In the circumstance where crease height asymmetry is significant enough that it cannot be corrected by skin excision, modification of the crease height is necessary. It is always easier to elevate crease height as opposed to decreasing height. Therefore, the surgeon should aim to elevate the low crease. This may not be possible, depending on the patient's lid preference.

Elevation of the crease height is accomplished by incising the previous scar, slightly undermining the inferior skin to release the supratarsal fold, and re-anchoring the skin edge at the new higher position. Lowering the crease is more difficult. If the analogous approach is used to lower the crease, the skin at the original (higher) location will tend to reattach to the aponeurosis again. This effectively eliminates the newly lowered crease as the crease will always form at the most superior point of dermal attachment. Therefore, the strategy of lowering the crease involves making an incision at a new (lower) crease location and excising an ellipse of the skin that includes the old incision and underlying scar. In order to prevent re-adhesion, the preaponeurotic lid fat is then teased out and laid into the area of the old crease. The presence of the fat sitting between the levator and skin prevents reattachment. The fat may need to be gently sutured into place to prevent it from shifting postoperatively. If no lid fat is available, an appropriate sized fat graft is harvested from elsewhere on the patient and used as a free fat graft. Crease lowering is generally less successful than crease elevation, and the patient should be warned of the potential for suboptimal correction.

12.14.4 Ptosis

Ptosis may occur from levator aponeurosis dehiscence or transection that is not recognized during surgery. This is managed by reopening the incision, locating the proximal aponeurotic edge, and attaching it back to the tarsal plate or distal end of the aponeurosis as the findings dictate. In unrecognized preoperative ptosis, the postoperative asymmetry occurs with the ptotic side having the more pretarsal show. Management consists of levator advancement on the ptotic side. Alternatively, removal of supratarsal skin from the non-ptotic side will increase the degree of pretarsal show. The ptosis will still remain, however, so this method is only useful for minor degrees of ptosis as only the pretarsal show is corrected.

12.14.5 Loss of Supratarsal Crease

Loss of the crease may occur within the first 6 months after surgery with the open approach. This is caused by the failure of scar adhesion to occur, usually due to placement of the anchoring sutures in the wrong structures, such as the septum, as opposed to the aponeurosis. It may also be due to an insufficient clearing of adipose and other tissue from the aponeurosis, which causes inadequate scar adhesion between the aponeurosis and dermis. Management involves opening the incision and re-anchoring the skin once the base is adequately prepared.

In the non-incisional method, loss of the crease is usually an inevitable outcome. The non-incisional method is not a permanent procedure because little scar tissue is formed. After a variable number of years, the crease becomes less defined as the sutures lose their hold and 'cheese wire' through the soft tissues. Eventually, the crease will completely disappear as there is little internal scar tissue to maintain the result. Management consists of repeating double lid surgery, either with incisional or non-incisional methods.

12.14.6 Visible Scars

Unsightly scarring occurs infrequently. When it does occur, it is usually in an area of increased skin tension, such as with epicanthoplasty scars, or in the presence of significant skin excision. Thicker scars can usually be managed with scar massage and the passage of time. Steroid injections can also be used sparingly beginning at 4–6 months post-surgery. Surgical scar revision is rarely required.

12.14.7 Multiple Folds

Multiple folds are caused by adhesions from the skin to the levator at multiple levels superior to the intended crease. This complication is a result of insufficient adipose tissue in the lid, either occurring naturally, due to surgical excision, or a combination of both. Management consists of fat grafting to the lid in the regions where the extra folds occur. Alternatively, hyaluronic acid fillers may be used as the source volume augmentation. When the folds are especially severe or tight, open release and transposition of preaponeurotic fat, or free fat grafting, may be required.

12.15 Results

Examples of results are shown in Figs. 12.21, 12.22, and 12.23. Case details are provided in the legend accompanying each figure. Figure 12.21 shows an example of bilateral double fold blepharoplasty performed on a patient with pre-operative asymmetry. Figure 12.22 shows an example of a patient with monolids who underwent bilateral double fold blepharoplasty. Figure 12.23 shows an example of a patient with pre-operative symmetry where unilateral right double-fold blepharoplasty was performed.

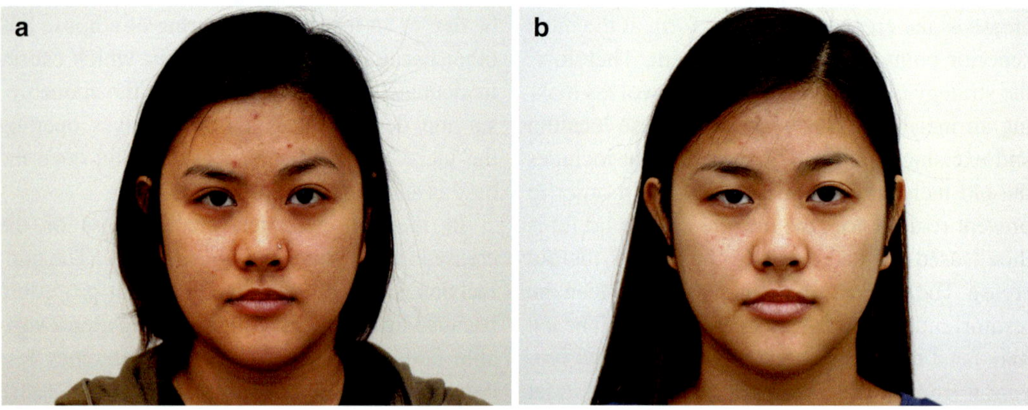

Fig. 12.21 A female patient with preoperative asymmetry, before (**a**) and after (**b**) bilateral double fold blepharoplasty. The patient requested that the post-operative pretarsal show remain similar to the left pre-operative distance. Correction of pseudoptosis on the right side is accomplished as part of the double fold procedure. A bilateral procedure was recommended because the existing (left) crease would occasionally fluctuate in appearance becoming less defined at times. Operating on the left side allowed for better stability of the crease and overall symmetry

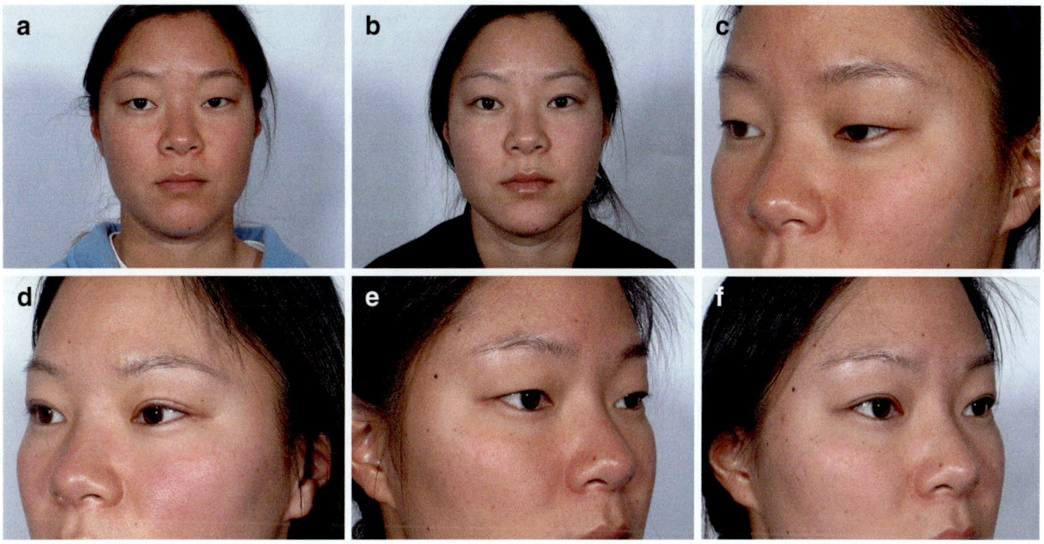

Fig. 12.22 A female patient with single folds, before (**a**-front view, **c**-left view, **e**-right view) and after (**b**-front, **d**-left, **f**-right) bilateral double fold blepharoplasty with approximately 2 mm of pretarsal show

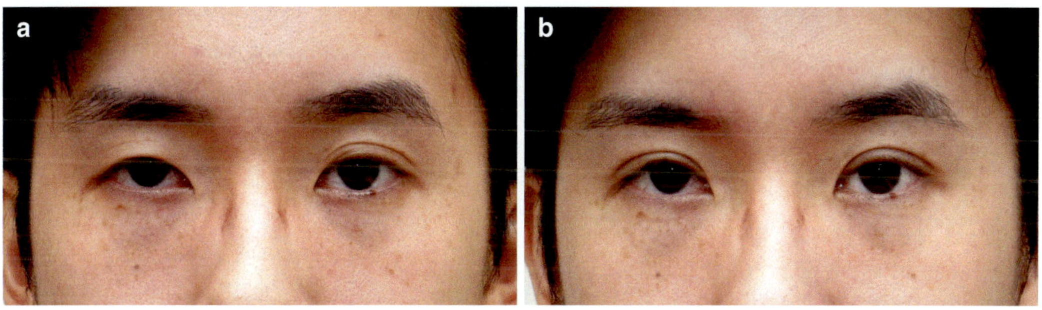

Fig. 12.23 A male patient with preoperative asymmetry, before (**a**) and after (**b**) bilateral double fold blepharoplasty. The patient requested that the pretarsal show remain the same as the pre-operative distance on the left. Note that the post-operative left lid fold definition is significantly improved. This example illustrates why bilateral surgery is performed even when the patient does not seek a change in the existing pretarsal show. Even though the pretarsal show would be symmetric, unilateral (right-sided) correction would have resulted in lid folds with asymmetric definition. Correction of pseudoptosis on the right side is accomplished as part of the double fold procedure

12.16 Conclusion

Asian blepharoplasty is one of the most sought-after cosmetic procedures worldwide. The surgery should no longer be viewed as a niche procedure as demand continues to increase inside and outside of Asia. Understanding the unique anatomy of the Asian upper lid is critical to understanding the underlying aesthetic issues and management of patients seeking Asian blepharoplasty. The keys to success are careful patient evaluation, formulation of an appropriate surgical plan, and flawless execution. Creation of a supratarsal crease is at the core of Asian blepharoplasty. The techniques described are straightforward, but despite this, near-perfect execution is usually required to minimize complications. Asymmetry is the most common complication, usually due to surgical imprecision. The learning curve is normally steep, but once a surgeon becomes proficient at it, Asian blepharoplasty is one of the most rewarding procedures for both surgeon and patient alike.

References

1. ISAPS international survey on aesthetic/cosmetic procedures performed in 2014.
2. Jang JW. Double-eyelid surgery: incisional techniques. In: Jin HR, editor. Aesthetic surgery of the Asian face. New York: Thieme; 2016. p. 162–72.
3. Fakhro A, Yim HW, Kim YK, Ngyuen AH. The evolution of looks and expectations of Asian eyelid and eye appearance. Semin Plast Surg. 2015;29:135–44.
4. Sayoc BT. Absence of superior palpebral fold in slit eyes; an anatomic and physiologic explanation. Am J Ophthalmol. 1956;42:298–300.
5. Jeong S, Lemke BN, Dortzbach RK, Park YG, Kang HK. The Asian upper eyelid: an anatomical study with comparison to the Caucasian eyelid. Arch Ophthalmol. 1999;117(7):907–12.
6. Zubiri JS. Subdermal placement of sutures in double eyelid surgery. Aesthet Surg J. 2013;33(5):722–32.
7. Kure K, Minami A. A simple and durable way to create a supratarsal fold (double eyelid) in Asian patients. Aesthet Surg J. 2001;21(3):227–32.
8. Park JI. Modified Z-Epicanthoplasty in the Asian eyelid. Arch Facial Plast Surg. 2000;2:43–7.

Male Rejuvenation of the Upper Face with Endoscopic Brow Lift

13

Ronaldo Righesso

13.1 Introduction

Aging forehead and eyes continue to be a common concern for patients worldwide [1]. In the recent past, men represented only 6% of patients, but over the last several years, this conservative trend seems to be changing [2–6]. As data show, there was a 273% increase in the number of cosmetic procedures performed on men between 1997 and 2014 [2].

The concepts of brow shape aesthetics are different between male and female [2, 3]. Glabellar sex differences are so pronounced that older methods of sex determination of skeletons relied on the width and projection at the glabella [2]. The male aesthetics seems to remain relatively constant throughout the decades, less affected by cultural trends and advances.

Several authors already described the female's brow shape aesthetics [2–20]. In general, for the female patient, the aesthetic brow begins medially at a position above the medial canthus and alar base. Laterally, the brow ends at an axis connecting the lateral canthus to the alar base. The peak of the brow should be at a position 5 to 10 mm superior to the lid margin and above the lateral limbus. In the 1980s, Ellenbogen asserted that the caudal margin of the medial brow should be 1 cm above the caudal extension of the supraorbital rim [2, 18, 19]. Cook changed concepts, suggesting that the classical positioning of the brow should sit at the level of the orbital rim for men, while it should arch well above the supraorbital rim in women. He suggested that the highest point of the brow should be positioned vertically at the level of lateral canthus instead of a more medial position which could result in an unnatural, surprised look to the face [2, 7].

During the 1990s, the preferred medial brow was at or below the supraorbital rim instead of the medial brow above the rim. At that time, it was established that the peak of the brow should rarely be 10 mm above the horizontal of the most caudal portion of the medial brow. It should be higher in women than men. The shape of the male eyebrow is usually less arched and flat or nearly horizontal [2], and the lateral brow is more prominent in men. Later, Roth and Metzinger made a comparison of shape and dimensions of female frontal photographs portrayed in magazines in 2001 and found the brow peak to be closer to the lateral canthus than to the limbus [2]. Griffin and Kim concluded that the ideal female brow is gradually becoming lower and flatter than it used to be, making it less different than the male eyebrow. This trend was regarded in part to be a response to the increasing parity between men and women in workplace [2, 7].

Current trends show thicker brows for men, with a more horizontal course, resting just along

R. Righesso (✉)
SBCP - Brazilian Society of Plastic Surgery, Bento Gonçalves, Rio Grande do Sul, Brazil
e-mail: contato@ronaldorighesso.com.br

K. Jeffords et al. (eds.), *Aesthetic Surgery for Men*, https://doi.org/10.1007/978-3-032-03840-1_13

or above the supraorbital rim without tapering [3, 13]. In general, the "golden ratio" remains a useful parameter which consists in a mathematical proportion relationship from 1 to 1.618. The distance between the superior and inferior lids and the distance from the superior lid margin to the eyebrow arch are embraced by this concept. In men, the golden ratio is inverted than in women, with a measure of 1.6 to the open eye, and 1 to the distance from the superior lid to the eyebrow arch (Fig. 13.1) [20]. This could be a guide, not a fixed rule, because the position of the eyebrows may vary quite from one patient to another. We advocate an individualized treatment, and the type of fixation here described promotes this. A surgeon must keep in mind that not always a higher brow elevation results in a superior aesthetic effect, mainly in men.

When men seek facial rejuvenation, they usually look for small modification, demanding such changes to be conservative and subtle, even not noticeable [2]. In this scenario, endoscopic brow lift seems appropriated, offering good and long-lasting results with almost inconspicuous scars [5, 11, 14, 15, 20–30]. There is a great number of male patients that could be benefited by endoscopic brow lift and for some reason are conducted to other therapies. In 2012, nearly 25,000 surgical forehead lift procedures were performed in the United States, along with nearly 5 million neuromodulator and filler injections, many of which were performed in the upper face [5]. The surgeon focused on male population should be prepared to offer the best treatment as possible keeping in mind these specific differences and requests.

13.2 Technique

Although Passot first described the brow lift procedure in 1919 [17, 20, 30], the modern coronal approach was not described until 1962 by Gonzalez-Ulloa [4, 5]. The early 1990s witnessed the introduction of the endoscope for brow lift surgery. Vasconez, Isse, and Chachir were among the first to describe their techniques [1, 4, 15, 23, 25, 31]. Several subsequent authors have since published various modifications and refinements [4–6, 8–10, 12, 17, 20, 21, 32]. The technique has evolved from an experimental curiosity to broad general acceptance [11] and its basic concepts were established. A subperiosteal dissection combined with the removal of the corrugator supercilii and procerus muscles and the release of the periosteum from the temporal line of fusion allows the surgeon to lift the brow to the desired degree [4, 5]. There is still some controversy around the ideal method of brow fixation. A great variety of techniques and devices, and even no fixation, was already suggested [27, 31]. The studies conducted by Boutros [33] and Romo [34] about periosteal adherence supported the importance of some kind of fixation. In an animal model, it takes 6 to 12 weeks to demonstrate adherence of the periosteum to calvarium [14]. Currently, it is generally accepted that a better fixation leads to less relapse [11, 12, 28]. Many

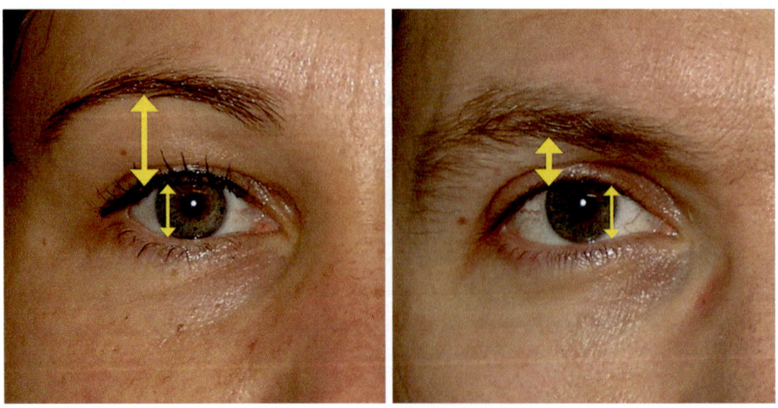

Fig. 13.1 "Golden ratio" differences between female (right) and male (left). The arrows show the distance from superior and inferior eyelids and the distance from the margin of the superior eyelid to the beginning of the eyebrow

opinions appeared based on this concept. Rohrich [12] divided the techniques for endoscopic fixation into endogenous and exogenous, in order to facilitate comparisons.

Since 2001, we have been using a combination of techniques previously described [20, 21]. The basic endoscopic brow lift is similar as proposed by Isse [1, 23, 25], and the fixation method is a composite of McKinney's [14] and Casagrande's techniques [17, 20, 23]. As suggested by Casagrande [17, 23], we use a Reverdin modified needle (Fig. 13.2) to grasp deep tissues, and we anchor it in a tunnel made on external cortical bone, as proposed by McKinney [14]. The tunnel should be made with a specific device at a proper location (Figs. 13.3 and 13.4) in order to guarantee the correct depth without tearing the dura mater membrane. This technique allows a precise suture exactly at the point where more traction is needed with the added advantage of allowing additional sutures as needed for the case, producing a very accurate elevation [16, 20, 22, 23, 25]. An additional suture is done superiorly, similar to that proposed by McKinney [14], taking the periosteum-galea about 2 cm in front of each paramedian incision. These sutures will be attached at the bone tunnel in the same way that the sutures taken closer to the eyebrows. At the lateral brow, the suture is done fixing the superficial temporal fascia to the deep temporal fascia, with a vector toward posterior and superiorly. Normally just one or two sutures are needed (Fig. 13.5); we use a 3–0 black nylon in all internal sutures.

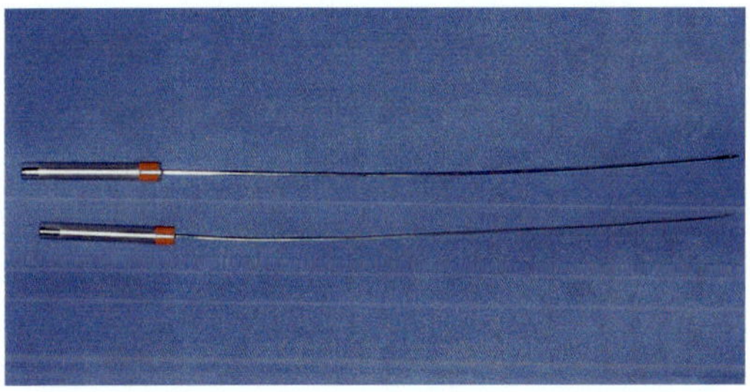

Fig. 13.2 A pair of Casagrande's needle: about 20 cm long with an eye to capture the thread at its ending

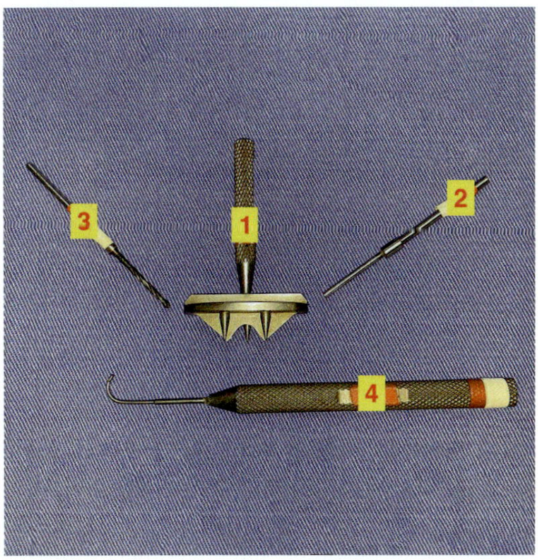

Fig. 13.3 Bone bridge system: (1) main piece, (2) pin, (3) drill, (4) grasp

Anesthesia includes regional facial nerve blocks and intravenous sedation conducted by an anesthesiologist. The entire forehead is tumescent, infiltrated with local anesthesia and epinephrine [22]. The endoscopic entry point consists of two temporal incisions placed 2 cm posterior to the hairline. Two additional 2 cm paramedian incisions ("zigzag" shaped at the skin and vertical at the deepest planes) are located 4 cm from the midline and will receive the device to construct the cortical bone tunnel. An additional "lazy-V" shaped incision at the midline is necessary (Fig. 13.6). For patients with anterior hairline recession, a 2-portal technique [13] may be performed only using the paramedian incisions. In these cases, care must be taken in order to avoid a bone tunnel more than 5 cm away from the midline as skull is usually thinner in this area. The temporal incisions are made as well.

Through the central scalp incision, initial blind subperiosteal dissection is performed just at the central portion and up to 2 cm above the superior orbital rims. The incision at the temporal area is done, and after a limited blind dissection, for less than 1 cm, the deep temporal fascia is identified. The endoscope (4 mm, 30 degrees) is introduced guiding the dissection all the way. The dissection proceeds inferiorly at an areolar plane just between the deep and superficial temporal fascia (Fig. 13.7). Great attention must be taken

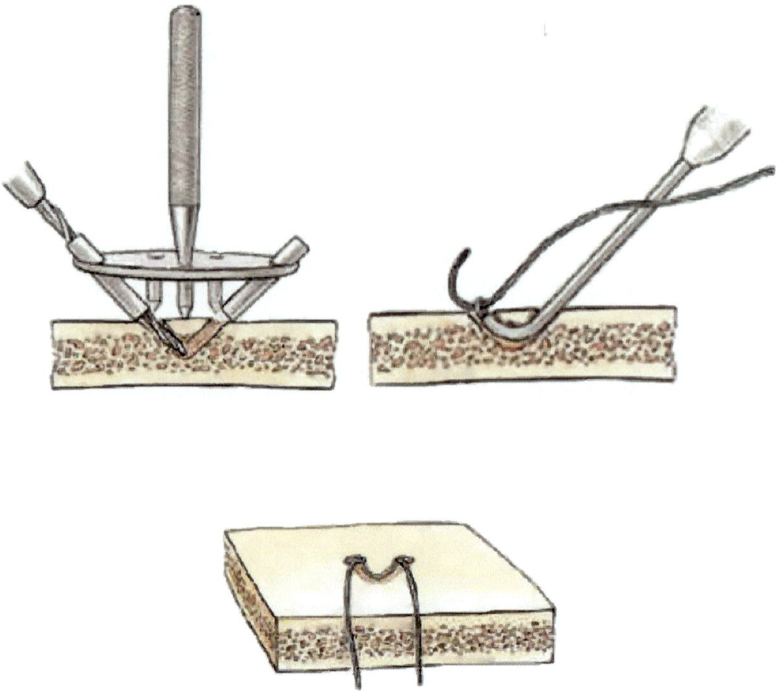

Fig. 13.4 Schematic use of Medtronic Xomed Brow Lift Bone System®

at this area in order to preserve the temporal branch of the facial nerve that runs within a thin fat pad on the underside of the superficial temporal fascia, considered to be in the ceiling of the dissection space. Damage to this nerve will result in ipsilateral weakness or paralysis of the frontalis muscle, superior portion of the orbicularis, and portions of the procerus and corrugator supercilii muscles, compromising the main surgical goal [5]. The sentinel vein (medial zygomaticotemporal vein) is the inferior limit of the temporal dissection and provides a relative landmark to the position of temporal branches of the facial nerve [29]. The sentinel vein (Fig. 13.6) should be preserved, except if the midface will be approached.

In order to keep the proper plane, the dissection goes from temporal to central area, releasing the temporal fusion line with a Joseph elevator. The endoscopic dissection returns to the forehead and focuses on superior orbital rim; the visualization of the supratrochlear and supraorbital nerve is accomplished. Its position is well known, laterally from midline 1.5 and 2.5 cm, respectively [24, 29, 36]. The orbital rim periosteal dissection is performed from medial to lateral. The sentinel vein is identified again. An extensive liberation at the lateral portion is done with special attention to the temporal adhesion. Vertical incisions are performed [20, 24] just lateral to the emergence of the supraorbital bundle. At the conclusion of the temporal release, both areas are connected, and the periosteum is completely separated from the superior and medial orbital rims, except in men, when medial dissection is conservative [21, 35]. An external maneuver of superior skin traction confirms adequate release of the structures.

Once the sensitive nerves are identified, the glabellar musculature is carefully dissected with a curved grasper and a portion of muscle is excised. Resection of procerus, corrugator, and depressor supercilii is performed, preserving the transverse head of the corrugator [21, 35]. In male population, muscle resection is a crucial step of surgical planning. Men used to have wider muscles that should be explored in order to reduce the glabellar wrinkles [17].

The fixation takes place after undermining and muscle resections are completed. The desired level of brow elevation and the points of traction are outlined at the beginning of the procedure with the patient in an upright position and are

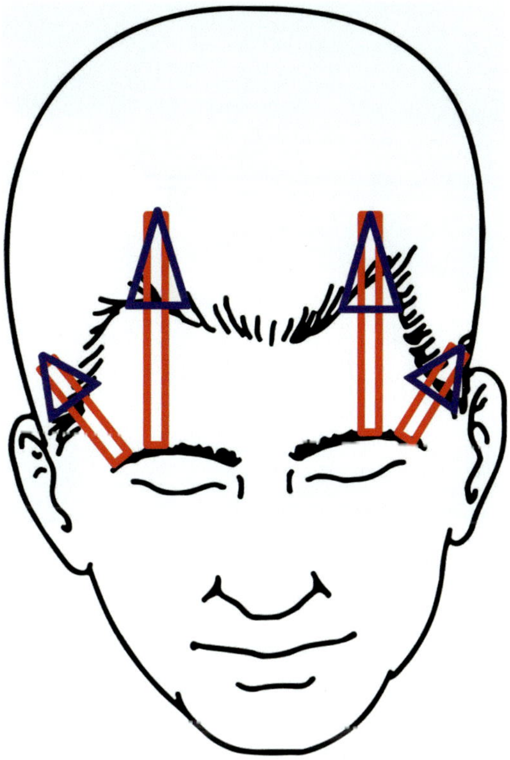

Fig. 13.5 Schematic representation of traction sutures to raise the brows. The rectangular shapes represent the loops made with Casagrande's needles at distant points, close to the brows. The triangular shapes represent sutures done by direct visualization at the periosteum superiorly and at the superficial temporal fascia at the temporal area. The sutures at the paramedian area should be knotted at the bony tunnel and at the temporal incision, attached at the deep temporal fascia

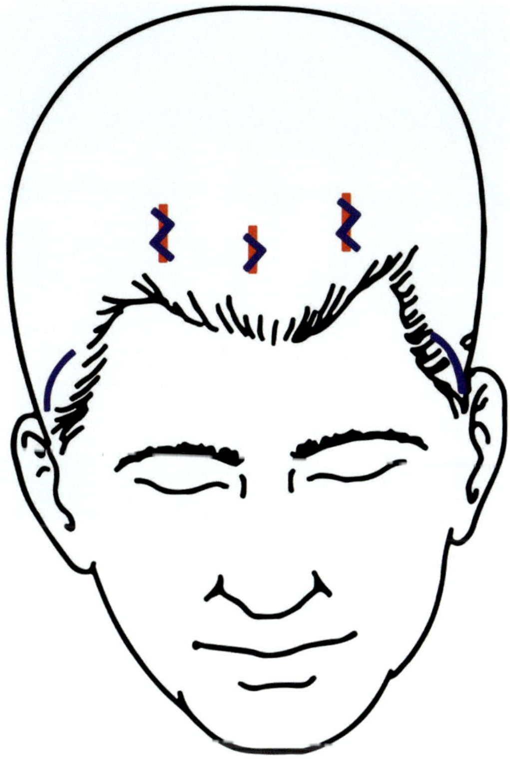

Fig. 13.6 Five incisions of the endoscopic brow lift. Thicker lines represent cutaneous incisions: two paramedian incisions are 4 cm far from midline and are "zig-zag" shaped, the median incision is "lazy-V" shaped, and two temporal incisions arch shaped. The thinner lines represent vertical incision at the deeper planes, periosteum, and galea

reassessed before the needle introduction. This step should be meticulously done, since most cases with brow collapse are due to an unappropriated fixation [18, 20, 23].

Transcutaneous fixation is performed using a Casagrande needle [17] (a long, fine needle with a hole at the end) (Fig. 13.2) entering the skin at the point defined at the beginning. After the introduction of the needle through the skin, endoscopic visualization allows direct observation of needle penetration in the optical cavity. The needle is then carefully drawn out through the paramedian incision, and the thread is introduced through the eye of the needle. The needle is passed back under the skin and, after a small trajectory through the soft tissues, the needle grasps some deep tissue at the periosteal free margin and advances cephalic approximately 1 cm, going vertically through the supraorbital adhesions without perforating the skin. The needle then exits at the same paramedian incision. The thread is released from the needle, and the resultant loop is attached to the periosteal margin and deep plane adjacent structures, without pinching the skin. A firm traction is exerted at this loop, monitored by endoscopic guidance in order to check if a good volume of tissue is captured and if the upright traction promotes the estimated elevation without creating a depression at the skin. If any failure is detected, the process is repeated until perfection is attained. Sometimes more than one suture is needed. An additional suture is done superiorly, with the

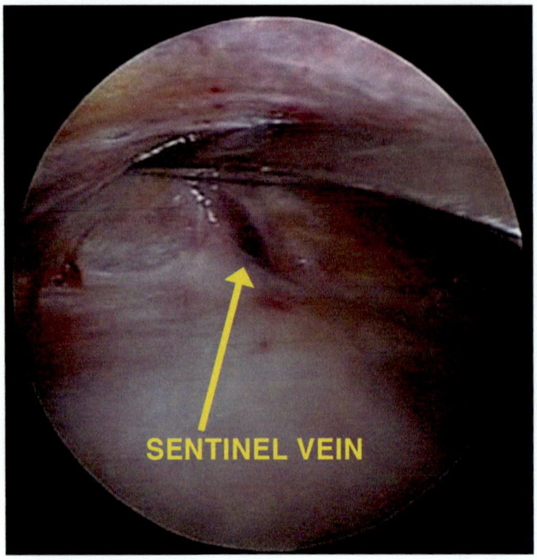

Fig. 13.7 Endoscopic visualization of the sentinel vein at the temporal dissection. A Joseph elevator pointed to the superficial temporal fascia, where the temporal branch of facial nerve runs

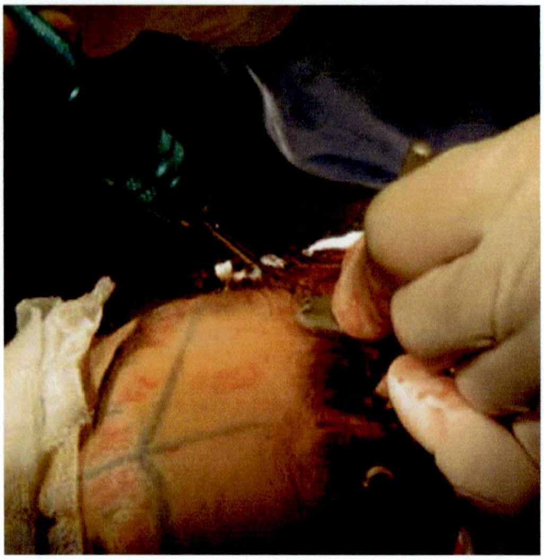

Fig. 13.8 Drilling the bone tunnel

same thread, nylon 3-0. This superior suture pinches the periosteum about 2 cm in front of the paramedian incision at two points, resulting in a "V" shape. This extra suture is done in order to promote additional strength to the elevation and conceal any redundancy from the deep structures brought superiorly [22]. The same number of sutures is made at the opposite site, if symmetry is the main purpose (Fig. 13.5).

With both sides prepared, the next step is drilling the bone tunnels. In order to avoid any dural lesion, "free hand" techniques are not recommended [28]. We use the Medtronic Xomed Brow-lift Bone Bridge System ® (Jacksonville, Fla.) [14] (Figs. 13.3 and 13.4) which minimizes the chance of penetrating the inner cranial plate and turns the procedure simple and fast. The main piece of the set has 3 tines to avoid glissade and should be adjusted at the paramedian incision that is made in a "zigzag" style in order to better fit the apparatus. With a 1.2 mm burr (included on the kit) on an air drill, the first hole is made. The burr has a limiter and penetrates just 3 mm at the bone at an inclination of 45 degrees (Fig. 13.8). The burr is removed, and a pin is inserted at the first hole, keeping the apparatus stable. The second hole is made. Finally, the apparatus is removed, and the 2 holes are checked. Each hole is perfectly aligned, resulting in a tunnel where the threads would be knotted. The next step is performing the bone tunnel at the other side. With both tunnels already done, a pair of Senn-Miller retractors is positioned, allowing precise vision (Fig. 13.9). An additional kit component is inserted into the tunnel to grasp and deliver the thread through the other tunnel. This component has a cleft at its border, and the thread should be inserted on it. The piece is retracted and the loop stays inside the bone tunnel (Fig. 13.9). The threads are knotted once all the stitches have been passed at the tunnels, starting with the loops coming from medial to lateral and from down to up [22]. Only after the first side is completed with all the stitches knotted, the other side will be assessed. The patient should be in sitting position in order to observe the result and symmetry. The traction sutures at the temporal area complete this step. The skin at the temporal incision is everted and a 3-0 nylon suture takes a bite at the superficial temporal fascia resulting in an additional loop. Traction is applied in order to check efficiency and then this loop is knotted to the deep temporal fascia. This suture produces a vector that directs toward cranial and posterior. The opposite temporal area will be assessed the same way.

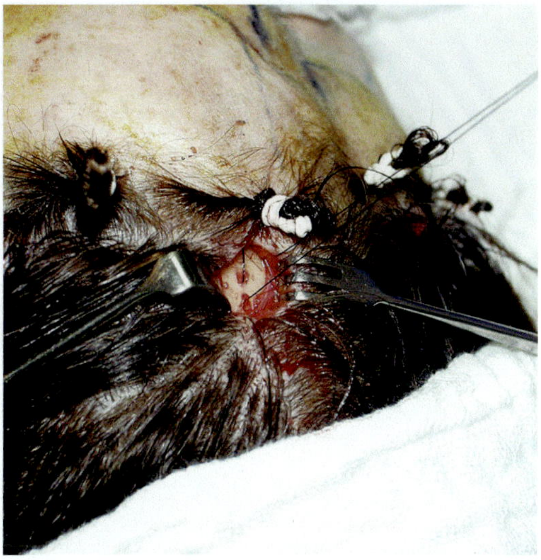

Fig. 13.9 A pair of Senn-Miller retractors showing the bone tunnel with one 3-0 nylon inside

The final step is skin closure. Regularly 4-0 nylon is used. The skin suture is performed without tension and addressed just to the superficial planes in order to avoid alopecia. It is not uncommon to see a skin redundancy at the paramedian portal caused by skin elevation, but the zigzag incision helps to deal with it. No skin is resected, and a bandage is not necessary.

If a superior blepharoplasty is planned, the skin markings are now reappraised.

13.3 Results

Three hundred forty-eight (348) patients had endoscopic brow lifts performed by the author with the reported technique between 2001 and 2017. In the first ten years, men corresponded just to 5% of the patients, but more recently, the men's group increased to 12% (overall mean, 10%). The men ranged in age from 44 to 71 years (mean age, 54 years), and the women ranged in age from 38 to 76 years (mean age, 48 years). About 50% of the male patients had receding hairlines, but no one was bald. Thirty percent of them had already undergone hair transplantation and just one was submitted to hair transplantation at the same time as the endoscopic brow lift. All patients were Caucasian. No smokers in the group. Forty percent had a history of prior cosmetic procedures.

All patients had additional procedures performed at the same time as their endoscopic brow lift. Upper lid blepharoplasty was performed in 50% of patients. The amount of skin removed was significantly shorter than in conventional cases. No fat was injected at the lateral eyebrow in order to produce a lifting effect. The fat injections were addressed to complementary areas of the face such as nasojugal groove, tear trough deformity, and perioral wrinkles.

Just minor complications were reported at the men's group. One patient experienced a weakness of the frontalis muscle, which was resolved within 40 days. Two patients reported knot extrusion at 3 months post-operative, one at the left temporal incision and other at the right paramedian incision. Both were removed under local anesthesia. Skin depression at the level of the needle entrance was observed in one case, unilateral and resolved spontaneously with massage. There were no cases of scar alopecia, paresthesia, uneven brows, or recurrent lateral hooding that demanded a new surgical procedure. No patient complained of an altered hairline position or forehead permanent decreased sensibility. A high index of satisfaction was achieved, according to Strasser's [37, 38] scale, and no complaints of severe pain or edema were observed.

13.4 Discussion

Many patients who search plastic surgery for facial rejuvenation or blepharoplasty present with forehead and eyebrow ptosis as part of their overall aesthetic appearance [23, 25]. It is up to the surgeon to make the correct diagnosis and clearly point this out to the patient [25]. At the consultation, the patient sits in front of a mirror with the face in complete repose, and the surgeon exerts traction to the lateral side of the brow and the skin redundancy is analyzed. A ptosis from the fronto-temporal region is detected if there is a skin fold beyond the superior lid margin that reaches the lateral periorbital area (Connell's positive signal) [20]. The precise diagnosis avoids treating redundancy at superior palpebral skin with an inappropriate blepharoplasty [17, 23, 25, 26]. If it is done, it will result in a diminished distance from the tarsal margin to the eyebrow, worsening the problem. This becomes more obvious during elevation of the brows by frontal muscle activation, resulting in an inadvertent superior eyelid opening.

Brow position can become lower with time and many patients may search for a secondary blepharoplasty in order to ameliorate this false skin redundancy at superior eyelid. The solution to this situation is a brow lift (Figs. 13.10, 13.11, 13.12, 13.13, 13.14, 13.15, 13.16, 13.17, and 13.18), which should be planned considering the cephalic elevation of the ptotic brow and if natural movements could expose the short eyelid producing a difficulty to completely close the eyes [20]. The patient should be aware that there is a difference between having some skin removed and achieving a rejuvenated face.

During some years, opinions about the endoscopic brow lift were diverse [39]. Some stated that the results would be ephemeral, with collapse after a year or so. Others blamed that an overcorrection would be produced lately, resulting in a "surprised look" [40] in women and a feminized face in men. Later, a lot of articles emerged in order to refute this misconception. Many series were conducted comparing pre- and postoperative results with extreme accuracy with the help of data processing [8, 11, 13–15, 20–22, 24, 26]. This strong evidence based on statistics regains credibility to endoscopic brow lift.

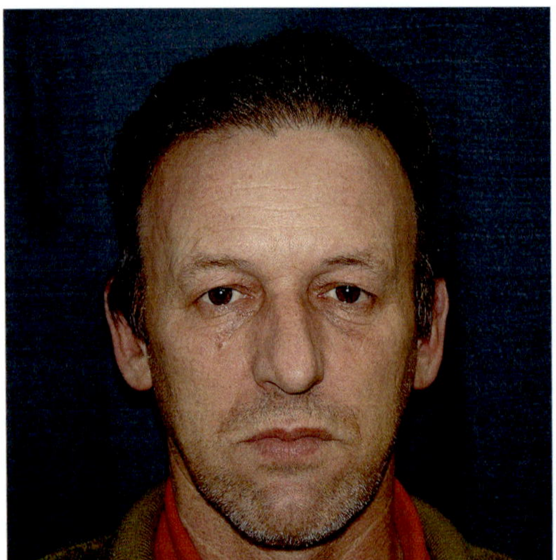

Fig. 13.10 Preoperative image. Male patient 54 years old, with previous hair transplantation surgery and superior blepharoplasty. Complaints about lateral sagging and excessive skin redundancy on superior and inferior lids

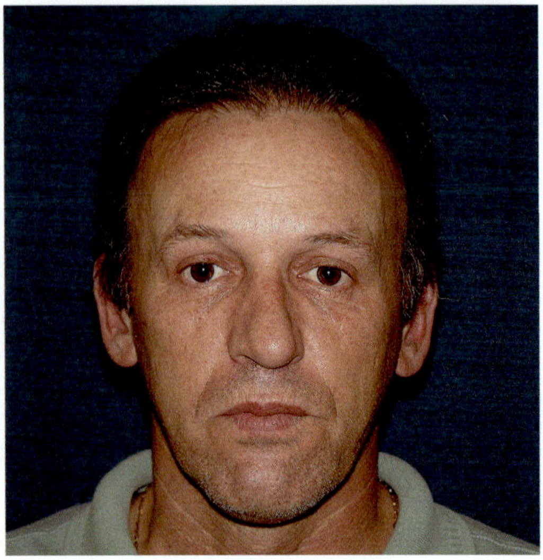

Fig. 13.11 Postoperative at 6 months after endoscopic brow lift, superior and inferior blepharoplasty

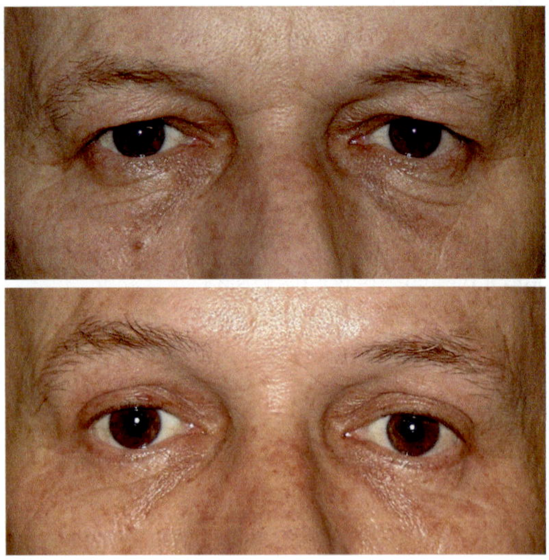

Fig. 13.12 Close comparison of preoperative and postoperative at 6 months

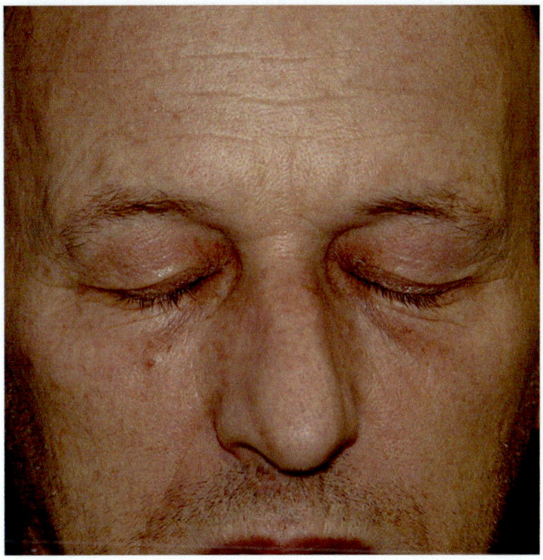

Fig. 13.13 Preoperative close, showing the skin redundancy and low brow position with the eyes closed

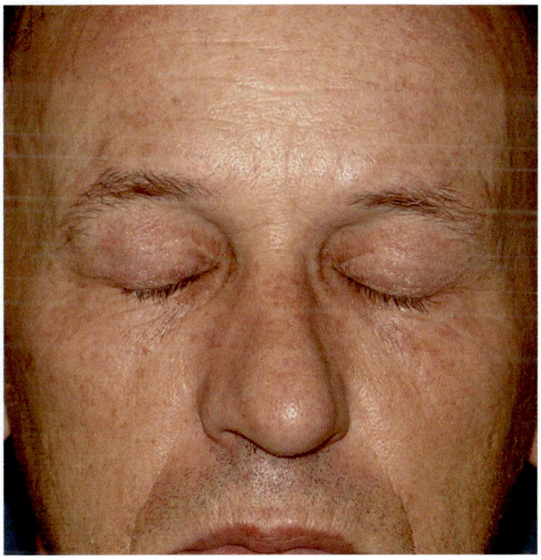

Fig. 13.14 Postoperative view at 6 months, showing the improvement at skin redundancy and adequate brow position with the eyes closed

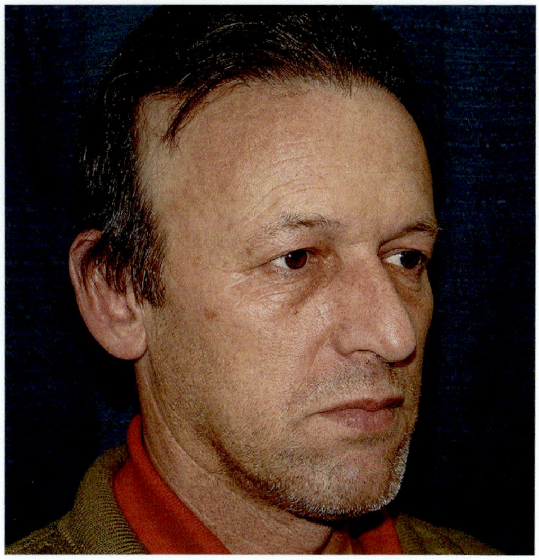

Fig. 13.15 Right oblique preoperative view

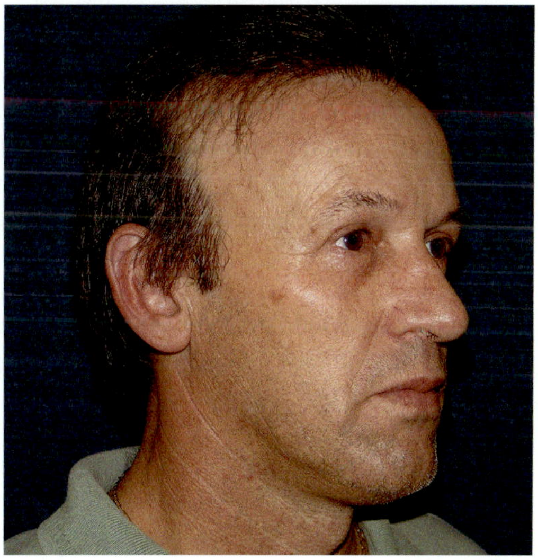

Fig. 13.16 Right oblique postoperative view at 6 months

In fact, when one looks back at the history of forehead lifts, some kind of controversy would be reasonable. The endoscopic surgery concepts were completely different from the conventional surgical basis at that time. The open approach relies mainly on soft tissue traction and resection demanding larger incisions. The only muscle mentioned as an eyebrow depressor was the corrugator supercilii muscle; no other muscles were named as responsible for lowering the eyebrows and frown line formation [30]. Suddenly, this concept changed abruptly, and the need of a new technology with a reasonable cost was a drawback. A different skill was necessary, since the convenience of the three dimensions applied at the open approach was no longer available at the endoscopic procedure limited to just two dimensions. This is an obstacle that still subsists

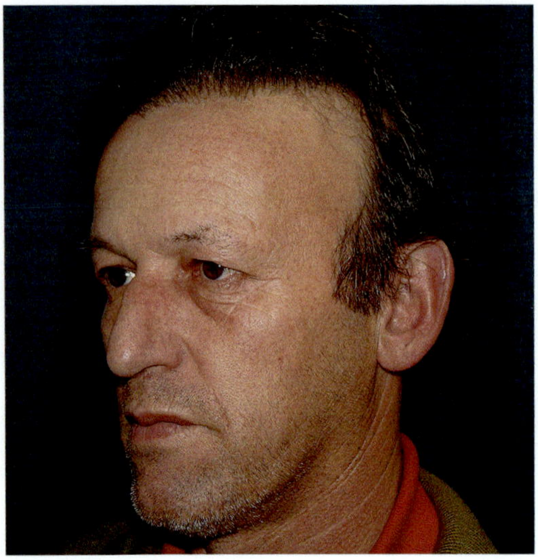

Fig. 13.17 Left oblique preoperative view

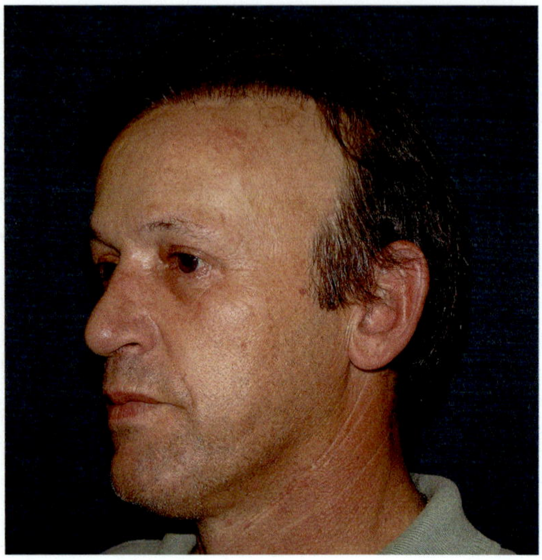

Fig. 13.18 Left oblique postoperative view

for many surgeons. Some other factors became of extreme relevance: periosteal and adhesions release; muscle modifications, including myotomies, myectomies, and detachment; and finally, several methods of flap fixation were considered of great value in order to achieve a consistent result [1]. These new concepts demanded a new investigation of the forehead's anatomy. The studies conducted by Moss and Mendelson [29] are key points of these actual understanding, but there are many others of great relevance [15, 16, 18, 21, 27, 28, 30].

In order to check our results, in 2004 we presented a retrospective study, published in 2006 [22]. A series of 20 consecutive patients was submitted to analysis. The measures at 2 and 6 months postoperative were compared with the preoperative data (Fig. 13.19). The measures were taken at 3 points, resembling the method used by Troilius [26]. A horizontal line is drawn at the midportion of the pupil; this line is represented as LP. At this horizontal line, three points are marked: first, at the most inner part of the

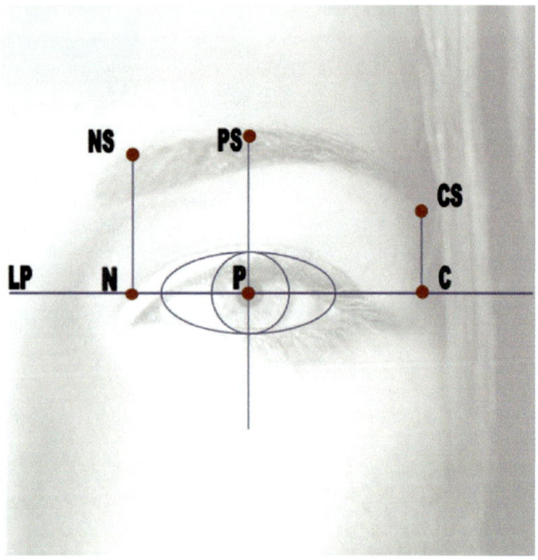

Fig. 13.19 Method used by the author to measure the distances between selected points. LP: horizontal line drawn at midpupil. N: point at line LP at the innermost part of canthal ligament. NS: vertical projection of point N at the top of the brow. P: point at line LP at the midpupil. PS: vertical projection of point P at the top of the brow. C: point at line LP corresponding at the last part of the brow (vertical projection inferiorly to the point CS). CS: point at the last part of the top of the brow

nasal canthus of the eye (N), second at the center of pupil (P), and the third at the most lateral part of the eyebrow, at the caudal portion of the brow (C). Three vertical lines will emerge from these three previous points till the uppermost point of the brow, resulting in three additional points: NS, PS, and CS. The distance between the points, N to NS, P to PS, and C to CS, results in three vertical lines. The process is repeated at the opposite side of the face. These lines were measured and respectively compared with the results observed at two and six months postoperative.

Our results were similar to other contemporary publication [14, 20, 21]. An elevation at all measured points at 2 and 6 months (Table 13.1) was achieved, with a statistical significance ($p < 0.001$) if compared with preoperative measures.

The elevation observed was according with the main brow lift's purpose: higher elevation at the lateral part of the brow, moderate at the center, and minimal at the internal portion. A little relapse occurred at the caudal portion when comparing measures at two and six months postoperative, but the elevation that lasted was still adequate, remaining a mean elevation of 4.103 mm at the caudal of the brows. McKinney [14] reported an elevation of 4.13 mm measured from the pupil center to the eyebrow apex. Jones and Groover [11] compared two groups with different types of fixation, one with fibrin glue and the other with cortical tunnels. Among the group with fibrin glue, the mean elevation was 3.79 mm, while in the other group, the mean elevation was 6.16 mm. The measures were collected from the mid-pupil to the peak of the brow, about 30 days after the procedure.

Table 13.1 Mean results of elevation achieved at the 3 points elapsed 2 and 6 months postoperative

Variable	Mean value (cm)
N-NS elevation:	
2 months	**0.2830**
6 months	**0.2871**
P-PS elevation:	
2 months	**0.3308**
6 months	**0.3656**
C-CS elevation:	
2 months	**0.4395**
6 months	**0.4103**

There is a consensus that some kind of fixation should be done [10, 32, 41]. The fixation here reported diverges from many others because the maximum point of traction is exerted exactly where it is needed (direct traction) and is fixed at a hard tissue. Methods that use a distant traction could not be so effective [16] in the presence of skin redundancy or a long forehead, for example. The low efficiency in producing traction over distant soft tissue is explained by the phenomenon called nonlinear elastic deformation [42].

Some controversy exists about the possibility to tear the inner cortical during a calvarial fixation resulting in a cerebrospinal fluid (CSF) leak [9, 12, 31, 41, 43]. The cadaveric studies conducted by Walden [41] didn't find any perforation caused by cortical tunnels at 45-degree angles. The thickest area of the cranium measured by Walden is the parietal bone behind the coronal suture, and the mean value for the entire population ranges from 6.80 to 7.72 mm. Cranial bone thickness increases posteriorly and medially, and women have thicker calvaria than men.

The wise advice when drilling the skull is to be cautious with bone fixation laterally and anteriorly. The safest place is at the paramedian position (4 cm from midline) [43].

Relative contraindications of any invasive brow fixation include situations in which internal fixation is otherwise contraindicated by infection, a thin atrophic scalp, and any sort of pathologic conditions of the bone including severe osteoporosis, cystic changes or hyperparathyroidism, Paget's disease, osteopenia or osteomalacia, osteonecrosis which may result from radiation, corticosteroid use, previous fracture, or surgery [41]. Of course, it is also prudent to avoid penetration of the sagittal sinus, so drill holes should not be made in the midline [41, 43]. For suspicious situations, a preoperative imaging study such as a computed tomography scan for assessing the thickness of the skull is mandatory.

Noninvasive methods such as botulinum toxin are easy to perform and cheaper if compared to a surgical procedure [3, 44]. Despite its growing popularity, very few studies about this subject have been published till now, and the recurrence and revision rates of the method are unknown [45, 46]. Very often, botulinum toxin is a useful tool to show the patient a glimpse of the improvement that brow elevation can grant. However, as in our experience, men generally seek a more definitive procedure. More efficient and lasting results can be achieved by endoscopic brow lift.

13.5 Conclusion

After a period of heavy use, the general indication of the endoscopic brow lift procedure declined. As reported by recent surveys, nonsurgical procedures increased significantly, including use of botulinum toxin, and this trend can be related to this [3, 45]. On the other hand, the number of endoscopic brow lift performed in our practice has increased in recent years, even in men.

Chances are some plastic surgeons are not suggesting to the male patient a surgical brow elevation fearing that scars could be visible in a bald patient or if any degree of hair loss gets accentuated [47]. Nevertheless, the indication can be done as the scars can be easily handled with the advanced techniques in hair restoration and endoscopic brow lift. In our practice, about 50% of male patients had the endoscopic brow lift at the recent years and 50% of them had been through previous hair restoration procedure.

Long-term follow-up has demonstrated that brow lift provides consistent and long-lasting results [8, 17, 20, 21, 23, 44, 45]. Besides several other advantages, this is the main reason to keep indicating this procedure to patients. From the surgeon's point of view, it is safe and smooth to perform as the brow can be reshaped through easy access to the depressor muscles and direct visualization and magnification of the supraorbital and supratrochlear neurovascular bundles. It is also minimally invasive, resulting in the least bleeding. As for the patients, the endoscopic approach is associated with very few scars, a short recovery time, and the rejuvenated fresh look. Many of these advantages are men's requirements.

References

1. Isse NG. Endoscopic facial rejuvenation: endoforehead, the functional lift. Case reports. Aesth Plast Surg. 1994;18:21–9.
2. Sedgh J. The aesthetics of the upper face and brow: male and female differences. Facial Plast Surg. 2018;34(2):114–8.
3. Keaney TC, Alster TS. Botulinum toxin in men: review of relevant anatomy and clinical trial data. Dermatologic Surg. 2013;39(10):1434–2.
4. Graham DW, Heller J, Kurkjian TJ, Schaub TS, Rohrich RJ. Brow lift in facial rejuvenation: a systematic literature review of open versus endoscopic techniques. Plast Reconstr Surg. 2011;128(4):335e–34.
5. Drolet BC, Phillips BZ, Hoy EA, Chang J, Sullivan PK. Finesse in forehead and brow rejuvenation: modern concepts, including endoscopic methods. Plast Reconstr Surg. 2014;134(6):1141–50.
6. Guyuron B. Evolving fixation methods in endoscopically assisted forehead rejuvenation: controversies and rationale (Discussion). Plast Reconstr Surg. 1997;100(6):1583–4.
7. Sclafani AP, Jung M. Desired position, shape, and dynamic range of the normal adult eyebrow. Arch Facial Plast Surg. 2010;12(2):123–7.
8. Jones BM, Lo SJ. The impact of endoscopic brow lift on eyebrow morphology, aesthetics, and longevity: objective and subjective measurements over a 5-year period. Plast Reconstr Surg. 2013 Aug;132(2):226e–38e.
9. Kobienia BJ, Van Beek A. Calvarial fixation during endoscopic brow lift. Plast Reconstr Surg. 1998;102(1):238–40.
10. Eppley BL, Coleman JJ, Sood R, Ha R, Sadove AM. Resorbable screw fixation technique for endoscopic brown and midfacial lifts. Plast Reconstr Surg. 1998;102(1):241–3.
11. Jones BM, Grover R. Endoscopic brow lift: a personal review of 538 patients and comparison of fixation techniques. Plast Reconstr Surg. 2004;113(4):1242–50.
12. Rohrich RJ, Beran SJ. Evolving fixation methods in endoscopically assisted forehead rejuvenation: controversies and rationale. Plast Reconstr Surg. 1997;100(7):1575–85.
13. Fisher O, Zamboni WA. Endoscopic brow-lift in the male patient. Arch Facial Plast Surg. 2010;12(1):56–9.
14. McKinney P, Sweis I. An accurate technique for fixation in endoscopic browlift: a 5-year follow-up. Plast Reconstr Surg. 2001;108(6):1808–10.
15. Ramirez OM. Anchor subperiosteal forehead lift: from open to endoscopic. Plast Reconstr Surg. 2001;107(3):868–71.
16. Stuzin JM, Baker TJ, Baker TM. Endoscopic foreheadplasty: a histologic comparison of periosteal refixation after endoscopic versus bicoronal lift. Plast Reconstr Surg. 2000;105(6):1118–21.

17. Casagrande C, Saltz R, Chem R, Pinto R, Collares M. Direct needle fixation in endoscopic facial rejuvenation. Aesthet Surg J. 2000;20(5):361–67.
18. Knize D. An anatomically based study of the mechanism of eyebrow ptosis. Plast Reconstr Surg. 1996;97(7):1321–33.
19. Gunter JP, Antrobus SD. Aesthetic analysis of the eyebrows. Plast Reconstr Surg. 1997;99(7):1808–16.
20. Badin AZ, Bittencourt LM, Balderrama CR. Lateral brow fixation in endoscopic forehead lift: long-term results with braided nylon percutaneous sutures. Aesth Plast Surg. 2010;34(1):78–87.
21. Graf RM, Tolazzi AR, Mansur AE, Teixeira V. Endoscopic periosteal brow lift: evaluation and follow-up of eyebrow height. Plast Reconstr Surg. 2008;121(2):609–16; discussion 617–9.
22. Righesso R. Mensuração da elevação das sobrancelhas no lifting endoscópico videoassistido. Rev Cient AMECS. 2006;11(2):11–22.
23. Casagrande C. Métodos de fixação em videocirurgia facial. In: Badin AZD, Casagrande C, Saltz R, editors. Rejuvenescimento Facial: cirurgia videoendoscópica e procedimentos ancilares. Rio de Janeiro: Revinter; 2003. p. 91–6.
24. Citarella EJR. Endoscopia da região frontal. Rio de Janeiro: Revinter; 1999.
25. Badin AZD. Ritidoplastia endoscópica frontal e periorbitária. In: Casagrande C. Plástica de face videoendoscópica. Rio de Janeiro:Dilivros; 2010, p. 151–77.
26. Troilius C. A comparison between subgaleal and subperiosteal brow lifts. Plast Reconstr Surg. 1999;104(4):1079–90.
27. Vasconez LO, Anastasatos JM. An accurate technique for fixation in endoscopic browlift: a 5-year follow-up (Discussion). Plast Reconstr Surg. 2001;108(6):1811.
28. Core GB. An accurate technique for fixation in endoscopic browlift: a 5-year follow-up (Discussion). Plast Reconstr Surg. 2001;108(6):1812–4.
29. Moss CJ, Mendelson BC, Taylor GI. Surgical anatomy of the ligamentous attachments in the temple and periorbital regions. Plast Reconstr Surg. 2000;105(4):1475–90.
30. Paul MD. The evolution of the brow lift in aesthetic plastic surgery. Plast Reconstr Surg. 2001;108(5):1409–24.
31. De Cordier BC, De la Torre JI, Al-Hakeem MS, Rosenberg LZ, Gardner PM, Costa-Ferreira A, et al. Endoscopic forehead lift: review of technique, cases and complications (Discussion). Plast Reconstr Surg. 2002;110(6):1569–70.
32. Stuzin JM, Baker TJ, Baker TM. Anchor subperiosteal forehead lift: from open to endoscopic (Discussion). Plast Reconstr Surg. 2001;107(3):872–3.
33. Boutros S, Bernard RW, Galiano RD, Addona T, Stokes B, McCarthy JG. The temporal sequence of periosteal attachment after elevation. Plast Reconstr Surg. 2003;111(6):1942–7.
34. Romo T, Scaflani AP, Yung RT, McCormick SA, Cocker R, McCormick SU. Endoscopic foreheadplasty: a histologic comparison of periosteal refixation after endoscopic versus bicoronal lift. Plast Reconstr Surg. 2000;105(3):111–22.
35. Sullivan PK, Salomon JA, Woo AS, Freeman MB. The importance of the retaining ligamentous attachments of the forehead for selective eyebrow reshaping and forehead rejuvenation. Plast Reconstr Surg. 2006;117(1):95–104.
36. Righesso R, Jaeger M. Anatomia cirúrgica da região frontal e temporal. In: Jaeger M, Grossmann E, editors. Anatomia cirúrgica da cabeça e do pescoço. Rio de Janeiro: Dilivros; 2013.
37. Strasser EJ. An objective grading system for the evaluation of cosmetic surgical results. Plast Reconstr Surg. 1999;104(7):2282–5.
38. Strasser EJ. Application of an objective grading system for the evaluation of cosmetic surgical results. Plast Reconstr Surg. 2002;1099(5):1733–40.
39. Chiu ES, Baker DC. Endoscopic brow lift: a retrospective review of 628 consecutive cases over 5 years. Plast Reconstr Surg. 2003;112(2):628–33.
40. Hidalgo DA. Discussion: finesse in forehead and brow rejuvenation: modern concepts, including endoscopic methods. Plast Reconstr Surg. 2014;134(6):1151–3.
41. Walden JL, Orseck MJ, Aston SJ. Current methods for brow fixation: are they safe? Aesth Plast Surg. 2006;30(5):541–8.
42. Finger R. A 5-year study of the transmalar subperiosteal midface lift with minimal skin and superficial musculoaponeurotic system dissection: a durable, natural-appearing lift with less surgery and recovery time. Plast Reconstr Surg. 2001;107(5):1273–83.
43. Harirchian S, Kuperan AB, Shah AR. Safety of cranial fixation in endoscopic brow lifts. Am J Otolaryngol. 2013;34(6):690–4.
44. Angelos PC, Stallworth CL, Wang TD. Forehead lifting: state of the art. Facial Plast Surg. 2011;27(1):50–7.
45. Cho MJ, Carboy JA, Rohrich RJ. Complications in brow lifts: a systemic review of surgical and nonsurgical brow rejuvenations. Plast Reconstr Surg Glob Open. 2018;6(10):e1943.
46. Maas CS, Kim EJ. Temporal brow lift using botulinum toxin a: an update. Plast Reconstr Surg. 2003;112(5 Suppl):109S–12S.
47. Rammos CK, Mardini S. Endoscopic browlift in the receding hairline patient. J Craniofac Surg. 2016;27:156–8.

Part III

Rhinoplasty

14 Male Rhinoplasty

Paul N. Afrooz, Bahar Abbassi, and Nima Khosravani

14.1 Introduction

Male patients seek rhinoplasty for a number of reasons, including injury or trauma, correction of nasal airway dysfunction, asymmetries, and a general improvement in nasal and facial aesthetics. Males are notoriously challenging rhinoplasty patients due to nonspecific complaints, inattentiveness during the consultation, and an overall poor understanding of what they would like to achieve [1–3]. Male rhinoplasty has a relatively low patient satisfaction rate, [4] and therefore, effective communication during the initial consultation will ensure that the patient has a strong understanding of the proposed changes, as well as the risks and benefits of the procedure [1]. In addition to understanding ethnic variations and patient-specific features, a thorough and comprehensive understanding of the principles and anatomic features that define a masculine nose is critical. Comprehensive preoperative planning, including photographs, thorough communication to understand goals and realistic post-operative outcomes, surgical planning, preservation of masculinity, and postoperative management, are keys to obtaining satisfactory outcomes in male rhinoplasty.

14.2 Analysis

The initial consultation is an important part of achieving patient and surgeon satisfaction. Navigating and identifying a patient's goals and post-operative expectations requires thoroughness and diligence. Frequently, male patients tend to have nonspecific complaints and difficulty conveying what they desire, and demonstrate a certain level of inattentiveness and disinterest during the consultation [1]. Therefore, it is imperative that surgeon is capable of assessing a patient's psychological motive in efforts to identify those with potentially unrealistic expectations [1, 2, 4]. Often, these patients are fixated on aesthetic flaws within themselves, which is heightened by their underlying psychological instability [5]. Plastic surgeons have used the SIMON profile (single, immature, male, obsessive, and narcissistic) as an additional level of screening to identify and filter potentially problematic patients [1, 3]. Photographs aid a surgeon in understanding the patient's desires by helping the patient point to and articulate specific features that are displeasing to them.

Computer-assisted facial analysis has allowed patients to become more involved in their consultation and provides a medium for which a surgeon

P. N. Afrooz · N. Khosravani (✉)
Coral Gables, FL, USA
e-mail: PNA@drpaulafrooz.com

B. Abbassi
Clark Institute for Aesthetics, Winter Park, FL, USA

K. Jeffords et al. (eds.), *Aesthetic Surgery for Men*, https://doi.org/10.1007/978-3-032-03840-1_14

can test a patient's understanding of the different components of surgery and their effects on the final outcome. However, while it is important for patients to be well-informed, they must also understand that these tools are merely used for educational and informative purposes and do not dictate or guarantee a final surgical outcome [1]. Males have a tendency to be vague during the consultation and struggle with articulating their chief complaints. Subsequently, postoperative dissatisfaction is often due to the patient's lack of insight into their condition and not due to technical error [4, 6]. In general, males tend to be less compliant postoperatively, contributing to a higher incidence of postoperative complications. Edema and ecchymosis tend to be more pronounced in male patients, and though these are normal postoperative findings, there is a tendency to fixate on these changes, leading to anxiety and sometimes depression. For these reasons, the importance of the preoperative consultation is once again emphasized. For patients that require increased reassurance and counseling, additional pre-surgical appointments can help build and strengthen the patient-physician relationship and provide the opportunity to improve communication. It is not uncommon for the surgeon to require preoperative clearance from mental health providers as part of their preoperative routine.

It is important for the surgeon to be candid with patients when it comes to expectations and realistic results, and these discussions should be well documented. Thorough informed consent is important for any surgical procedure, but in-depth discussion of what to expect during the recovery period is equally important.

The surgeon must have a strong understanding of masculine features. Therefore, it is also necessary to apply techniques that will preserve or enhance masculinity—and conversely, anticipate and avoid changes that will lead to feminization. In addition to preserving masculinity, all efforts must be taken to produce harmonious subtle changes that maintain and obey the principles of aesthetic facial proportions.

14.3 Masculine Features

14.3.1 Radix

The radix (Fig. 14.1) is the area where the forehead connects with the nasal dorsum through a soft, concave curve [7]. With the eyes in a natural gaze, the radix is found between the upper eyelash line and supratarsal fold [1]. The radix is shallower in males (4 mm) in comparison to females (6 mm) [7].

14.3.2 Nasolabial Angle

The nasolabial angle (Fig. 14.2) is defined as the angle between the midpoint of the nostril aperture and a line perpendicular to the Frankfurt horizontal, intersecting the subnasale [7, 8]. Brown and Guyuron described the nasolabial angle as the intersection of a line traversing through the most anterior and posterior edges of the nostril and a plumb line perpendicular to the horizontal facial plane [9]. A nasolabial angle of 90–120 degrees is often cited; however, this range fails to distinguish the gender specific differences, as men (95–100 degrees) tend to have a slightly more acute angle than women (103–108 degrees) [1, 2, 7–9]. Although an "ideal range" for the nasolabial angle has been described, the surgeons must use their own discretion while keeping these ranges in mind [7, 8].

14.3.3 Nasal Dorsum

The male dorsum (Fig. 14.3) tends to be longer, stronger, wider, and straighter than the female counterpart [1, 5, 7]. The dorsum should be centered along a line from the radix to the tip defining points (Fig. 14.4) [1].

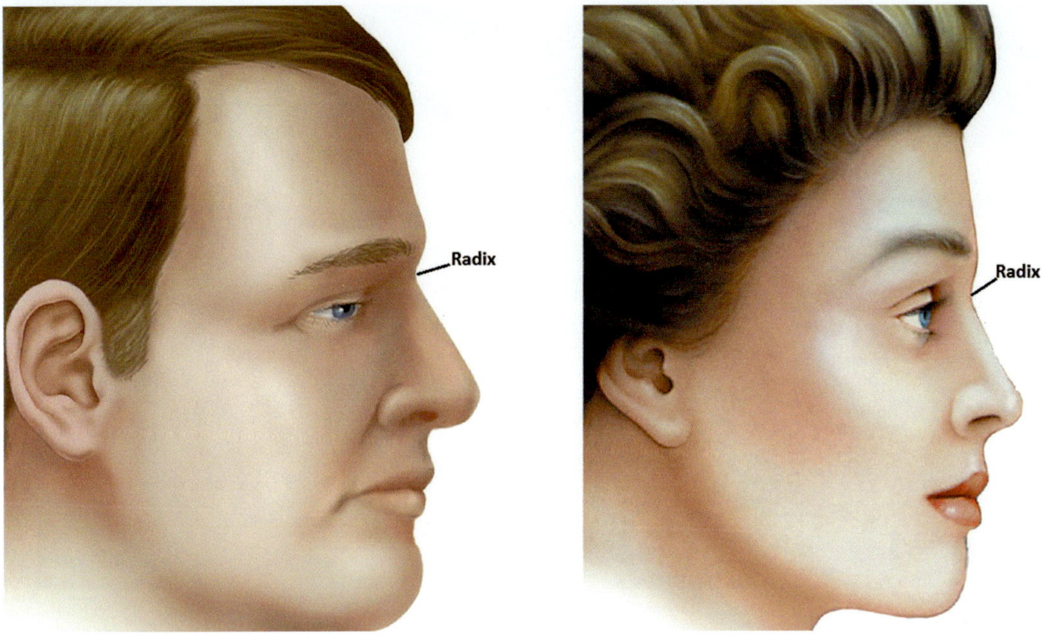

Fig. 14.1 Radix

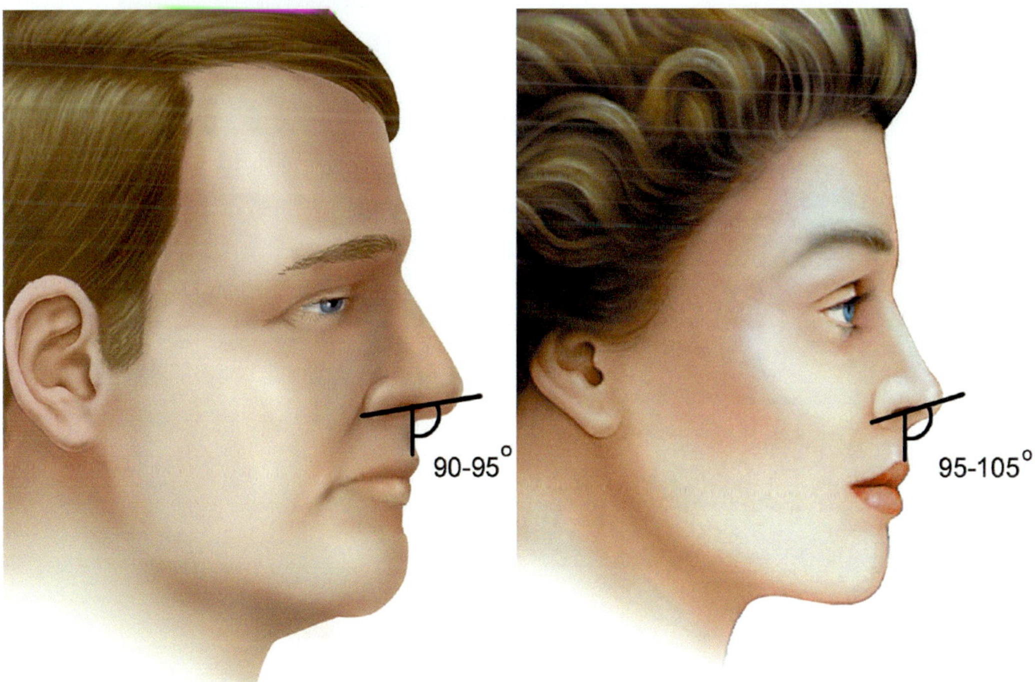

Fig. 14.2 Nasolabial angle

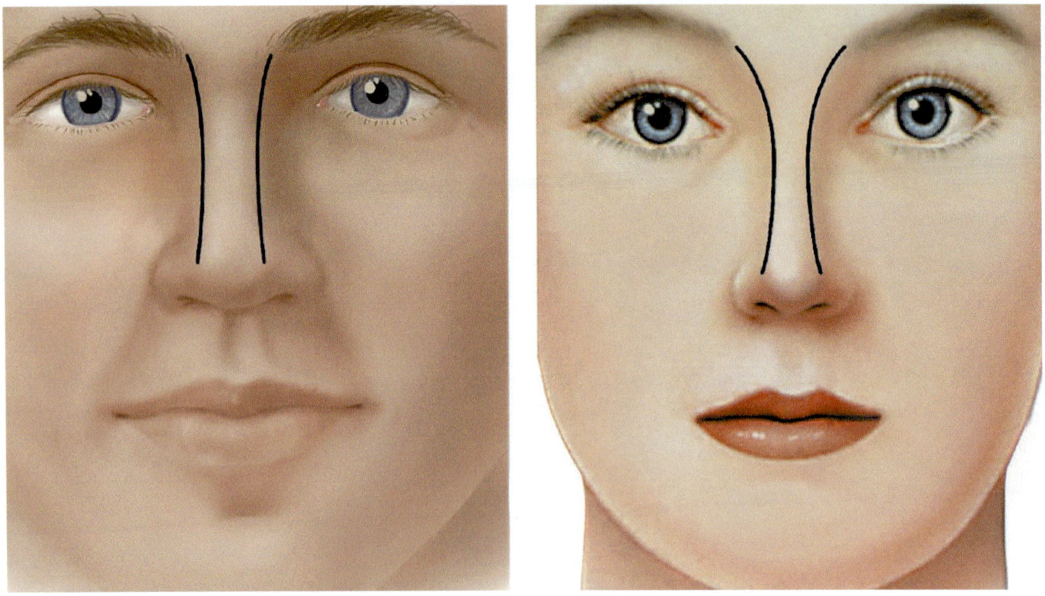

Fig. 14.3 Nasal dorsum

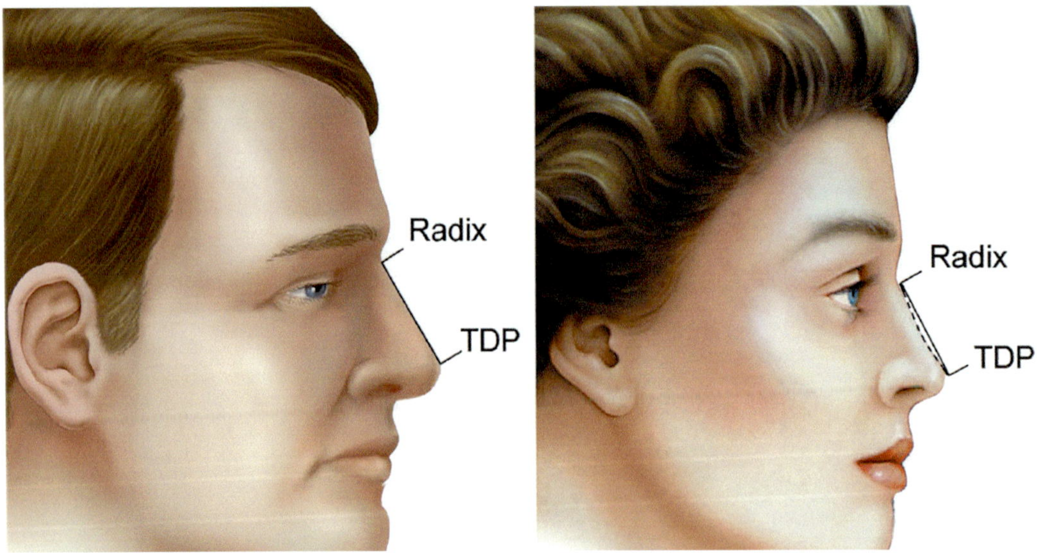

Fig. 14.4 Radix and tip defining points

14.3.4 Nasal Tip

The male nose has greater tip projection (Fig. 14.5) and slightly less tip rotation (90–95 degrees, as opposed to 95–105 degrees in females). It is also broader (Fig. 14.6) and more bulbous with little to no supratip break (Fig. 14.7) [1, 2, 7].

14.3.5 Skin

The male nose generally has thicker glabrous skin, which can mask alterations in the underlying framework [1, 2, 5]. In patients with thicker skin, conservative debulking of subcutaneous fat and removal of interdomal fat, in conjunction with creating a firm cartilaginous frame, will

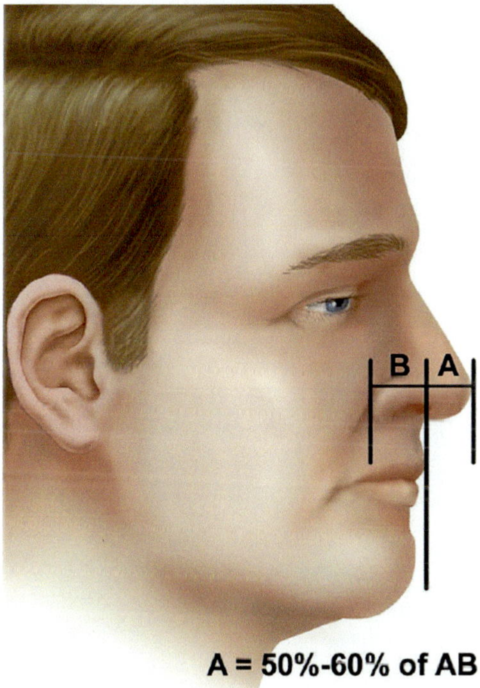

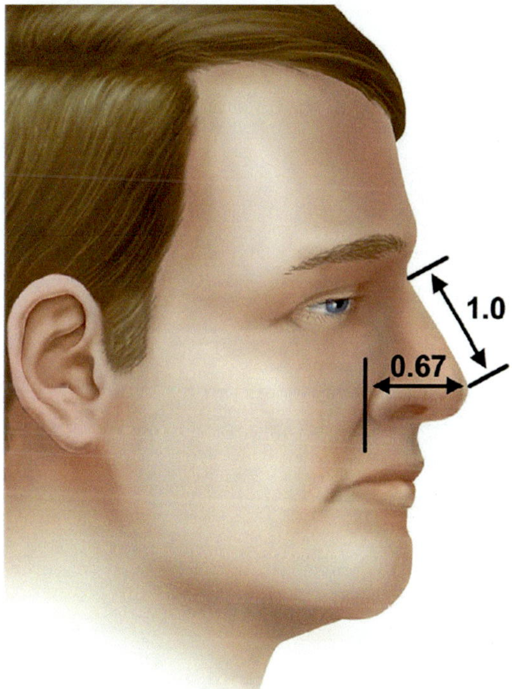

Fig. 14.5 Tip projection

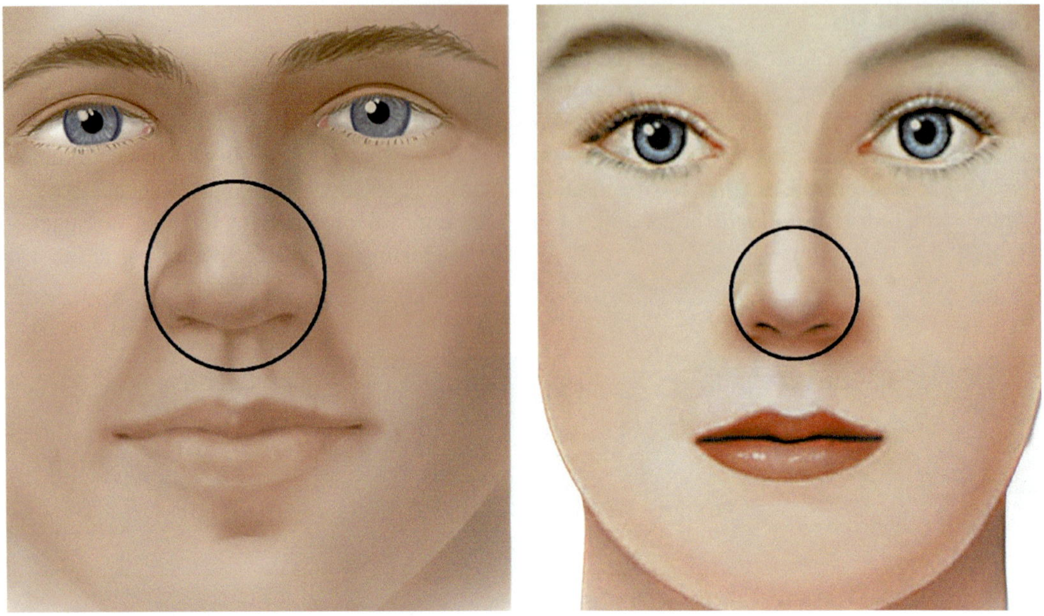

Fig. 14.6 The male tip is broader and less defined

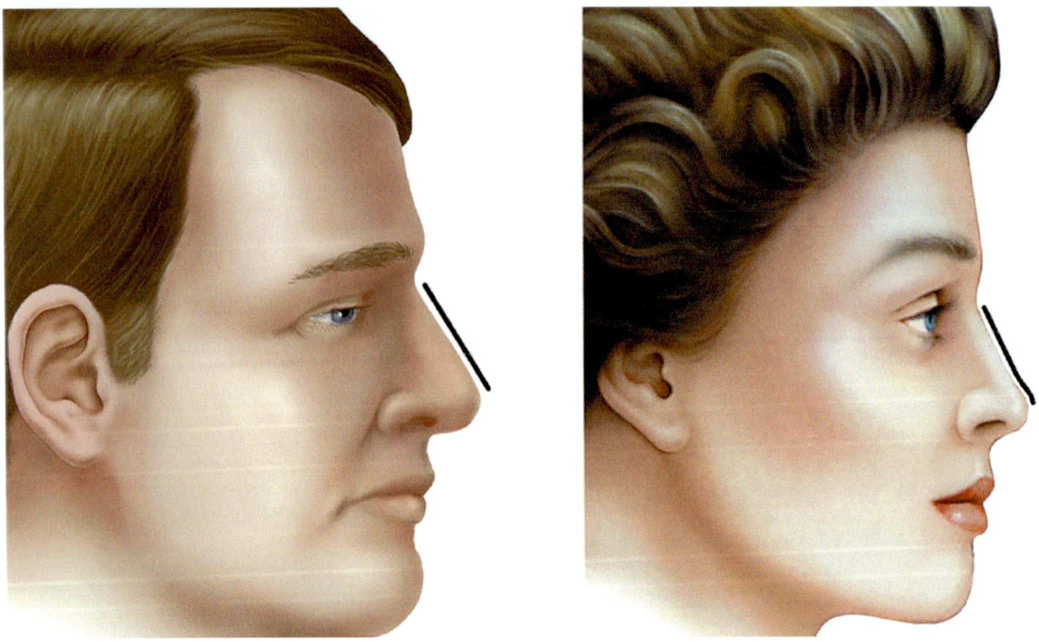

Fig. 14.7 Supratip break

facilitate the desired definition and intended aesthetic changes. Additionally, eliminating dead space and trimming redundant skin can also enhance tip definition and the final aesthetic outcome [10].

14.4 Technique

The key to successful male rhinoplasty is preservation of masculinity while maintaining symmetry and harmony of personal unique and ethnic features. Common reasons for male rhinoplasty include dorsal hump reduction and tip modification [5].

14.5 Dorsal Hump Reduction

Following elevation of the skin envelope and periosteum overlying the dorsum, a component dorsal hump reduction is carried out. A weighted retractor or an Aufricht retractor is placed to retract the skin envelope and facilitate adequate exposure. Alar retractors are placed in the domes of the lower lateral cartilages to facilitate exposure of the anterior septal angle (ASA) (Fig. 14.8). The prominence of the ASA is usually easily palpated. The ASA is defined, and the mucoperichondrium of the septum is scored with a number 15 blade to initiate the dissection in the proper plane. A Cottle septal elevator is used for this part of the dissection. The proper plane is verified by the blue/gray color of the cartilaginous septum, as well as the relative ease of mucoperichondrial elevation. Dissection proceeds most easily in a posterior direction and is then directed superiorly and anteriorly (Fig. 14.9). As dissection proceeds anteriorly toward the junction of the septum and ULC, the septal elevator is rolled gently under the ULC in an effort to dissect mucoperichondrium from the overlying ULC for several millimeters. This will ensure that the nasal lining is not violated with the forthcoming separation of the ULCs from the dorsal septum. The mucoperichondrial dissection is then carried out on the contralateral side. Following mucoperichondrial dissection, the ULCs are separated from the dorsal septum. An Aufricht retractor is used for accurate visualization of the dorsum up to the level of the keystone. A number 15 blade is placed underneath the ULC-septal junction. With the knife blade flush against the septum, the ULC-septal junction is separated up to the level of the nasal bones. The upper lateral cartilages are gently retracted, and the dorsal septum is trimmed incrementally to the desired height.

The bony dorsum is then rasped incrementally to the desired level. Rasping is performed carefully and in an oblique fashion in order to avoid disruption of the cartilaginous septum from the perpendicular plate of the ethmoid at the level of the keystone. A meticulous effort is made to ensure a smooth transition from the bony dorsum to the cartilaginous dorsum.

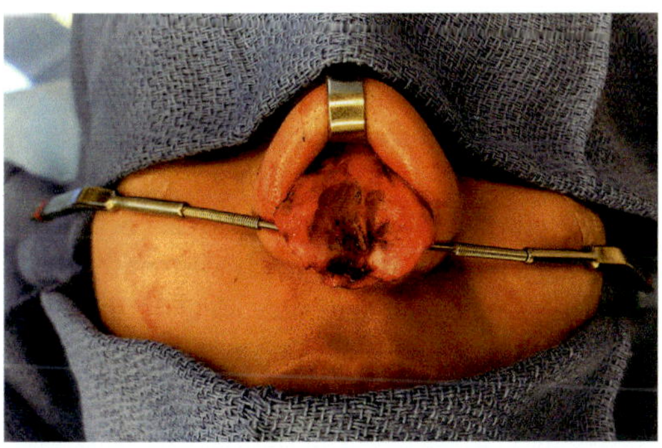

Fig. 14.8 Placement of lower lateral cartilage retractors for adequate exposure of the anterior septal angel

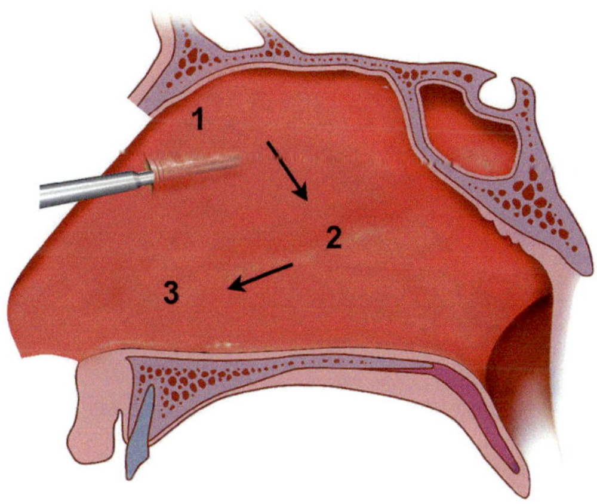

Fig. 14.9 Elevation of the mucoperichondrium is most easily performed in a posterior, inferior and anterior direction

14.6 Septoplasty and Harvesting Septal Cartilage

A nasal speculum is placed on one side of the septum to retract the upper lateral cartilage and gently push the septum to the opposing side. This maneuver facilitates visualization and accurate design of the dorsal L-strut. We prefer leaving an L-strut of at least 15 mm dorsally and 10 mm caudally in order to ensure stability of the dorsum. Furthermore, at the cephalic portion of the cartilaginous septum, at the articulation with the perpendicular plate of the ethmoid, the cut is directed in a posterior-oblique direction in order to maximize the remaining articulation between the cartilaginous septum and the perpendicular plate of the ethmoid (Fig. 14.10). Caudally, at the incision transition from dorsal to caudal septum, the cut is designed in a rounded manner rather than as a sharp angle. This reduces the risk of fracture of the L-strut at this transition point. The cartilaginous septum to be harvested is carefully freed using a septal elevator to dislodge the posterior and caudal portion of the septum from the perpendicular plate of the ethmoid and the vomer. Deviations of the vomer bone, or spurs, are removed with a rongeur.

The septal L-strut is assessed for residual deviation or irregularities. If the caudal portion of the septum is to be dislodged to one side of the maxillary crest, it is freed from the maxillary crest, trimmed of any redundant excess, and secured to the midline with a 5–0 PDS suture.

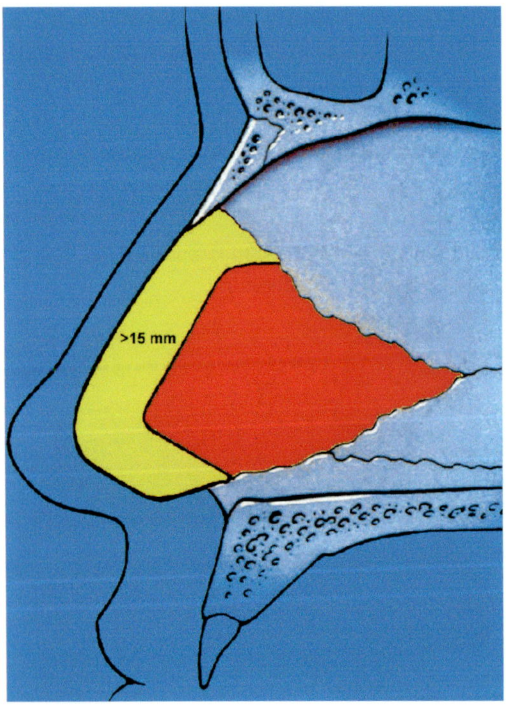

Fig. 14.10 Design of the L-strut of the cartilaginous septum. Cephalically, the incision aims posteriorly in order to maximize the surface area of the articulation between the perpendicular plate of the ethmoid and the cartilaginous septum

14.7 Osteotomies

Nasal osteotomies are performed to narrow a wide bony vault at the base or at the dorsum. They are also performed to close an open roof or to straighten deviated nasal bones. To address a wide bony base, we prefer a low-to low percutaneous perforated lateral osteotomy using a 2 mm osteotome through a lateral stab incision [11]. The incision is placed at the nasofacial junction, and a discontinuous low-to-low lateral osteotomy from the pyriform aperture to the level of the medial canthus is carried out. If narrowing the bony dorsum is desired, a medial osteotomy is performed in a superior oblique direction using a 4 mm osteotome. Following osteotomies, gentle digital pressure is used to mobilize the nasal bones into the desired position.

14.8 Midvault Reconstruction

Repositioning the nasal bones following osteotomies will highlight any residual asymmetries of the ULCs, particularly when correcting significant nasal bone deviation. Asymmetries between the ULCs are trimmed as necessary. Reconstitution of the cartilaginous midvault is performed in order to achieve ideal aesthetics of the dorsum and create a graceful transition between the bony vault and the cartilaginous midvault [12, 13]. Furthermore, this will optimize long-term stability and avoid an inverted-V deformity. To ensure a smooth transition and equalization of width between the bony dorsum and the cartilaginous midvault, spreader grafts may be used [14] (Fig. 14.11). If excess ULC is available, autospreader flaps may be utilized by folding the excess anterior portion of the ULCs over [15] (Fig. 14.12). Otherwise, spreader grafts approximately 4 mm wide are carved from septal cartilage and sutured to each side of the dorsal septum. The spreader grafts can be placed just cephalad to the caudal end of the nasal bones to control the width of the nasal bones, and they usually span to the caudal end of the ULCs. The spreader grafts are secured to the dorsal septum with 5–0 PDS horizontal mattress sutures. The upper lateral cartilages are then secured to the spreader graft-septal complex to reconstitute the cartilaginous midvault with 5–0 PDS horizontal mattress sutures.

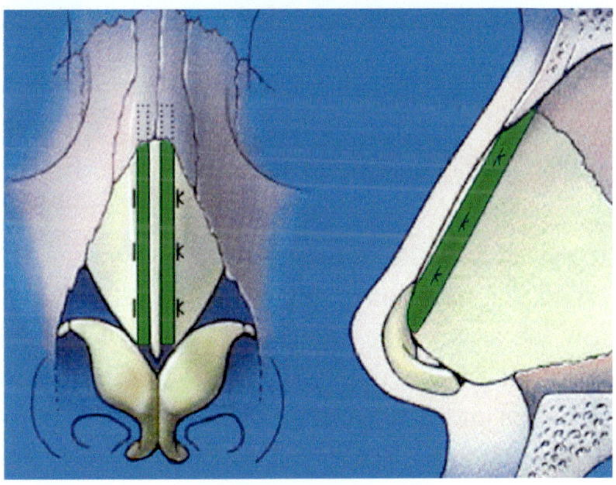

Fig. 14.11 Spreader grafts

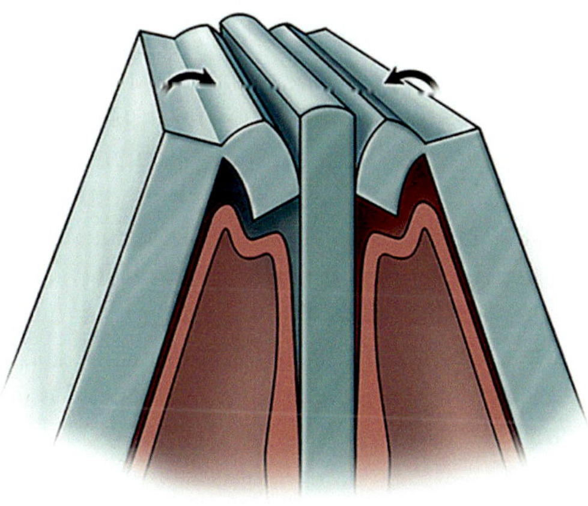

Fig. 14.12 Autospreader flaps

14.9 Columellar Strut

Sometimes a columellar strut is necessary to increase projection, or fortify and straighten the columella (Fig. 14.13). In males with thick skin, a strut is routinely used to create a firm underlying framework. The strut is carved from the longest and sturdiest portion of autologous cartilage, measuring approximately 4 mm wide. A pocket is created within the soft tissue between the medial crura. The pocket is not extended all the way to the nasal spine, thereby maintaining a pad of soft tissue between the posterior end of the strut and the nasal spine in order to prevent the strut from directly contacting the nasal spine. Contact between the columellar strut and the nasal spine is frequently reported to cause a "clicking" sensation. Furthermore, the soft tissue pad between the posterior end of the strut and the nasal spine provides a small amount of recoil. Because the strut is not contacting the unyielding nasal spine, the tip complex has a more natural dynamic with facial animation.

The strut is secured to the medial crura at the base of the columella with a 5–0 polydiaxanone horizontal mattress suture. This horizontal mattress suture is initiated between the medial crura on one side of the strut in order to bury the knot between the medial crura. Additional sutures are placed in a similar fashion between the strut and the middle crura while monitoring the angle of divergence between the middle crura.

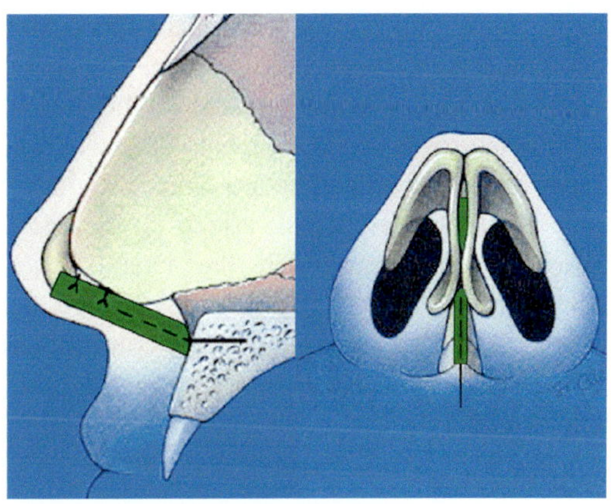

Fig. 14.13 Columellar strut

14.10 Tip Shaping

The shape of the nasal tip is evaluated and correlated with the preoperative photographs. Bulbosity of the nasal tip is a frequent motivating factor in primary rhinoplasty. A cephalic trim of the lateral crura will partially address the bulbosity of the nasal tip [16]. The cephalic trim is marked based on the excess portion contributing to bulbosity, while also maintaining a minimum of 5 mm anteriorly and 6 mm posteriorly. This will ensure adequate residual cartilaginous support. After the markings have been made, the portions of the lateral crura to be resected are injected to facilitate the dissection of the nasal lining. Next, the cartilage is incised, carefully dissected from the underlying nasal lining, and removed.

14.10.1 Interdomal Suture

If the distance between the two domes is excessive or if the distance between the tip-defining points is too wide, an interdomal suture is used to narrow the interdomal distance [17] (Fig. 14.14). Using a 5–0 PDS, the interdomal suture is placed from lateral to medial through one dome, and again from medial to lateral through the opposite dome as a loop stitch. If the domes are misaligned, or if they overlap with use of a simple loop stitch, a figure-of-eight suture can be used such that the suture is placed from lateral to medial through one dome and then lateral to medial through the opposite dome. The figure-of eight suture will prevent overlap of the domes and will serve to properly align them. The suture is tightened incrementally to achieve the desired interdomal distance. The cephalo-caudal placement of the interdomal suture along the domes may also have considerable effects on the orientation of the domes and the lateral crura. Therefore, depending on the desired change, the orientation of the domes and lateral crura should be carefully monitored when placing the interdomal suture.

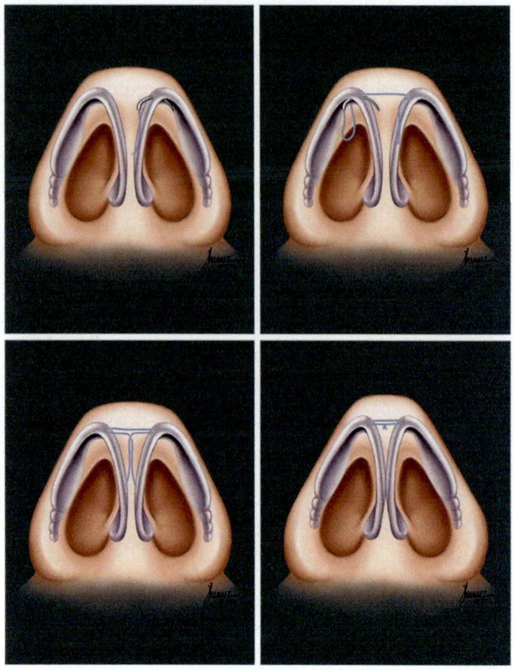

Fig. 14.14 Interdomal suture

14.10.2 Transdomal Suture

If the arch of the domes is excessively wide or broad, the transdomal suture can be used to narrow the arch of the domes [17] (Fig. 14.15). As the arch of the dome is narrowed, the dome becomes more projected. Therefore, the transdomal suture slightly increases nasal tip projection, and the sharper contour of the apex of the dome increases tip definition. A 5–0 PDS suture is placed from medial to lateral across the dome in a horizontal mattress fashion and tied on the medial aspect of the dome, making sure the suture does not violate the nasal lining. The suture is tightened incrementally until the desired shape is achieved. Similar to the interdomal suture, the cephalo-caudal placement of the transdomal suture can have a significant impact on the orientation of the domes and the lateral crura. Therefore, these dynamics must be anticipated and monitored during placement of transdomal sutures.

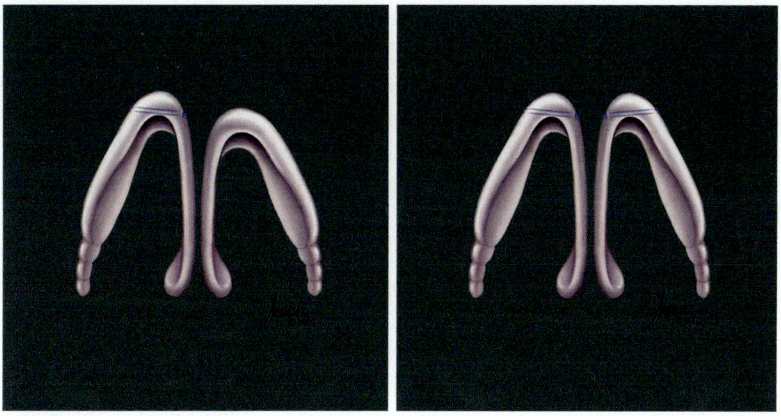

Fig. 14.15 Transdomal suture

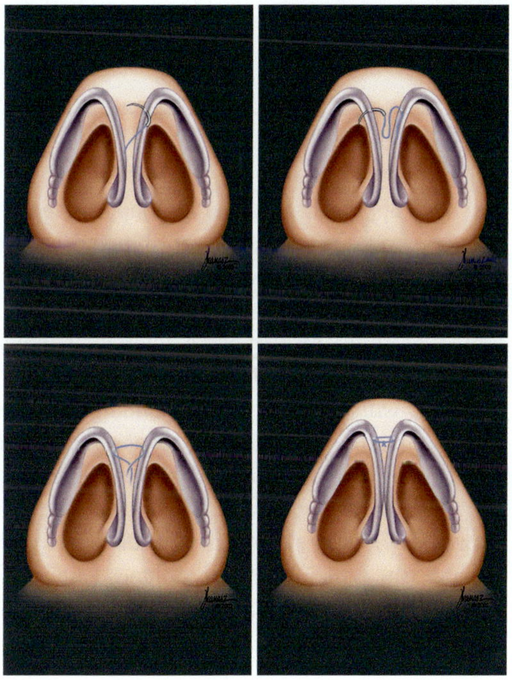

Fig. 14.16 Middle crura suture

14.10.3 Middle Crura Suture

The middle crura suture is used to control the angle of divergence between the middle crura [17] (Fig. 14.16). Depending on the length of the columellar strut, the middle crura suture may incorporate the strut. By reducing the angle of divergence between the middle crura, this suture will increase tip projection, increase tip support, narrow the anterior columella, and reduce the interdomal distance. Similar to the aforementioned tip-shaping sutures, the middle crura suture may have additional effects on the infratip lobule size. The position of the domes and lateral crura should be monitored during suture placement.

14.11 Alar Contour Grafts

To correct or prevent retraction of the alar rim, alar contour grafts are placed along the alar rim margin in a vestibular pocket [18]. A hook is placed in the nostril apex and gently retracted. Using a pair of iris scissors, a vestibular pocket is dissected along the alar rim toward the alar facial junction. A cartilage graft measuring 2–3 mm wide and approximately 15 mm long is fashioned and placed within the vestibular pocket along the alar rim.

14.12 Closure

The transcolumellar incision is closed with meticulous realignment using 6–0 nylon interrupted sutures. Within the vestibule, the infracartilaginous incision is closed using interrupted 5–0 chromic gut sutures. The infracartilaginous incision is best exposed by placing a double hook using slight eversion similar to the exposure used in making the incision initially. Generally, three interrupted sutures are placed in the lateral aspect of the incision. Medially, two to three interrupted sutures are placed. Suture placement near the soft tissue triangle and nostril apex is avoided, as these sutures frequently distort the contour of the soft-tissue triangle, nostril apices, and alar rim. As a general rule, the suture bites within the infracartilaginous incision are made as small as possible in order to avoid distortion or retraction of the alar rim.

14.13 Splinting

Following meticulous closure, mupirocin-coated Doyle splints are placed within the nostrils and sutured in place using a 3–0 nylon horizontal mattress suture through the membranous septum. The nasal skin is cleaned, and steri-strips are placed in an overlapping fashion along the dorsum and to the level of the supratip breakpoint. A metal splint is then placed over the steri-strips. Finally, a surgicel hemostatic wrap is cut into several pieces of approximately 4 x 4 mm in dimension. Several pieces are coated in mupirocin ointment and packed within the nostril apices to provide internal support and splinting of the nostril apices and soft-tissue triangles during the acute healing phase.

14.14 Postoperative Regimen

Primary rhinoplasty patients receive intraoperative antibiotics, followed by 24 h of postoperative antibiotics. Patients are instructed to clean incisions daily with dilute hydrogen peroxide in the postoperative period, followed by application of antibiotic ointment. Columellar sutures are typically removed at 7 days. If alar base surgery is performed, these sutures are usually left in place for 10–14 days due to dynamic activity at the alar-cheek junction and potential for wound dehiscence. Internal and external splints are removed at 7 days, followed by nighttime taping of the supratip area with steri-strips for 4–6 weeks.

14.15 Conclusion

The open approach in primary rhinoplasty facilitates accurate visualization of the underlying anatomy in order to precisely correct anatomic deformities and enhance nasal shape and function. Gratifying results begin with meticulous preoperative analysis of the deformities in conjunction with a clear understanding of the patient's goals. Once realistic expectations are set, thorough preoperative preparation is essential to operative execution. While the level of complexity among rhinoplasty patients is highly variable, the principles and techniques herein are fundamentally comprehensive and will serve as a solid foundation for the rhinoplasty surgeon.

References

1. Rohrich RJ, Janis JE, Kenkel JM. Male rhinoplasty. Plast Reconstr Surg. 2003;112(4):1071–85.; quiz 1086, Sep 15 2003. https://doi.org/10.1097/01.prs.0000076201.75278.bb.
2. Tanna N, et al. Evidence-based medicine: current practices in rhinoplasty. Plast Reconstr Surg. 2018;141(1):137e–51e. https://doi.org/10.1097/prs.0000000000003977.
3. Nassif PS. Male revision rhinoplasty: pearls and surgical techniques. Facial Plast Surg. 2005;21(4):250–70. https://doi.org/10.1055/s-2006-939504.

4. Khansa I, Khansa L, Pearson GD. Patient satisfaction after rhinoplasty: a social media analysis. Aesthet Surg J. 2016;36(1):1–5. https://doi.org/10.1093/asj/sjv095.
5. Daniel RK. Rhinoplasty and the male patient. Clin Plast Surg. 1991;18(4):751–61.
6. Blackburn VF, Blackburn AV. Taking a history in aesthetic surgery: SAGA--the surgeon's tool for patient selection. J Plast Reconstr Aesthet Surg. 2008;61(7):723–9. https://doi.org/10.1016/j.bjps.2007.09.049.
7. Sajjadian A, Guyuron B. Primary rhinoplasty. Aesthet Surg J. 2010;30(4):527–39.; quiz 540, Jul–Aug. https://doi.org/10.1177/1090820x10380388.
8. Armijo BS, Brown M, Guyuron B. Defining the ideal nasolabial angle. Plast Reconstr Surg. 2012;129(3):759–64. https://doi.org/10.1097/PRS.0b013e3182402e12.
9. Brown M, Guyuron B. Redefining the ideal nasolabial angle: part 2. Expert analysis. Plast Reconstr Surg. 2013;132(2):221e–5e. https://doi.org/10.1097/PRS.0b013e3182958b40.
10. Guyuron B, Lee M. An effective algorithm for Management of Noses with thick skin. Aesth Plast Surg. 2017;41(2):381–7. https://doi.org/10.1007/s00266-017-0779-1.
11. Rohrich RJ, Krueger JK, Adams WP Jr, Hollier LH Jr. Achieving consistency in the lateral nasal osteotomy during rhinoplasty: an external perforated technique. Plast Reconstr Surg. 2001;108(7):2122–30.; discussion 2131–2.
12. Roostaeian J, Unger JG, Lee MR, Geissler P, Rohrich RJ. Reconstitution of the nasal dorsum following component dorsal reduction in primary rhinoplasty. Plast Reconstr Surg. 2014;133(3):509–18. https://doi.org/10.1097/01.prs.0000438453.29980.36.
13. Afrooz PN, Rohrich RJ. The keystone: consistency in restoring the aesthetic dorsum in rhinoplasty. Plast Reconstr Surg. 2018;141(2):355–63. https://doi.org/10.1097/prs.0000000000004091.
14. Sheen JH. Spreader graft: a method of reconstructing the roof of the middle nasal vault following rhinoplasty. Plast Reconstr Surg. 1984;73(2):230–9.
15. Byrd HS, Meade RA, Gonyon DL Jr. Using the autospreader flap in primary rhinoplasty. Plast Reconstr Surg. 2007;119(6):1897–902. https://doi.org/10.1097/01.prs.0000259196.02216.a5.
16. Rohrich RJ, Ahmad J. Rhinoplasty. Plast Reconstr Surg. 2011;128(2):49e–73e. https://doi.org/10.1097/PRS.0b013e31821e7191.
17. Guyuron B, Behmand RA. Nasal tip sutures part II: the interplays. Plast Reconstr Surg. 2003;112(4):1130–45.; discussion 1146–9,. https://doi.org/10.1097/01.prs.0000076505.83375.74.
18. Rohrich RJ, Raniere J Jr, Ha RY. The alar contour graft: correction and prevention of alar rim deformities in rhinoplasty. Plast Reconstr Surg. 2002;109(7):2495–505.; discussion 2506–8,.

15 Multi-cultural Ethnic Rhinoplasty: An Emphasis on Hispanic, Middle Eastern, African-American, and Asian Noses

Ali Sajjadian and Kiana Panbechi

15.1 Introduction

In any race or culture, balance between facial features is a standard marker of beauty. Beautiful noses are harmonious with other facial components, and are symmetric, vertically aligned, and between the eyes [1]. As social media, Hollywood, and pop culture continue to shape standards of beauty, the Caucasian or Western look has been universally accepted as the ideal to attain [2]. The Western nose is moderately thin, tapered, angular, and slightly projecting [2]. This specific phenotype may have evolved to become a marker for genetic fertility and health [3]. Today, it has become the ultimate goal in rhinoplasty for immigrants of ethnic backgrounds who wish to achieve a nose more similar to their Caucasian counterparts. In the United States, "ethnic rhinoplasty" has been traditionally thought as a procedure to reshape the nose of an African-American or Asian nose. However, Hispanics are now the largest minority population in the United States and rhinoplasty in this population has increased over time. Morphology of the Hispanic nose is also similar to Mediterranean/Middle Eastern noses: dorsal hump, long nasal bones, poor tip projections, and moderate tip bulbosity [4]. Both Hispanic and Middle Eastern Rhinoplasty can be categorized as ethnic rhinoplasty along with procedures done on the African-American and Asian populations. In all four, Hispanic, Middle Eastern, African-American, and Asian cases, the variability in anatomical features create challenges to rhinoplasty, and the surgeon must have a deep understanding of these differences in order to perform a successful procedure. The Hispanic nose is complex due to the irregularity across patients caused from differences in racial mixture. Similarly, difficulties intrinsic to the nasal anatomy among the Middle Eastern population can make surgical results less predictable and, in some cases, less enduring. The Middle Eastern nose offers challenges in the heavy, thick skin envelope, an over-projecting osseocartilaginous vault, weak alar cartilages, and short medial crura [5–7]. Facial malformations that can arise from these intrinsic features include a large bulbous nose, a drooping and poorly defined tip, a broad and bony middle vault, and a short columellar labial angle [5–7]. The African-American nose is typically described as flat, round with flared alae and little dorsal projection [8]. The Asian nose typically exhibits thick sebaceous skin, a low dorsum and inadequate projection and blunted nasal contours [9]. The purpose of this chapter is to provide information on the anatomic features, treatment goals, operative techniques, and potential problems of Hispanic, Middle Eastern, African-American, and Asian rhinoplasties that will lead to successful and pleasing surgical results.

A. Sajjadian (✉) · K. Panbechi
Newport Beach, CA, USA

K. Jeffords et al. (eds.), *Aesthetic Surgery for Men*, https://doi.org/10.1007/978-3-032-03840-1_15

15.2 Anatomical Features

15.2.1 Hispanic Nose Anatomical Features

Due to the various racial combinations of the Hispanic community, the Hispanic nose is complex to describe. Nevertheless, studies have shown that a "typical" Hispanic nose varies from a Western nose in that it has a tip which projects to a lesser extent, a wider base than a Western nose, and alae that depend on lateral view [10]. One measure of the difference in nasal features between the races is the nasal index. Nasal index is an anthropometric technique that compares the width of the base of the nose with the height of the nose [100 Å ~ (nasal breadth)/(nasal height)]. In Caucasians, the index value is approximately 70; in African-Americans, the index value can range from 85 to 95; and in Hispanics, the index value of the Mestizo nose is approximately 75 (as is the Asian nose) [10]. Hispanic noses can be classified into four types of deformities to provide surgeons a practical way of analyzing and formulating surgical treatment plans [11]. According to Daniel's 2003 paper, Hispanic Rhinoplasty in the United States, with Emphasis on the Mexican American Nose, categorizes the nasal deformities (and their familiar older terminology) as follows:

Type I (the Castilian nose) is characterized by normal radix height, a high-arched osseocartilaginous vault, and a tip with nearly normal projection. This surgically indicates no need for a radix graft and incremental reduction of the hump. Lateral osteotomies can be done to correct the wide nasal width, and a columellar strut can correct the lack of tip definition.

Type II (the Mexican American nose) is characterized by a low radix height and upper dorsum, a nearly normal bridge, and a dependent tip (an under-projecting tip), which creates the illusion of a major dorsal hump. For surgical correction, minimal soft tissue defatting can be utilized, radix graft used for the hypoplastic radix, and multiple tip sutures to correct the lack of tip definition.

Type III (the Mestizo nose) is characterized by a dorsum-base disproportion attributable to a heavy, wide/broad base with minimal definition and a wide tip (under-projection of the tip), which is complicated by a thick skin envelope. A reduction of the extremely wide nasal base can be implemented using sills and alar wedges.

Type IV (the Creole nose) is similar to the African-American nose with an inter-alar width > 45 mm, an exceedingly flat dorsum, and an under-projecting tip. The necessity for a full-length dorsal augmentation differentiates these cases from the Type III Mestizo nose.

15.2.2 Middle Eastern Nose Anatomical Features

Familiarity of Middle Eastern nasal anatomy is essential in order to create an operative plan that will ensure balanced and optimal aesthetic results. Some anatomical features generally found in Middle Eastern Noses are normal to thick soft tissue, wide and asymmetric nostrils, wide nasal vaults, and under-projected and under-rotated tip morphology. The highlighted features, which will be described in further detail, are the skin envelope, the dorsum, the upper lateral cartilages, and the alar base/nostrils.

15.2.2.1 Skin Envelope

The degree of skin and soft tissue thickness varies in the Middle Eastern population based on their origin. Clinical experience shows that only 36% of Middle Eastern patients have relatively thick skin and soft tissues with Fitzpatrick skin types III-V [12]. This observation is based upon a scale ranging from +3 to −3, with N at the "zero" position representing normal thickness [13, 14]. Those from more northern areas, however, such as northern Iran, Turkey, and Armenia, often have thinner and lighter skin, ranging from +1 to −1 in skin thickness. The surgical implication is that one must identify those with thick skin and consider skin envelope defatting and open structure tip grafts to achieve tip definition [12]. Conversely, one should avoid tip-destructive techniques, such as domal division or Goldman tip, in two-thirds of Middle Easterners with thinner skin.

15.2.2.2 The Dorsum

A common procedure in Middle Eastern rhinoplasty is reduction of prominent dorsal hump. The nasal dorsum is typically composed of approximately equivalent amounts of bone and cartilage in majority of Middle Eastern patients, although primary cartilaginous or bony (least common) dorsum may also be observed. The greatest reductions are done in the cartilaginous hump. This makes the use of spreader grafts an essential technique to avoid an inverted V deformity [12].

15.2.2.3 Upper Lateral Cartilages

One unique anatomical feature of Middle Easterners is the extreme width of the upper lateral cartilages at their junction with the alar cartilages. The extended lateral junction between upper lateral cartilage and lower lateral cartilage is a unique feature of Middle Eastern patients [12].

15.2.2.4 Alar Base/Nostrils

Many Middle Eastern rhinoplasty patients have a wide alar base that requires excision. This observation has caused surgeons in the past to design their tip surgery based on the assumption that the alar cartilages are massive and require extreme excision or division of the alar cartilages as the solution. However, this approach can lead to a critical loss of support [12]. Thus, conservation management is essential to prevent unnatural morphology of ala and alar crease [15].

15.2.2.5 Septal Deviation and Asymmetry

More than half Middle Eastern rhinoplasty patients present with significant deviation of the caudal septum [12]. Septal deviation is an important element of asymmetry often found in a background of pervasive facial asymmetry in Middle Eastern Patients. In order to achieve realistic results, it is important that the patient recognizes and accepts the limitations of their preexisting facial asymmetry. However, the septum plays an important role in providing tip support and maintenance of nasal tip position and shape [15].

15.2.3 African-American Nose Anatomical Features

The African-American nose can vary due to the multi-racial background of the population. There are certain features, however, that differ from the Caucasian or Western nose. Bone and cartilage support is often found to be lacking in African-American patients. This results in a wide dorsum with poor anterior projection and a wide pyriform aperture [16]. Generally, most African-Americans have thick skin with a prominent subcutaneous fibrofatty pad. This leads to a droopy tip with little definition. The nasal alae tend to be wider than the Caucasian nose and tend to flare as well. This feature of their nasal anatomy can contribute to nasal valve physiology. A study in 1997 comparing the total nasal resistance of Caucasian and African-American healthy adults found a statistically significant decrease in the mean total airway resistance in African-Americans in comparison to Caucasians (0.136 Pa/cm^3/s in African-Americans and 0.176 Pa/cm^3/s in Caucasians by the anterior method) [17]. The premaxillary area for African-American patients is often hypoplastic. Septal cartilage can often be lacking, and structural augmentation material is required to provide functional and long-lasting results.

15.2.4 Asian Nose Anatomical Features

The word "Asian" encompasses people from many different ethnic origins, including Southeast Asia, India, and Eastern Asia. This results in a variety of aesthetic features and anatomical characteristics. Despite these variations, three broad morphological categories have been created to describe the typical "Asian" nose. The first group is the leptorrhine nose (tall and thin), typical of those from a Caucasian or Indo-European descent. The second group is the platyrrhine nose (broad and flat), which is associated with those from an African origin. The last group is the mesorrhine nose (intermediate), which has features between the leptorrhine and platyrrhine types. The most common morphology is the mesorrhine nose with a low dorsal projection, a rounded and under-projected tip, and flared nasal base and wide nostrils [18]. The typical Asian nose tends to have thicker skin than Caucasian noses. Asian noses have substantial subcutaneous soft tissue with weak lower lateral cartilages, and a small and thin septal cartilage. This makes it difficult to use the septal cartilage for graft use, and oftentimes surgeons have to resort to other autologous or alloplastic materials for augmentation [19]. Furthermore, Asian noses typically have a shorter distance between the cephalic area of the upper lateral cartilages and the caudal area of the nasal bone than Caucasians. This area, referred to as the keystone area, is typically 4–5 mm on average in the Caucasian population [20]. Asians also tend to have weak nasal bones. The protruding part of the premaxilla, which is attached to the caudal part of the septal cartilage edge, is known as the anterior nasal spine (ANS). Among Asians, the ANS is not fully developed, and even missing in some patients [21]. Overall, the shorter and lower dorsum and rounder tip of the Asian nose call for augmentation techniques to ensure an aesthetically pleasing result [19].

15.3 Treatment Goals

The main goal of the surgeon is patient satisfaction in conjunction with a long-lasting and structurally sound nose. The surgeon's goal is to comply with the patient's desires as much as possible and obtain harmony and a natural-looking result. The nose should not look "operated" and should be balanced with the patient's other facial features. The surgeon must therefore take into account the patient's racial characteristics and limitations. Proper communication is key in order to ensure the patient understands what is a realistic goal, and for the surgeon to understand what the patient envisions. For this, computer imaging can be an extremely useful tool to allow the patient to receive a concrete visualization of the surgeon's vision and what is realistically possible. Computer imaging can also promote discussion of the specifics (i.e., "I want a nose like this picture.") rather than just generalities (i.e., "I want a thinner nose.") and can prevent misunderstandings [15]. An important note is that nasal function should never be compromised in the interest of aesthetics.

15.3.1 Hispanic Treatment Goals

An important aspect of communication between patients and the surgeon is the language. English may be a second language for many Hispanic patients. Many of these Hispanic patients may not speak English at home. In fact, some may even need to use an interpreter. The surgeon's role is to ensure that the patient is fully educated and can express his or her goals effectively.

15.3.2 Middle Eastern Treatment Goals

While functional preservation along with a significant size reduction is a main concern for the surgeon, for most Middle Eastern patients, aesthetics are the focus [12]. Middle Eastern patients are knowledgeable and highly opinionated about the aesthetic goals of rhinoplasty due to their cultural attraction and commonality in their population to this procedure.

The majority of older female patients (25–55 years) want their noses refined and made more feminine for they feel that their noses are too large and bulky, while their tips are too wide and droopy [12]. Younger female patients (15–25 years) have similar complaints but want more significant change that will result in a "cute" nose [12]. They prefer natural looks and ala as opposed to the surgically "operated" look of their older female relatives with pinched tips, nostril show, and inverted V deformities. Surgeons have to keep in mind that a Western nose on an individual with Middle Eastern facial features does not always look natural and gives the impression of a surgical alteration. For instance, the goal for correction of the nasolabial angle (and columellar-labial angle) should be 95° or less, with an approach to less correction being preferable [15]. A good method for finding balance for natural-looking nasal proportions is to use the standard nasal ratios as a guide. Examples include moderate dorsum reduction, narrowing of wide nasal bones, correction of alar flaring, and conservative debulking of fibrofatty tissue. Common nasal tip procedures include creating definition and correcting an under-supported nasal tip. Specific operative techniques will be discussed in the next section.

15.3.3 African-American Treatment Goals

African-American patients want a procedure that will improve their aesthetic appearance but preserve their heritage. Compared to Caucasian patients, African-American patients prefer a wider alar width and a more acute nasolabial angle [22]. Common goals usually discussed in this ethnic rhinoplasty discussion are increased tip definition, decreased width, dorsal adjustment (either augmentation or reduction), increased nasal tip projection, and decreased nasal tip edema [23].

15.3.4 Asian Treatment Goals

While most Caucasian patients and other ethnic groups are seeking to reduce the overall size and dorsal hump of the nose, Asian rhinoplasty patients seek the opposite. Due to the low dorsum typical of most Asian noses, the most commonly addressed issue in both primary and secondary Asian rhinoplasty is dorsal augmentation. This can be achieved by using autologous cartilage to structure the tip, followed by using implant material to augment the dorsum [24]. Nasal lengthening can also be a goal for some patients. It is advisable to discuss the affects this can have on the overall balance of the face with the patient in order to have a common understanding of the possible results.

15.4 Operative Techniques

The surgeon should prefer surgical techniques that are more conservative and less invasive, and that produce longer-lasting results [25]. The goal is to achieve a natural-looking result where no part of the face dominates. For this, systematic planning is recommended in which it is important to consider balance (the symmetry of the face in the frontal view), harmony (the relationship of the facial elements in profile), condition of the dorsal profile, tip inclination and projection of the nose from the face, and condition of the nasal base (which includes the relationship of the columella to the nostril edge [15, 26–29].

15.4.1 Operative Techniques in Hispanic Rhinoplasty

15.4.1.1 General Techniques

Due to their anatomic tendencies and variations that arise from different racial mixtures, Hispanic noses often require extensive work on their internal structures to create the desired aesthetic result. Hispanic noses often require augmentation such as surgical grafts. The surgeon must carefully decide what graft material is needed to obtain the desired results. The surgeon must first decide whether rigid or soft reconstruction methods are needed. Less rigid methods have recently been favored [20]. Autologous materials such as septal cartilage, conchal cartilage, and costal cartilage have proven to be the best graft material [30, 31]. An alternative is harvested calvarial (parietal) bone. Using diced and wrapped cartilage or crushed and shaved cartilage can obtain the optimal rigidity between cartilage and bone. Furthermore, it is important to note that although synthetic implant material, such as polyethylene, can be used, there is a risk of extrusion. For instance, Gore-Tex mesh, which has been used in rhinoplasties in the past, is now a less preferred choice due to the risk of infection and extrusion [25, 26].

15.4.1.2 Specific Techniques

Due to the variety of shapes presented in Hispanic patients, the key to achieving successful results is an individualized plan for each patient. This section will present the surgical techniques recommend by Daniel for each of the four main deformities found in Hispanic noses [11] (Fig. 15.1):

Type I (Castilian): The Hispanic Castilian nose typically has a prominent osseocartilaginous vault and nearly normal tip projection; therefore, the basic surgical goal is to perform a "functional reduction rhinoplasty"—this gives the patient the smaller nose they want and retains or improves their respiratory function.

Type II (Mexican American): Altering the Hispanic Mexican American nose can be extremely challenging; it requires maximal surgical finesse. There is normal dorsal height over the cartilaginous vault and decreased projection in both the adjacent radix area and the tip. The basic goal is to perform a "finesse rhinoplasty."

Type III (Mestizo): The typical Hispanic Mestizo nose needs to have the dorsum-base disproportion corrected—augment the dorsum and reduce the base. Additionally, the distal end of the nose may be large and covered in thick skin. The basic goal is to perform a "balanced rhinoplasty."

Type IV (the Creole nose): The Hispanic Creole nose is like the African-American nose, and recommended operative procedures are similar.

15.4.2 Operative Techniques in Middle Eastern Noses

15.4.2.1 Skin

Considerations for operative techniques should begin with the skin. As discussed earlier, about one-third of patients have thick, heavy skin. For these patients, a conservative defatting of the skin envelope should be done. The undersurface should never be trimmed past the level of the subdermal plexus. In addition, open structure tip grafts will be needed to provide tip definition in those individuals who have thick skin. Due to the large and heavy skin envelope, along with the significant reduction, a wide array of grafts is required. The goal is to use spreader grafts, columellar struts, tip grafts, and even alar rim grafts in order to provide adequate structure to the nose [12]. Operative techniques for the majority of Middle Eastern patients who have normal skin thickness are less variable. For these patients, debulking of the skin envelope and major tip alteration techniques that are destructive or divisional should be avoided altogether. Since the treatment for patients with thick versus normal skin is very different, preoperative assessment and planning are essential [15].

15.4.2.2 Dorsum

Most of the dorsal reduction is completed in the cartilaginous vault. To achieve moderate dorsal reduction, an incremental approach is preferred. Reduction may be achieved with a rasp for bony regions and scissors for cartilaginous regions of the vault. For predominately bony humps that are cephalically dominant, reduction may average 2.5 mm or more and will extend into the radix area. In these patients, burr can be used to establish appropriate height of radix region. Reduction of anterior cartilage is usually minimal [15]. Dorsal humps that are osseocartilaginous will require greater reduction of cartilage (approximately 3.5 mm) than bone (approximately 1.5 mm). Accordingly, cartilaginous humps will require very little bone reduction (<0.5 mm) but may require cartilage resection of 4 mm or greater. Due to the significant amount of cartilage removed, spreader grafts or Byrd's "auto-spreader flap" [32] are used to stabilize the internal valve angle in cartilaginous vaults. This added support helps prevent collapse of the midvault, resulting in the displeasing inverted-V deformity, and ensures a patent internal valve. These supportive grafts will also prevent this deformity in bony or osseocartilaginous humps

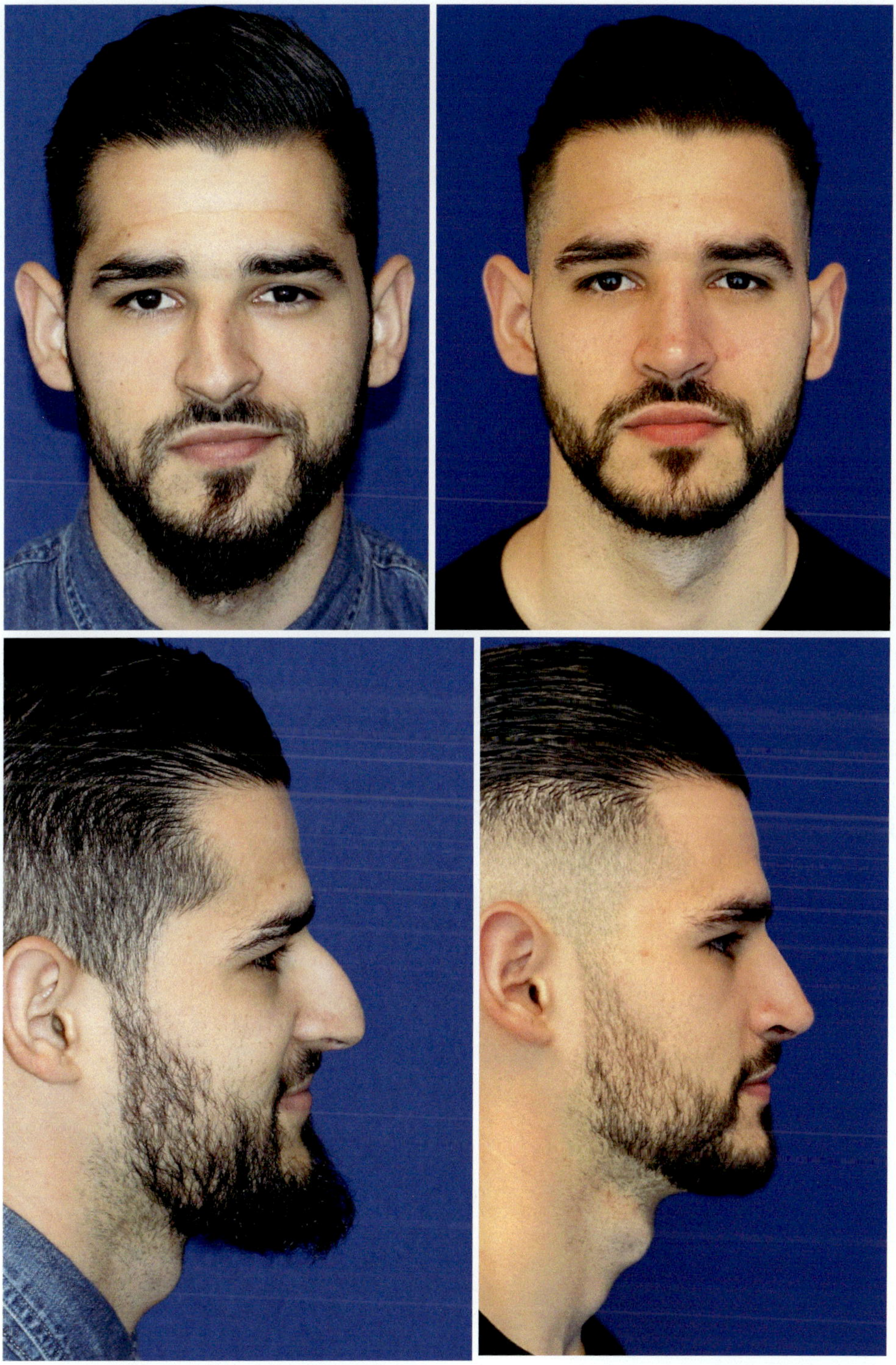

Fig. 15.1 Preoperative photographs of a 28-year-old Hispanic male patient, displaying a characteristic type 1 (Castilian nose) with a moderately arched osseocartilaginous vault and deviation of the nasal tip and lower nose, are shown in Fig. 15. The postoperative image demonstrates surgical correction achieved through incremental hump reduction and a columellar strut to refine tip definition. The dorsum was reconstructed using spreader flaps and centralized with septal rotation sutures. Nasal tip contour, projection, and rotation were enhanced with a columellar strut and bilateral alar rim grafts

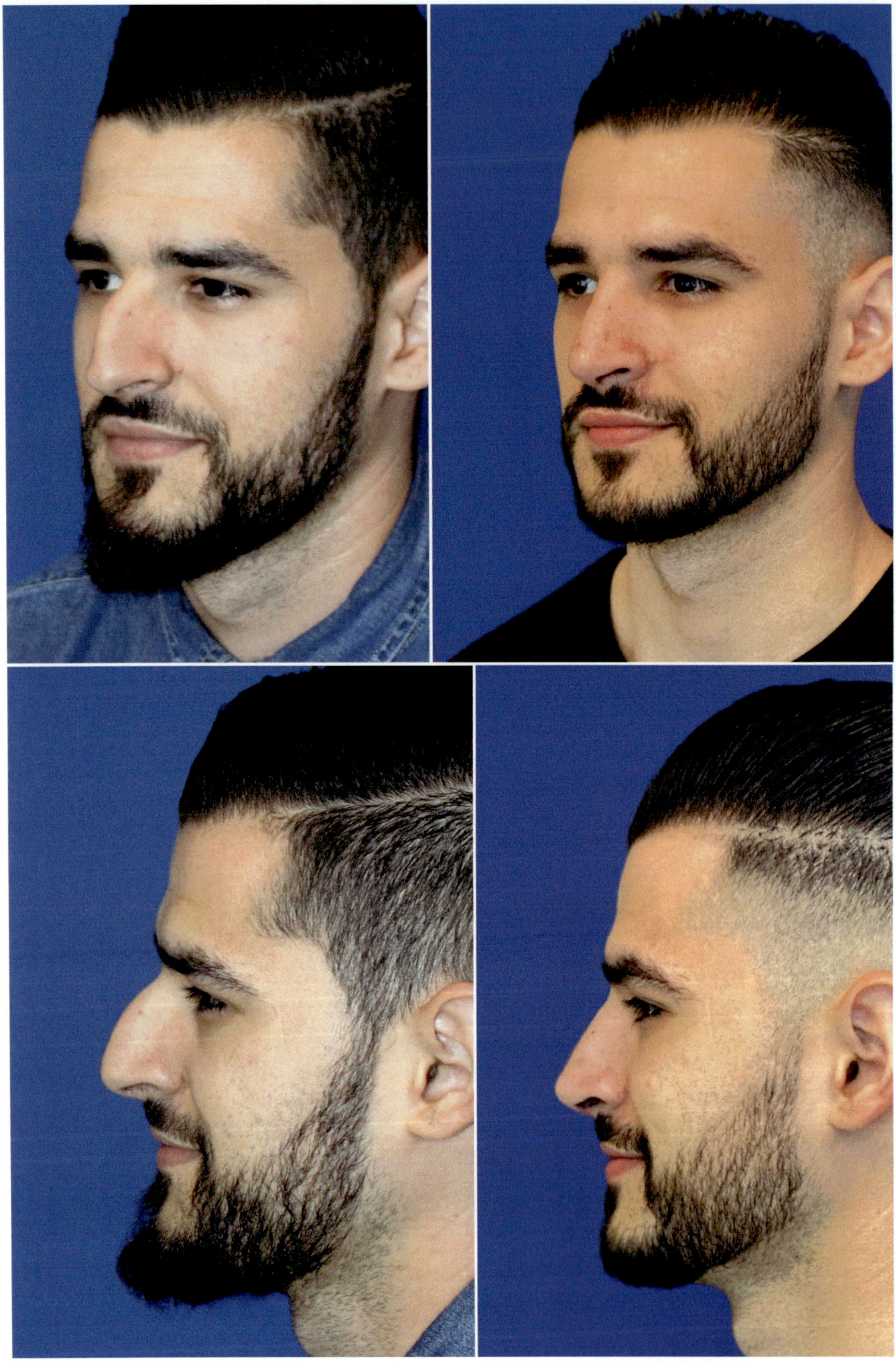

Fig. 15.1 (continued)

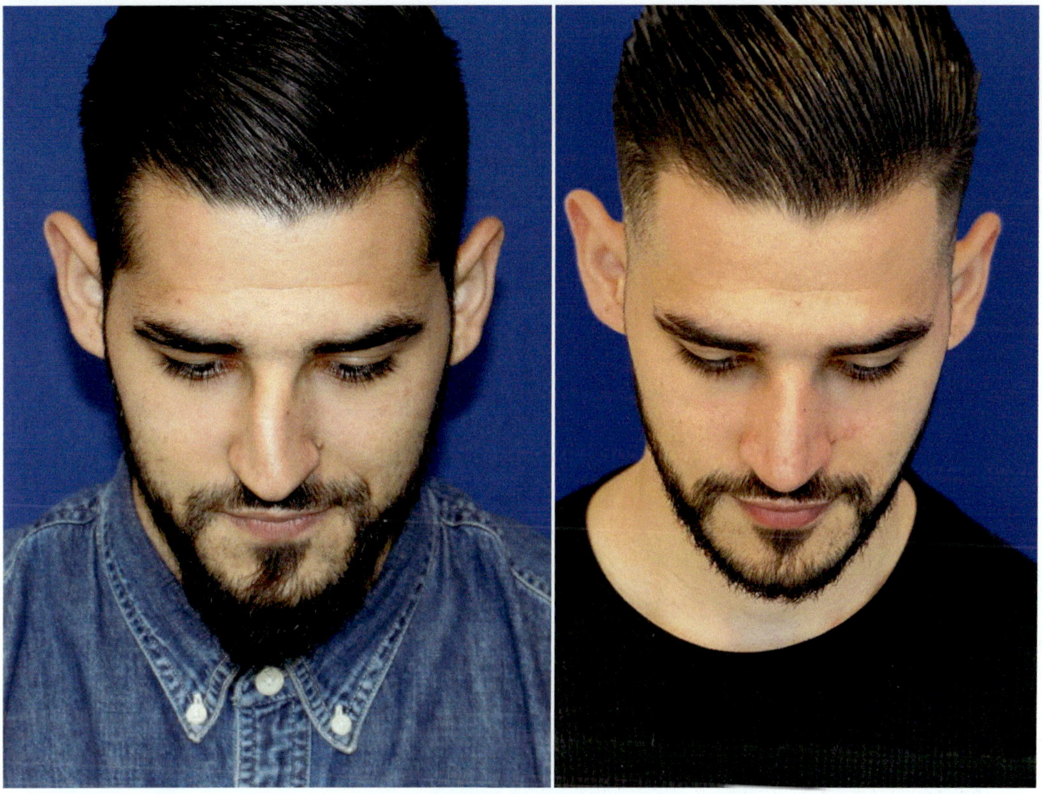

Fig. 15.1 (continued)

where there has been an extensive amount of reduction (Fig. 15.2).

15.4.2.3 Alar Base/Nostrils

In over half of Middle Eastern rhinoplasty patients, in order to enhance nostril shape, the alar base width needs to be reduced, along with narrowing of the nostril sills [33]. To minimize any visible scars, nostril sill excision extending into the alar crease can be used. A preferred nostril-to-tip ratio is 60:40 for an aesthetically pleasing appearance [15]. To address alar flaring with a large nostril size, complete wedge excision may occasionally be required. This operative technique involves an incision that extends into the vestibule and reduces the flaring. Similarly, vestibular sill excision can be used in patients with wide nostril width. Excessive alar base narrowing should be avoided as it can lead to racial incongruity. To address undesirable tip position (poor projection and/or droopy tip) commonly found in Middle Eastern rhinoplasty patients, a strong columnar strut is needed to support and reconfigure weak alar cartilages. Columellar strut is essential for creating a favorable platform to maintain tip shape and position in the long term.

In addition, columellar strut will also prevent tip droop upon smiling, especially when open structure rhinoplasty approach is utilized. Other procedures that will establish proper tip position include removal of excess tissues by performing caudal septal resection and excision of redundant lining.

15.4.2.4 Lateral Cartilages

Middle Eastern rhinoplasty patients often present with extreme width of the upper lateral cartilages at their scroll junction with alar cartilages [12]. It is necessary to surgically disrupt the lateral junction between upper lateral cartilage and lateral crura by either resecting the excess cephalic lat-

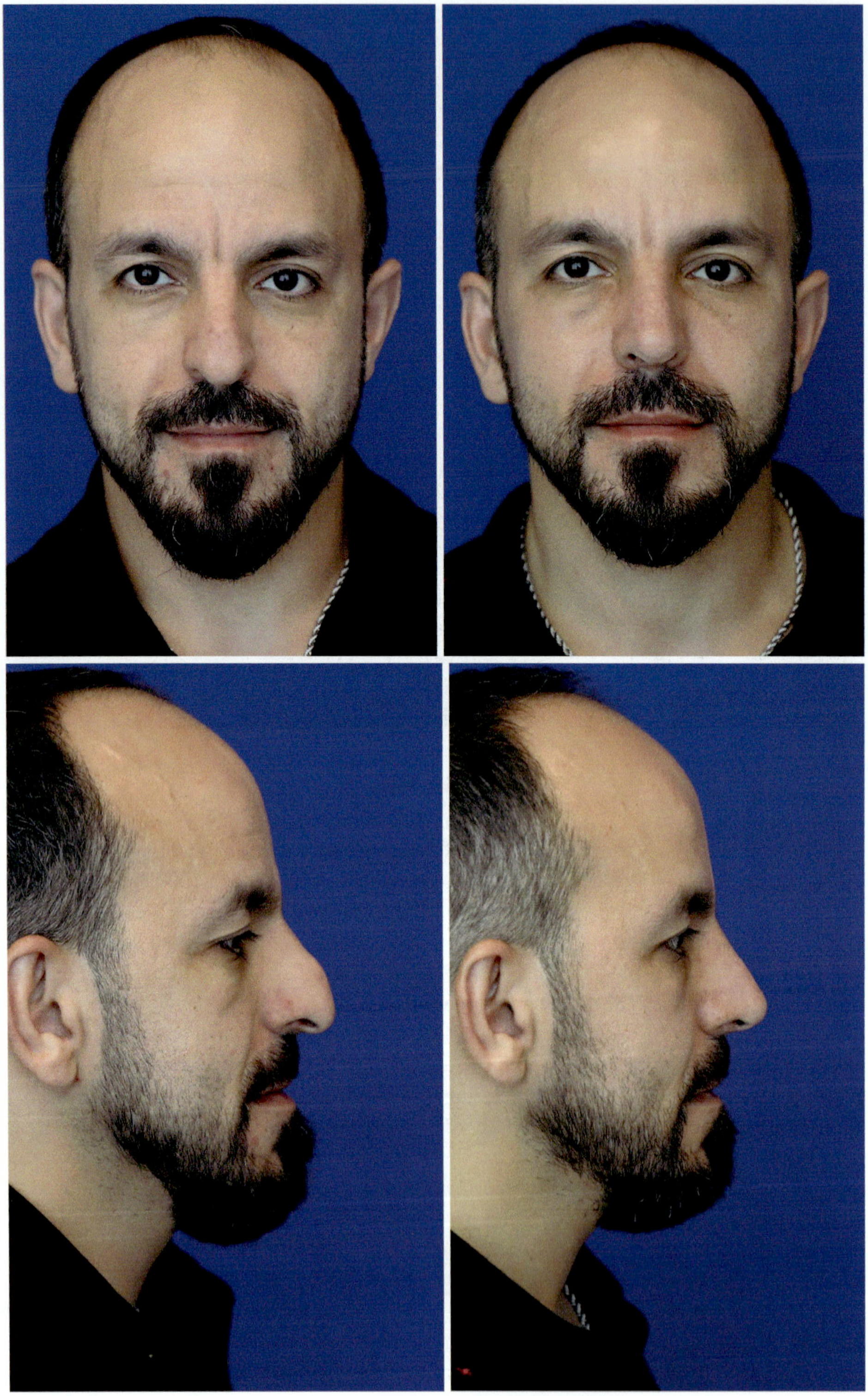

Fig. 15.2 Preoperative images of a Middle Eastern male, 35 years old patient, with a deviated septum to the left, with a high-arched osseocartilaginous vault and under-projected, and under-defined tip. The after image shows surgical correction with caudal septal relocation, septal extension graft tip support, and multiple sutures in the tip to stabilize and support the position of the nasal tip. The dorsum was reduced with component reduction and reconstructed with the aid of bilateral spreader flaps and bilateral spreader grafts

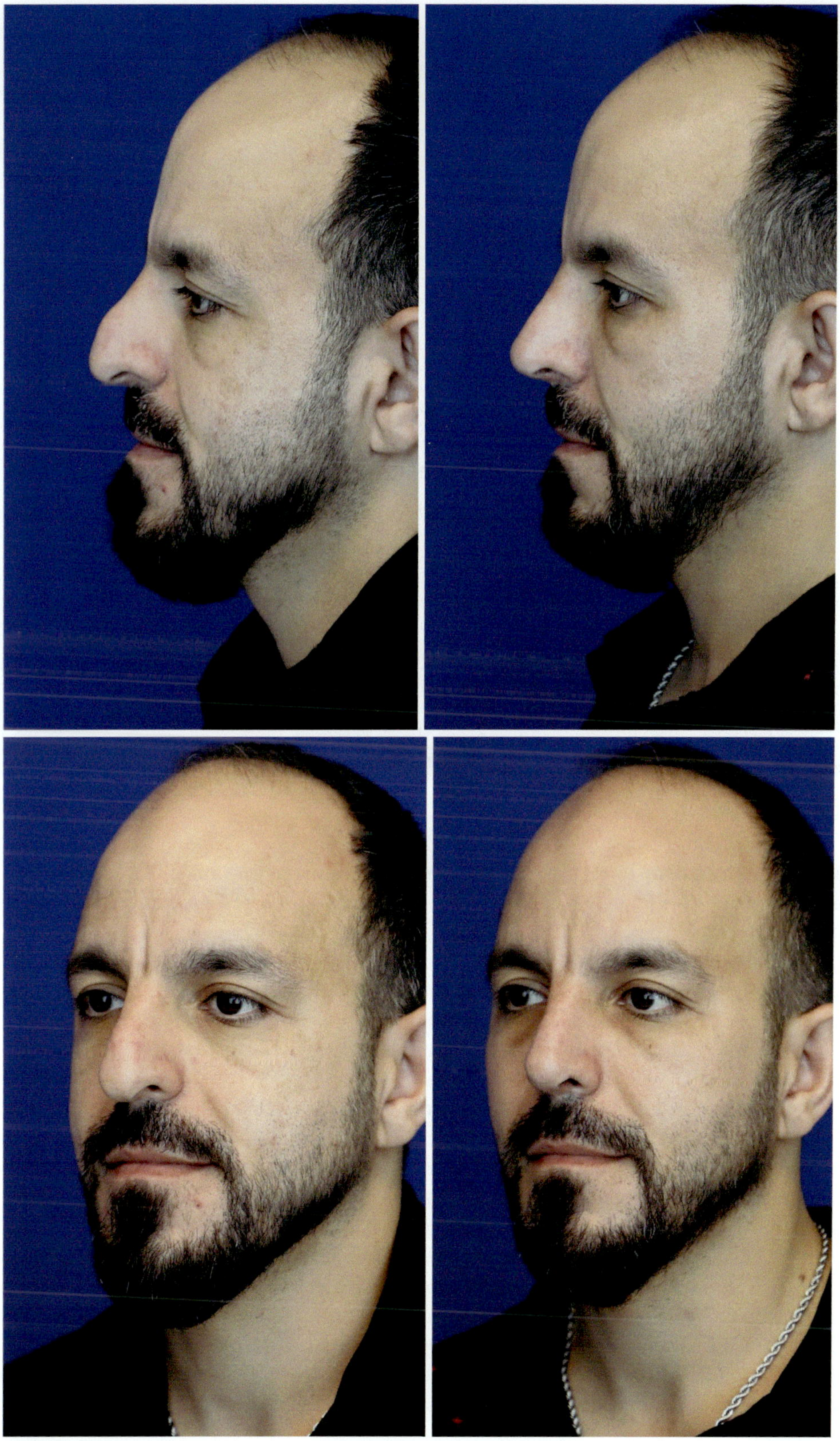

Fig. 15.2 (continued)

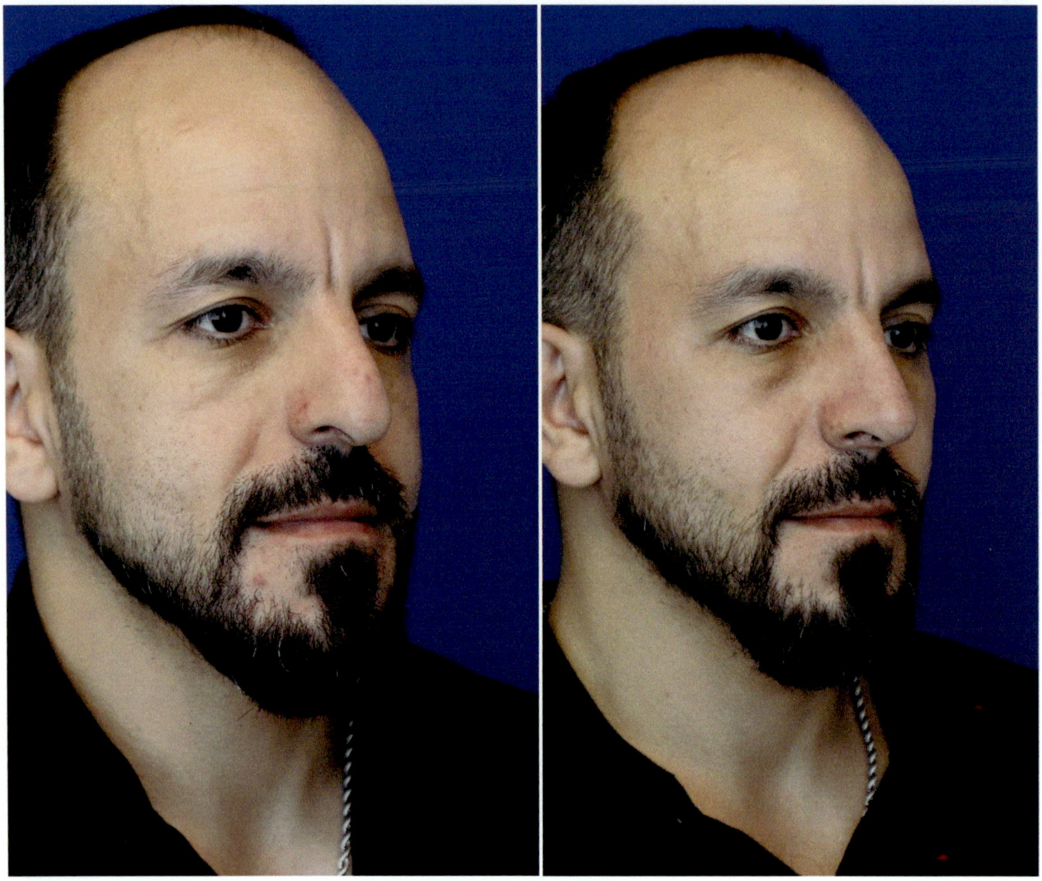

Fig. 15.2 (continued)

eral crura or by a sharp direct division with cartilage preservation [12].

15.4.2.5 Septum

Most Middle Eastern rhinoplasty patients have severe septal deviation that can create significant functional and aesthetic deformities. Caudal septal relocation is commonly performed for over half of Middle Eastern patients to address and correct this anatomical issue. Because septal deviation in Middle Eastern patients is often in conjunction with overall asymmetry in the face, the patient must in informed of the limitations to correcting septal deviation. Due to the importance of the septum in providing tip support, caudal septal vestibular resection and suturing may be required to maintain tip position. In addition, a cartilaginous septum that contributes significantly to the dorsal hump may require alteration. When septal resection is performed, the surgeon may harvest excess cartilage for use as grafts as needed.

15.4.3 Operative Techniques in African-American Rhinoplasty

15.4.3.1 Nasal Tip

Increased tip definition is a common request for any patient of rhinoplasty regardless of background. This is no exception for African-American patients. However, the achievability of the result is due to the skin thickness of the patient. To successfully achieve narrowing of the nasal tip, domal and inter-domal sutures can be utilized [26].

Permanent sutures can be used for long-lasting results. For patients with thick skin, lateral crura strut grafts or a shield-shaped tip graft can be used for further definition [26].

Nasal tip projection may be lacking in many patients as well, who present with an acute nasolabial angle and alar columellar disproportion. Nasal tip projection should be counterbalanced with augmentation or reduction of the nasal dorsum as the structure to support the tip can be heavy. To improve nasal tip projection, a cap graft can be used from conchal cartilage. For patients who do not have thick skin, a columellar strut can be combined with lateral crura steal [26]. For those patients with heavy, thick skin, a shield-shaped tip graft and cap graft is the better option to increase tip projection. For patients with a short nose or a nose with a foreshortened caudal septum, a caudal extension graft can be used instead of columellar struts to provide tip support. This method also reorients vertically oriented lower lateral cartilages as it provides a more caudal position to the lateral aspect of the cartilages in relation to the dome [26].

15.4.3.2 Nasal Width

In many cases, patients prefer a width adjustment in the upper, middle, or lower thirds of the nose. A challenge to adjusting the upper third of the nose is short splayed nasal bones, and medial and lateral osteotomies that can narrow this portion. In this case, intermediate osteotomies can be utilized to medialize the upper third of the nose. For patients who can tolerate augmentation, addition of septal cartilage can also provide a visual image of a narrower nose [26]. For patients with a wide alar base, alar base reduction with internal wedge excision can be used to adjust the alar width. Excision of vestibular skin, along with preservation of a medial skin flap, will reduce nostril size and decrease the likelihood of nasal sill notching. It is important to note that alar base reduction should not be performed when the nostrils are wide but not flared, as this will cause a pinched appearance of the nose due to decreasing the angle between the alae and the nasal base [16].

15.4.3.3 Dorsum

Most African-American rhinoplasty patients present with deficient nasal structural support. Therefore, it is important to consider augmentation in addition to reduction methods in order to ensure functionality as well as aesthetically pleasing results [16].

African-American patients fall into three categories regarding dorsal adjustment needs as classified by Ofodile in 1995. The first is those African Americans who have dorsal convexity and require reduction [34]. The second type is said to have "low" nasal dorsum and will require augmentation. Septal cartilage, auricular cartilage, or rib cartilage can be used to achieve the desired effect. It is important to note that due to poor scar formation, many African-American patients should be consulted and informed preoperatively if rib cartilage is to be harvested for the procedure.

15.4.4 Operative Techniques in Asian Rhinoplasty

Since augmentation techniques are used to achieve results for Asian rhinoplasty, this section will discuss the methods of harvesting graft material, as well as addressing the primary concerns for Asian rhinoplasty patients: tip refinement, dorsal adjustment, and alar base adjustment.

15.4.4.1 Graft Material

Both autologous and alloplastic materials can be used to achieve augmentation results. Common autologous tissues used for dorsal augmentation include septal cartilage, conchal cartilage, and costal cartilage. Although it is easy to harvest and shape septal cartilage, due to the small septal cartilage of Asian patients, it is difficult to harvest sufficient septal cartilage to achieve the desired augmentation results. In this case, conchal cartilage can be harvested through a retroauricular incision, as opposed to an anterior incision, which would present a visible anterior scar [20].

Costal cartilage can also be used but the risk of scarring on the chest should be explained to the patient. Various alloplastic materials can also be utilized in Asian rhinoplasty, although they are traditionally condemned in Caucasian rhinoplasty. Indeed, due to the thick skin and weak cartilaginous framework found in Asian patients, alloplastic implants used in Asian rhinoplasty can be highly beneficial, but need to be nontoxic, nonimmunogenic, and be able to maintain their original texture and shape [24]. Traditionally, the most commonly used alloplastic materials have been Gore-Tex and Silicone. Considerations for extrusion and infection should be carefully considered, and whenever possible, autologous materials should be used in favor of alloplastic implants.

15.4.4.2 Nasal Tip Refinement

For Asian nasal tip refinement, the goal is to lengthen the short columella and reorient the round nostrils in a more vertical format [20]. Three tip graft techniques are discussed in this section.

15.4.4.3 Cartilage Graft Technique

This technique is the most common for improving tip support, projection, and definition. Autologous graft material is preferred. When septal cartilage is insufficient, conchal or costal cartilage can be utilized. It is important to note the risk of over-rotation of the tip from a blunting of the columellar lobular angle. In addition, the thick skin of Asian patients will likely compress and bend the cartilage when the nose is covered again with skin. Thus, to achieve the desired tip adjustment and appropriate projection, it is recommended to utilize a shield supporting graft cephalically [24].

15.4.4.4 Shield Graft Technique

A shield graft is positioned above the middle and medial crus of the lower lateral cartilages, and shaped, rightfully so, in the shape of a shield. This will lengthen the infra-tip lobular segment and help obtain optimal tip projection. It is important to note that vertically and horizontally oriented shield grafts depend on the shape and orientation of the underlying lower lateral cartilage. If an Asian patient presents with an under-projected tip with a round contour, a vertically oriented shelf graft or only graft can worsen the overall nasal shape and should be avoided. In this case, a multilayer tip graft can be a more beneficial alternative. In this method, caudal extension of the septum, modification of the lower lateral cartilages, columellar strut placement, and dome suturing are performed before the first shield graft is placed on the dome [24]. The number of graft layers used depends on the overall tip projection desired.

15.4.4.5 Onlay Graft Technique

Onlay grafting is a procedure that places horizontally oriented grafts at the dome of the tip. This method is only beneficial to patients with proper tip support to increase their tip projection or camouflage irregularities. It is favorable to place a columellar strut to project the middle crus and strengthen the tip support before positioning the onlay graft on the dome. This method is called an umbrella graft and prevents the infra-tip lobule area from appearing excessively long when viewed from the basal side [24].

15.4.4.6 Dorsal Augmentation

The thickness of the patient's skin should be taken into consideration when creating a surgical plan for dorsal augmentation. For patients with thin skin, excessive dorsal augmentation can create a risk of implant visibility or extrusion. Thus, soft implant materials such as fascia or morselized cartilage should be used. Conversely, for patients with thick skin, stronger implant material such as silicone or costal cartilage should be used. The preferred choice of costal cartilage is the fifth or sixth rib accessed through an inframammary incision [20].

Asian patients often present with weak and mal-positioned alar cartilages, with a wide alar base. The goal is to transform the round nostrils into an oval shape. To prevent scarring and weakening of the alar rim, a modified nostril sill excision should be performed by angulating the excision so it tapers on the alar crease for 3–4 mm [20]. Alar rim support grafts should be used to support rim strength and nostril shape [20].

15.5 Potential Problems

Correction of deviated nose

Correction of a deviated nose typically involves an open approach and releasing of all the attachments of mucoperichondrial and mucoperiosteal attachments as well as removal of the posterior part of the septum attachments to the vomer and perpendicular plate of the ethmoid. The key is always to create a straight midline septum and parallel dorsal aesthetic lines. Typically, scoring and suturing via horizontal and vertical mattress sutures are used to achieve this goal, along with the placement of spreader grafts. (Fig. 15.3)

15.5.1 Potential Problems in Hispanic Rhinoplasty

Due to the variety in racial mixture, no single technique can be used for the correction of a Hispanic nose. Type II (Mexican American) noses can be especially challenging and require a strong surgical plan and finesse. Surgeons can maximize their success by carefully studying their patients and analytically organizing a pre-surgical analysis rather than assuming that what is present in a Hispanic nose is similar to a Caucasian nose. For example, the mid-dorsal humps seen in some Hispanic noses may not be

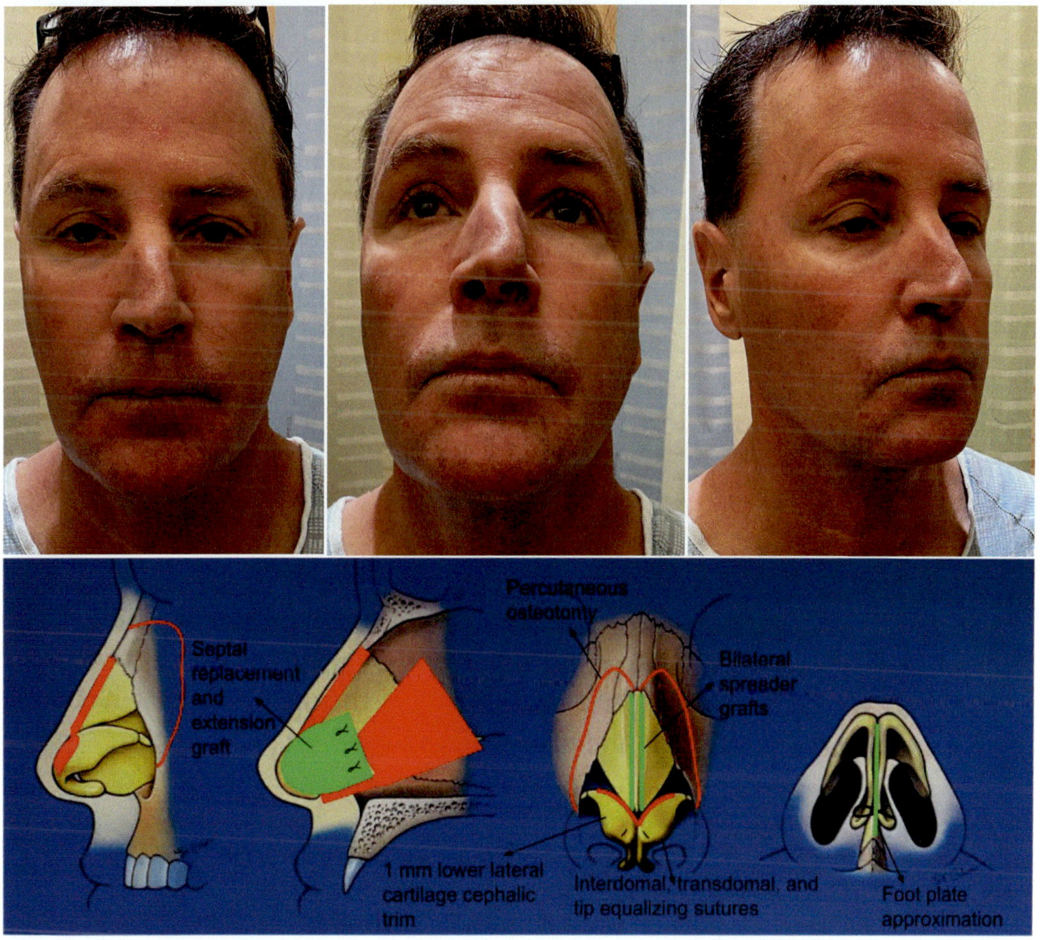

Fig. 15.3 Preoperative and postoperative view of a patient with long-standing nasal deviation and nasal airway obstruction. Rhinoplasty procedure included component reduction, septoplasty, and reconstruction, including caudal septal replacement and placement of septal extension graft and bilateral spreader grafts. Tip suturing included hem-domal, dome-equalizing, and intermodal sutures. Postoperative views show correction of deviation and asymmetry as well as improvement of the dorsum and nasal tip

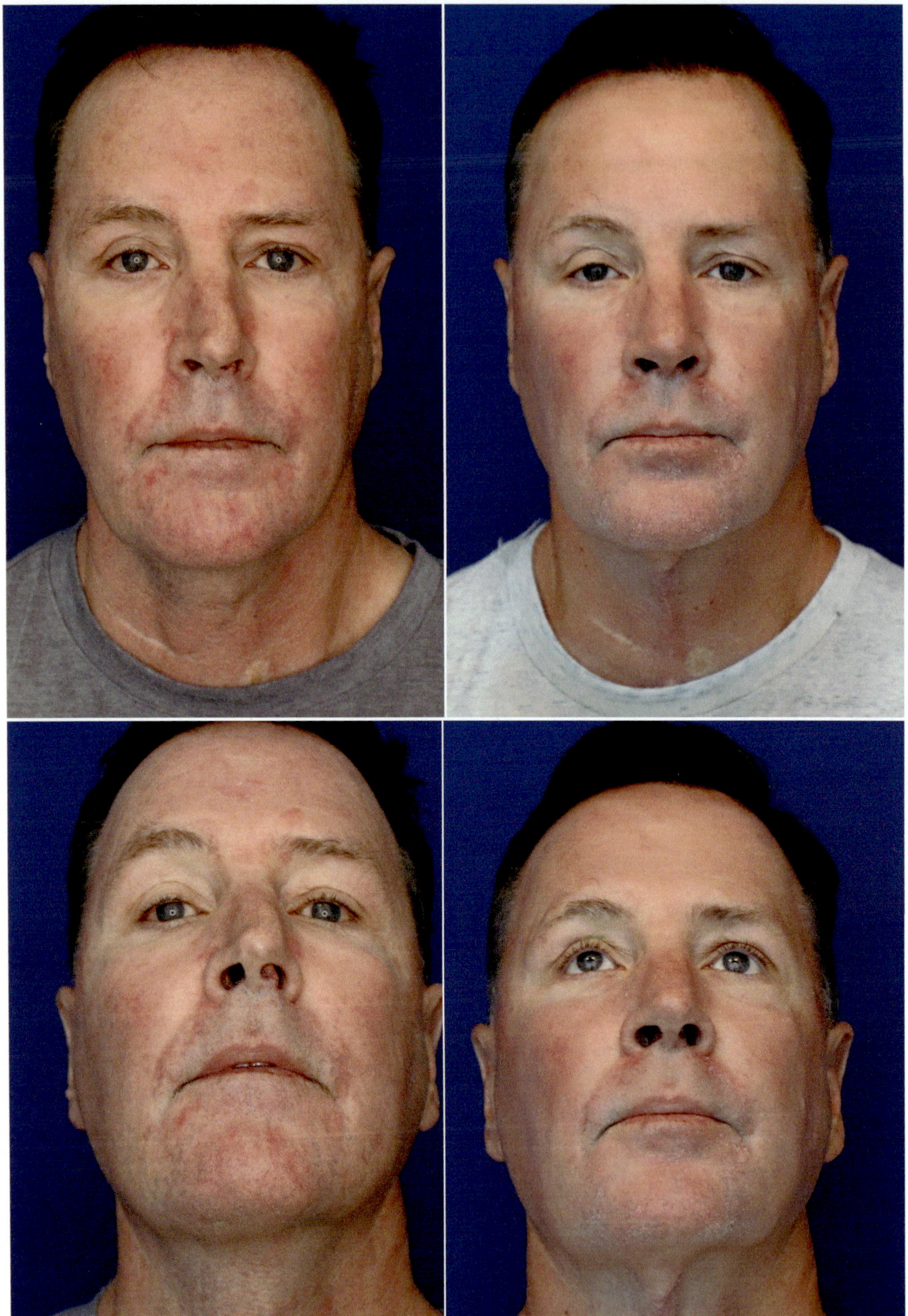

Fig. 15.3 (continued)

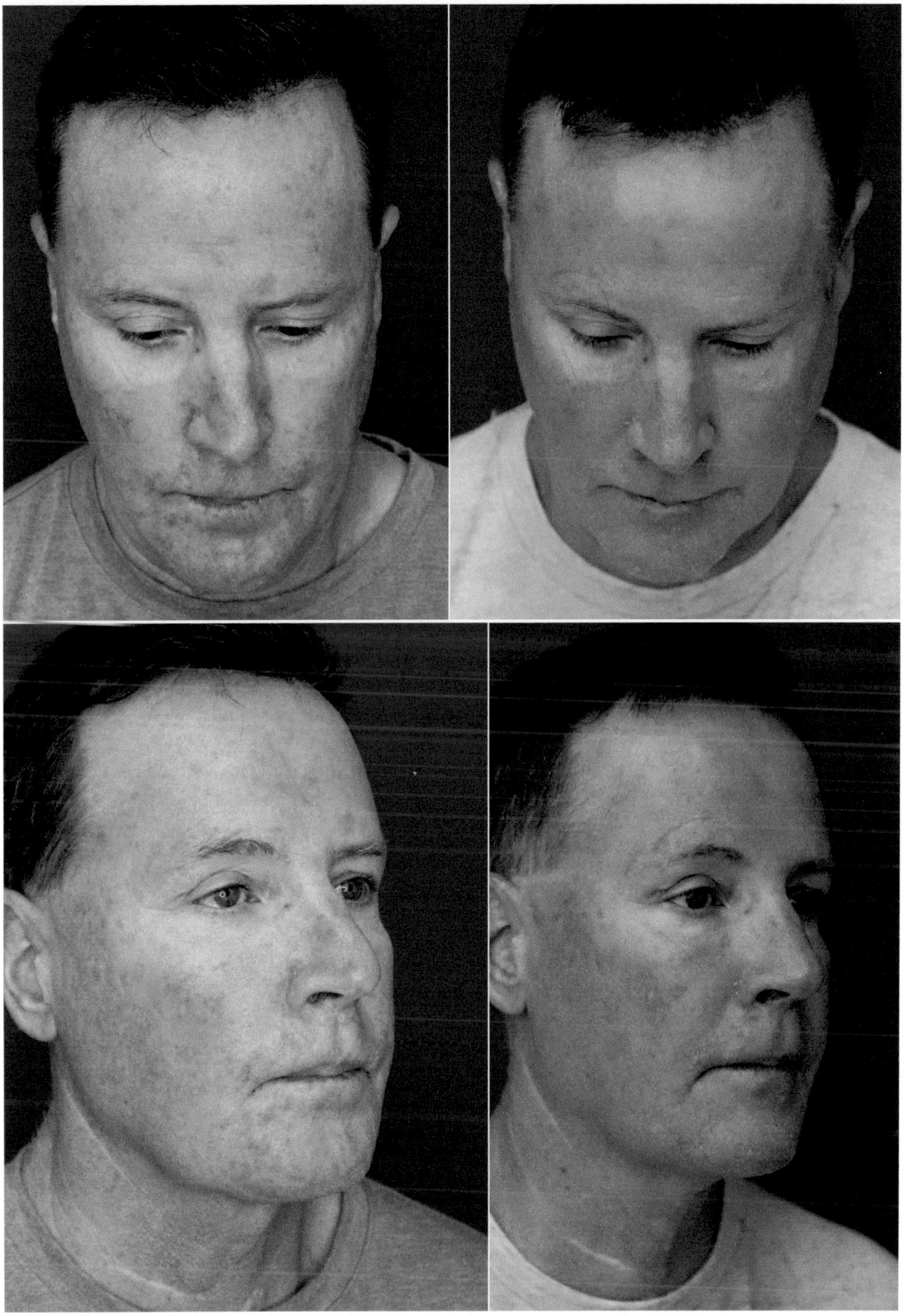

Fig. 15.3 (continued)

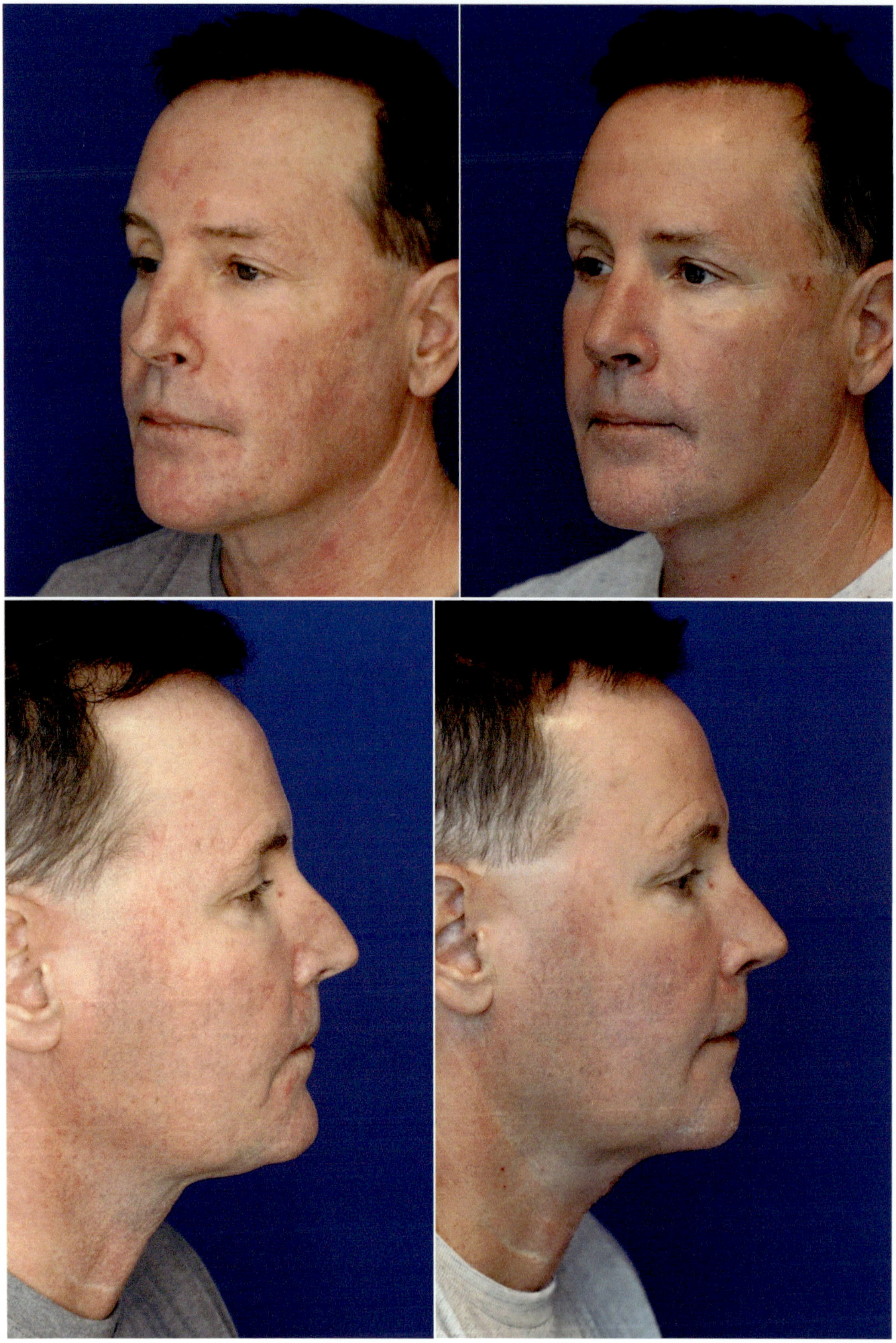

Fig. 15.3 (continued)

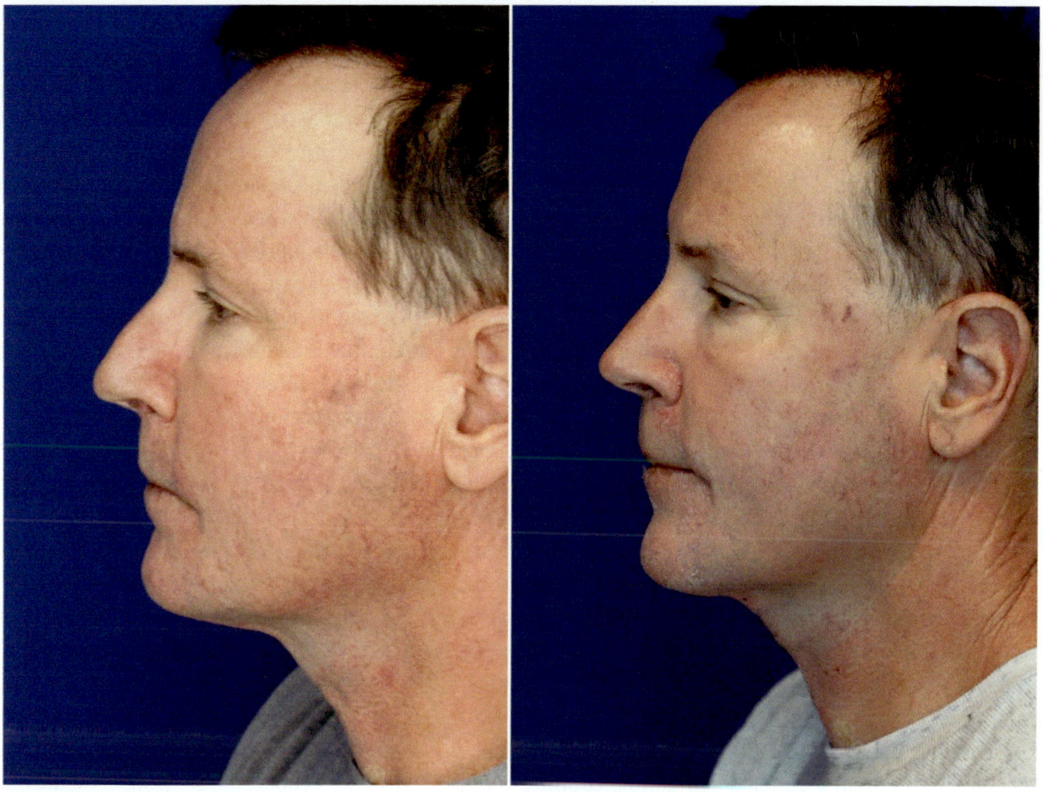

Fig. 15.3 (continued)

true humps at all, but rather "pseudo-humps" due to the lack of tip protrusion and the low nasal starting points in that population. Female patients are more likely to exhibit this dorsal pseudo-hump. Increasing the tip projection can reduce the necessity and extent of dorsal hump reduction [26]. Another example is how the prominence of the Hispanic premaxilla can make it appear as if the patient has a ptotic appearance of the Hispanic nasal tip [11]. Furthermore, for the inside nasal framework to be seen on the outside, the overlying skin must be thin and pliable so that it can drape over the framework. Due to the thicker skin of Hispanic patients, this draping can be harder to accomplish, and thinning the nasal skin to conform to the underlying framework is not always effective. Because the Hispanic nasal cartilage tends to be weak, a good plan is to augment and strengthen the underlying skeleton with cartilage grafts to achieve this draping effect [11]. This is important to note, as previous misconceptions believe that reducing the nasal skeleton should make thick noses more delicate and refined. However, the Hispanic skin is so thick and the cartilages so weak that forming a defined, angular nasal tip by trimming cartilages is not recommended. Due to the thick and oily quality of skin, Hispanics tend to take longer to heal than Caucasian patients, and grafting can cause prolonged swelling. Scars can take longer to mature and the patient needs to be educated regarding the timing of their healing process. Expectations need to be discussed between surgeon and patient as studies have demonstrated that surgery on Hispanic noses did not bring either tip definition or skin thickness to within Western standards [11].

15.5.2 Potential Problems in Middle Eastern Rhinoplasty

Middle Eastern patients who request secondary surgery can be categorized by the patient's presenting complaints five main groups by Daniel's 2009 paper "Middle Eastern Rhinoplasty in the United States: Part II. Secondary Rhinoplasty":

Group 1 patients had an acceptable "natural result," but wanted a smaller and more refined nose and tip. The original surgeon was pleased with the results, but the patient could not be counseled to be satisfied. Group 2 patients felt that their primary deformity had not been completely corrected and that their nose was still too long and too droopy. The dorsal hump reduction combined with a failure to respect the caudal septum had produced a nose that appeared longer. Group 3 patients felt they had unnatural results, and wanted to eliminate the visible surgical stigmata that arise from tip bosses, alar retraction, inverted-V deformity, and an over-resected dorsum [25]. Group 4 patients had major secondary deformities along with functional limitations. Group 5 patients had multiple aggressive procedures that required rib grafts to make the essential aesthetic reconstructions [35]. With the Middle Eastern community being a relatively more knowledgeable patient population in regard to rhinoplasty, their attention to detail and demand for Western yet natural aesthetic results can be challenging to accommodate. This requires communication and patient education from the surgeon in regard to what is realistic both aesthetically and functionally.

15.5.3 Potential Problems in African-American Rhinoplasty

There is a psychosocial implication to African-American rhinoplasty. Often, African American patients reveal during the history taking process that they will feel stigma when sharing their decision to undergo rhinoplasty with their community, as it can be seen as a denial of their heritage. Patients often clearly state that they do not want to look operated on. Many patients do not have another person in their community or direct contact that has had the procedure done. Therefore, oftentimes, they base hopes and desires on inaccurate bases of information [17]. Although in general the African-American patient is usually well adjusted and has reasonable expectations, a discussion should be had with the patient to insure there is transparency with what outcome is possible. Occasionally, it is important to explain to the patient that they may need to undergo other facial plastic procedures such as mentoplasty and maxillary augmentation in conjunction with rhinoplasty to achieve the desired result. The difficult nose type to operate on is the short nose with thick skin, recessed caudal septum, and weak cartilages [26]. In this case, the thick skin envelope proves a challenge as it has tissue memory. Furthermore, the thick skin is often paired with soft lower lateral cartilages. Great preoperative attention to detail, additional structure, and alternative sources for augmentation will allow for a successful surgery and the intended outcome. Another concerning issue regarding African-American rhinoplasty is the potential donor site for autologous cartilage, which is frequently needed to achieve results when structural augmentation is needed. Many African-American patients are hesitant to have auricular or costal cartilage harvested, as there is a great concern for hypertrophic scars, keloids, and post-inflammatory hyperpigmentation. The surgeon should discuss the history of healing and counsel the patient on the possibility of keloid formation at the donor site.

15.5.4 Potential Problems in Asian Rhinoplasty

A possible complication with Asian rhinoplasty arises from the use of alloplastic implants. Although most patients can accept the implant, there is a risk of displacement, extrusion, infection, and thinning of the skin over the implant [36]. It is important to note that the L-shaped silicone implant cannot maintain nasal length and causes shortening of the nose over time [37].

Another consideration is that many Asian women have difficulty consenting to the use of costal cartilage due to the scars it leaves on the chest. Furthermore, the use of costal cartilage presents the risk of warping and graft visibility and requires the utmost precision and skill to create aesthetically and functionally pleasing results. For this reason, the use of costal cartilage for augmentation material is associated with a 15% risk of revision surgery [38]. Another common reason for dissatisfaction with rhinoplasty results is discordance between the expectations of the patient and surgeon. Careful preoperative communication is key to avoiding unrealistic goals that can lead to disappointment.

15.5.5 Preservation Rhinoplasty

Preservation rhinoplasty is a less invasive alternative to traditional rhinoplasty techniques, focusing on preserving the nasal structures (S-ULC, ligaments and soft tissue as well as Lower lateral cartilages) while refining the profile. It is ideal for patients with minor or moderate deformities and well-defined nasal anatomy, or patients with axis deviation of the nose offering natural results with minimal disruption of the septum-upper lateral cartilage (S-ULC) junction.

In comparison to structural rhinoplasty, which involves major reshaping through separation of S-ULC junction or extensive resection of bone, cartilage, and soft tissue, preservation rhinoplasty focuses on maintaining the nasal dorsal framework. It is most effective for patients with minor to moderate deformities such as dorsal humps or asymmetries. The goal is to achieve subtle refinement without removing large amounts of tissue, ensuring both aesthetic and functional outcomes.

Various techniques are employed in preservation rhinoplasty. Surface techniques are the least invasive, focusing on subtle reshaping of the dorsum to improve the profile. Subdorsal reduction is effective for mild humps, preserving the nasal structure while smoothing the profile. Impaction techniques, like the push down and let down methods, are ideal for moderate deformities. Push down involves applying downward pressure to flatten prominent humps, while let down releases tension by removing small fragments of ascending process of maxilla or nasal bones allowing cartilage to settle naturally for a smoother transition. High strip subdorsal reduction removes a strip of cartilage from the upper dorsum, correcting moderate to large humps while maintaining the overall nasal framework. Low strip reduction removes part of the lower septum, gradually lowering the dorsum and providing predictable results for significant deformities. (Fig. 15.4)

Overall, preservation rhinoplasty offers a less invasive approach for refining the nose with subtle adjustments. It is particularly effective for patients with moderate deformities and well-preserved nasal anatomy, with specific technique selection playing a key role in achieving optimal results. (Fig. 15.4)

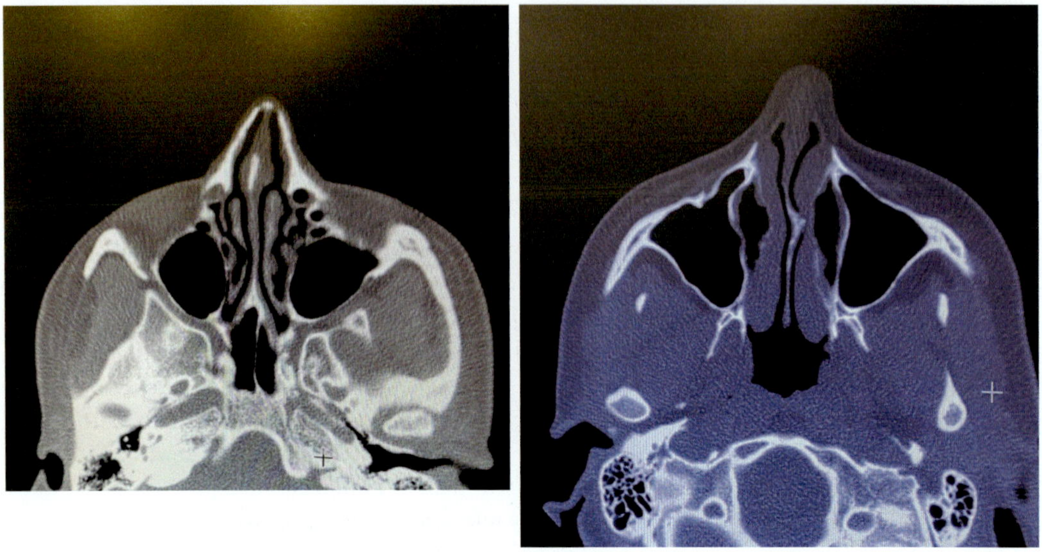

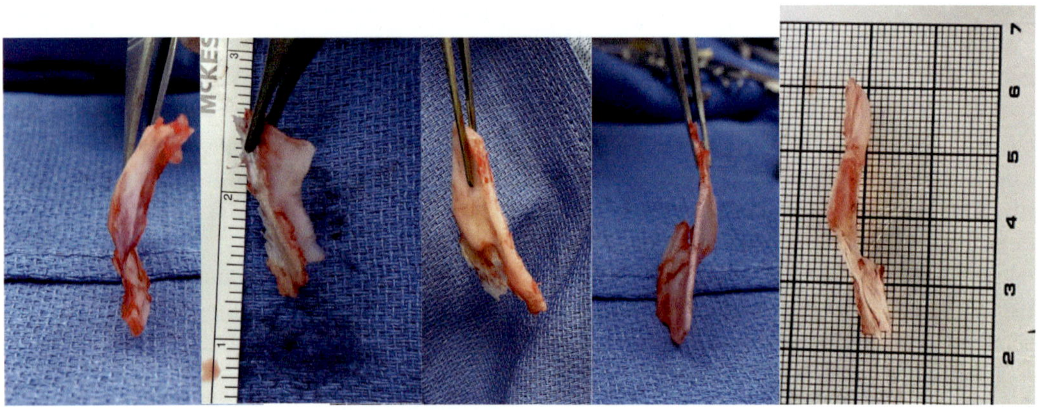

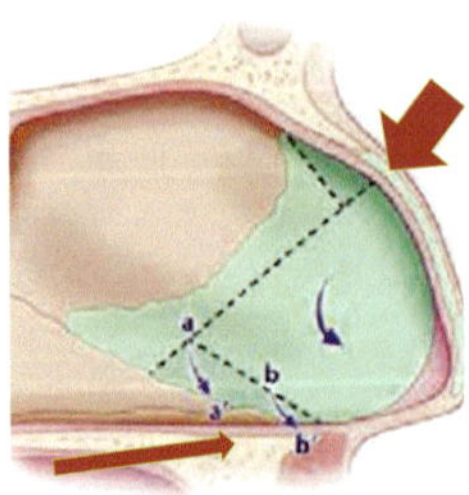

Fig. 15.4 Preoperative photographs of an 18-year-old with congenitally deviated and asymmetric nose with significant overprotection and dorsal hump. Postoperative views after a 5 mm cartilaginous dorsum reduction using preservation rhinoplasty techniques (Cottle- low strip letdown technique) with deprotecting the dorsum and reducing the dorsal hump. A 5 mm osteotomy of the lateral nasal wall and ascending process of the maxilla was done on the left side with dorsal root osteotomy, and lateral percutaneous osteotomy allowed centralization of the nasal pyramid and improved harmony of the nasal and facial features. Tip columellar strut and alar rim grafts were used to improve support and contour of the nasal tip

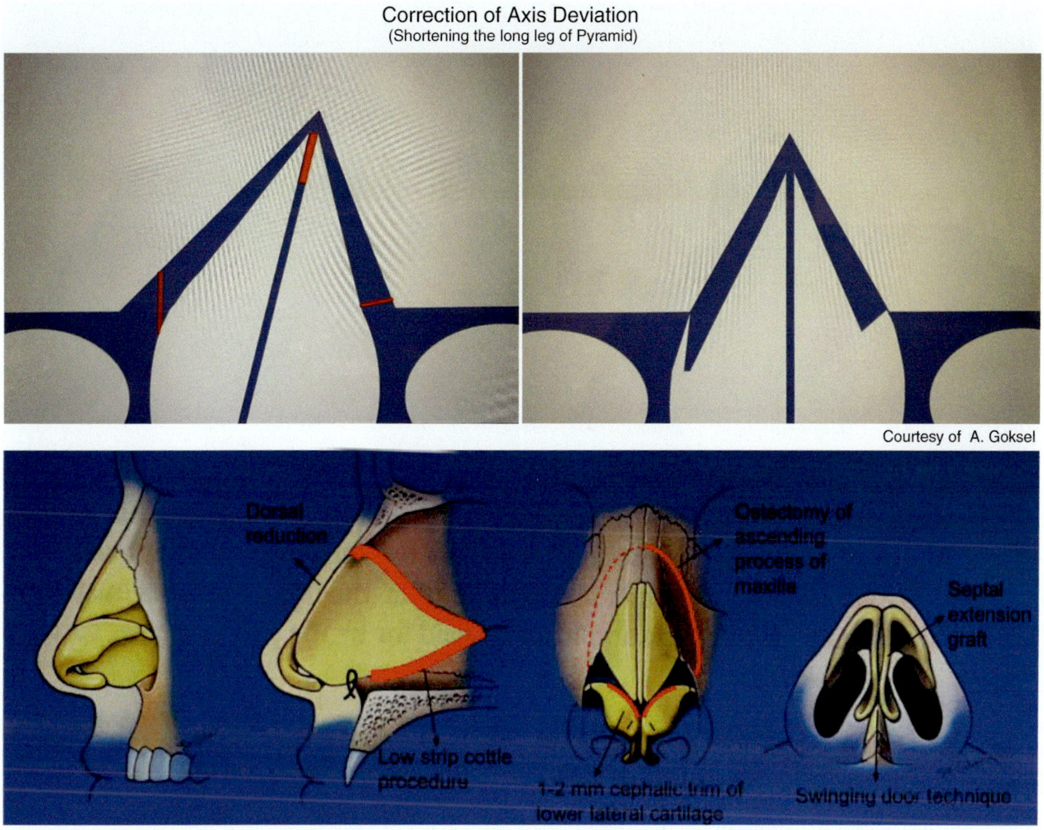

Fig. 15.4 (continued)

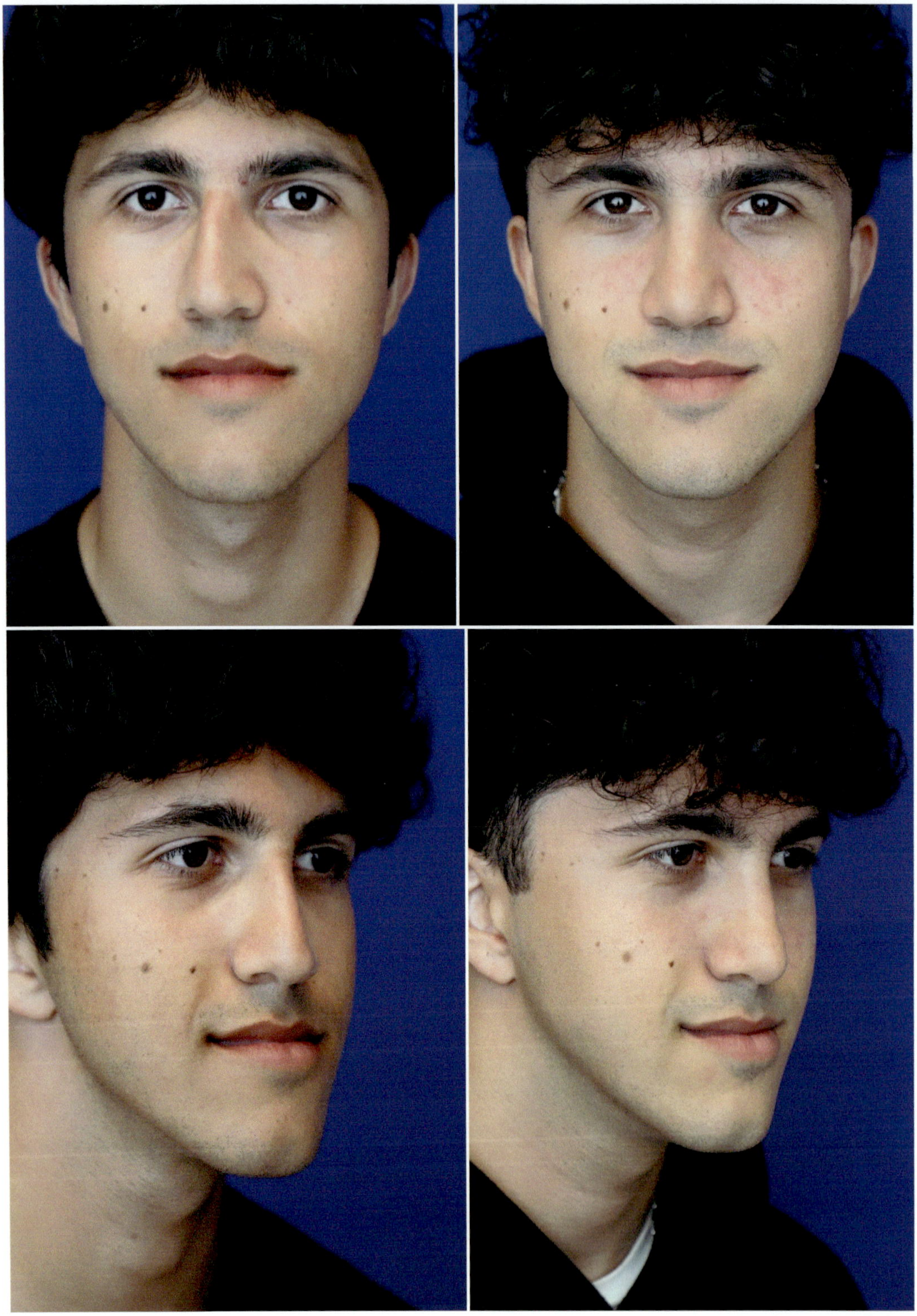

Fig. 15.4 (continued)

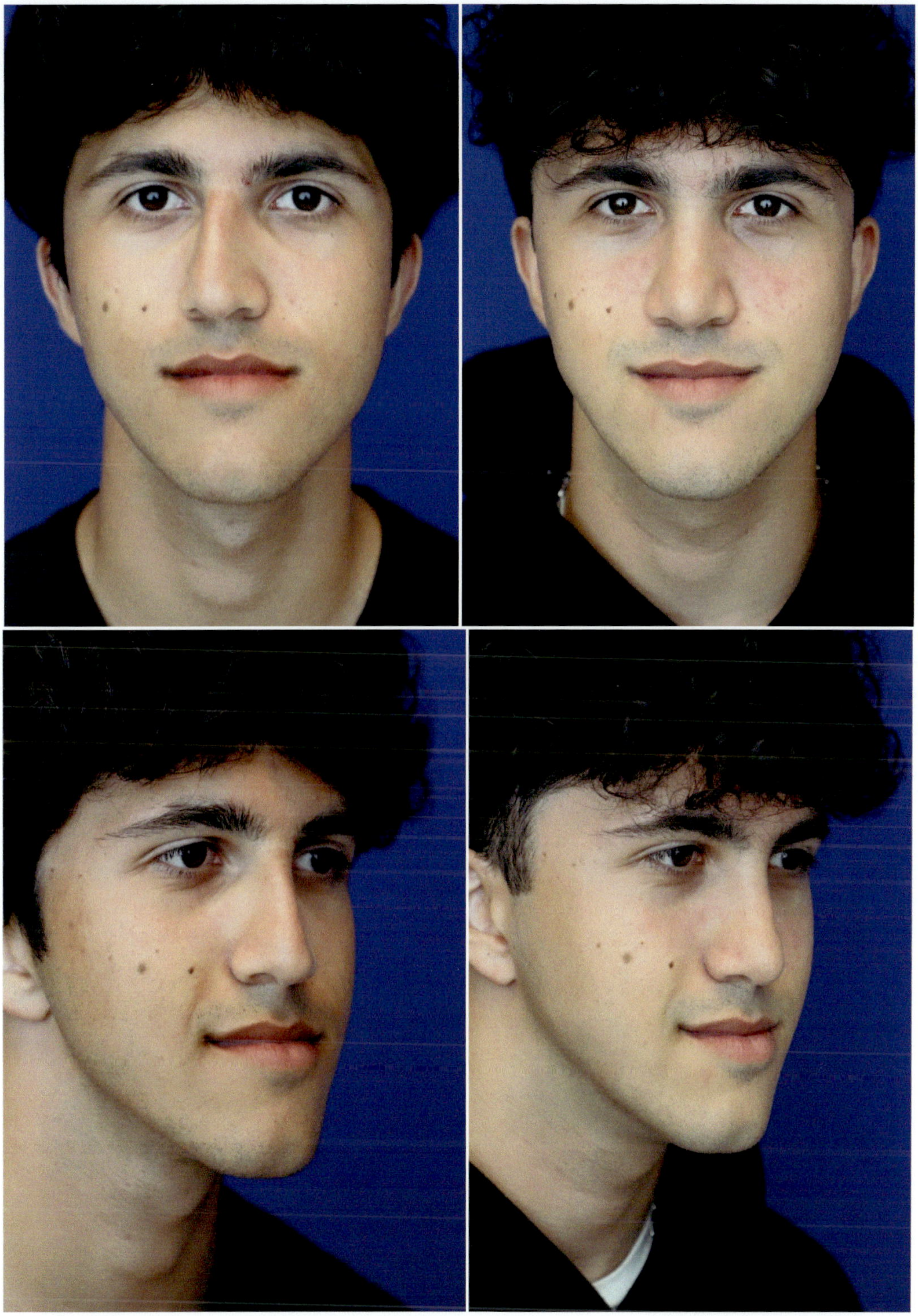

Fig. 15.4 (continued)

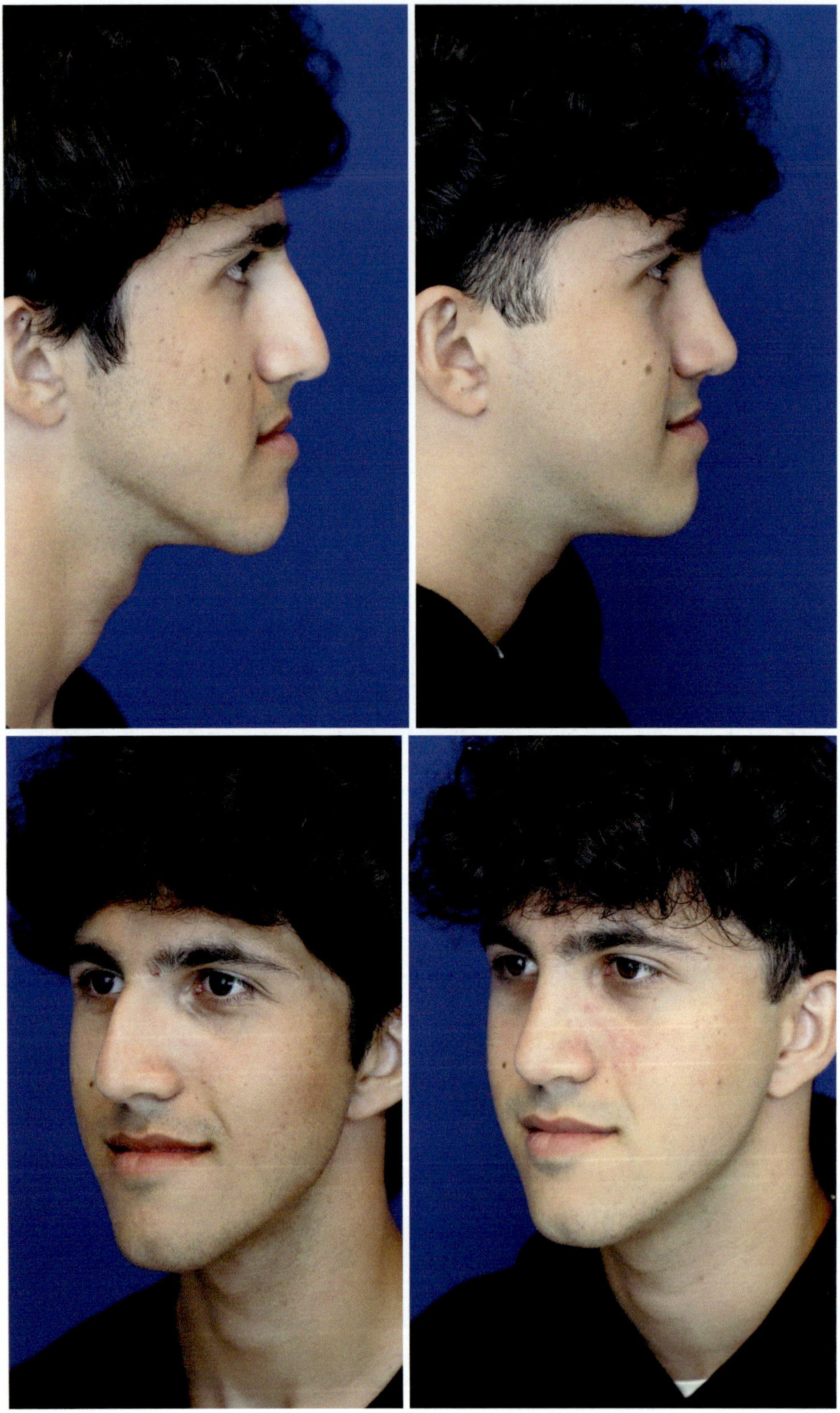

Fig. 15.4 (continued)

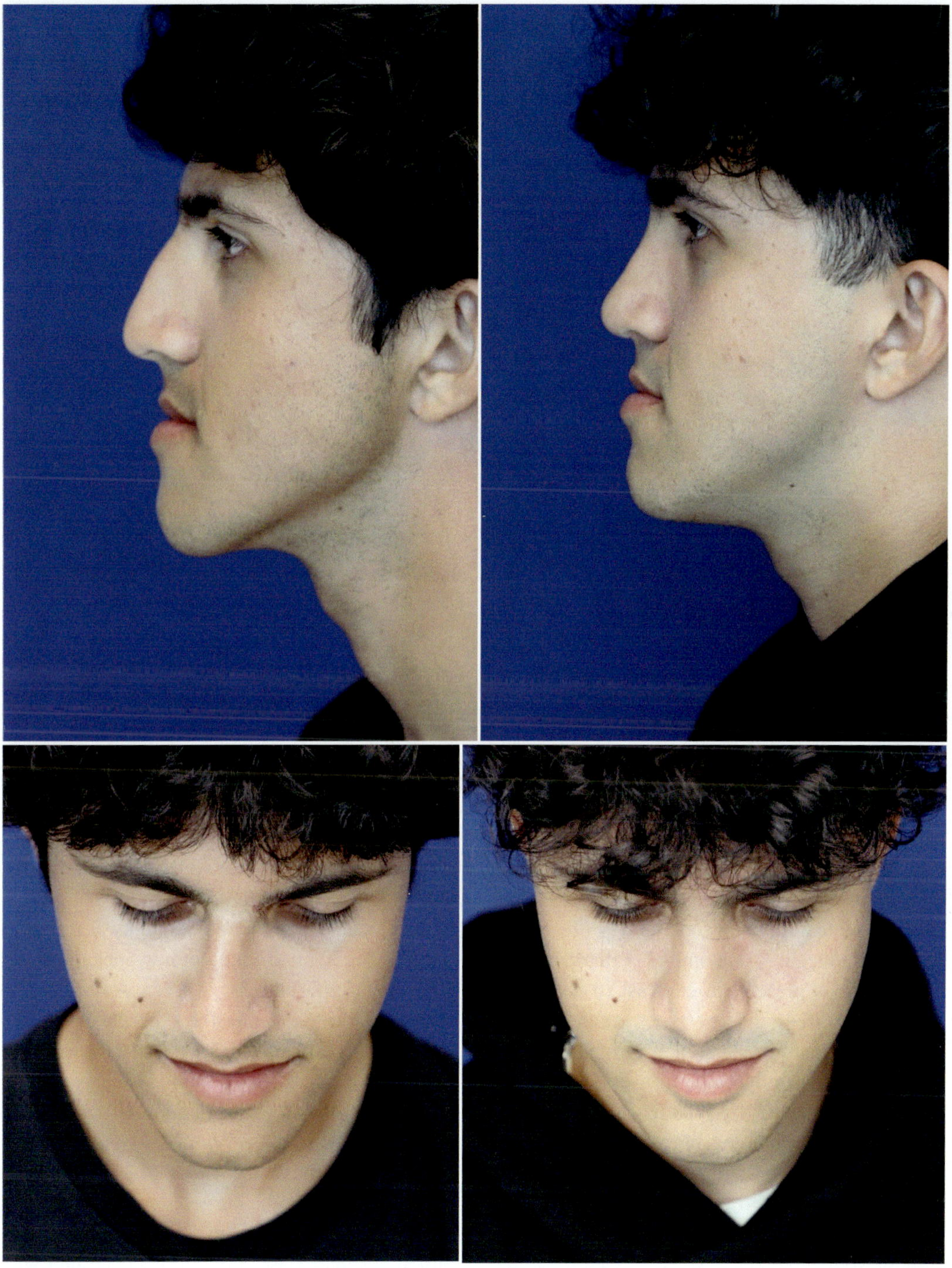

Fig. 15.4 (continued)

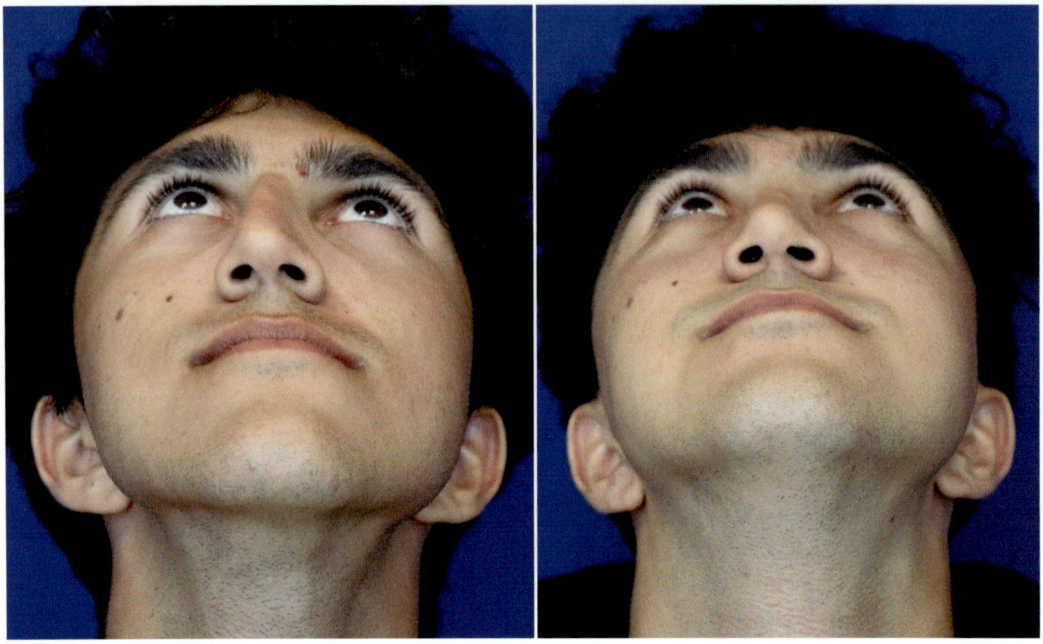

Fig. 15.4 (continued)

15.6 Conclusion

In this chapter, the anatomical features and related operative techniques for Hispanic, Middle Eastern, African-American, and Asian rhinoplasty are described in order to provide insight on the complexities and variations present in these ethnic patient groups. In respect to Hispanic rhinoplasty, the following conclusions are important: significant anatomical diversity of deformities is present, in contrast to Asian and black noses; four distinct types of deformities have been identified, and each requires its own specific surgical approach; conservative dorsal reduction is essential for type II and III noses. As the Hispanic population grows and becomes more prosperous, plastic surgeons in the United States can expect to encounter an increasing number of Hispanic patients requesting rhinoplasty.

Moreover, Middle Eastern rhinoplasty offers a challenging subset of nasal deformities. The variety of anatomical characteristics such as skin envelope, lateral cartilages, nostrils/alar base, and septum deviation all contribute to making surgical planning an essential component for a successful procedure. Operative techniques include: reducing the specific component of the dorsal deformity and using a balanced approach of augmentation and reduction. It is important to note that tip shape is achieved optimally through structural support and not excision. Similarly, when analyzing African-American rhinoplasty, augmentation and reduction must be balanced in regard to dorsum and tip adjustments. It is important to try to maintain their ethnic appearance, as it is very important for African Americans to maintain and represent their heritage through their facial features. In regard to Asian rhinoplasty, it is unique in its common use of augmentation techniques to achieve a larger dorsum and more refined tip.

Not surprisingly, the focus of rhinoplasty is often different for the surgeon compared to that of the patient. Whereas the patient's primary concern is aesthetics, the surgeon is concerned with balancing size reduction and preserving nasal function. Surgeons need to spend a great deal of time communicating realistic expectations with patients given their facial asymmetry and anatomical features. Natural-looking rhinoplasty can be accomplished by avoiding aggressive maneuvers and by creating a thorough and analytical surgical plan, along with understanding the ethnic anatomical features of each individual patient [12, 15, 26, 35].

References

1. Sajjadian A, Guyuron B. Primary rhinoplasty. Aesthet Surg J. 2010;30:527–39.
2. Cobo R. Mestizo rhinoplasty. Facial Plast Surg. 2003;19(3):257–68.
3. Patel AD, Kridel RW. Hispanic-American rhinoplasty. Facial Plast Surg. 2010;26:142–53.
4. Aston S. Aesthetic plastic surgery. Philadelphia: Saunders/Elsevier; 2009.
5. Guyuron B. The middle eastern nose. In: Matory Jr WE, editor. Ethnic considerations in facial aesthetic surgery. Philadelphia: Lippincott-Raven; 1998.
6. Sajjadian A, Guyuron B. Primary rhinoplasty. Aesthetic Surg J. 2010;30:527.
7. Daniel RK. Middle eastern rhinoplasty in the United States: part I. Primary rhinoplasty. Plast Reconstr Surg. 2009;124:1630.
8. Schultz AH. Relation of the external nose to the bony nose and nasal cartilages in Whites and Negroes. Am J Phys Anthropol. 1913;1:329–39.
9. Toriumi DM, Swartout B. Asian rhinoplasty. Facial plastic surgery. Clinics. 2007;15:293–307.
10. Leach J. Aesthetics and the Hispanic rhinoplasty. Laryngoscope. 2002;112:1903–16.
11. Daniel RK. Hispanic rhinoplasty in the United States, with emphasis on the Mexican American nose. Plast Reconstr Surg. 2003;112.244–56. discussion 257–258
12. Daniel RK. Middle eastern rhinoplasty: anatomy, aesthetics, and surgical planning. Facial Plast Surg. 2010;26:110.
13. Daniel RK. Middle eastern rhinoplasty in the United States: part I. Primary rhinoplasty PlastReconstr Surg. 2009;124:1630.
14. Daniel RK. Rhinoplasty: an atlas of surgical techniques. New York: Springer; 2002.
15. Sajjadian A. Advanced aesthetic rhinoplasty. New York: Springer; 2013. p. 187–95.
16. Romo T III, Abraham M, Pafford W. Advanced aesthetic rhinoplasty. New York: Springer; 2013. p. 197–206.
17. Canbay EI, Bhatia SN. A comparison of nasal resistance in White Caucasians and Blacks. Am J Rhinol. 1997;11:73–5.
18. Byron JB, Jonas TJ, Shawn DN. Surgical anatomy of nose, head and neck surgery. Otolaryngology. 2006;2:2530.
19. Kim JS, Khan NA, Song HM, Jang YJ. Intraoperative measurements of harvestable septal cartilage in rhinoplasty. Ann Plast Surg. 2010;65:519–23.
20. Kim EK, Daniel RK. Operative techniques. Aesthet Surg J. 2010;32:1018–30.
21. Zingaro EA, Falces E. Aesthetic anatomy of the non-Caucasian nose. Clin Plast Surg. 1987;14:749–65.
22. Porter JP, Olson KL. Anthropometric facial analysis of the African American female. Arch Facial Plas Surg. 2001;3:191–7.
23. Porter JP. Rhinoplasty in the African-American nose. Advanced therapy in facial plastic and reconstructive surgery. Shelton: People's Medical Publishing House; 2001. p. 347–63.
24. Jang YJ. Advanced aesthetic rhinoplasty. New York: Springer; 2013. p. 163–73.
25. Daniel RK. Mastering rhinoplasty. New York: Springer; 2009.
26. Sajjadian A. Advanced aesthetic rhinoplasty. New York: Springer; 2013. p. 176–86.
27. Guyuron B, Behmand RA. Nasal tip sutures part II: the interplays. Plast Reconstr Surg. 2004;112:1130–45. discussion 1146–1149
28. Sajjadian A, Guyuron B. An algorithm for treatment of the drooping nose. Aesthet Surg J. 2009;29:199–206.
29. Pearlman SJ. Surgical treatment of the nasolabial angle in balanced rhinoplasty. Facial Plast Surg. 2006;22:28–35.
30. Sajjadian A, Rubinstein R, Naghshineh N. Current status of grafts and implants in rhinoplasty: part I. Autologous grafts Plast Reconstr Surg. 2010;125:40e–9e.
31. Sajjadian A, Naghshineh N, Rubinstein R. Current status of grafts and implants in rhinoplasty: part II. Homologous grafts and allogenic implants. Plast Reconstr Surg. 2010;125:99e–109e.
32. Byrd HS, Meade RA, Gonyon DL Jr. Use of the autospreader flap in primary rhinoplasty. Plast Reconst Surg. 2007;119:1897.
33. Daniel RK. Middle eastern rhinoplasty: anatomy, aesthetics, and surgical planning. Facial Plast Surg. 2006;26:110.
34. Ofodile FA, Bokhari F. The African American nose: part II. Ann Plast Surg. 1995;34:123–9.
35. Daniel RK. Middle eastern rhinoplasty in the United States: part II. Primary rhinoplasty. Plast Reconstr Surg. 2009;124:1640–8.
36. Pak MW, Chan ES. Van Hasselt CA. Late Complications of Nasal Augmentation.
37. Deva AK, Merten S, Chang L. Silicone in nasal augmentation rhinoplasty: a decade of clinical experience. Plast Reconstr Surg. 1998;101:1230–7.
38. Bateman N, Jones NS. Retrospective review of augmentation rhinoplasties using autologous cartilage grafts. J Laryngol Otol. 2000;114:514–8.

Rhinoplasty: The Old Fractured Athletic Nose

16

Christian L. Stallworth, Jaime R. Garza, and Kelly Kafka

16.1 Introduction

Surgical correction of the old fractured nose is a challenging problem in rhinoplasty. Post-traumatic etiologies may include assault, motor vehicle accidents, falls, and sports injuries [1]. Nasal bone fracture is the most common fracture associated with blunt facial trauma, with sport-related injuries and assaults topping this list. Sports-related nasal fractures occur most commonly in males and are associated with all sports, including non-contact sports such as basketball, soccer, and softball [2]. As the most projecting structure of the face, nasal bone fractures account for 50% of all sports-related injuries, and 15% of all sports-related nasal fractures are repeat fractures [3]. These fractures result in a range of symptom severity from asymptomatic to significant functional and aesthetic morbidity. A nasal fracture sustained during sporting activities can often have ramifications on immediate as well as future performance, resulting in avoidance behaviors and lack of confidence [4].

Injuries sustained in childhood become more apparent as the child ages and the dorsum and septum grow [5]. Fracture patterns are generally dictated by the direction of force at the time of injury. The most common is the lateral blow resulting in displacement of the nasal and maxillary bones from the midline in the direction opposite that of the impact. A direct trauma to the dorsum of the nose results in an "open book" type of nasal fracture with splaying of the nasal bones away from the midline resulting in a depression of the dorsum. Fracture patterns are also influenced by the patient's age. Patients who are adults at the time of injury are predisposed to comminuted fractures due to demineralized and inelastic nasal bones, whereas younger patients generally present with more straightforward fractures or dislocations, given the elasticity of the structures [2]. Closed treatment in the acute setting is associated with a high rate of recurrence of structural deformities, as posttraumatic nasal deformity requiring subsequent rhinoplasty or septorhinoplasty remains in as many as 50% of these cases [6].

C. L. Stallworth (✉)
Department of Otolaryngology—Head & Neck Surgery, Division of Facial Plastic and Reconstructive Surgery, Long School of Medicine, University of Texas Health Science Center, San Antonio, TX, USA
e-mail: jrgmd@txps.net

J. R. Garza
University of Texas Health-San Antonio, San Antonio, TX, USA

Tulane University School of Medicine, New Orleans, LA, USA

K. Kafka
Brooke Army Medical Center, Fort Sam Houston, TX, USA

K. Jeffords et al. (eds.), *Aesthetic Surgery for Men*, https://doi.org/10.1007/978-3-032-03840-1_16

16.2 Patient Selection and Evaluation of the Crooked Nose

Surgical principles of rhinoplasty for aesthetic and functional concerns apply to the correction of the post-traumatic crooked nose. Evaluation of the crooked nose should include a systematic analysis of all components of the nasal structures, including the dorsal and caudal septum, bony pyramid, frontal bone, ethmoid, vomer, upper and lower lateral cartilages, and the skin envelope. The surgeon should also recognize the potential for each of these components to exert forces on and impact the position and integrity of neighboring components. If a damaged area is not addressed, this may lead to a recurrent deformity. A methodical evaluation also provides the opportunity to identify coexisting or pre-existing problems that are particularly concerning for the patient. Physical examination must include manual palpation of the nose and caudal septum, along with external and internal inspection of each of the aforementioned nasal components. Doing so will not only allow for the assessment of the septum and nasal valves but also help identify septal disruptions or other cartilaginous and dynamic perturbations not detected by radiologic examination. The nose should be examined from the anterior, lateral, oblique, and base views [1]. Diagnostic nasal endoscopy can be very useful for diagnosing subtle damage as well. With a full assessment, the repair of the post-traumatic crooked nose can be performed in a similar stepwise fashion as an elective septorhinoplasty.

The fracture pattern at the time of injury can influence the sequelae in the patient with delayed presentation. While a thorough history of events is important for the complete evaluation, this might not be possible in a patient who presents in a delayed fashion with an aged crooked nose. The history of multiple nasal fractures or previous functional problems should be elicited [7]. A simple fracture involving only one segment of the bony pyramid does not often result in septal deviation, while involvement of multiple segments can lead to destabilization of the system and result in significant airway obstruction. Displacement of multiple segments is often associated with a septal fracture [5]. A thorough physical exam is critical in the acute setting, too, as disruption of internal structures is often overlooked at the time of injury. Proper evaluation and treatment in the acute setting, including closed reduction, meticulous repair of skin lacerations, and incision and drainage of a septal hematoma, help lessen future functional and aesthetic problems. Failure to diagnose and treat a septal hematoma can cause significant deterioration of the septal cartilage, leading to a saddle nose deformity or septal perforation [5]. Cartilage necrosis and loss can also be seen after infection resulting from significant mucosal disruptions [8].

Treatment in the acute setting is associated with a high rate of recurrence of structural deformities, sometimes requiring multiple operations for adequate correction. Some advocate repair of the acute nasal fracture within 7–14 days to facilitate the repositioning of malpositioned segments. Closed reduction of nasal bone fractures in the emergency department or office can be performed under local anesthesia, but adequate reduction of a septal fracture with deviation is often more difficult. Initial inadequate treatment can lead to future recurrent deviation [7]. Internal and external splints are useful in the post-reduction period. Hippocrates first described the importance of post-reduction bandages and splints for preservation of form and function in the fifth century BC with similar variations used today [9].

Factors such as concomitant injuries or desire for correction of unrelated aesthetic or functional problems would lend toward a delayed approach to surgical correction. Also, significant swelling present in the acute setting can mask an inadequate closed reduction. In the pediatric patient, acute problems such as airway obstruction should be addressed initially, but definitive repair should be approached judiciously as removal of bony and cartilaginous septum components can lead to stunted facial growth. This must be weighed in the setting of a complete nasal obstruction due to bony and/or cartilaginous fractures or dislocations as, untreated, these can lead to significant chronic sinus and nasal obstruction disorders.

A thorough evaluation of the old fractured nose is important because chronic bony and cartilaginous deformities can lead to the development of hypertrophic inferior turbinates, synechiae between the septum and the lateral nasal wall components, sinus ostia obstruction, and mucosal changes.

16.3 Techniques for Repair

Nasal deviation can be categorized into different types, and a full understanding of the injury is needed before embarking on repair. [10] Caudal septal deviation is most common and can lead to airway compromise due to obstruction of the external nasal valves as well as deviation of the nasal tip from the midline. A patient may have a C-shaped or S-shaped septal deviation that is either oriented in the anteroposterior or cephalocaudal direction [10]. Pre-operative photo documentation is essential for the diagnosis of existing deformities such as distortion of dorsal aesthetic lines, deviations of the nasal pyramid from its midline orientation, presence of a fractured bony pyramid leading to a prominent, widened or deviated dorsum, deviations of the caudal septum, or a combination of these injuries. Photographs are also essential for the preoperative planning, intraoperative reference, and post-operative comparison that comprise the stages needed for the planning and execution of nasal reconstruction. It is only by these steps and attention to detail that nasal reconstruction may provide both a functional and aesthetically ideal nose that fits the individual patient.

An open approach with wide exposure of all nasal septal components is most often utilized via bilateral marginal or infra-cartilagenous incisions and an inverted "V"- shaped trans-columellar incisions [11]. Careful sharp dissection of the soft tissue envelope of the underlying nasal architectural components is recommended to help disrupt extrinsic forces carried from areas of injury through the dermal attachments. Dissection over cartilaginous structures should leave perichondrium in place. The subperiosteal plane is appropriate for exposure of the bony pyramid. The upper lateral cartilages are exposed through a vertical incision along the dorsum and sharply separated from the septum in a submucoperichondrial plane. The lower lateral cartilages should be separated from the upper lateral cartilages to release any contorting forces exerted by cartilaginous fractures of mid-vault. Wide exposure of the septum is necessary to assess for evidence of old fractures and subsequent deviations and spur formation. This can be accomplished via an incision directly on the stratified squamous epithelium overlying the caudal septum (hemitransfixion incision) or directly through the tip and mid-vault exposure from the open approach from above. This requires sharp and blunt separation of the mucoperichondrial and mucoperiosteal flaps from the dorsal aspect of the septal structures, back to the vomer and perpendicular plate of the ethmoid down to nasal floor with elevation on either side of the maxillary crest. This allows similarly for release of external forces on the septum. Intrinsic forces affecting the septum such as altered portions and prominent spurs of the vomer, perpendicular plate of the ethmoid and maxillae and distorted cartilaginous septal fractures that are contributing to deviation may be addressed. Imperative that a concerted attempt at septoplasty be performed and not a septal resection of all deviated structures. When addressing the ethmoid portion of the septum, it is important to make a transverse cut across the ethmoid bone with septal scissors just above the deviation to prevent any untoward injury to the attachments of the ethmoid bone at the skull base that could lead to a cerebrospinal fluid leak. The overriding goal is to restore adequate room for airflow through the nasal passages but also to preserve as much of the bony and cartilaginous structures as possible in case of future injuries. Understanding that repeat nasal fractures, as previously stated, are all too common in the athlete only leaving the traditional 8–10 millimeter dorsal and caudal strut is counterproductive [10]. However, this must be tempered with the need to harvest septal cartilage and bone for grafting of the crooked nasal components. When harvesting septal cartilage for grafting, an L-strut comprised of at least 10 millimeters each of dorsal and caudal cartilage should be retained for structural support. If the caudal septum is deviated from the midline, release from its attachment to the maxillary crest and any subsequent scar tissue is necessary for adequate mobilization and to prevent recurrent deformity. Fixation with a 4–0-polydioxanone suture utilizing a figure of eight configuration can be used to anchor the caudal septum in the midline position to the periosteum at the anterior nasal spine [11]. Further, in the setting of fixed bowing or fracture of the caudal septum, extracorporeal septoplasty may be required. Fixation to the anterior nasal spine using a drill hole is also reliable [10]. Judicious cartilage scoring of the concave surface can be used, but most often resection of the crooked cartilaginous septum leaving an adequate strut is utilized. The resected cartilage can then be carved on the back table with a scalpel blade to correct any deformities and place it back into position. Alternatively, an extracorporeal approach can be used in severe cases of septal deformity. This is accomplished by removing the entire septum and performing corrective measures on the back table including scoring, resection, and grafting to straighten the septum, and then the entire septum is placed back into position and fixated to the rhinion or remnant dorsal septal cartilage and the anterior nasal spine with sutures. As the septum provides the foundation of the entire nasal pyramid, adequate correction of a deviated septum is often considered the most integral part of correction of the crooked nose [12]. External nasal deformity cannot be treated without concurrent evaluation and correction of the septum [8].

Cartilage grafts are useful to restore structural integrity or the nose. In the old fractured nose due to septal cartilage damage, it is often necessary to harvest additional cartilage for reconstructing the nasal skeleton. In our hands, rib cartilage grafts are our first choice followed by auricular cartilage. L-strut reinforcement and tip support can be achieved with septal extension grafts. These can help augment the internal valve in the form of spreader grafts, sutured to the dorsal septum. The midvault of the nose is typically collapsed on either side of the dorsal midline due to disruption of the attachments of the upper lateral cartilages to the septum. This compromises the internal nasal valves and leads to nasal obstruction. Reconstruction of the internal nasal valves requires the placement of cartilaginous spreader grafts on either side of the dorsal septum with mattress suture fixation and then elevation of the upper lateral cartilages and suture fixation of those structures to the newly restored dorsal midvault [13]. 4–0 and 5–0 polydioxanone (PDS) absorbable sutures are used for fixation of these structures. There is no need to introduce permanent sutures, as they will only serve as a potential nidus for infection and serve no long-term purpose.

Spreader grafts also serve to even out dorsal asymmetry and recreate the dorsal aesthetic lines. A septal extension graft modification of the spreader graft can also provide tip projection and support in the traumatically shortened nose. Tip distortion is common after fracture of any cartilaginous portion of the nose due to intrinsic pulling forces. Creating tip support with a columellar strut graft can be achieved in the case of deviated medial crura. This should be placed in a pocket between the medial crura and sutured to the medial/middle crura with horizontal mattress 5–0 PDS sutures or transcutaneous 4–0 plain gut sutures [5]. The tip can be reconstructed with the use of lateral crural strut grafts for deformed lateral crura that thereby support the external nasal valves and add to the aesthetic result of a pleasing tip. Further tip refinement is accomplished with Daniel's three-suture technique and the possible addition of cartilaginous shield or onlay tip grafts for tip projection and definition based on preoperative photographic planning [14].

Correction of the malpositioned nasal bony pyramid will influence the position and direction of the septum, and vice versa. Complex injuries resulting in disruption of both bony and cartilaginous components require deconstruction at their juncture with suture and percutaneous pinning techniques to reposition after the lateral walls are repositioned with osteotomies [5]. Lateral and/or radix percutaneous osteotomies can be used to create a greenstick fracture to reposition a deviated dorsum [11]. A prominent dorsum can be addressed with either ostectomy or rasping. Any septal resection should be performed after dorsal hump reduction to prevent over-resection of the dorsal supporting strut. For more complex injuries with asymmetry associated with the dorsal deviation, both medial and lateral osteotomies may be used to allow full mobility of the nasal bones, as well as grafting with shaped remnants of resected ethmoid and vomer bones. This is especially useful for the concave nasal bone. To prevent displacement of fragments when double-level osteotomies are performed, the higher osteotomy should precede the lower. Finally, intermediate osteotomies are often required to help equalize the side wall length in cases of a deviated nasal pyramid [15].

Dorsal collapse with saddle nose deformity, often the result of an untreated septal hematoma with subsequent cartilage loss, can also lead to retraction of the columella. Dorsal augmentation and medial crural suture fixation can help to correct this deformity. Dorsal onlay grafts may be used to augment an anatomic reconstruction. To help reduce visibility, a dorsal onlay graft of finely diced cartilage wrapped in temporoparietal fascia should be the first choice for dorsal height restoration and camouflage of dorsal irregularities [6].

Complementary techniques, including camouflage grafting on the concave side of a deviated nose, can augment anatomic reconstruction. Camouflage grafting using morselized cartilage can be useful for filling small concave defects of the dorsum [13]. Judicious use is important for these camouflage techniques to avoid widening of the dorsal aesthetic lines or creating an overly prominent dorsum [11]. A combination of surgical approaches using principles of anatomic reconstruction and augmentation with cartilage grafts helps overcome shortcomings of purely reconstructive techniques, which can lead to weakening of structural support [11]. Synthetic implants and injections, including Mersilene mesh and injectable silicone, were once used for recreation of nasal architecture. Their use is no longer considered standard of care due to long-term complications, including extrusion, infection, and dislocation. Cadaver allograft can be used as a substitute when native cartilage is not available, but it is unpredictable and not highly recommended.

Timing of reconstructive structural rhinoplasty can be critical for success as well. Revision rhinoplasty should be timed 10–12 months after initial operation or trauma unless there is a significant functional issue or obvious displacement of graft material. Delay from the onset of injury or surgery allows for tissues to solidify and scarring to mature, thereby providing a more solid and stable framework to work with and decreasing the risks of intraoperative and postoperative hemorrhage. The surgeon must set expectations with each patient and thoroughly discuss the risks and benefits of these aggressive techniques. This is especially true when the correction of minor deformities is considered. Acceptance of a small persistent deformity is sometimes necessary to avoid structural collapse [5]. Return to sports is not recommended until 6–8 weeks after closed reduction or surgical repair due to the risk of reinjures. When return to play cannot be delayed, a protective facial mask should be worn [16].

Surgical correction of the old athletic crooked nose starts with a thorough evaluation of all affected components with the realization that one injured component will exert forces on others. An open approach to repair is recommended to allow full exposure and improved manipulative control of all anatomic components. Anatomic deconstruction and realignment of the nasal bones, septum, upper and lower lateral cartilages, and management of hypertrophic internal nasal structures, release of synechiae, and repair of septal perforations are often necessary to help prevent recurrent deviation and functional problems. Camouflage techniques with cartilage grafts should be used judiciously to augment anatomic repair. Patients should be counseled that acceptable correction might require a staged approach.

References

1. Nina Lu G, Humphrey CD, Kriet JD. Correction of nasal fractures. Facial Plast Surg Clin North Am. 2017;25(4):537–46.
2. Cox AJ. Nasal fractures—the details. Facial Plast Surg. 2000;16(2):87–94.
3. Cannon CR, Cannon R, Young K, Reploge W, Stringer S, Gasson E. Characteristics of nasal injuries incurred

during sports activities: analysis of 91 patients. Ear Nose Throat J. 2011;90(8):E8–12.
4. Lennon P, Jaber S, Fenton JE. Functional and psychological impact of nasal bone fractures sustained during sports activities: a survey of 87 patients. Ear Nose Throat J. 2016;95(8):324–32.
5. McCollough EG. Nasal plastic surgery. W B Saunders Company. 1994;1994:221–46.
6. Higuera S, Lee EI, Cole P, Hollier LH, Stal S. Nasal trauma and the deviated nose. Plast Reconstr Surg. 2007;120(7 Suppl 2):64S–75S.
7. Mondin V, Rinaldo A, Ferlito A. Management of nasal bone fractures. Am J Otolaryngol. 2005;26(3):181–5.
8. Rees TD, Baker D, Tabbal N. Rhinoplasty: problems and controversies, a discussion with the experts. The C.V: Mosby Company; 1998. p. 392–6.
9. Lascaratos JG, Segas JV, Trompoukis CC, Assimakopoulos DA. From the roots of rhinology: the reconstruction of nasal injuries by Hippocrates. Ann Otol Rhinol Laryngol. 2003;112(2):159–62.
10. Cerkes N. The crooked nose: principles of treatment. Aesthet Surg J. 2011;31(2):241–57.
11. Byrd HS, Salomon J, Flood J. Correction of the crooked nose. Plast Reconstr Surg. 1998;102(6):2148–57.
12. Kienstra M. Secondary rhinoplasty: revising the crooked nose. Facial Plast Surg. 2011;27(5):491–6.
13. Daniel RK, Calvert JW. Diced cartilage grafts in rhinoplasty surgery. Plast Reconstr Surg. 2004;113(7):2156–71.
14. Daniel RK. Rhinoplasty: a simplified, three stitch, open tip suture technique. Part 1: primary rhinoplasty. Plast Reconstr Surg. 1999;103(5):1491–502.
15. Bloom JD, Immerman SB, Constantinides M. Osteotomies in the crooked nose. Facial Plast Surg. 2011;27(5):456–66.
16. Marston AP, O'Brien EK, Hamilton GS. Nasal injuries in sports. Clin Sports Med. 2017;36(2):337–53.

Otoplasty in the Male Patient

17

Jeffrey L. Lisiecki and Robert H. Gilman

17.1 Introduction

Prominauris, the prominent ear deformity, is a common concern for which patients present to the plastic surgeon. It is present in 5% of the Caucasian population and has autosomal dominant inheritance [1]. Men and women are affected equally by prominauris and seem to undergo otoplasty at similar rates [2, 3]. By proportion, however, this means that greater number of males, adult and child, undergo otoplasty relative to most other cosmetic surgical procedures [2]. Prominauris can have a negative impact on the psyche and quality of life of patients. It is associated with decreased self-esteem, increased anxiety, behavioral problems, and social avoidance, even in adult patients [4]. Otoplasty has been shown to improve quality of life using validated, patient-reported outcome measures [4]. The improvements in health-related quality of life after otoplasty appear to occur regardless of patient gender [5].

Otoplasty for correction of the prominent ear was first described by Dieffenbach in 1845 [6]. Over the subsequent decades, numerous different methods of suturing, scoring or rasping the cartilage, and tissue resection have been described and applied to the problem of prominent ears. The goals of the operation have remained consistent, however, and are best articulated by McDowell in 1968: the removal of protrusion of the upper third of the ear, the helix being visible beyond the antihelix on anterior view, a smooth helical contour, a postauricular sulcus that is not decreased or distorted, the ear not being too close to the head, and symmetry between the two ears to within 3 mm at any measured point [7]. Beyond these, creation of an antihelical fold where it is absent or under-developed, as well as positioning and contour of the lobule, are critical considerations [6]. While these goals are generally applicable to both genders, there are unique anatomic, developmental, and aesthetic factors that must be considered in the male otoplasty.

17.2 Auricular Growth, Patient Selection, and the Timing of Surgery

Growth and development of the auricle have been studied extensively and differ between men and women. Ear width approximates mature size at age 7 in boys, and length approximates the mature size at age 13 typically; this is a full year later than what is observed in females [6]. The lobule itself grows over time, both as the individual develops into adolescence, and again later into adulthood with a period of relative stagnation in early adulthood [8]. The gender differences

J. L. Lisiecki · R. H. Gilman (✉)
Department of Surgery, Section of Plastic Surgery, University of Michigan, Ann Arbor, MI, USA
e-mail: gilmanr@med.umich.edu

K. Jeffords et al. (eds.), *Aesthetic Surgery for Men*, https://doi.org/10.1007/978-3-032-03840-1_17

in ear development appear to apply somewhat across ethnicities, as a Chinese study also found ear width matured later in males than females (7 versus 5 years), while length matured at 14 years in both genders [9].

Men and women appear to time their otoplasties differently. In a large retrospective study, Baker and Converse found that men tended to have surgery earlier in life than women, while women were more likely to have otoplasty later in adulthood than men [10]. They hypothesized that men become more adjusted to their prominent ears with age, while women may become more aware of them. More recent research has supported this finding [11]. The reason for this is unclear, though it is notable that men tend to undergo aesthetic operations that are not gender-specific (such as otoplasty) at a younger age than women overall [12].

In our clinical experience, there is also a second wave of men seeking otoplasty later in life. This appears to be related to the development of androgenic alopecia with age, and the increased ability to perceive pre-existing prominent ears as a result. Finally, there are highly individual and patient-specific reasons for seeking otoplasty that may defy the usual trends of surgical timing. One study describes soldiers, most of whom were men, who sought and underwent otoplasties to be able to more comfortably wear their standard-issue field helmets [13]. Otoplasty becomes increasingly difficult with age, as the cartilage becomes stiffer and more calcified, and therefore less amenable to certain techniques [6].

17.3 Anthropometry of Male and Female Ears

The anatomic differences between the male and female ear have been well-characterized (Fig. 17.1). Men have larger heads than women, so the root of the helix is positioned a greater distance from the lateral palpebral fissure than in women [14]. The ideal position of the ear appears to be with the upper edge level with the lateral point of the brow [15, 16]. The height of the pinna is 6.5% larger in men than in women and does not change in adulthood [17]. The width of the ear is approximately 50–60% of the height, so accordingly the ear is also wider in men than in women [16]. Indeed, all measurements of the auricle are larger in men than in women [18].

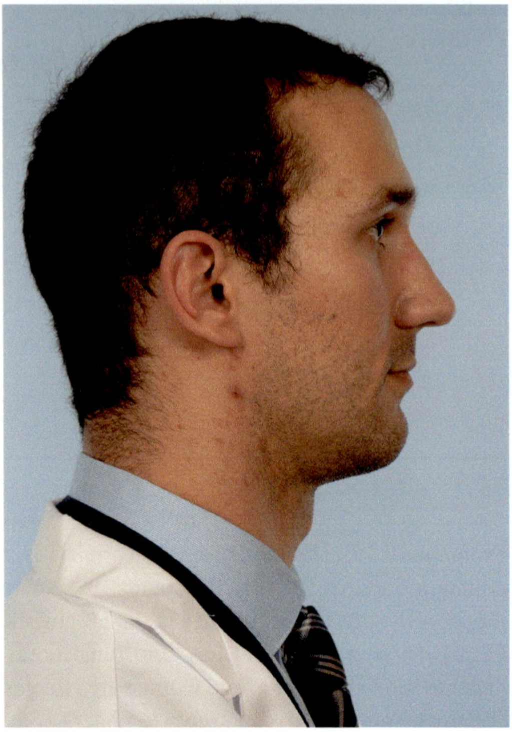

Fig. 17.1 Normal external ear anatomy

The relative dimensions of the lobule in men compared to women are less clear. Some studies say that the height and width of the lobule are the same in men and women, while others report that men have longer lobules than women [17, 19]. What is clear is that the earlobe becomes longer with age in men, and that age is the primary predictor of earlobe length in men [8, 17, 19]. The primary differences between men and women in the aging of the lobule appear to be related to piercing status; as women are more likely to have pierced lobules, this is a more significant predictor of lobule length in women [19].

A key anatomical difference between the male and female ear is the degree of protrusion between the auricle and the mastoid skin, often termed the cephaloauricular angle. Mean protrusion is measured as the line from the helical root to the most lateral aspect of the helix and the plane of the mastoid skin [14]. The often-cited normative values are 25 degrees in males and 21 degrees in females [20]. That is, a less-projecting ear is a more feminine facial feature.

There are ethnic differences in the size of the ear lobule, which seems to be smaller in Indian individuals than the reported measurements in Caucasian and East Asian populations [8]. Ethnicity may also negate or augment the differences in ear morphometry between men and women. One study of Han Chinese individuals found similar dimensions of the auricle between adult men and women [21].

17.4 Patient Education and Awareness

There may be a difference in patient education and awareness regarding otoplasty as well. Of plastic surgeon's websites that offered male plastic surgical procedures in 2015, only a small fraction discussed otoplasty [22]. Furthermore, men seeking aesthetic procedures in general tend to be younger, have a higher BMI, and are more likely to be smokers than women [12]. It is therefore incumbent on plastic surgeons to ensure that patients are educated about this procedure and its benefits, and that patients seeking this procedure are properly optimized and counselled on the risks and potential complications of the procedure.

17.5 Aesthetic Differences in Male Otoplasty, Technique, and Its Advantages

While the overall aesthetic goals for correction of prominent ear are similar between the genders, there are subtle but definite differences. McDowell noted that it is especially important not to make the ear too close to the head in the male patient [7]. He recommended a helix to postauricular skin distance of 10–12 mm at the top of the auricle, 16–18 mm in the middle third, and 20–22 mm in the lower third [7]. In terms of degrees of projection between the auricle and the plane of the mastoid skin, a good goal for correction is less than 35 degrees in general, but ideally around 25 degrees for men, as opposed to a lesser angle (around 21 degrees) in women [14]. Decreasing projection too much may be overly feminizing or simply look unnatural, or distort the helix so it lies less prominent than the antihelical fold on the anterior view. All of these are unfavorable cosmetic results in the male patient. Furthermore, it is especially important not to obliterate or distort the postauricular sulcus in men, as shorter hair makes this deformity more noticeable.

The preferred method for otoplasty used by the senior author of this chapter (RHG) involves the following steps:

Marking the position of the present or proposed position of the antihelical fold (see Fig. 17.2).
Marking the postauricular sulcus and a conservative lenticular postauricular skin excision centered on the postauricular sulcus (see Fig. 17.3).

Marking the planned Mustarde suture positions, typically three per side, which will help to re-form the antihelical fold [23]. A helpful technique for precise placement of Mustarde sutures is the use of methylene blue, in a 1 mL syringe with a 30 gauge hypodermic needle, to tattoo the position of the planned Mustarde sutures onto the

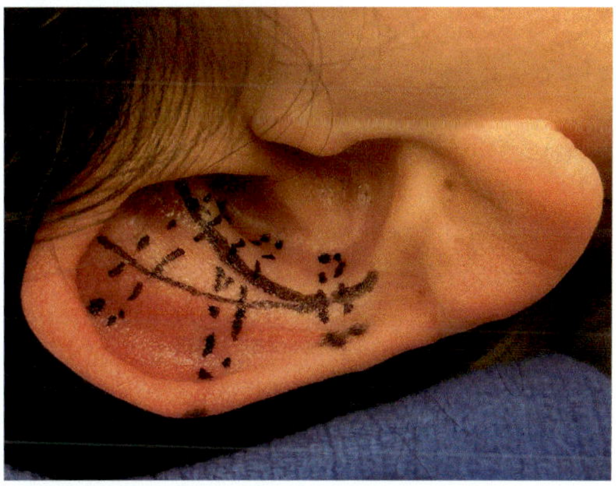

Fig. 17.2 Preoperative marking; planned position of the antihelical fold and Mustarde sutures

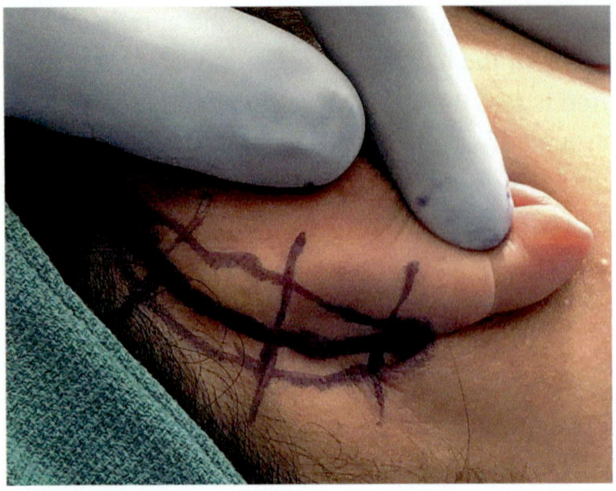

Fig. 17.3 Postauricular incision plan

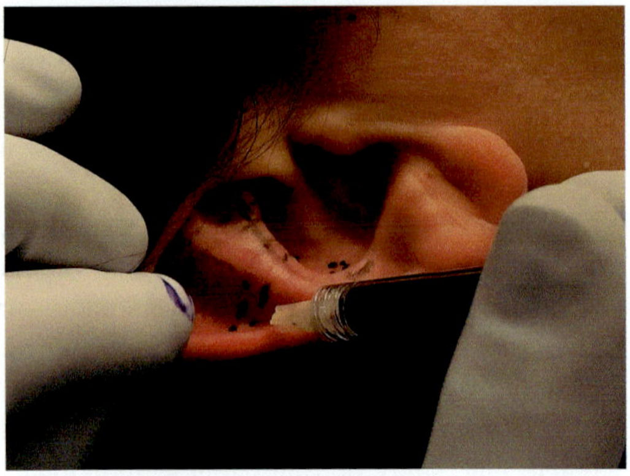

Fig. 17.4 Using methylene blue to tattoo the position of the Mustarde sutures on the cartilage

cartilage itself. Each side of the mattress suture must be placed wide enough apart to insure a gentle and natural antihelical fold. When elevating the skin off the postauricular cartilage, the surgeons then can identify the tattoo on the cartilage and ensure proper placement (see Figs. 17.4 and 17.5).

The planned postauricular skin excision is made, and a conservative lenticle of skin is excised from the auricular cartilage and supraperiosteal tissue on either side of the postauricular sulcus. Soft tissue consisting of skin, subcutaneous fibrofat, and postauricular muscle can be removed from the underlying mastoid bone down to periosteum to facilitate insetting the ear (see Fig. 17.6).

The cauda helicis is identified (see Fig. 17.5) and used to access the anterior surface of the cartilage. Iris or tenotomy scissors are used to create a sub-perichondrial tunnel on the anterior surface of the cartilage (see Fig. 17.7). The anterior surface is abraded at the planned anti-helical fold using a Dingman otoabrader (see Figs. 17.8 and 17.9). Mattress-type Mustarde sutures are made with 4–0 PDS but clamped and not tied down yet. Many surgeons have used permanent, undyed Prolene sutures. The use of such a permanent suture is unnecessary and can lead to late suture abscess and annoyingly palpable postauricular

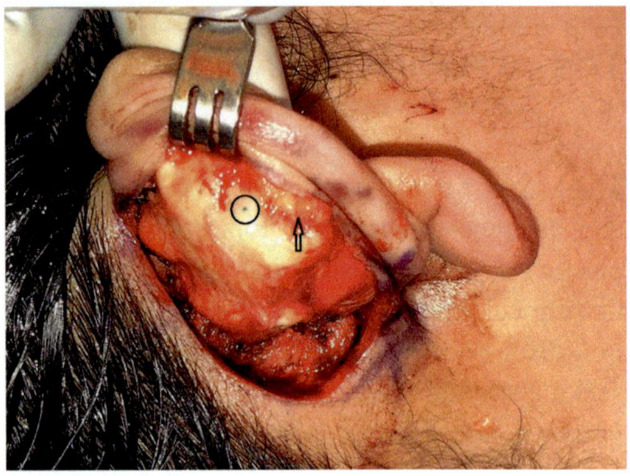

Fig. 17.5 Exposed cartilage with Methylene Blue Tattoo (circle), access to the anterior surface of the ear via the cauda helices (arrow)

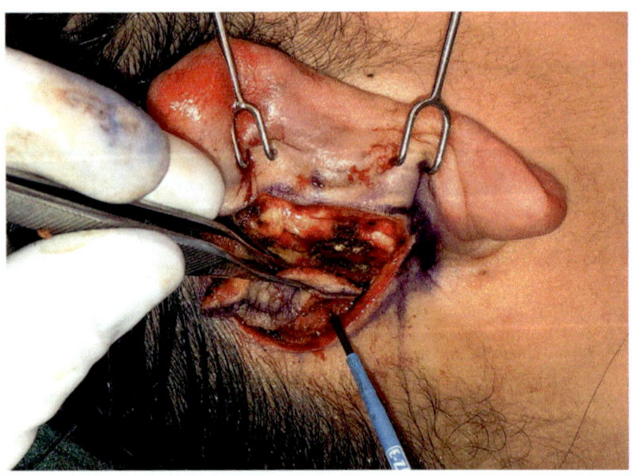

Fig. 17.6 Removal of postauricular soft tissue

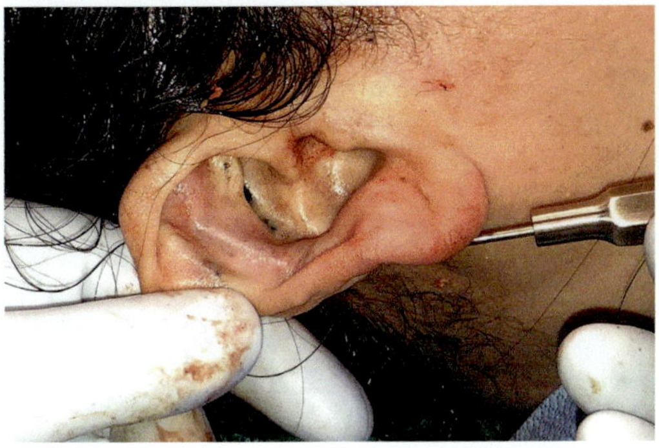

Fig. 17.7 Creating anterior antihelical tunnel with scissors

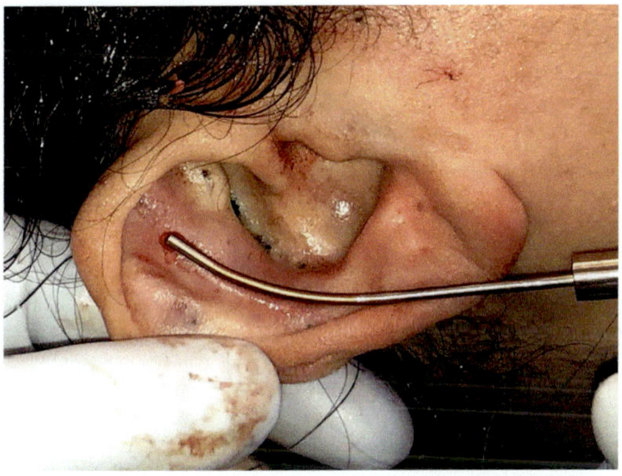

Fig. 17.8 Cartilage abrasion using a Dingman Otoabrader positioned external to the area to be abraded

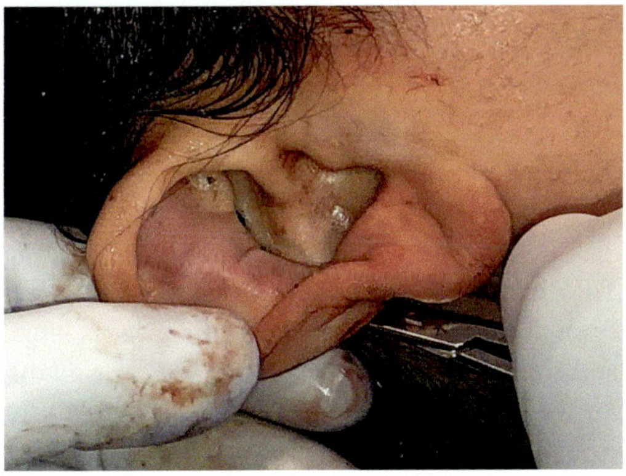

Fig. 17.9 Cartilage abrasion using a Dingman Otoabrader

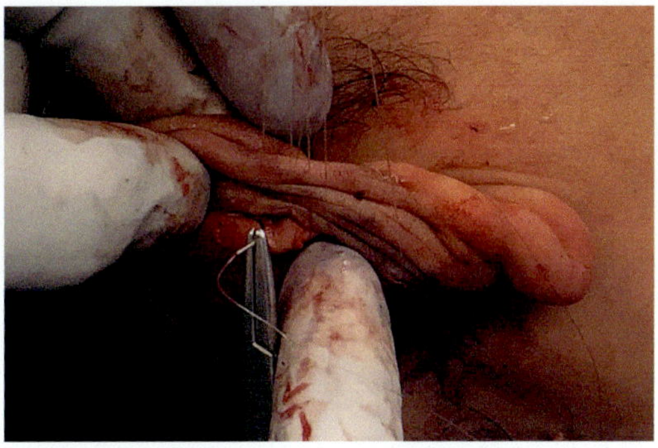

Fig. 17.10 Placement of Mustarde suture

irregularities. When placing the sutures, care is taken not to puncture the skin on the anterior surface of the pinna (see Fig. 17.10). Three of these sutures are used with the first at the midpoint of the ear, approximately 1 cm superior to the cauda helicis. The second is placed at or just inferior to the bifurcation of the helical crura, and the third is placed between the second suture and the superior helical rim spanning the superior crus of the antihelix. If the ear is still protruding due to prominence of the conchal bowl, the conchal eminentia may be shaved in the manner described by Webster [24].

One or two Furnas sutures from the posterior and superior wall of the concha are made to the mastoid fascia, taking care not to distort the external ear canal [25]. The Mustarde sutures are then tied down, from inferior to superior, making sure the antihelical fold is smooth and the cephaloauricular angle is appropriate (see Figs. 17.11, 17.12, and 17.13). Careful hemostasis should be assured prior to tying the sutures to prevent auricular hematoma. The incision is closed with a running 4–0 chromic gut suture. While placing the suture, a bite is taken at the depth of the sulcus as well as at the skin edges to preserve and not obliterate the sulcus. Skin glue is helpful to seal the incision and to adhere the pinna to the mastoid skin temporarily, to protect the repair in the

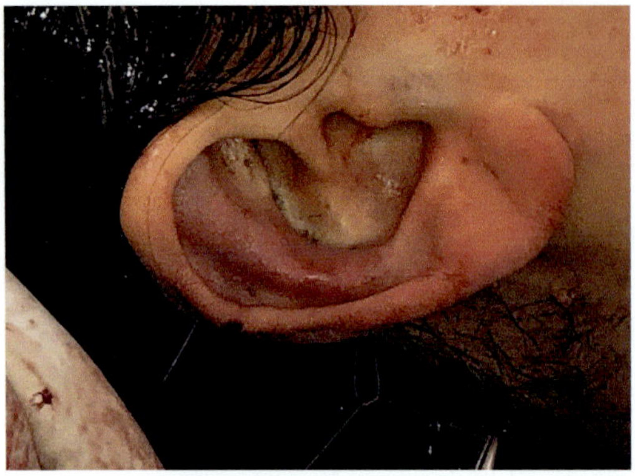

Fig. 17.11 Tying Mustarde suture

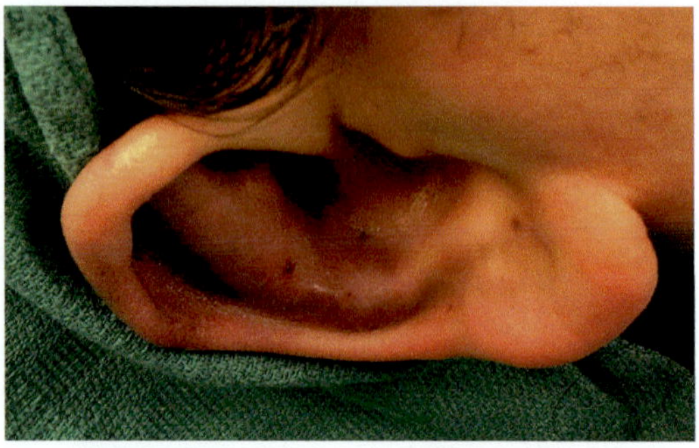

Fig. 17.12 Postoperative ear position with all sutures in place and tied

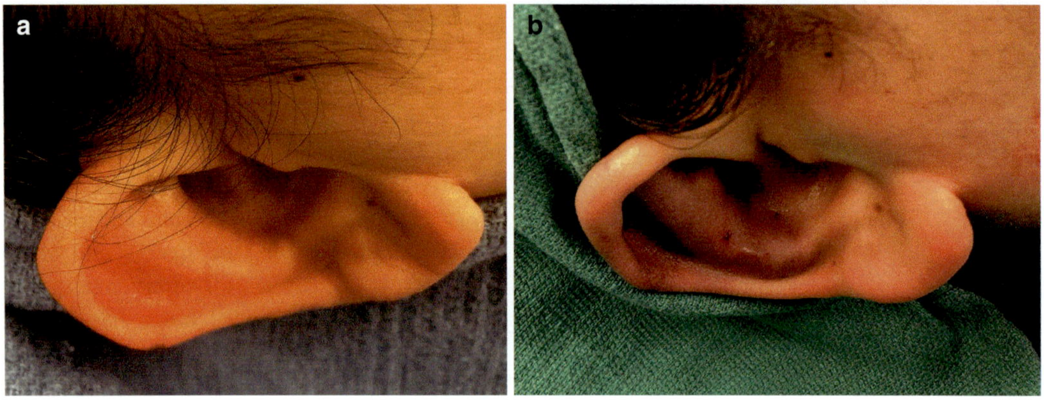

Fig. 17.13 Preoperative (**a**) and postoperative (**b**) position of the ear

immediate postoperative period. Moistened cotton balls are packed into the contours of the auricle following the procedure, and a padded otologic wrap is placed around the head to secure them.

The dressing can be removed in 3–5 days. The patient is asked to wear a "ski band" style headband at night for 4–6 weeks after the operation and to sleep on several pillows with 30–45 degrees of head elevation for 2–3 weeks post op. The patients are warned that there will be ecchymosis for at least 2 weeks post op and warned against strenuous activity for 2–3 weeks and contact sports for 8 weeks post op.

The most common otoplasty complication is auricular hematoma necessitating evacuation and through-and-through bolster dressing to prevent late cartilage distortion. Infection, sensory loss, early relapse, obliteration of the postauricular sulcus, and overcorrection (telephone ear) have been reported.

17.6 Conclusion

The male otoplasty is distinct in several ways from the female otoplasty. The male ear is larger and more prominent than the female ear, and this difference must be respected in otoplasty. Acknowledging this difference, as well as the developmental and patient-specific considerations that drive men to undergo otoplasty, is critical to success. Respecting these differences, male otoplasty is a sound procedure with a long history, which stands to provide significant benefit to patients.

References

1. Adamson PA, Strecker HD. Otoplasty techniques. Facial Plast Surg. 1995;11(04):284–300.
2. Limandjaja G, Breugem C, van der Molen AM, Kon M. Complications of otoplasty: a literature review. J Plast Reconstr Aesthet Surg. 2009;62(1):19–27.
3. Holcomb JD, Gentile RD. Aesthetic facial surgery of male patients: demographics and market trends. Facial Plast Surg. 2005;21(4):223.
4. Schwentner I, Schmutzhard J, Deibl M, Sprinzl GM. Health-related quality of life outcome of adult patients after otoplasty. J Craniofacial Surg. 2006;17(4):629–35.
5. Bermueller C, Kirsche H, Sebert A, Rotter N. Quality of life and patients' satisfaction after otoplasty. Eur Arch Otorrinolaringol. 2012;269(11):2423–31.
6. Janis JE, Rohrich RJ, Gutowski KA. Otoplasty. Plast Reconstr Surg. 2005;115(4):60e–72e.
7. McDOWELL AJ. Goals in otoplasty for protruding ears. Plast Reconstr Surg. 1968;41(1):17–27.
8. Sharma A, Sidhu NK, Sharma MK, Kapoor K, Singh B. Morphometric study of ear lobule in northwest Indian male subjects. Anat Sci Int. 2007;82(2):98–104.
9. Zhao S, Li D, Liu Z, Wang Y, Liu L, Jiang D, et al. Anthropometric growth study of the ear in a Chinese population. J Plast Reconstr Aesthet Surg. 2018;71(4):518–23.
10. Baker DC, Converse JM. Correction of protruding ears: a 20-year retrospective. Aesth Plast Surg. 1979;3(1):29–39.
11. Kajosaari L, Pennanen J, Klockars T. Otoplasty for prominent ears–demographics and surgical timing in different populations. Int J Pediatr Otorhinolaryngol. 2017;100:52–6.
12. Kaoutzanis C, Winocour J, Yeslev M, Gupta V, Asokan I, Roostaeian J, et al. Aesthetic surgical procedures in men: major complications and associated risk factors. Aesthet Surg J. 2017;38(4):429–41.
13. Salgado CJ, Mardini S. Corrective otoplasty for symptomatic prominent ears in US soldiers. Mil Med. 2006;171(2):128–30.
14. Kelley P, Hollier L, Stal S. Otoplasty: evaluation, technique, and review. J Craniofacial Surg. 2003;14(5):643–53.
15. Posnick JC, Al-Qattan MM, Whitaker LA. Assessment of the preferred vertical position of the ear. Plast Reconstr Surg. 1993;91(7):1198–203. discussion 204–7
16. Tolleth H. Artistic anatomy, dimensions, and proportions of the external ear. Clin Plast Surg. 1978;5(3):337–45.
17. Sullivan PK, Brucker MJ, Patel J. A morphometric study of the external ear: age and sex related differences. 2010.
18. Sforza C, Grandi G, Binelli M, Tommasi DG, Rosati R, Ferrario VF. Age-and sex-related changes in the normal human ear. Forensic Sci Int. 2009;187(1–3):110.
19. Azaria R, Adler N, Silfen R, Regev D, Hauben D. Morphometry of the adult human earlobe: a study of 547 subjects and clinical application. Plast Reconstr Surg. 2003;111(7):2398–402.
20. Farkas L, editor. Growth of normal and reconstructed auricles. Symposium on reconstruction of the auricle St Louis: Mosby; 1974.
21. Wang B, Dong Y, Zhao Y, Bai S, Wu G. Computed tomography measurement of the auricle in Han population of North China. J Plast Reconstr Aesthet Surg. 2011;64(1):34–40.
22. Sinno S, Lam G, Brownstone ND, Steinbrech DS. An assessment of gender differences in plastic surgery patient education and information in the United States: are we neglecting our male patients? Aesthet Surg J. 2015;36(1):107–10.
23. Mustarde J. The correction of prominent ears using simple mattress sutures. Plast Reconstr Surg. 1963;32(4):486.
24. Webster GV. The tail of the helix as a key to otoplasty. Plast Reconstr Surg. 1969;44(5):455–61.
25. Furnas DW. Correction of prominent ears by concha-mastoid sutures. Plast Reconstr Surg. 1968;42(3):189–94.

18 Orthognathic Surgery for the Male Patient

Eduardo Nicolaievsky and Jeff Rothenberg

18.1 Diagnosis

> The beginning is most important part of the work.—Plato

Orthognathic surgery is an art and science that encompasses a thorough understanding of multiple concepts, incorporating them as a unit in order to achieve optimal esthetic and functional results [1–3].

The definition of diagnosis, according to Dorland's Medical Dictionary, is the determination of the nature of a case of disease [4]. In orthodontics, the disease is the malocclusion. This often leads to facial disharmony and esthetic imbalance. With Class III patients, the facial imbalance results from maxillary deficiency, mandibular prognathism, or a combination of the two.

The clinical exam begins from the moment the clinician introduces themself to the patient. Facial imbalances can be recognized from one's speaking, smiling, and even head posture.

Frontal photographs should be taken both intra and extra-orally. These allow you to identify facial and dental midlines, lip competence, and incisor display both in the relaxed position as well as in a dynamic smile. An evaluation of tooth display in the buccal corridors should also be considered for ideal transverse esthetics (Figs. 18.1, 18.2, 18.3, 18.4, 18.5, and 18.6).

From the anteroposterior perspective, considerations of facial height, lip projection, soft tissue convexity, or concavity are all factors that are affected by underlying hard tissue positions.

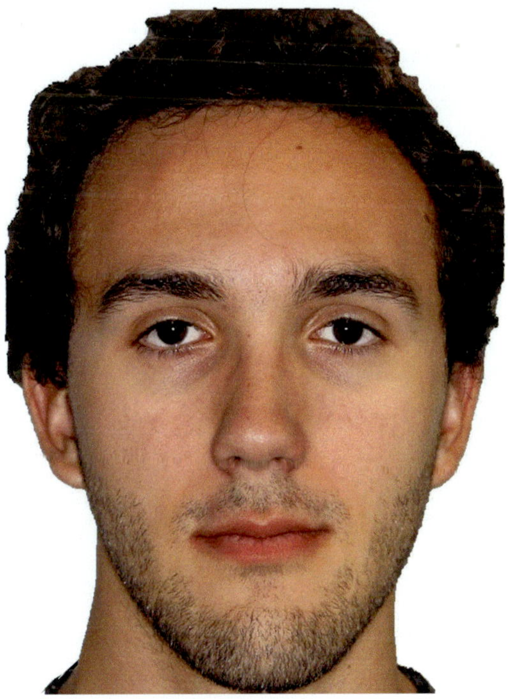

Fig. 18.1 26-year-old male with mid-face concavity and poor upper lip support; repose position

E. Nicolaievsky (✉) · J. Rothenberg
Division of Oral/Maxillofacial Surgery, Mount Sinai Hospital, Miami Beach, FL, USA
e-mail: enico@blumnico.com

K. Jeffords et al. (eds.), *Aesthetic Surgery for Men*, https://doi.org/10.1007/978-3-032-03840-1_18

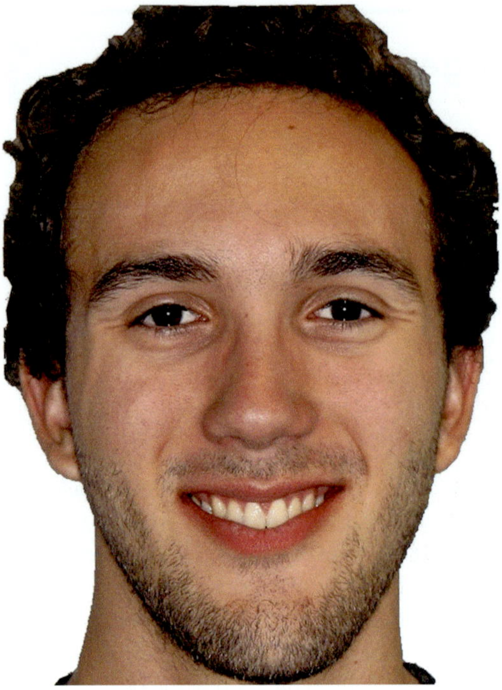

Fig. 18.2 Full labial mobility with complete dental exposure and discrepant dent-gingival margins

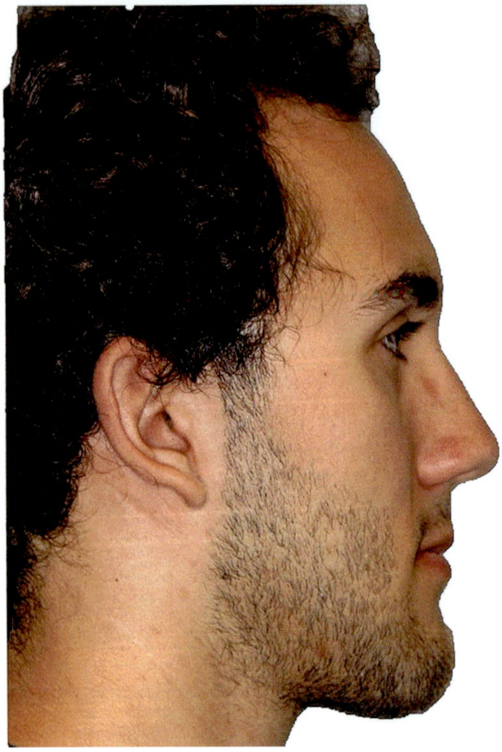

Fig. 18.3 Lateral view demonstrating maxillary deficiency, acute naso-labial angle, and negative facial convexity, and Wits angle

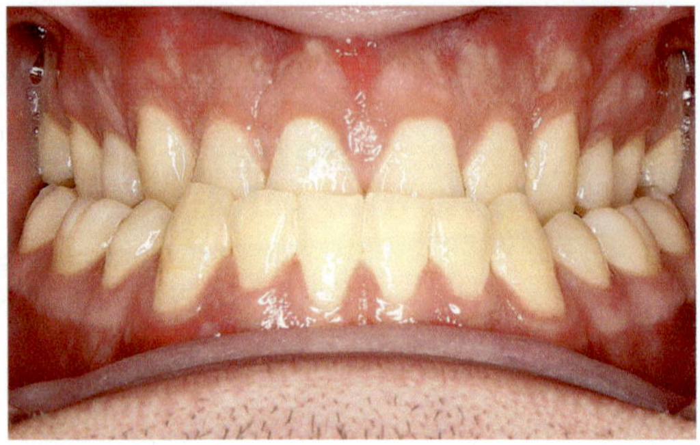

Fig. 18.4 Class III malocclusion, posterior crossbite

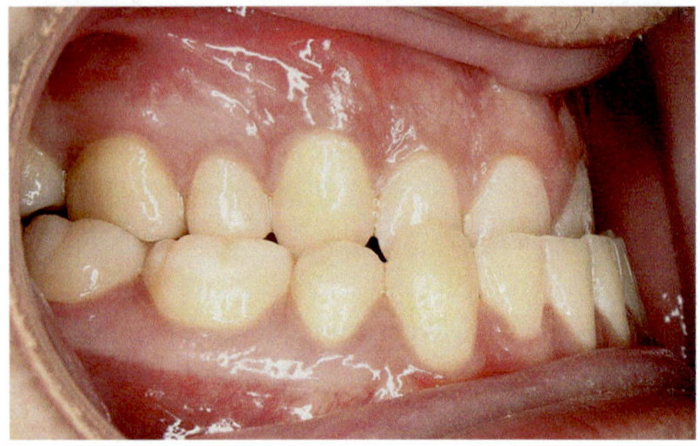

Fig. 18.5 Right lateral view, Class III cuspid/molar occlusion, partial dental compensation

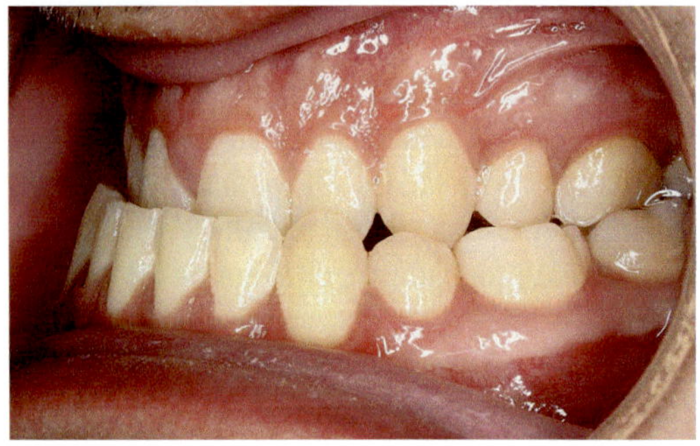

Fig. 18.6 Left lateral view, Class III cuspid/molar occlusion, partial dental compensation

Angle's classification system is a guideline used by all orthodontists when evaluating the dentition and malocclusion. This classification system utilizes the dentition to determine the anteroposterior position of the dental bases. This is not the only area for obtaining an esthetic outcome. The soft tissue profile characterized with each Angle classification also has significant importance to facial esthetics (Figs. 18.7, 18.8 and 18.9).

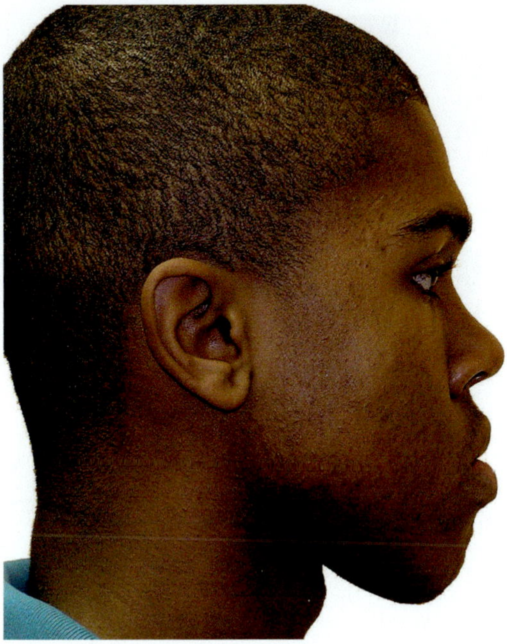

Fig. 18.7 Concave profile, Class III

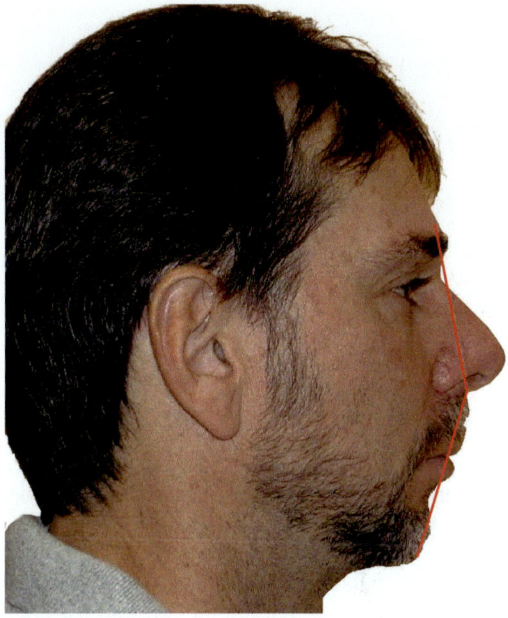

Fig. 18.9 Convex profile, Class II

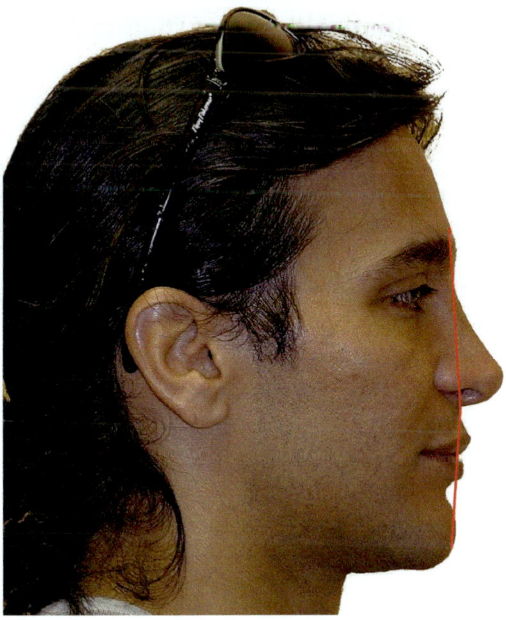

Fig. 18.8 Balanced profile, Class I

A complete diagnosis should include:

- Comprehensive medical history.
- Physical examination.
- Cephalometric/cone beam computed tomography (CBCT), 3D analysis and prediction.
- Intraoral digital scan, virtual and physical models, maxillary, mandibular arches, and inter-occlusal record.
- Intraoral and extraoral photography.
- CBCT and photographic superimposition, orthognathic software.

The clinical exam begins from the moment the clinician introduces themself to the patient. Facial imbalances can be recognized from one's speaking, smiling, and even head posture.

Cephalometric norms are a useful tool and have been obtained from many years of observation. These norms can be used for both gender and ethnic considerations and should be used as

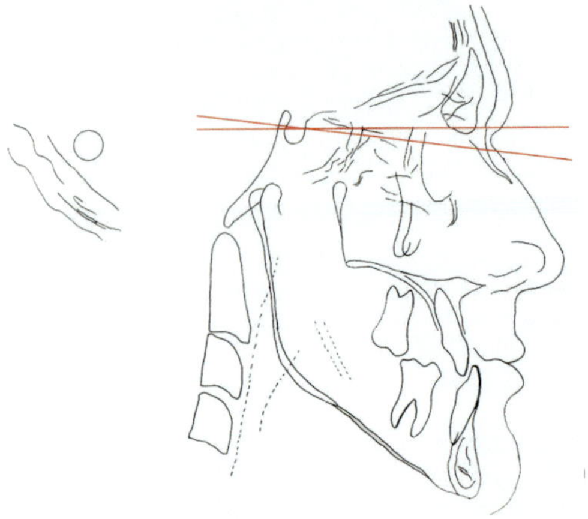

Fig. 18.10 Conventional lateral cephalogram; reference planes, Frankfort plane (Po-Or), SN plane (Sn-N point)

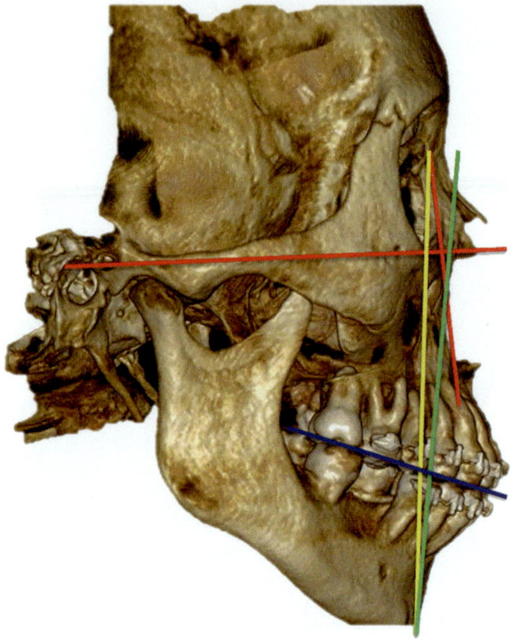

Fig. 18.11 Cone beam computed tomography cephalogram with multiple planes and angles

an aid or guideline, but not an absolute for positioning all patients (Figs. 18.10 and 18.11).

Cephalometric norms are a useful tool and have been obtained from many years of observation. These norms can be used for both gender and ethnic considerations and should be used as an aid or guideline, but not an absolute for positioning all patients.

During facial growth and development, it is not uncommon to see compensations in the dentition due to the underlying skeletal discrepancy. For Class III patients, one can expect some degree of dental compensation resulting in proclination of the maxillary incisors as well as upright or retroclined mandibular incisors. For an ideal esthetic outcome that is supported by hard tissue, decompensation of the dentition to the ideal tooth position should be achieved for greater skeletal movements and long term stability.

18.2 Spatial Planes of Diagnosis

The coronal visualization of the face should not be isolated in the diagnosis of the deformity. Rather, it should be considered in conjunction with the remaining planes of dimension. Head orientation is of outmost importance in preventing misdiagnosis [1].

The concept of natural head position has been controversial in the literature [5].

Natural head positioning techniques for accurate clinical photography and scan acquisition have been described. The inter-pupillary and inter-tragal planes should be parallel to the horizon. Likewise, vertical orientation lines that are perpendicular to the horizontal lines at the level of the mid-portion of the inter-canthal region, pupillary area, and mid-zygomatic regions should be compared in an analytical manner. The use of 3D imaging has substantially changed the accuracy and understanding of facial deformities. In the author's opinion, one of the most important applications of this technology is in orthodontic and surgical planning, including the facilitation of pre-operative laboratory splint fabrication and the incorporation of the spatial relationship in the practitioner's visualization of the craniofacial anatomy (Figs. 18.12, 18.13, 18.14 and 18.15; Table 18.1) [6].

Reliance on cephalometric analysis and treatment planning can sometimes lead to esthetic concerns.

Some practitioners do not systematically examine the face prior to making treatment planning decisions [7].

The dentition should be analyzed in a thorough manner. It is imperative to have an ideal occlusal relationship to be able to achieve the surgical goals. All disciplines in dentistry should be considered as needed in the specific cases. Orthodontist, prosthodontist, periodontist, endodontist, and oral and maxillofacial surgeons are all valuable contributors to a team approach.

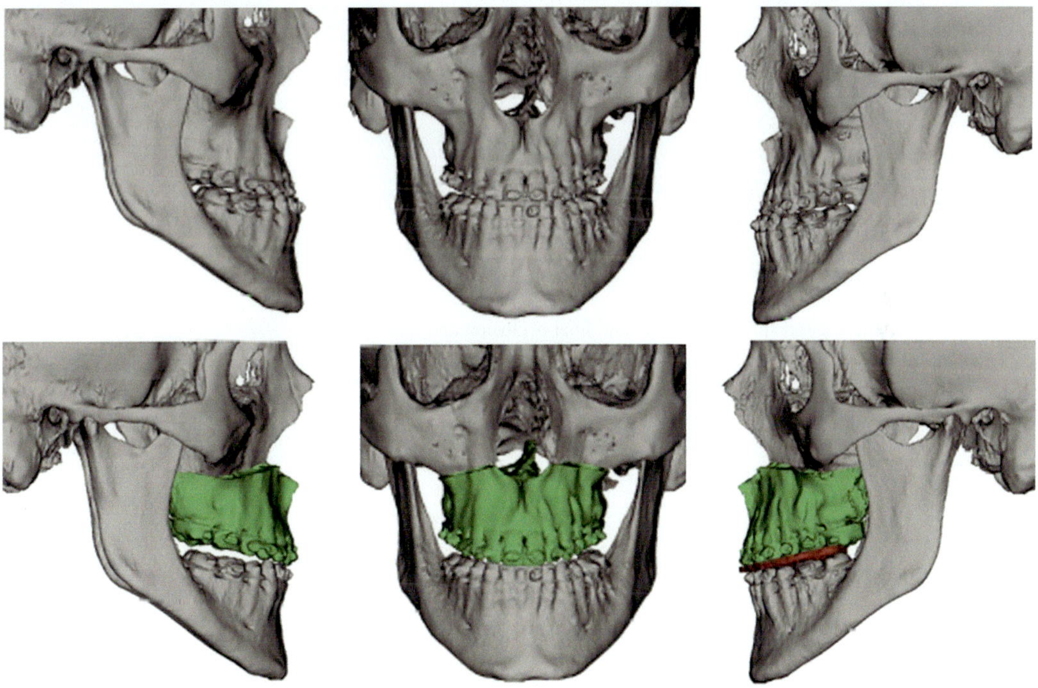

Fig. 18.12 Virtual digital planning; pre-op and post-op 3D changes

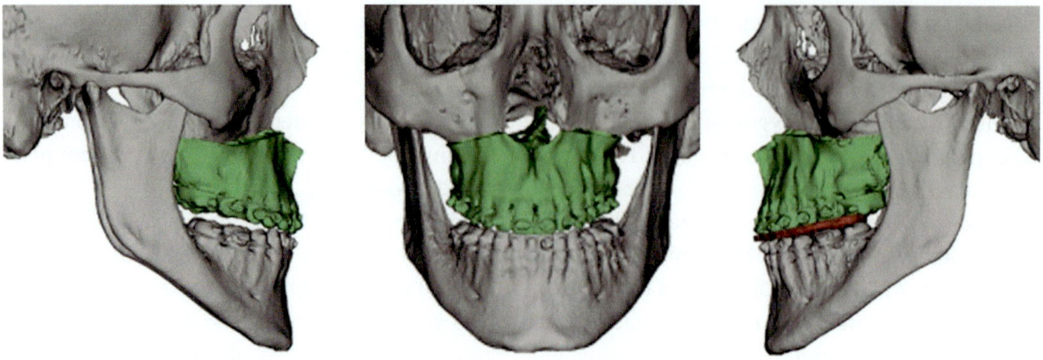

Fig. 18.13 Virtual planning; Le-Fort I Maxillary Osteotomy with surgical splint

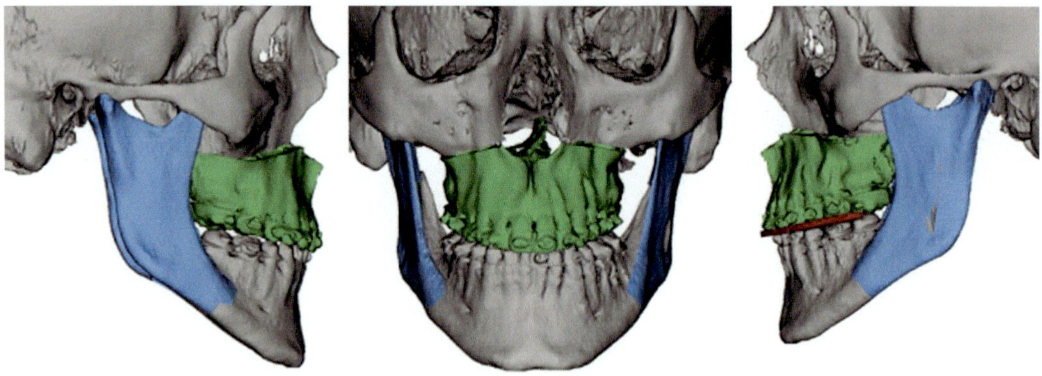

Fig. 18.14 Bilateral sagittal split osteotomy with final occlusion and final splint

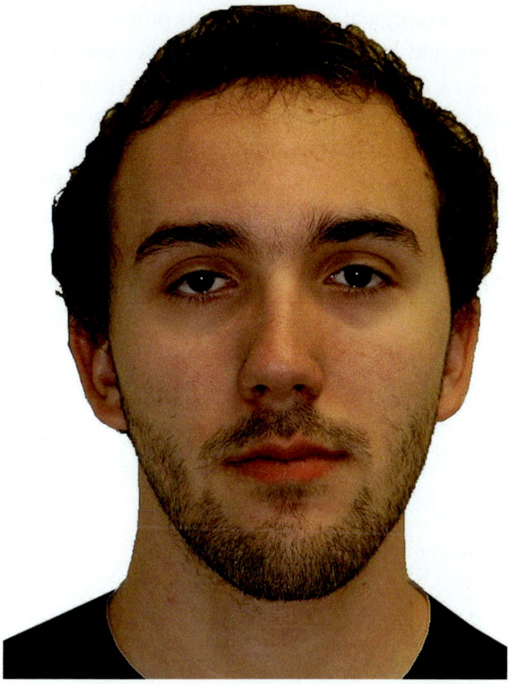

Fig. 18.15 Pre-orthodontic preparation; frontal facial view, relaxed labial position

18.3 Orthodontics

The objectives of orthodontics in orthognathic surgery are to enable maximal surgical correction of the deformity, to facilitate segmental surgery if needed, and to enable the production of an ideal stable occlusion.

The preoperative positioning of the teeth determines the nature and extent of the surgical procedure and influences the final esthetic result.

If indicated surgical odontectomies should be performed to meet orthodontic goals and objectives.

18.3.1 Presurgical Orthodontic Objectives

Orthodontic goals:

- Alignment of the dentition.
- Leveling the occlusal plane as needed.

Table 18.1 Measurements demonstrating actual changes in the facial skeleton after bi-maxillary surgery

Point	Name	Anterior/posterior	Left/right	Up/down
ANS	Anterior nasal spine	4.81 mm anterior	1.50 mm right	1.65 mm down
A	A point	4.37 mm anterior	1.50 mm right	1.49 mm down
ISU1	Midline of upper incisor	3.50 mm anterior	1.50 mm right	1.50 mm down
U3L	Upper left canine	3.58 mm anterior	1.50 mm right	1.08 mm down
U6L	Upper left anterior molar (meiobuccal cusp)	37.73 mm anterior	1.50 mm right	0.54 mm down
U3R	Upper right canine	3.59 mm anterior	1.50 mm right	1.12 mm down
U6R	Upper right anterior molar (meiobuccal cusp)	3.73 mm anterior	1.50 mm right	0.60 mm down
ISL1	Midline of lower incisor	3.69 mm posterior	1.74 mm right	0.11 mm down
L6L	Lower left anterior molar (mesiobuccal cusp)	2.90 mm posterior	1.05 mm right	0.06 mm up
L6R	Lower right anterior molar (mesiobucal cusp)	4.38 mm posterior	1.11 mm right	1.07 mm up
B	B point	4.41 mm posterior	2.16 mm right	0.06 mm down
Pog.	Pogonion	5.02 mm posterior	2.68 mm right	0.19 mm down

- Incisor de-compensation.
- Buccal segment de-compensation.
- Inter-arch coordination.

18.3.2 Providing a Means for Intra-Operative Fixation

Traditionally, dental decompensation is performed prior to surgical correction. The objectives of dental decompensation are to position the dentition within the alveolus at an ideal inclination for long-term health and stability. At this time, both arches are treated individually for ideal tooth positioning without the concern for occlusion [8]. Often this will worsen the bite until surgical movements are performed thus resulting in ideal tooth position in the dental housing and ideal esthetics based on proper support to the soft tissue from both the dentition and the skeletal structure (Figs. 18.16, 18.17, 18.18, 18.19, 18.20, and 18.21) [9].

Orthodontic objectives have traditionally been to complete the majority of dental movement prior to surgical correction. This process of alignment and leveling traditionally takes on average from 1 to 2 years. In the more recent years, surgical intervention is being performed early in treatment, surgery-first approach (SFA), to utilize the regional acceleratory phenomenon (RAP) as there is a rapid turnover of bone and cellular healing, thus leading to faster tooth movement [10, 11]. Elimination of the presurgical orthodontic

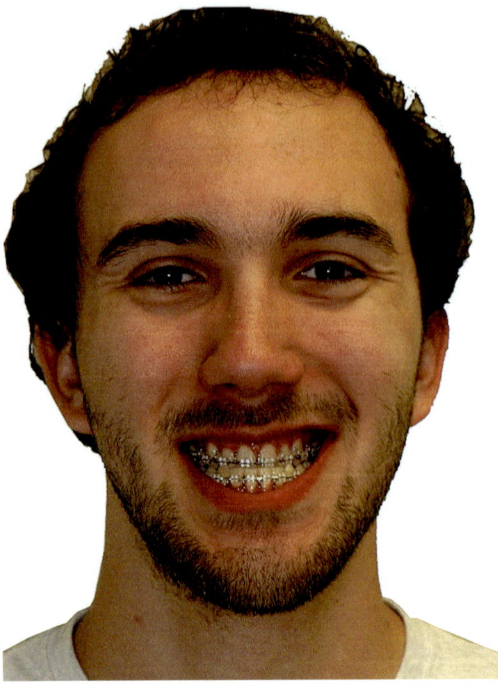

Fig. 18.16 Labial motion, frontal view; appliances in place

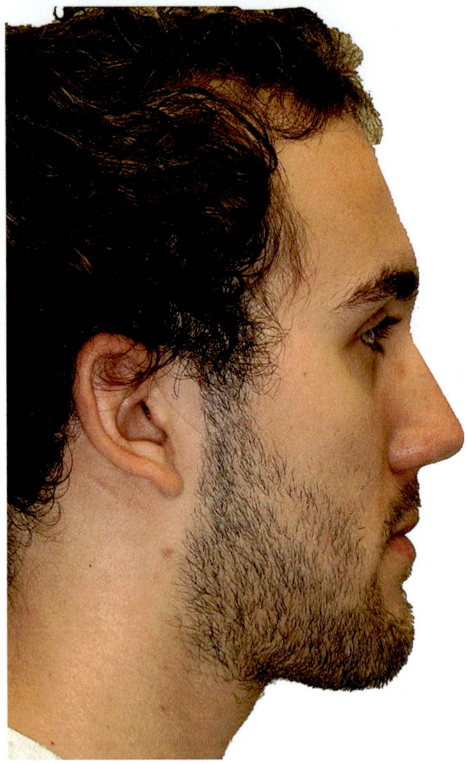

Fig. 18.17 Pre-orthodontic right lateral facial view

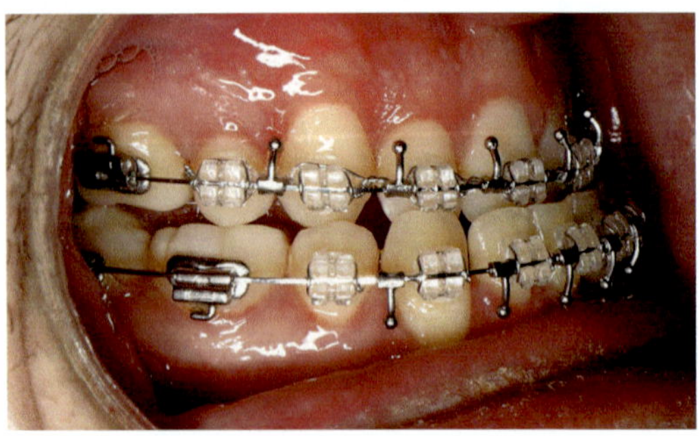

Fig. 18.18 Right lateral occlusal view; orthodontic preparation with increased overjet de-compensation

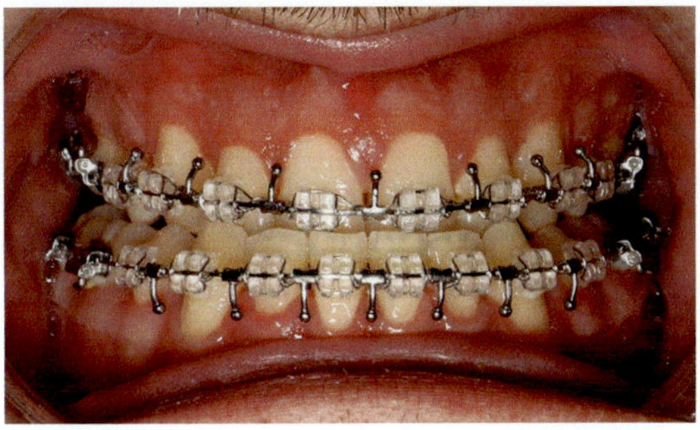

Fig. 18.19 Antero-posterior occlusal view; surgical hooks within the orthodontic passive arch wire, immediately pre-op

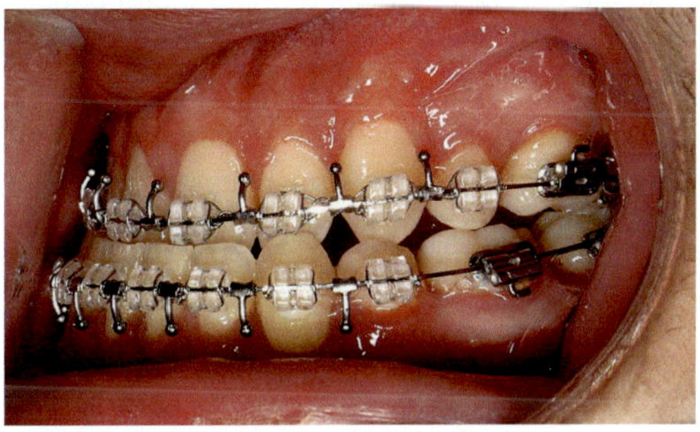

Fig. 18.20 Left lateral occlusal view; orthodontic preparation with increased overjet de-compensation

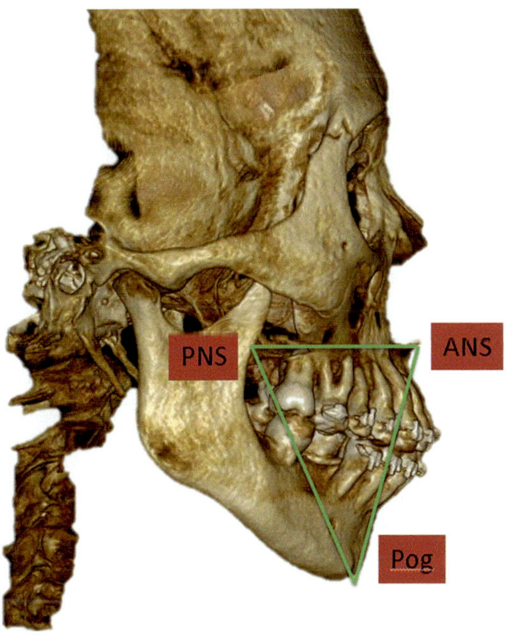

Fig. 18.21 ANS/PNS/Pog triangle. Reference triangle for evaluation of maxilla-mandibular complex rotation

phase has been found to significantly reduce treatment duration [12]. This is a major benefit when the dentition is compromised by decalcifications or even root resorption. Careful considerations should be taken prior to this approach. The criteria suggested for the SFA approach consist of well-aligned dentition, normal-to-mild crowding, minimal axial inclination discrepancies of the anterior dentition, minimal transverse determines, and a flat-to-mild curve of spee. When an SFA approach is chosen, patients are bonded within weeks of their surgical procedure. Interarch elastics are given immediately after surgery to aid in both stabilization and seating of the occlusion. Surgical splints will not be indicated post-surgery unless the transverse relationship is addressed and usually will remain from four to six weeks.

Orthognathic surgery should be performed after growth has ceased for Class III patients when the malocclusion is due to excessive jaw growth. Patients with deficiencies in growth can consider surgical correction prior to cessation, but latency growth should be considered.

18.3.3 Skeletal Anchorage

Anchorage should always be a consideration when devising a proper mechanics plan for orthodontic treatment objectives. In modern orthodontics, skeletal anchorage has become another possibility to better deliver an ideal result, limiting unwanted side effects. The use of endosseous implants, temporary anchorage devices (TADs), and skeletal bone plates are all viable options when seeking the skeletal structure to push off versus the dentition.

The first documented case utilizing endosseous implants was in the early 1970s by Dr. Tom Horton and Dr. Hilt Tatum. Dental implants once fully integrated are found to be the most predictable source for skeletal anchorage [13, 14]. Either in provisionalization or a cemented final restoration, brackets can be placed traditionally and used to limit unwanted side effects associated with orthodontic tooth movement.

The use of TADs is a conservative approach to utilizing the skeletal structure for anchorage. TADs are often placed and removed by the treating clinician chairside with either a topical or local anesthetic. The composition of TADs is titanium or a titanium alloy covered by a smooth surface. Unlike conventional dental implants, TADs are designed specifically not to osseointegrate as removal is to be planned for once no longer needed. There is an initial stabilization period of four to six weeks prior to utilization.

The use of surgical plates, skeletal anchorage system (SAS), is another option for skeletal anchorage but should be considered as a more invasive procedure. These surgical plates will require an appointment for both placement and removal by an oral surgeon. In 1992, Dr. Junji Sugawara first developed the use of miniplates and the SAS system [6]. A pioneer in orthodontic achievements utilizing skeletal anchorage, Dr. Sugawara has utilized SAS for correcting skeletal discrepancies often without the need for orthognathic surgery. The SAS approach should be considered for the correction of Class III malocclusions as well as skeletal openbites, depending on the severity and the knowledge of the treating clinician.

Hugo De Clerck has also utilized skeletal bone plates in orthodontics. His approach and philosophy have been directed toward midfacial deficient Class III patients in their adolescent years. Surgical plates are placed in the maxilla at the infrazygomatic crest and the mandibular canine region for intermaxillary elastic use [15]. Treatment objectives are to stimulate midfacial remodeling with minimal dental compensations and dental movement. Correction has been statistically noted for skeletal versus dental change as seen in traditional facemask therapy [16]. If excessive mandibular growth takes place, this approach can reduce the surgical correction to only the mandible for setback for Class III correction.

Mandibular third molars in particular have been a controversial subject. Some practitioners recommend to perform their removal six to eight months prior to mandibular osteotomies to facilitate rigid fixation procedures. Others have demonstrated that it is perfectly safe to do the odontectomies at the time of the sagittal split osteotomy by designing the cut as usual and performing the actual dental extraction after proximal segment separation. Then the alveolus site is evaluated to select the appropriate fixation methods (Bicortical screws vs. monocortical screws with plate placement).

Profitt has described the limitations of conventional orthodontic tooth movement. However, the technique of pre-orthodontic selective alveolar de-cortication can be helpful in preparing the patients orthodontically for orthognathic surgery [17].

Selective alveolar decortication initiates normal healing processes and stimulates trabecular bone turnover adjacent to the surgical injury.

18.4 Male Consideration

As in all of medicine and surgery, the patient's presenting complaint is very important. The clinician should be aware that patients often attend their first consultation with mixed emotions, and many find it difficult to convey their reasons for seeking advice or treatment. It is recommended to have the first appointment dedicated to the interview and acquisition of records. This will allow the surgeon to better understand the deformity and the psychological status.

Proportionality of the facial thirds is a key determinant of successful orthognathic treatment.

Many studies have investigated the phenotype of the masculine gender in facial appearance. Empirical evidence for the association of facial phenotypes in humans remains scarce and inconsistent.

Modern morphometrics and image analysis have opened an array of new possibilities.

The regression of facial shape on masculinity indicated that male facial features tend to have a wider face, wider inter-orbital distance, a wider nose, thinner lips, and larger more rounded lower facial outline [18].

Differences in cephalometric values based on age and gender have been published extensively in the past.

In the correction of a dental deformity, the clinician's vision should be based on (1) fundamental aesthetic principles, (2) the biologic realities of the tissues, (3) patient-specific dysfunctions, and (4) individual treatment preferences.

18.5 Airway Considerations

The continuous flow of air through the upper airway system is thought to be a stimuli for maxillary lateral growth. Clinical detection of structural narrowing of the upper airway could allow early recognition of developing dental and skeletal discrepancies as well as atypical facial morphology and/or obstructive sleep apnea (OSA) [19].

The measurement of the axial cross-sectional area of the pharyngeal lumen can play an important role in evaluation of OSA [20].

A triangle involving the anterior nasal spine (ANS), posterior nasal spine (PNS), and pogonion (Pog) is constructed during the treatment-planning phase to assist in selecting the rotation point and developing a surgical cephalometric visual treatment objective with airway space changes [6] (Figs. 18.22, 18.23 and 18.24).

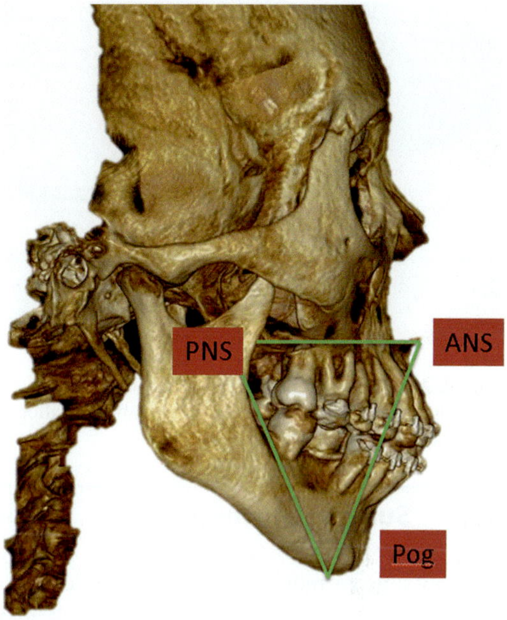

Fig. 18.22 Clockwise rotation of the maxillo-madibular complex with decreased chin projection

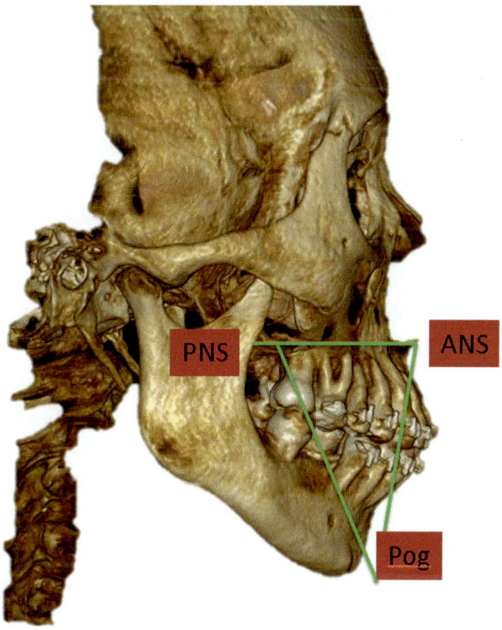

Fig. 18.23 Counter-clockwise rotation of the maxilla-mandibular complex with increased projection of the chin projection

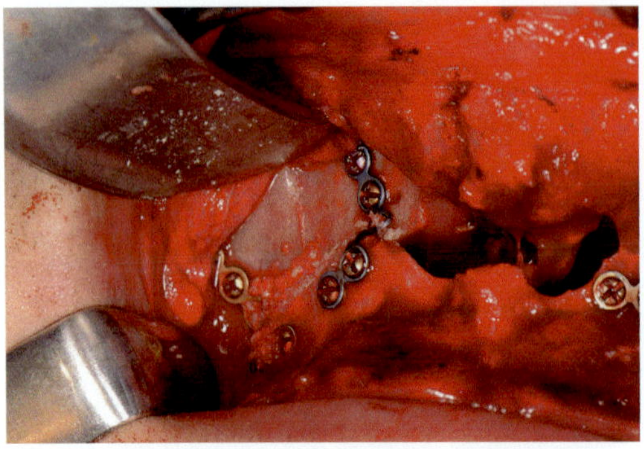

Fig. 18.24 Right side Lefort I maxillary osteotomy with application of rigid fixation with downdraft with allogeneic graft material

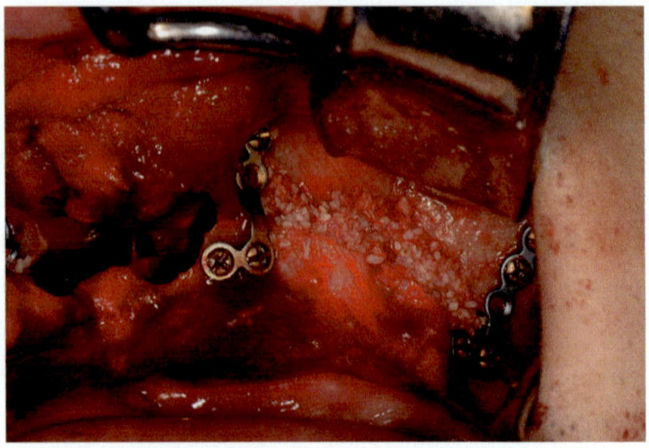

Fig. 18.25 Left side Lefort I osteotomy with advancement and down graft with rigid internal fixation and graft material at the osteotomy site

18.6 Surgical Techniques

It is possible to mobilize the facial skeleton to achieve a total symmetric multi-plane result, and with the application of pre-fabricated surgical guides, it is possible to transport the plan in the operating room.

Rigid fixation has changed the stability of the case and has eliminated the need for maxillomandibular fixation for the initial 4–6 week period in most cases.

Fixation techniques allow the surgeon to select the type of hardware to be used in every case, including mono-cortical, bi-cortical screws, lag screws, and plates, remembering that biomechanical and physiological principles be used in order to obtain a stable position of the maxillofacial complex while bone healing is taking place.

It is important to mention that surgical hooks should be incorporated into the orthodontic arch wire to facilitate the temporary inter-arch fixation and provide the ability to allow for elastics application as needed to guide the occlusal position and start performing minor dental movements, posterior occlusal closure as the patient's dental relationship requires.

Maxillary (Lefort I, II, III, segmented, rapid palatal expansion), mandibular, (sagittal split osteotomies, intraoral vertical osteotomies, modified osteotomies), anterior horizontal osteotomies, (genioplasty), ostectomies, osteoplasties, and application of alloplastic implants have proven to allow the surgeon to achieve the different surgical goals in a safe manner (Figs. 18.25 and 18.26).

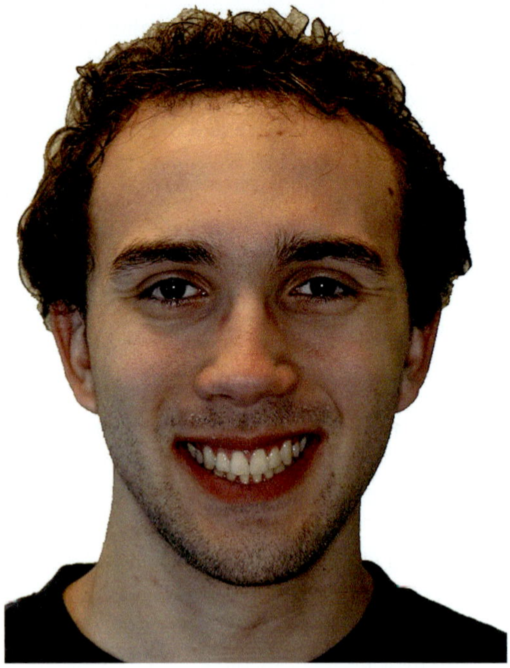

Fig. 18.26 Post-op coronal view with adequate facial balance and soft tissue support

The surgeon should try to minimize the amount of surgical procedures to minimize morbidity in every sense. However, some deformities require multiple surgical, orthodontic, and restorative procedures to achieve the needed facial projection.

Ancillary facial plastic surgery procedures can be added as well as part of the treatment (rhinoplasties, cheiloplasties, liposuction, injection of botox/fillers).

Hypotensive anesthesia is utilized in a routine fashion during orthognathic surgery by minimizing intraoperative blood loss and maintaining adequate blood and oxygen supply to vital organs. A mean arterial pressure of 50–65 mm of Hg is perfectly tolerated in most instances. Deliberate hypotensive anesthesia (DHA) decreases blood pressure by decreasing cardiac output, by decreasing peripheral vascular resistance, or by decreasing a combination of both. Cardiac output must remain sufficiently high not only to provide adequate oxygen supply to the vital organs as well as remove metabolic waste products before any accumulation can cause tissue damage.

It is also believed that patient's head position and attention to ventilation significantly influence venous return and minimizing blood loss in some circumstances, anti-hypertensive medications are also required.

Blood transfusions in the intraoperative and postoperative phases of treatment are infrequently required. Patient selection (medical history, laboratory values), anesthesia management, and meticulous hemostatic surgical techniques are applied.

It has been well documented that with consistent anesthesia techniques, the two factors of greatest importance for blood loss are (1) surgeon's experience and (2) operative time [21].

For individuals undergoing orthognathic surgery with combined maxilla-mandibular procedures, published studies indicate that blood replacement is required in 2.5–75% of the cases [2].

In the authors' experience, blood transfusion with controlled operative variables has been needed in 1.5% of cases.

It has been recommended to prepare the patient with autologous blood donations, but the actual criteria for blood transfusion should be the same as for those for allogeneic blood transfusions [2].

Surgical techniques have been routinely utilized in a predictable fashion since 1960. Bilateral sagittal split osteotomies and Maxillary Lefort I osteotomies are the most common procedures utilized in orthognathic surgery patients.

Multiple scientific papers have demonstrated the biological basis in terms of vascular supply and healing capacity. The versatility of the movements able to achieve of the maxillo-mandibular complex is unlimited.

Intraoral vertical ramus osteotomies are utilized ocassionally in some instances having the disadvantage of boney contact surface but indicated in some asymmetric cases because of limited boney interferences [22].

The transverse dimension should be evaluated and addressed, as segmental surgeries are indicated in some instances [8, 11]. It can be performed simultaneously with the additional movements or in a staged manner with distraction osteogenesis, including surgically assisted rapid palatal expansion and mandibular midline expansion.

18.7 Discussion

The objectives of orthognathic surgery should include aesthetics, function, and stability [23].

It is a multidisciplinary sub-specialty requiring the incorporation of team members, from the diagnosis to the execution of the case, to fulfill the treatment goals in a satisfactory manner. Orthodontic preparation is mandatory in some cases to position the dental arches in such a way that the desired jaw movement can be maximized. In other cases, the "surgery first" concept may be applied, reducing the orthodontic treatment due to bony physiological changes induced by the osteotomies [24–26].

Postoperative results have clearly demonstrated a significant benefit in esthetics, function, and psychological behavior of patients over the years. Self-esteem and personality changes are evident in these cases (Figs. 18.27, 18.28, 18.29, 18.30, 18.31 and 18.32) [27].

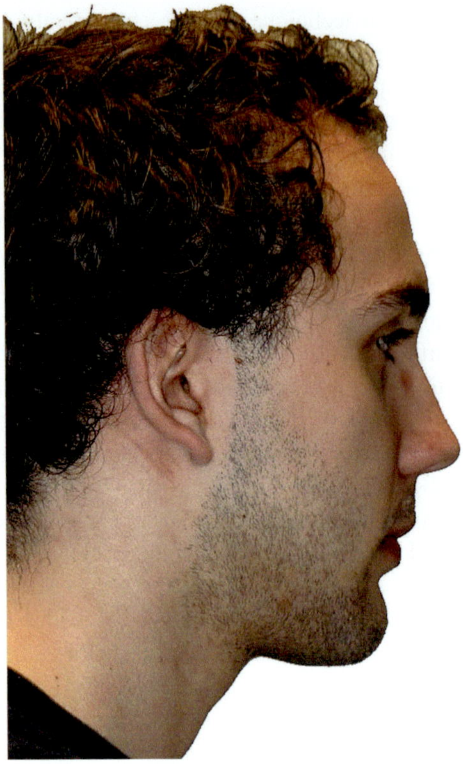

Fig. 18.27 Post-op, right lateral facial view with balanced features and nasal projection

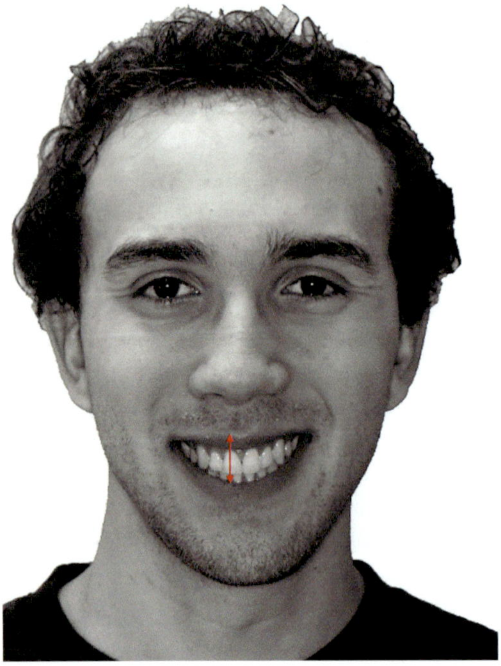

Fig. 18.28 Final dento-labial frame

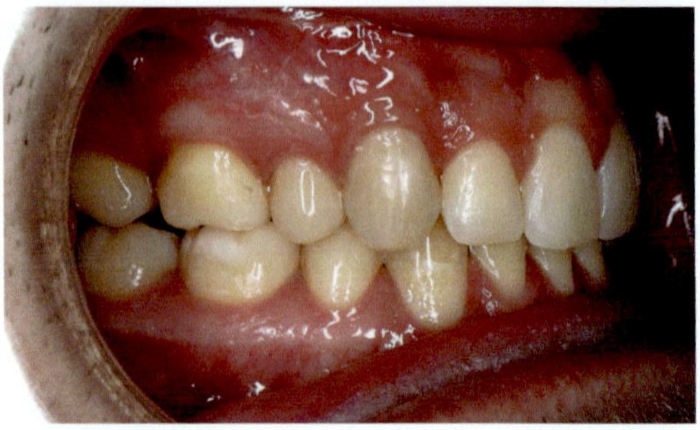

Fig. 18.29 Final occlusion, right lateral dental view, Class I occlusion

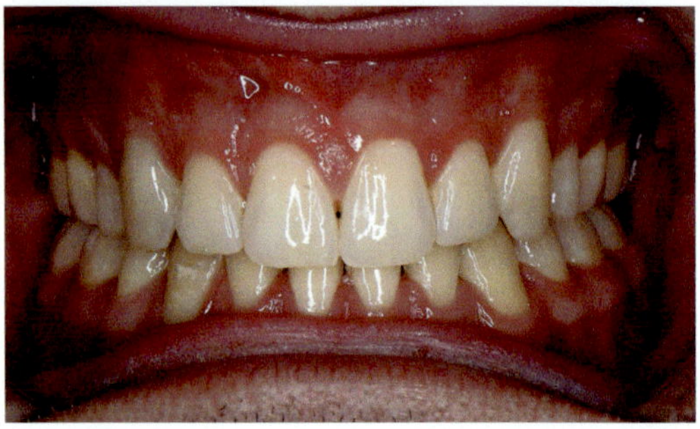

Fig. 18.30 Final occlusion, frontal view with excellent Class I occlusal contacts

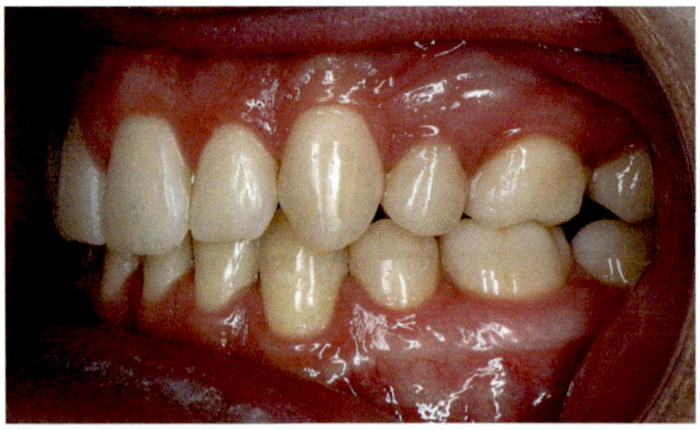

Fig. 18.31 Final occlusion, left lateral dental view, Class I occlusion

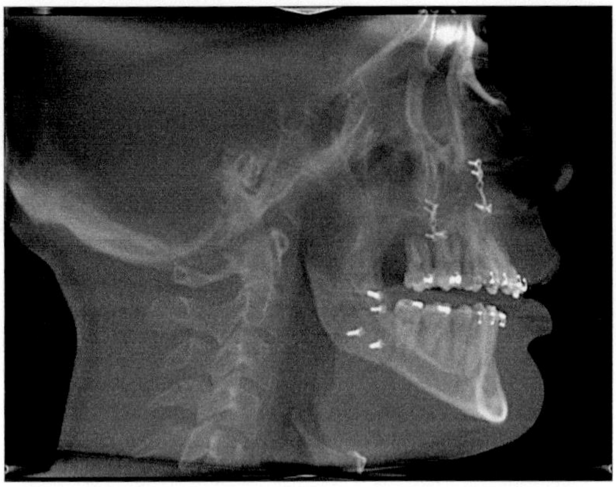

Fig. 18.32 Post-operative lateral cephalogram in relaxed position, rigid internal fixation is demonstrated

18.8 Conclusion

Orthognathic surgery is a multidisciplinary modality that requires meticulous diagnosis and planning. When performed correctly, the final results are extremely beneficial to the patients in an esthetic, functional, and psychological manner [28–30].

References

1. Albrektsson T, Branemark PI, Hansson HA, et al. Osseointegrated titanium implants: requirements for ensuring a long-lasting, direct bone-to-implant anchorage in man. Acta Orthop Scand. 1981;52(2):155–70.
2. Albrektsson T, Jacobsson M. Bone-metal interface in osseointegration. J Prosthet Dent. 1987;57(5):597–607.
3. Arnett GW, Gunson MJ, McLaughlin R. Three dimensional facial treatment planning. In: In Bell WH, Guerrero CA, editors. Distraction osteogenesis of the Facila skeleton. Hamilton: B.C. Decker Inc.; 2007.
4. Avrahami E, Englender M. Relation between CT axial cross-sectional area in the oropharynx and obstructive sleep apnea syndrome in adults. Am J Neuroradiol. 1995;16:135–40.
5. Cevidanes L, Baccetti T, Franchi L, McNamara JA Jr, De Clerck H. Comparison of two protocols for maxillary protraction: bone anchors versus face mask with rapid maxillary expansion. Angle Orthod. 2010;80(5):799–806.
6. De Clerck HJ, Cornelis MA, Cevidanes LH, Heymann G, Tulloch CJF. Orthopedic traction of the maxilla with miniplates: a new perspective for treatment of midface deficiency. J Oral Maxillofac Surg. 2009;67:2123–9.
7. Dorland's Illustrated Medical Dictionary, 30th ed. Philadelphia: WB Saunders, 2003.
8. Finn MD. Surgical assistance of rapid orthodontic treatment and temporary skeletal Anchorage. Oral Maxillofac Surgery Cl N Am. 2014;26:539.
9. Frost HM. The regional acceleratory phenomenon: a review. Henry Ford Hosp Med J. 1983;31:3–9.
10. Ghali GE, Sikes JW. Intraoral vertical ramus osteotomy as the preferred treatment for mandibular prognathism. J Oral Maxillofac Surg. 2000;58:313.
11. Guerrero CA. Surgical orthodontics in mandibular widening. In: In Bell WH, Guerrero CA, editors. Distraction osteogenesis of the facial skeleton. B.C. Decker Inc; 2007.
12. Harris M, Hunt N. Fundaments of orthognathic surgery and non surgical facial esthetics. World Scientific Publishing Co.; 2018.
13. Kula K, Ghoneima A. Cephalometry in orthodontics:2D and 3D. Quintessence Publishing Co.; 2018.
14. Mitteroecker P, Windhagers S, Mueller GB, Schaefer K. The morphometrics of masculinity in human faces. PLoS One. 2015;10:2.
15. Naini FB, Gill DS. Orthognathic surgery, principles, planning and practice. Wiley Blackwell; 2017.
16. Nanda R. Biomechanics and esthetic strategies in clinical orthodontics. St Louis: Elsevier; 2005.
17. Nanda R, Uribe F. Temporary anchorage devices in orthodontics. St Louis: Elsevier; 2009.
18. Nanda R, Uribe F. Atlas of complex orthodontics. St Louis: Elsevier; 2017.
19. Nicolaievsky E. Asymmetric mandibular deformity. In: Carlson ER, McDonald JJ, NIcolaievsky E. The luckiest man: a festschrift in on honor of Robert E, Marx, DDS. Hanover Park: Quintessence Publishing Co; 2016.
20. Posnick JC. Orthognathic surgery. St Louis Mo: Principles & Practice. Elsevier Saunders; 2014.
21. Proffit W, Fields H. Contemporary orthodontics. 3rd ed. St Louis: Mosby; 2000.
22. Reyneke JP. Essentials of Orthognathic surgery. 2nd ed. Chicago, Ill: Quintessence Publishing Co.; 2010.
23. Rumasak D, Apipan B, Kaewpradup P. Factors that determine intra-op blood loss in bi-maxillary osteotomies and the need for operative blood loss. J Oral Maxillofac Surg. 2011;69:456.
24. Sharma V, Yadav K, Tandon P. An overview of surgery-first approach: recent advances in orthognathic surgery. J Orthod Sci. 2015;4(1):9–12.
25. Shindol JM, Matsumoto Y, Sato Y, et al. Soft tissue cephalometric norms for orthognathic and cosmetic surgery. J Oral Maxillofac Surg. 2013;71:24–30.
26. Sugawara J. JCO interviews, Dr. Junji Sugawara on the skeletal anchorage system. J Clin Orthod. 2000;33:689–96.

27. Swennen GRJ. 3-D virtual treatment planning of orthognathic surgery. Berlin: Springer Publishing; 2017.
28. Uribe F, Adabi S, Janakiraman N, Allareddy, Steinbacher D, Shafer D, Villegas C. Treatment duration and factors associated with the surgery-first approach: a two-center study. Prog Orthod. 2015;16:29.
29. Wilcko WM, Wilko T, Bouquout JE, et al. Rapid orthodontics with alveolar reshaping. Int J Periodontics Restorative Dent. 2001;21:9.
30. Wolford L, Perez DE. Surgical management of congenital deformities with temporomandibular joint malformation. Oral Maxillofac Surg Clin North Am. 2015;27:137–54.

Genioplasty: Osteoplastic vs. Implant

19

Faisal Al-Mufarrej and Keith Jeffords

19.1 Introduction

Chin augmentation can be performed either in isolation or in combination with orthognathic procedures or rhinoplasty. A physician's training and background often play a great role in how chin augmentation is performed. Otolaryngologists and plastic surgeons may be more likely to perform implant surgery; oral surgeons and craniofacial surgeons are more likely to offer osteoplastic advancement; and dermatologists only offer filler techniques. While there is a great deal of personal bias amongst surgeons, when choosing between the type of genioplasty for any given patient, one must consider the advantages and disadvantages of each technique in their selection and perform the procedure that is best suited to each patient's specific needs. The provider must be comfortable in evaluating the patient and performing the procedure that is best suited.

19.2 Evaluation

When evaluating the chin, it is important to do so in the context of a full facial analysis, including orthognathic and nasal relationships. In the case of maxillary retrusion and/or malocclusion, orthognathic surgery may be necessary with or without chin surgery. Chin retrusion should be assessed three dimensionally. The distance from the subnasale to mentum should ideally represent the lower third of the face with the lower lip and chin representing two-thirds of that height. The anteroposterior dimension of the chin should be assessed in relation to the nasion (Gonzalez-Ulloa zero meridian), alar groove (Goode meridian), lower lip vermilion (Silver method), and both the cervicomental (121–126 degrees) and mentocervical angles (110–120 degrees) [1].

19.3 Osteoplastic Advancement

19.3.1 Technique

This can be performed under general anesthesia or local anesthesia with sedation. If general anesthesia is performed, nasotracheal intubation is preferred unless a simultaneous rhinoplasty is performed. The surgeon is at the head of the table with the patient's neck in a slight extension. A gingivobuccal sulcus incision extending from canine to canine is performed, leaving a wide

F. Al-Mufarrej (✉)
The Michael and Marian Ilitch Department of Surgery, Wayne State University School of Medicine, Detroit, MI, USA
e-mail: falmufar@wayne.med.edu

K. Jeffords
Private Practice, Paramount Plastic Surgery, Smyrna, GA, USA

K. Jeffords et al. (eds.), *Aesthetic Surgery for Men*, https://doi.org/10.1007/978-3-032-03840-1_19

enough mucoperiosteal cuff for final closure. Subperiosteal dissection is performed, taking care to leave a lingual soft tissue pedicle centrally (including genioglossus and geniohyoid) to maintain blood supply to the distal bone segment. The midline is best marked vertically with a side-cutting burr prior to starting the osteotomy to maintain the alignment of the advanced bony segment. With the aid of a reciprocating saw, a bicortical horizontal osteotomy is performed on either side. Use of a piezoelectric saw may reduce the likelihood of bleeding and asymmetry, as well as intraoperative nerve and dental injury [2]. This can be performed lateral to medial or vice versa. The osteotomy is completed with digital downfracture of the bony segment.

A more oblique osteotomy may be performed if vertical height changes, in addition to advancement, are necessary. A wedge osteotomy or graft placement is performed if more significant shortening or lengthening is necessary, respectively. A jumping genioplasty, where the distal bony segment is placed in front of the mandible like an implant, also allows for significant simultaneous advancement and shortening. A two-tiered step-ladder osteotomy with two bony segments allows for significant advancement without a change to vertical height.

It is important to place the osteotomy 5 mm below the roots of the canines [3] and at least 6 mm below the mental nerve to prevent injury. The nerve typically dips inferiorly before exiting the mental foramen [4, 5]. Measuring with calipers and marking the intended osteotomy line prior to making the osteotomy may assist in ensuring a symmetric cut. Asymmetric osteotomies, however, may be performed to correct chin asymmetries, keeping in mind that soft tissue changes do not follow bony changes to the same extent. Once repositioned, the bone segment is fixed with a screw and/or adaptation plates. Figure 19.1 demonstrates the steps to the procedure. Figures 19.2, 19.3, and 19.4 demonstrate preoperative (a) and postoperative (b) images of sample patients undergoing osseous advancement genioplasty.

19.3.2 Advantages

While both techniques have been shown to result in high patient satisfaction, advancement genioplasty has a slightly higher satisfaction rate than alloplastic augmentation (96.3% vs 87.5%) [6] with a trend toward higher self-esteem and more likely to recommend the procedure.

The soft tissue response is also more predictable for the osteoplastic genioplasty. Guyron et al. note an 85% average soft tissue to hard tissue response, compared to 66% for alloplastic procedures by the same surgeon. Other studies have noted a 46–90% [7–9] response rate with alloplastic technique and 95–100% for osteoplastic [10–13]. The poorer soft tissue response rate seen with implants is likely multifactorial (bone resorption, lower implant material density compared to bone, capsular contracture, less rigid fixation, and implant displacement).

In addition to improved soft tissue response, the cervicomental angle improves more with the

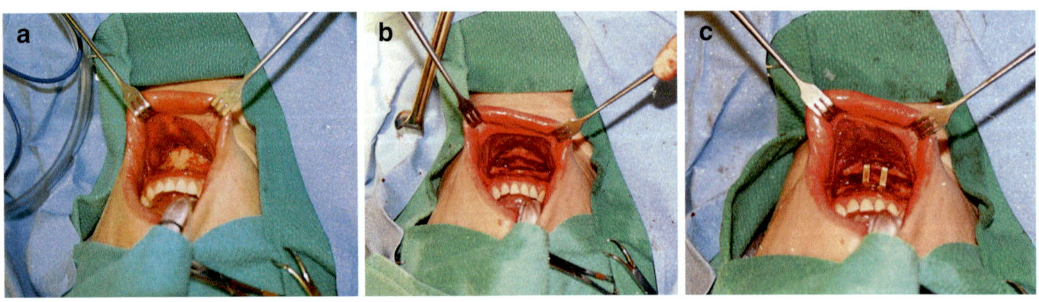

Fig. 19.1 Intraoperative view of osseous genioplasty after initial exposure (**a**), horizontal osteotomy (**b**), advancement and fixation (**c**)

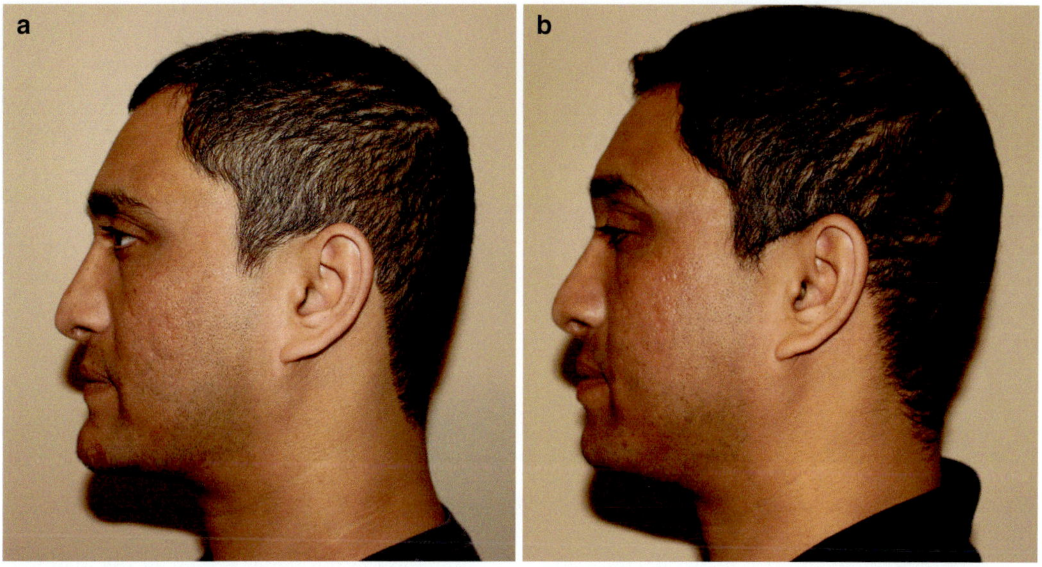

Fig. 19.2 Osseous genioplasty: Preoperative (**a**) and postoperative (**b**)

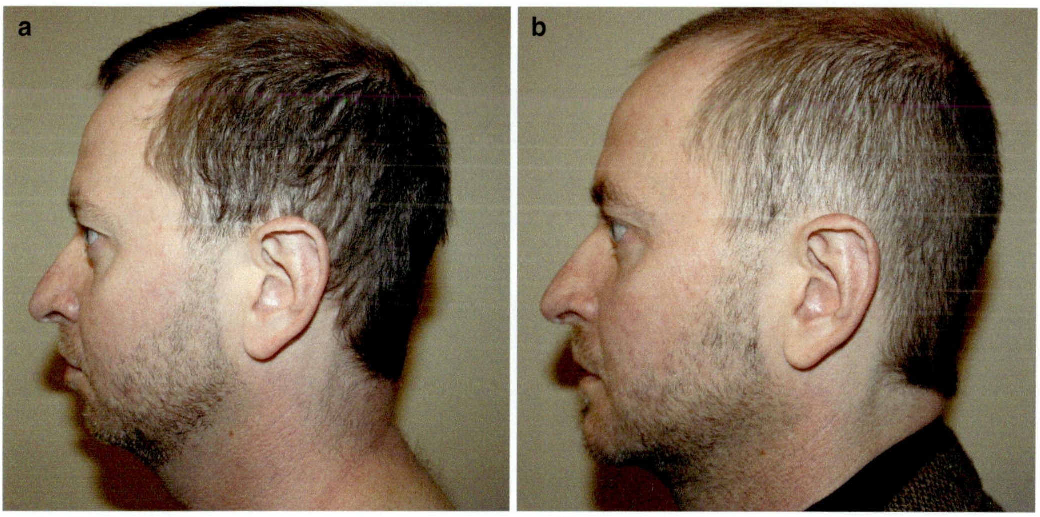

Fig. 19.3 Osseous genioplasty: Preoperative (**a**) and postoperative (**b**)

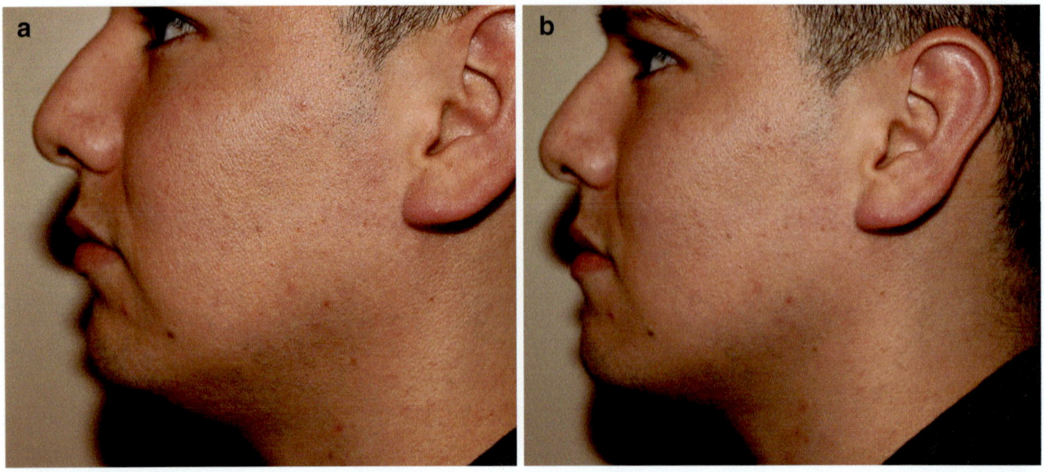

Fig. 19.4 Osseous genioplasty: Preoperative (**a**) and postoperative (**b**)

osteoplastic genioplasty [6]. Osteoplastic genioplasty also allows for three-dimensional correction of microgonia as well as correction of asymmetries.

19.3.3 Disadvantages

Osseous genioplasty is considered by some to be more invasive and as such requires a longer postoperative recovery with more postoperative swelling. Bleeding from osteotomy site and the potential for a floor-of-mouth hematoma is also more likely. Rare mandibular fractures have been reported [14].

Mental nerve injury is a recognized complication of the procedure, occurring at a rate of 10–20% in some studies [15, 16]. While some report complete nerve recovery at 12 months [17], others note around 6–7% permanent deficits [4, 18]. Rates of nerve injury can be reduced with careful placement of the incision, gentle retraction, and correct osteotomy.

Resorption of bone, typically at the inferior border of the advanced segment, even avascular necrosis, can rarely occur if the soft tissue pedicle is detached from the bone segment intraoperatively and the bone is advanced as a free graft [19–21]. Relapse rates ranging from 2.6% to 30% have also been documented [22].

Notching at the lower border of the mandible can occur in up to 72.5% patients, compromising the final aesthetic result, especially in older patients with preexisting jowling [15]. A witch's chin deformity (genial ptosis) can also occur if the mentalis is overstripped and not resuspended at the end of the case.

Malposition of bone segment, malunion, and nonunion can occur particularly with semirigid fixation using wires [23]. Hardware-related pain and discomfort are rarely seen, especially if it is loose.

19.3.4 Indications

Patients who need three-dimensional correction of microgenia are typically best suited to undergo osseous genioplasty. Also, patients with vertically long chins should not undergo implant augmentation as it may lengthen the chin further. Additionally, since standard implants do not fix asymmetries, patients who have asymmetric microgenia should undergo osseous rearrangement. Patients who are high risk for implant infection, including those with previous infections, periodontal disease, or heart valve disease, are better suited for osseous advancement.

Patients with failed implant genioplasties should not undergo repeat implant placement but instead undergo osseous genioplasty. In fact, an osseous genioplasty should be considered for every patient with a failed implant to prevent delayed soft tissue deformities. Cohen et al. reported a high rate of soft-tissue chin deformities in patients for whom implants were removed without repeat genioplasty: chin ptosis, bunching, dimpling (90%); asymmetrical motion of the lower lip (50%); and pogonial tenderness (20%). These deformities, once established, are virtually uncorrectable and should be prevented with osseous genioplasty [24].

In addition to the above-noted absolute indication, there are many relative indications for this approach. While some surgeons have used large implants with good results, patients who require >4–6 mm advancement [25] or need for concomitant improvement in the cervicomental angle should be considered for osseous genioplasty. Matarosso et al. [26] believe that patients with labial incompetence and lip strain are not good candidates for implants and are better with osteoplastic advancement because of the excessive labial force placed on the implants with resultant bone resorption. Hyperactivity of the chin musculature may also displace the implant or produce a constant source of irritation [27].

Based on their retrospective comparative study, given the more predictive result obtained with osteoplastic genioplasty, Guyuron et al. actually recommend that the osteoplastic technique be performed for every patient, except older patients, particularly those with a small degree of microgenia [6].

19.4 Alloplastic Augmentation

19.4.1 Technique

The procedure can be done under general anesthesia or local anesthesia (mental nerve block and local infiltration). The cutaneous midline should be marked prior to injecting local anesthetic or starting the procedure. A submental or intraoral approach can be done.

When an intraoral approach is selected, a limited gingivobuccal sulcus incision is made, the mentalis muscle is divided, and either a central subperiosteal or supraperiosteal pocket is developed. The mental nerves are identified and protected.

With a submental approach, a 2–3 cm incision is placed just behind the submental crease, and a central subperiosteal plane is developed. While a subperiosteal pocket increases implant stability, it may be more likely to cause bony erosion. For long anatomic implants, surgeons may opt to have a central supraperiosteal pocket that is extended subperiosteally laterally. The implant should be placed along the lower border of the mandible and below the mental nerves. Unless the subperiosteal pocket is tight, the implant should be fixed with either a suture or a unicortical titanium screw. The mentalis muscle is then repaired.

The skin or gingiva is then closed, and the patient is placed in a chin strap postoperatively for 5–7 days. While the very first implant genioplasty described used metal, there have been many materials used since, including: Teflon, hydroxyapatite, Gore-Tex (W.L. Gore and Associates Inc., Flagstaff, AZ), porous polytetrafluoroethylene carbon (Proplast; Vitek Inc., Houston, TX), hard tissue replacement (HTR) polymer, polyamide mesh (Supramid; J. Jackson Inc., Alexandria, VA), and high-density polyethylene (Medpor; Porex Surgical Inc., College Park, GA). Custom-made implants (using Mersilene mesh) have also been reported [28]. Preferably, the implant should have an anatomic configuration with a posterior surface that contours to the surface of the mandible and tapered margins that blend with the mandibular border. Silastic implants (made of solid medical-grade silicone) are probably the most used nowadays, with well-documented success [29–33]. Silastic implants are ideal because they are inert, comfortable, nonpalpable, malleable, resistant to infection, and nontoxic.

19.4.2 Advantages

Implants are quicker, easier, with less swelling and bleeding risk. Even though many advocate osseous genioplasty for large advancements, implants offer flexibility in size and shape. One can achieve a smoother, cleaner jaw line with no risk of bony malunion or nonunion. There is also less risk of nerve injury. This is especially true with the submental approach, which also carries no risk of chin ptosis.

19.4.3 Disadvantages

In general, while both techniques are safe in expert hands with similar overall morbidity [1–6], when complications arise, they tend to be more severe with alloplastic augmentation. Implants are associated with 5–7% infection rate [34–37]. Infection can present with tenderness, erythema, swelling, drainage, or intraoral fistula. This can be reduced with use of nonporous implants (Silastic), sterile submental approach, careful handling of soft tissues, avoidance of oral contamination, and use of systemic antibiotics and antibiotic irrigation. Implant salvage can be attempted with washout and antibiotics, but implant removal is often necessary [29]. Delayed rejection of the implant can also occur and present in a manner similar to that of an infection. In delayed rejection, a foreign body reaction occurs with granuloma formation and negative microbacterial cultures. While there is always a risk of seeing this with new implant materials, this is rare with the inert Silastic implants.

Other complications related to alloplastic augmentation include misalignment, malposition, displacement, extrusion, bony encapsulation, and soft tissue capsular contracture [38, 39]. Proplast implants are associated with 86% rate of posterior settling of >1 mm and an almost 20% rate of bony encapsulation [39]. The rounded, thicker implants are more likely to be associated with these complications than the newer anatomic implants. The use of porous implants allows for tissue ingrowth and stabilizes the implant. A submental approach also keeps mentalis intact and prevents superior displacement. Migration is also minimized by avoiding big implants, limited pocket dissection, layered closure, and suture or screw fixation to bone or periosteum [40].

Bone resorption can occur due to the pressure of the soft tissue and the implant against the bone, which may be accompanied by a foreign body reaction along the bone surface [39]. Resorption is seen in almost all patients with Proplast I and Proplast II (Vitek Corp) implants [6, 39], with average resorption of 1.25 mm (range 0.0–3.3 mm). Resorption occurs in the first 12 months and affects young patients and males more often, especially if performed concomitantly with maxillary surgery [39]. The size of the implants makes no difference in the amount of bone resorption, although there is slightly less soft tissue change when larger implants are used [39]. Resorption rates of 50–85% have been reported with the use of Silastic (Dow Corning, Midland, MI) implants [41–43]. No resorption is seen with porous block hydroxyapatite (PBHA) [39] or hard tissue replacement polymer implants [36]. Compared with Proplast implants, PBHA demonstrates greater soft tissue changes at pogonion relative to the implant size (average 86.8% versus 83.0%) [39]. The absence of detectable resorption and the excellent soft tissue change make PBHA an attractive alternative as a chin implant material, although it is technically more difficult to use.

It is important to note that despite implant-related bone resorption, no secondary dental or mandibular sequelae have ever been reported with implants. In multiple series, bone resorption has not necessitated the removal of implant [27, 44, 45]. One case of removal due to alveolar bone erosion into the tooth root was reported in Pitanguy's series of 600 patients. Additionally, concomitant soft tissue changes are often not seen with bone absorption. Less resorption is seen when the implant is placed over the hard bone of the lower mandible, rather than the thinner bone closer to the alveolus [42]. Supraperiosteal placement of implants may result in less resorption than subperiosteal placement, which strips the bone of its blood supply [33, 46]. Also, most of the data on bone resorption is published at a time when large centrally placed rounded implants were popular instead of the newer, extended, softer anatomic implants. Such implants produce more pressure on bone and are more likely to migrate superiorly, where bone resorption is more likely.

It is important to note that while there is a great deal of literature on implant-related complications, most of the literature is older when less optimal implants were used and surgeons had much less experience with alloplastic augmentation.

19.4.4 Indications

Implants should be considered if the surgeon has limited experience with the osseous genioplasty or when the patient desires a less invasive procedure with a faster recovery time. Since implants augment in a mainly symmetric anteroposterior dimension, alloplastic augmentation is the best fit for patients with symmetric anteroposterior chin deficiencies and no need for vertical change. This is especially true if transverse widening and squaring of the chin are needed or desired.

Osseous advancement without vertical shortening often tapers the chin. Transverse widening is more easily achieved with an implant. As such, implants should be strongly considered in patients with tapered faces, especially males who often desire a more prominent squared chin.

Furthermore, implants, especially extended anatomic ones, may be better for older patients with jowling as the inferior mandibular notching seen with osteotomy can deepen their prejowl sulcus.

Implants may be considered when one is already performing a submental incision for platysmal tightening and/or submental liposuction/lipectomy or during a facelift [15, 47]. While osseous genioplasties are routinely done with split sagittal osteotomies, implants should be considered instead when an anterior mandibular osteotomy is being performed along with a genioplasty—in order to avoid having two close osteotomies, secondary difficulties with stabilization, and risks of nonunion, malunion, and bone resorption.

Implants should also be considered in revision surgery after previously failed bony advancement [48]. In rare, severe cases of microgenia (>15 mm needed), often in patients with other orthognathic or craniofacial needs, implants may be a necessary adjunct to osseous genioplasty in order to achieve the necessary advancement [49].

19.5 Non-alloplastic Augmentation

Fat grafting to the chin is another approach to chin augmentation. It requires little downtime with minimal risks and cost. While fat grafting may augment the chin sagittally, it is often ineffective in increasing chin height and only provides a modest amount of augmentation [50]. With a maximum volume of 10 cc, percutaneous multilayered fat-injection can provide up to 11 mm increase (7 mm on average) in sagittal projection in 6 months postoperatively [51]. Microgenia has to be overcorrected intraoperatively by 1-2 mm (often with about 1 cc of extra fat) to account for postoperative fat resorption. In addition to treating mild microgenia, fat grafting can correct chin rhytids, chin fat ptosis, lateral chin hollowing, various degrees of soft tissue asymmetry, bifid chins, and deep labiomental sulcus [52]. As such, fat grafting can be a powerful adjunct tool to osteoplastic or alloplastic genioplasty.

Fillers can also be used, though temporary. 1–2 mL of high G prime HA or CaHA filler may be injected through a needle (28 G or 25 G, 1-inch) or cannula (blunt-tipped 22–25 G, 1.5-inch) into the supraperiosteal plane (with or without subdermal injection). Needle injections are performed as 0.1–0.2 cc vertical depots at the gnathion with smaller depots slightly lateral to the gnathion on either side. Injections below and above that level may be performed to adjust the vertical height of the chin and the menotocervical angle, respectively. Augmentation using a cannula is performed using a fanning technique through an entry site at the gnathion. While anterior projection of the pogonion and menton is more easily achieved using needles, cannulas may reduce the risk of bruising [53]. Needles can be safely used with HA fillers because of the ease of their reversibility in the case of rare intra-arterial injection. In an 18-month open-label study of rejuvenation using an HA filler, 98.3% of patients injected were satisfied or very satisfied with their chin results [54].

Swelling, bruising, delayed nodules, granuloma, and infection are possible and should be treated as necessary. Contour irregularities are rare with supraperiosteal injections given the thickness of the chin soft tissues. However, superficial injections may cause contour deformities, especially with animation [53].

19.6 Conclusion

There are various approaches to chin augmentation. A physician's training and background may bias his or her approach, but one must only perform the procedure that is best suited to each patient's specific needs. When selected appropriately and performed correctly, all approaches are safe and effective. While there is a great deal of literature on the advantages and disadvantages of each approach, there is no strong evidence that one approach is truly superior to the other, and surgeons should be familiar and comfortable with each procedure.

References

1. Arroyo HH, Olivetti IP, Lima LF, Jurado JR. Clinical evaluation for chin augmentation: literature review and algorithm proposal. Braz J Otorhinolaryngol. 2016;82(5):596–601.
2. Bertossi D, Albanese M, Mortellaro C, Malchiodi L, Kumar N, Nocini R, et al. Osteotomy in genioplasty by piezosurgery. J Craniofac Surg. 2018;29(8):2156–9.
3. Spear SL, Mausner ME, Kawamoto HK Jr. Sliding genioplasty as a local anesthetic outpatient procedure: a prospective two-center trial. Plast Reconstr Surg. 1987;80(1):55–67.
4. Ousterhout DK. Sliding genioplasty, avoiding mental nerve injuries. J Craniofac Surg. 1996;7(4):297–8.
5. Ritter EF, Moelleken BR, Mathes SJ, Ousterhout DK. The course of the inferior alveolar neurovascular canal in relation to sliding genioplasty. J Craniofac Surg. 1992;3(1):20–4.
6. Guyuron B, Raszewski RL. A critical comparison of osteoplastic and alloplastic augmentation genioplasty. Aesth Plast Surg. 1990;14(3):199–206.
7. Dann JJ, Epker BN. Proplast genioplasty: a retrospective study with treatment recommendations. Angle Orthod. 1977;47(3):173–85.
8. Kent JN, Westfall RL, Carlton DM. Chin and zygomaticomaxillary augmentation with Proplast: long-term follow-up. J Oral Surg (American Dental Association: 1965). 1981;39(11):912–9.
9. Karras SC, Wolford LM. Augmentation genioplasty with hard tissue replacement implants. J Oral Maxillofacial Surg. 1998;56(5):549–52.
10. Bell WH, Gallagher DM. The versatility of genioplasty using a broad pedicle. J Oral Maxillofacial Surg. 1983;41(12):763–9.
11. Gallagher DM, Bell WH, Storum KA. Soft tissue changes associated with advancement genioplasty performed concomitantly with superior repositioning of the maxilla. J Oral Maxillofacial Surg. 1984;42(4):238–42.
12. McDonnell JP, McNeill RW, West RA. Advancement genioplasty: a retrospective cephalometric analysis of osseous and soft tissue changes. J Oral Surg (American Dental Association: 1965). 1977;35(8):640–7.
13. Krekmanov L, Kahnberg KE. Soft tissue response to genioplasty procedures. Br J Oral Maxillofac Surg. 1992;30(2):87–91.
14. Goracy ES. Fracture of the mandibular body and ramus during horizontal osteotomy for augmentation genioplasty. J Oral Surg (American Dental Association: 1965). 1978;36(11):893–4.
15. Lindquist CC, Obeid G. Complications of genioplasty done alone or in combination with sagittal split-ramus osteotomy. Oral Surg Oral Med Oral Pathol. 1988;66(1):13–6.
16. Westermark A, Bystedt H, von Konow L. Inferior alveolar nerve function after mandibular osteotomies. Br J Oral Maxillofac Surg. 1998;36(6):425–8.
17. Hohl TH, Epker BN. Macrogenia: a study of treatment results, with surgical recommendations. Oral Surg Oral Med Oral Pathol. 1976;41(5):545–67.
18. Nishioka GJ, Mason M, Van Sickels JE. Neurosensory disturbance associated with the anterior mandibular horizontal osteotomy. J Oral Maxill Surg. 1988;46(2):107–10.
19. Mercuri LG, Laskin DM. Avascular necrosis after anterior horizontal augmentation genioplasty. J Oral Surg (American Dental Association: 1965). 1977;35(4):296–8.
20. Spear SL, Kassan M. Genioplasty. Clin Plast Surg. 1989;16(4):695–706.
21. Ellis E 3rd, Dechow PC, McNamara JA Jr, Carlson DS, Liskiewicz WE. Advancement genioplasty with and without soft tissue pedicle: an experimental investigation. J Oral Maxill Surg. 1984;42(10):637–45.
22. Polido WD, de Clairefont RL, Bell WH. Bone resorption, stability, and soft-tissue changes following large chin advancements. J Oral Maxill Surg. 1991;49(3):251–6.

23. Davis WH, Davis CL, Daly BW, Taylor C 3rd. Long-term bony and soft tissue stability following advancement genioplasty. J Oral Surg. 1988;46(9):731–5.
24. Cohen SR, Mardach OL, Kawamoto HK Jr. Chin disfigurement following removal of alloplastic chin implants. Plast Reconstr Surg. 1991;88(1):62–6. discussion 7–70
25. Ward JL, Garri JI, Wolfe SA. The osseous genioplasty. Clin Plast Surg. 2007;34(3):485–500.
26. Matarasso A, Elias AC, Elias RL. Labial incompetence: a marker for progressive bone resorption in silastic chin augmentation. Plast Reconstr Surg. 1996;98(6):1007–14. discussion 15
27. Binder WJ, Kamer FM, Parkes ML. Mentoplasty—a clinical analysis of alloplastic implants. Laryngoscope. 1981;91(3):383–91.
28. Zeph RD. Custom-designed chin augmentation. Facial Plast Surg Clin North Am. 2008;16(1):79 85. vi
29. Mahler D. Chin augmentation--a restrospective study. Ann Plast Surg. 1982;8(6):468–73.
30. Beekhuis GJ. Practical suggestions on facial plastic surgery—how I do it. Augmentation mentoplasty using polyamide mesh. Laryngoscope. 1976;86(10):1602–5.
31. Dmytryshyn JR. Mentoplasty. J Otolaryngol. 1981;10(3):181–4.
32. Snyder GB, Courtiss EH, Kaye BM, Gradinger GP. A new chin implant for microgenia. Plast Reconstr Surg. 1978;61(6):854–61.
33. Parkes M. Avoiding bone resorption under plastic chin implants. Archiv Otolaryngol (Chicago, Ill: 1960). 1973;98(2):100–1.
34. Adams JS. Grafts and implants in nasal and chin augmentation. A rational approach to material selection. Otolaryngol Clin N Am. 1987;20(4):913–30.
35. Epstein LI. Clinical experiences with Proplast as an implant. Plast Reconstr Surg. 1979;63(2):219–23.
36. Eppley BL, Sadove AM, Holmstrom H, Kahnberg KE. HTR polymer facial implants: a five-year clinical experience. Aesth Plast Surg. 1995;19(5):445–50.
37. Turvey TA, Epker BN. Soft tissue procedures adjunctive to orthognathic surgery for improvement of facial balance. J Oral Surg (American Dental Association: 1965). 1974;32(8):572–7.
38. Guyuron B, Kadi JS. Problems following genioplasty. Diagnosis and treatment. Clin Plast Surg. 1997;24(3):507–14.
39. Moenning JE, Wolford LM. Chin augmentation with various alloplastic materials: a comparative study. Int J Adult Orthodon Orthognath Surg. 1989;4(3):175–87.
40. Gubisch W, Kotzur A. Our experience with silicone in rhinomentoplasty. Aesth Plast Surg. 1998;22(4):237–44.
41. Bell WH. Correction of the contour-deficient chin. J Oral Surg (American Dental Association: 1965). 1969;27(2):110–5.
42. Friedland JA, Coccaro PJ, Converse JM. Retrospective cephalometric analysis of mandibular bone absorption under silicone rubber chin implants. Plast Reconstr Surg. 1976;57(2):144–51.
43. Robinson M, Shuken R. Bone resorption under plastic chin implants. J Oral Surg (American Dental Association: 1965). 1969;27(2):116–8.
44. Pitanguy I, Martello L, Caldeira AM, Alexandrino A. Augmentation mentoplasty: a critical analysis. Aesth Plast Surg. 1986;10(3):161–9.
45. Flowers RS. Alloplastic augmentation of the anterior mandible. Clin Plast Surg. 1991;18(1):107–38.
46. Jobe R, Iverson R, Vistnes L. Bone deformation beneath alloplastic implants. Plast Reconstr Surg. 1973;51(2):169–75.
47. Glasgold AI, Glasgold MJ. Intraoperative custom contouring of the mandible. Archives of otolaryngology—head & neck surgery. 1994;120(2):180–184.
48. Mohammad S, Dwivedi CD, Singh RK, Singh V, Pal US. Medpore versus osseous augmentation in genioplasty procedure: a comparison. Nat J Maxill Surg. 2010;1(1):1–5.
49. Findikcioglu K, Sibar S, Gulsen A. Treatment approach to severe microgenia cases: combined use of osseous and implant genioplasty. J Craniofac Surg. 2018;29(2):e175–e9.
50. Wang Q, Guo X, Wang J. Autogenous fat grafting for Chin augmentation: a preliminarily clinical study of cosmetic outcome. J Craniofac Surg. 2015;26(7):e625–7.
51. Basile FV, Basile AR. Prospective controlled study of Chin augmentation by means of fat grafting. Plast Reconstr Surg. 2017;140(6):1133–41.
52. Rohrich RJ, Sanniec K, Afrooz PN. Autologous fat grafting to the Chin: a useful adjunct in complete aesthetic facial rejuvenation. Plast Reconstr Surg. 2018;142(4):921–5.
53. Rho NK, Chang YY, Chao YY, Furuyama N, Huang PY, Kerscher M, et al. Consensus recommendations for optimal augmentation of the Asian face with hyaluronic acid and calcium hydroxylapatite fillers. Plast Reconstr Surg. 2015;136(5):940–56.
54. Talarico S, Meski AP, Buratini L, Manela-Azulay M, Simpson H, Sidou F, et al. High patient satisfaction of a hyaluronic acid filler producing enduring full-facial volume restoration: an 18-month open multicenter study. Dermatol Surg. 2015;41(12):1361–9.

20 Alloplastic Premandible Chin-Jaw Contouring

Edward O. Terino

20.1 Facial Contouring with Alloplastic Implants

20.1.1 Introduction

At no time in history has the quest for health and beauty been more intense and more widespread than in this millennium. The proliferation of jogging, walking, outdoor and indoor sports, day spas, fitness clubs, and weight control clinics all attest to this phenomenon. The Greek and Roman ideals of physical beauty are evoking renewed enthusiasm. Bold and dramatic facial bone structure, accented by a strong nose, significant malar-midface configuration, and a sharp, well-defined jawline are now the hallmarks of fashion models and the idols of cinema and television. Men are looking for the Brad Pitt, Johny Depp, Tom Cruise, George Clooney, and Tom Brady's chins and jawlines (Fig. 20.1).

Facial aesthetic surgery has presently evolved to the highest level possible with the three-dimensional restructuring of facial form. Repositioning of the deep soft tissue planes from the neck to the zygoma, as well as subperiosteal, upper, and midface elevation, has become commonplace [1].

Alloplastic implant contouring is not only a useful adjunct but should be a fundamental tool standardly used with a variety of new facial aesthetic techniques.

The earliest American explorations into alloplastic chin and mandible aesthetic alterations in the USA were in the 1950s [2, 3].

It is now possible for the aesthetic surgeon to restore, rejuvenate, or enhance facial forms that originate from either hereditary or aging origins. In a point of fact, infinite variations in facial contour are now possible. By using alloplastic techniques based on concepts of zonal anatomy and aesthetic volume deficiency typing, facial contours can be created or modified with a minimum of complications. The use of alloplastic implants on the "fourth skeletal plane" can produce optimum, significant three-dimensional contours of both mass and volume to improve contours of both the soft tissue and the skeletal anatomic elements of the face volume.

My plastic and reconstructive surgery training was in the 1960s. I entered private practice in Southern California in 1971. No one dreamed that cosmetic surgery would expand into a commercially flourishing, prominent medical industry that would capture middle-class America. The

E. O. Terino (✉)
Plastic Surgery Institute of Southern California, Agoura Hills, CA, USA

K. Jeffords et al. (eds.), *Aesthetic Surgery for Men*, https://doi.org/10.1007/978-3-032-03840-1_20

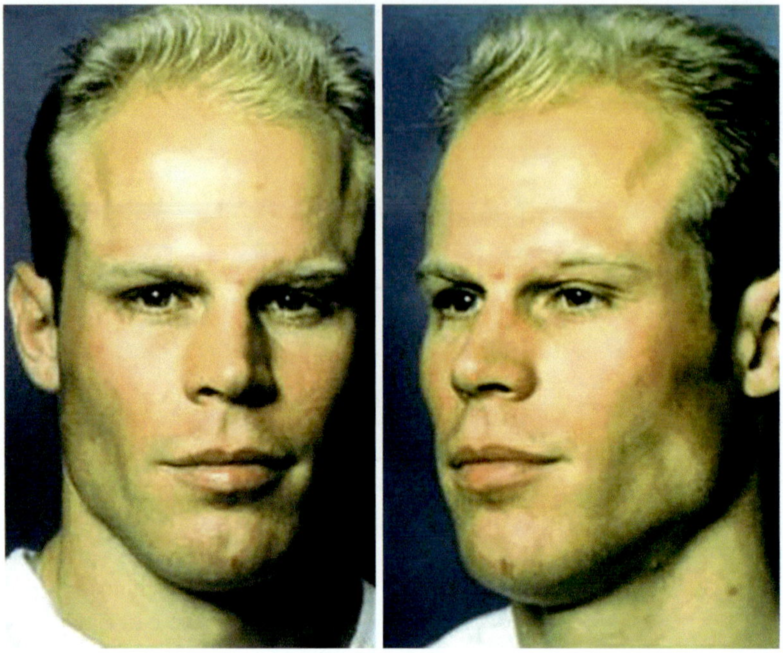

Fig. 20.1 Today's ideal "totally" male facial cheek-chin-jawline contours

idea that physicians would be interested in altering faces and bodies strictly for the sake of appearance, as opposed to illness, injury, or deformity, was beyond belief. The early practitioners of aesthetic surgeries for the face catered only to famous, eccentric, or entertainment world clientele. These plastic surgeons were professors at major universities. Even they did not foresee the exploding evolution in aesthetic surgery techniques or the enormous public demand for such surgical changes, which were about to occur.

In the 1970s, middle-class Americans with a Hollywood dream migrated in great numbers to Southern California. No wonder, then, that they expressed a strong interest in altering their appearance to look better at cocktail and dinner parties, beauty salons, health clubs, department stores, emergency rooms, and anywhere else a young plastic surgeon would be frequenting. Women's social clubs were always eager to hear lectures on new and exciting subjects. At that time, the majority of plastic surgery experience related to reconstructions of defects caused by birth, trauma, burns, and cancers. There was no promotional data or visual aids available to educate the public about plastic surgery in general or cosmetic procedures specifically.

Thirty years ago, the use of chin implants was relatively uncommon. The only available shapes were small, oval, round, or pointed. They were nearly always used as an adjunct to the rhinoplasties of that time period, which commonly resulted in an overly reduced dorsum. The advantages of a good profile were obvious, but the large majority of these cases possessed a genetically deficient mandibular-jawline lower third aesthetic segment, which necessitated more correction than the existing small implants could produce. Instead, they resulted in abnormal, artificial, unattractive lumps or bumps and a round, protuberant chin mound (Fig. 20.2).

Nonetheless, the striking improvement in facial aesthetics which resulted from rhinoplasties combined with even these early and now archaic implants was an impetus for me to create anatomic modifications of implant shapes and sizes for placement into the entire premandible chin and jawline region that would produce a natural and significantly greater enhancement of a contour (Fig. 20.3).

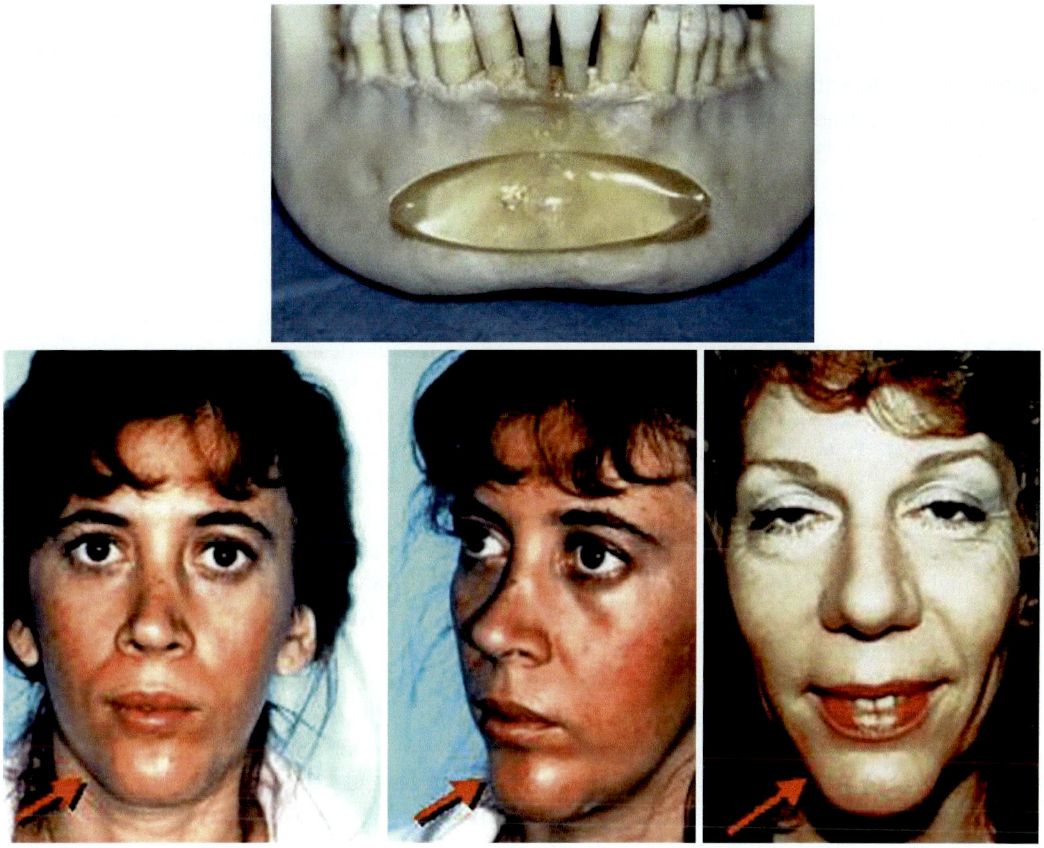

Fig. 20.2 Traditional CIRCA 1970s central oval implants produced an abnormal round protuberance

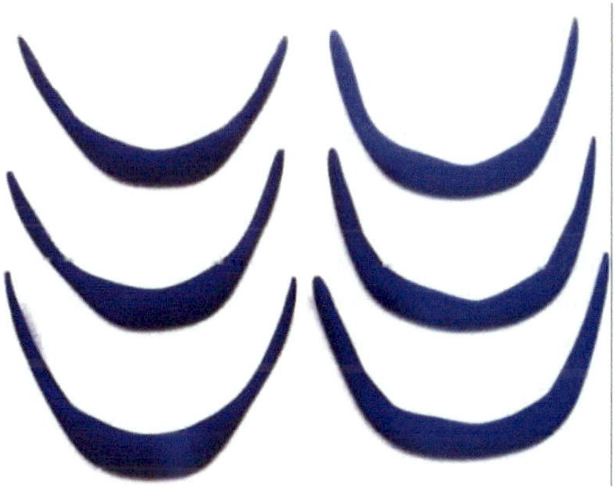

Fig. 20.3 Two new premandible implants (Terino square style 1 and 2) have varying dimensions and length that will augment the anterior and midlateral jawline variably

20.2 Facial Contouring with Alloplastic Implants

20.2.1 The Face

A person's attractiveness is really determined by the shape and form of their face. Shape and form are three-dimensional representations of volume and mass. In the context of a human face, these consist of both skeletal and soft tissue contours. These contours are judged attractive according to both their underlying bony characteristics and their overlying subcutaneous soft tissue substance.

The facial skeleton represents the underlying foundation. The overlying subcutaneous is the upholstery padding that creates a fashionable or unfashionable appearance. Finally, the overlying skin becomes the "canvas" over the face. In youth, it is distributed over the bony and soft tissue entities in a smooth manner that presents a youthful appearance [4].

20.2.2 Significance of Facial Contouring

Skeletal facial contouring originated 20 years ago when craniofacial surgeons, under the leadership of Dr. Paul Tessier, developed maxillofacial techniques that could correct severe congenital facial defects by radical alteration of the facial skeleton. Since 1980, the author has developed reliable procedures to alter facial shape with anatomic chin and malar-midface implants. The term "facial contouring" embodies all of these procedures.

Three-dimensional "sculpturing" procedures using only the soft tissue layers were a new development in facial plastic surgery. In the 1980s, these techniques included jowl and neck fat removal, as well as repositioning of the malar fat pad. In addition, subperiosteal and endoscopic mid- and upper-lifting techniques to alter facial contour were rapidly gaining in popularity. These techniques attempted to create three-dimensional changes in facial structure through soft tissue manipulations only and consequently suffered from a lack of permanence as well as precision.

In contrast, alloplastic facial augmentation produces permanent, effective three-dimensional alterations in facial contour with low risk and minimal morbidity. Moreover, the advantages of alloplastic techniques versus craniofacial autologous osseous engineering include their ready modifiability, exchangeability, and reversibility when implants are used. This feature alone provides a generous margin of safety and flexibility because variations in surgical judgment, as well as many imprecisions in physician-patient communications, can produce final appearances that are sometimes dissatisfying to patients, but can be easily corrected if necessary. Today's particular patients demand their "ideal scene" to be satisfied.

Strong skeletal contours enhance beauty. Redraping, reshaping, and redistributing the soft tissues over a strong facial skeleton enhance restoration and rejuvenation of the face and jawline. Augmentation of the lower third facial aesthetic segment of the chin and jawline with implants of permanent volume can enhance male faces to create today's desired well-defined, architectural chin-jaw structure.

I decided to label alloplastic skeletal augmentation to be known in the specialty of reconstructive and aesthetic surgery as "surgery of the fourth plane" since it is performed on the basic bone foundation above which lie the other three planes: (3) SMAS, (2) subcutaneous fat, and (1) skin. This fourth plane surgery of the face depends on the implantation of uniquely and anatomically configured volumetric alloplastic implants of different shapes and sizes. When placed in differing positions, they alter facial contours in a designated and controlled fashion, which produces predictable results. Dividing the facial skeleton into specific zones of anatomy and identifying common types of facial aesthetic contour volume deficiencies in these zones enable the surgeon to both choose appropriate implants and place them properly for achieving a desired effect.

20.2.3 Ideal Facial Implants

Alloplastic implants for facial contour alterations should have several optimal ideal features. Primarily, they must be conformable to the facial skeleton. Their design must include a posterior surface that contours to the external surface of the mandible and maxilla, as well as an external shape that imitates a desired and selected natural anatomic configuration. When the margins of the implant are tapered to blend onto the bony surface, they will be nonpalpable, as well as nonvisible through the overlying soft tissue envelope (Fig. 20.4). My anatomic design facial implants are readily exchangeable and suitable for most

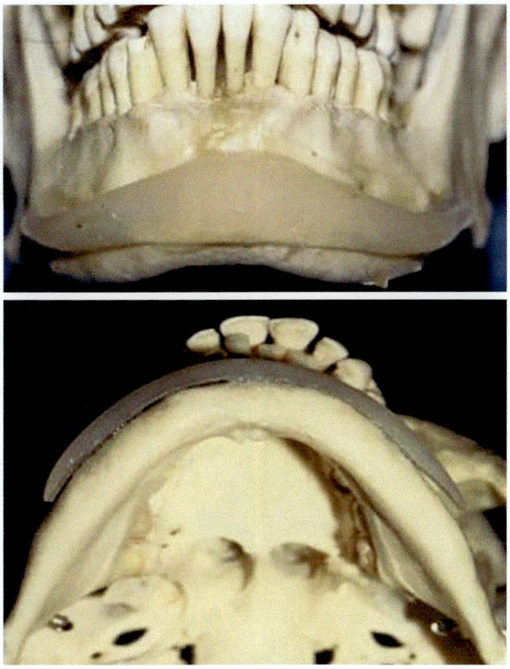

Fig. 20.4 Anatomic design implants that contour to the mandible and create a completely natural appearance

patients' needs. There is more precise computer technology that can give the surgeon and the patient exact dimensions of implants necessary to precisely predict a desired contour. However, they are extremely expensive at the present time and probably for another 10–15 years.

Facial contouring by alloplastic implant augmentation is still an art form that requires considerable experience. Facial implants should have no fixation patches, fenestrations, or fabrics to immobilize them on the bony plane. Biologic collagen fibrotic encapsulation completely ensures their immobility. They should be malleable enough to insert through relatively small soft tissue apertures. Implants should optimally have high host acceptability and a high resistance to infection so that the need for removal is rare. They should be easily modifiable by the surgeon before, during, or after the procedure.

Silicone rubber implants fully meet the above ideal qualifications. They are readily exchangeable and modifiable by open capsulotomy when desirable or necessary.

Porous implants such as hydroxyapatite and porex, and fenestrated implants which permit scar tissue ingrowth, are difficult to remove or exchange, especially through small operative entrance sites. Moreover, these materials have a significant incidence of infection which necessitates removal. Silastic rubber implants can survive the presence of inflammation and gross purulence. Treatment by drainage and possibly even irrigation procedures, along with the use of appropriate antibiotics, can often resolve infectious processes without necessitating removal.

Both soft tissue augmentations, as well as skeletal deficiencies, should be performed on the subperiosteal bone level. The natural encapsulation process biologically immobilizes a silicone implant so that it becomes firmly fixed both during muscle activity and with attempts at manual external manipulation. The contours will appear completely natural, providing the implant design is appropriate and the margins of the implant are tapered to blend along the bony surface.

Any segment of the premandible region can be augmented individually and differentially to create chin/jawline contours according to the surgeon's and the patient's preference.

20.2.4 Facial Aesthetics and Volume-Mass Interrelationships

The essential principle of facial aesthetics is the three-dimensional restructuring of form. It involves the appreciation of fundamental laws that govern an aesthetic balance of volume-mass relationships of the face. These laws are straightforward.

The most important facial promontories are (1) the malar/midface prominence, (2) nasal size and projection, (3) the entire mass of the lower third facial segment (jawline and mandible segment), and (4) of lesser significance are the supraorbital brow ridges (Figs. 20.5 and 20.6).

Altering any one of the three facial bony promontories directly and inversely affects the aesthetic importance of the others. When one structure is larger and takes up more space, another appears relatively diminished. As nasal

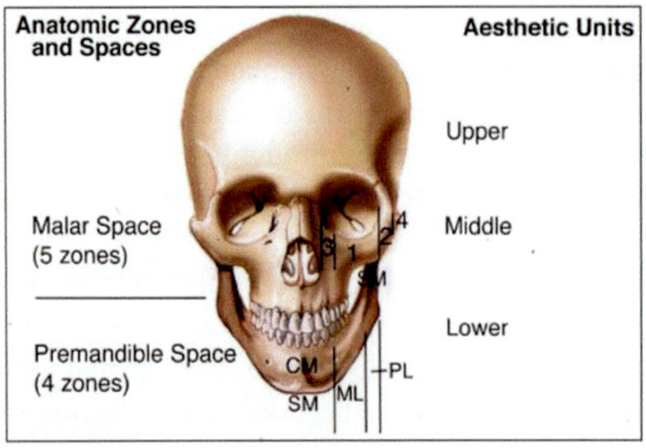

Fig. 20.5 An illustration showing the three aesthetic segments of the face: (1) upper, (2) middle, (3) lower. The anatomic zones of the midface and premandible–jawline are also indicated

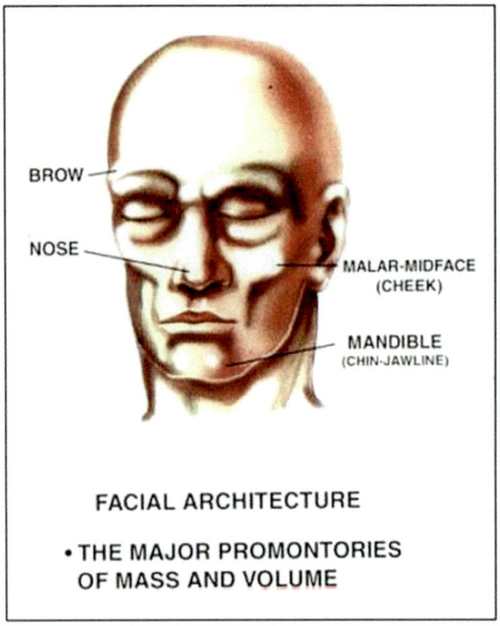

Fig. 20.6 The major promontories of mass and volume, which establish the major elements of external facial contour

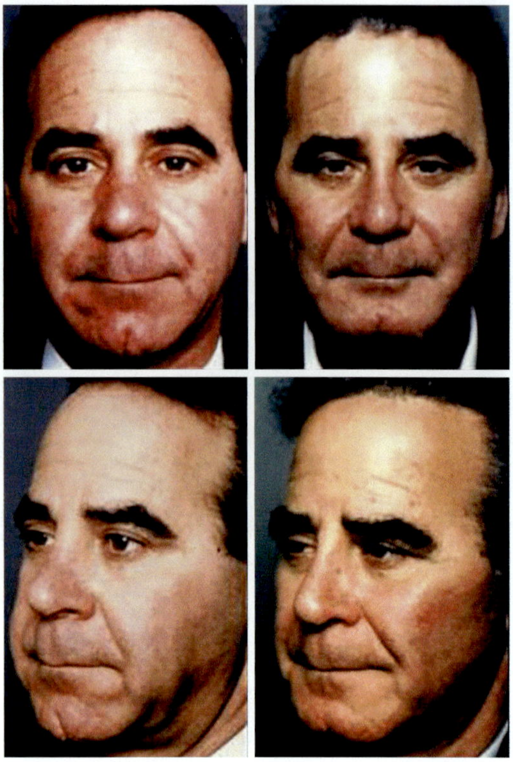

Fig. 20.7 44-year-old male, who in 1987 underwent revision rhinoplasty with conchal cartilage dorsal augmentation, malar augmentation with extra-large Terino malar shells, and large Terino square 1 chin implant (8 mm. projection)

significance is reduced, malar and mandibular volume and projection assume more importance. Two or more significant masses further reduce the size significance of the third (or fourth). By accenting the malar/submalar midface complex, the surgeon diminishes the significance of the nose and chin. By enhancing both the mandibular and malar areas, the surgeon effectively reduces the relative magnitude of the nose. Thus, the architectural laws of proportion dictate that the strength of the mass and volume characteristics of each promontory affects the relative balance of one to the other. Simultaneous changes in more than one have even greater significance than altering one alone.

20.2.5 Applications of Facial Balance

Patients with round, full, fleshy facial contours and an abundance of subcutaneous tissues and fat rarely appear beautiful by contemporary standards (Fig. 20.7). Lean-faced individuals with a long facial contour often have inadequate skeletal promontories in the malar and/or mandibular region, as well as deficient midfacial submalar soft tissues. These faces have an aesthetic imbalance.

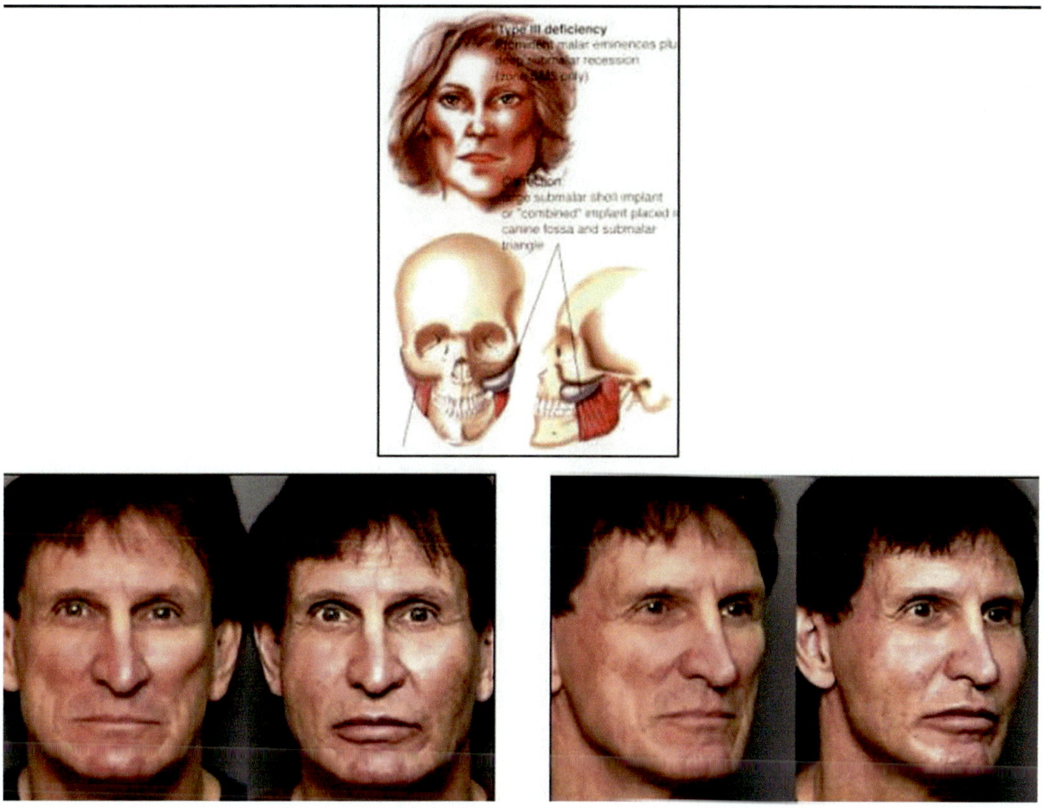

Fig. 20.8 Type 3 aesthetic facial volume deficiency consists of a very prominent malar bone structure and severe submalar zone deficiency. This occurs from aging or heredity. Example: 62-year-old patient who has a combined aging and hereditary submalar volume deficiency corrected by a jumbo malar shell (Right: post op view 8 months)

Both of these facial types (Fig. 20.8), and persons with combinations of these deficiencies, can be improved significantly by rearranging the volume-mass balance of the skeletal and soft tissue contours by alloplastic skeletal onlay techniques.

The author's extensive experience has conclusively demonstrated that alloplastic implants with a much larger surface area than were previously utilized are necessary to produce significant appearance change in the malar, midface, and premandible regions. Additionally, alterations in the size, shape, and positioning of these implants, even to a minor degree, create a significant or even subtle nuances of change in the appearance of the human face.

20.3 Facial Contouring with Alloplastic Implants

20.3.1 Analysis by Zonal Principles

To analyze the aesthetics of a specific patient's face, zonal principles of skeletal anatomy in the malar/midface and premandible regions have been developed.

Zonal analysis enables the surgeon to choose implant size and shape and determine positioning with certainty and prediction. This precision is even further enhanced by incorporating data that identifies several common types of facial aesthetic deficiencies in volume mass contours.

The premandible space is that location in the face which when augmented appropriately produces a variety of aesthetic changes to the chin and jawline contour [5]. To determine how to augment that space in a specific desired fashion, it is useful to think of the premandible jawline aesthetic unit in four distinct anatomic zones (Figs. 20.9 and 20.10).

20.3.2 Zonal Anatomy of the Lower Face

The entire mandibular contour can be altered. Lateral extensions on a conventional chin implant create a lateral widening to the lower third of the face (Fig. 20.11). Traditional implants placed centrally between the mental foramina in many patients produces abnormal central protuberance (Fig. 20.12).

Knowing and understanding the significance of mandibular zonal anatomy determines precise implant selection.

Zone 1 or CM consists of the central mentum between the mental nerves. Zone 2, the midlateral zone (ML), extends to the middle of the mandibular body (Fig. 20.13). A third zone (posterolateral zone or PL) overlies the posterior aspect of the mandibular body, including the angle of the mandible, as well as the lower third of the ascending ramus. Augmentation of this posterolateral zone widens the face at the posterior jawline and gives sculptured definition to the mandibular angle (Fig. 20.14). A fourth zone exists beneath the inferior border of the central mandible. This can be referred to as the submandibular zone (SM). Traditional chin implants have lacked the ability to extend the chin in a vertical direction. I invented a new implant design, however, which is now avail-

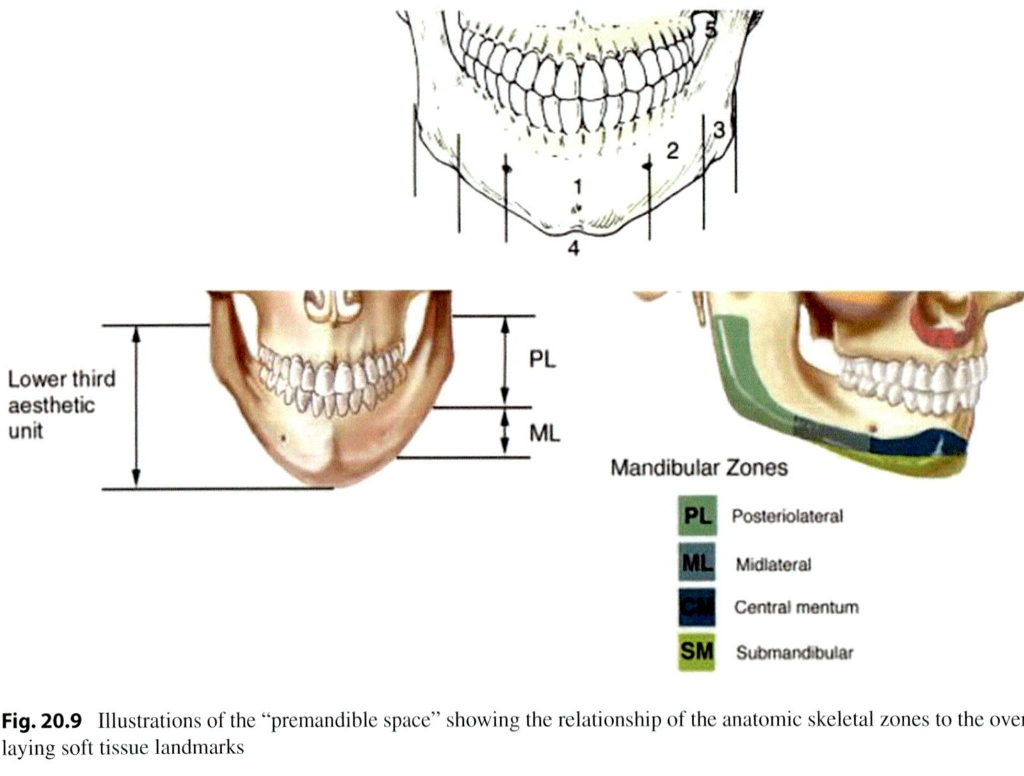

Fig. 20.9 Illustrations of the "premandible space" showing the relationship of the anatomic skeletal zones to the overlaying soft tissue landmarks

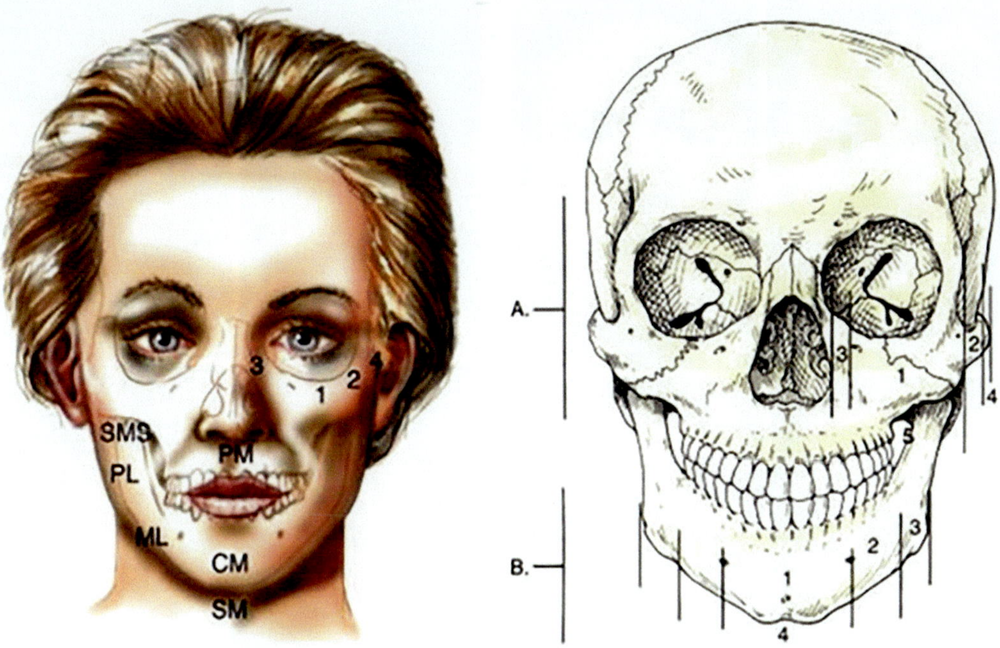

Fig. 20.10 Illustrations of the "premandible space" showing the relationship of the anatomic skeletal zones to the overlaying soft tissue landmarks

able and wraps around the inferior bony margin of the chin (Figs. 20.15 and 20.16). It increases the vertical height of the face from the lower lip to the inferior border of the bony chin (Fig. 20.17).

20.3.3 General Guidelines for Implant and Patient Selection

Even for the most experienced surgeon, the precise selection and positioning of implants, particularly when everyone universally has facial asymmetry, is difficult. General guidelines do exist, however. In the central premandible region, 5–7 mm of projection are most suitable for the majority of patients. Eight to ten millimeters are necessary for severe microgenia.

It should be noted that once the intended augmentation reaches 10 mm, the patient may better be served by an advancement osteotomy. The posterior angle (PL) is usually contoured adequately with an 8–10 mm lateral thickness, which gives the patient a total increase in lateral facial width of 1.6 cm.

As in all aesthetic procedures, preoperative evaluation and planning are essential. Precision communication with the patient is critical to success. Since it is imperative that the surgeon knows exactly what facial images the patient desires, it is mandatory to have the patient bring in old photographs of themselves or images from fashion magazines and other sources to help in this determination. Some patients want bold, well-defined features and classic contours (Fig. 20.18). Other, prefer more subtle changes.

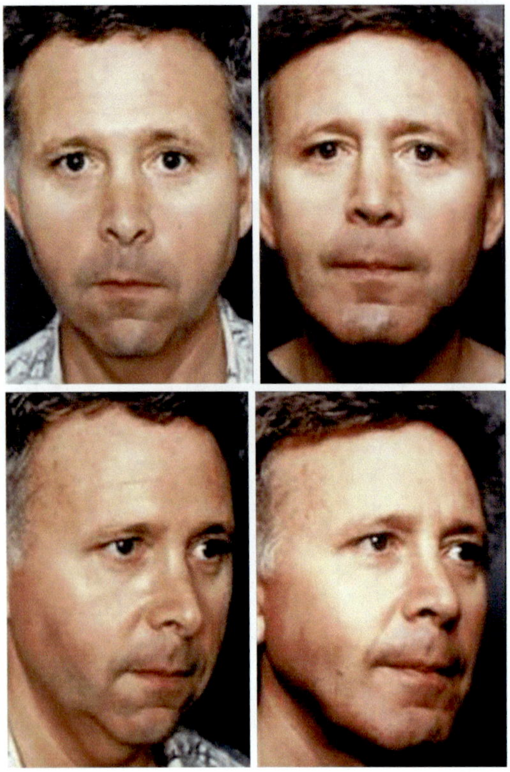

Fig. 20.11 A 52-year-old male who demonstrated widening of the midlateral zones of the mandible through the use of a large extended anatomic implant (post op results on the right)

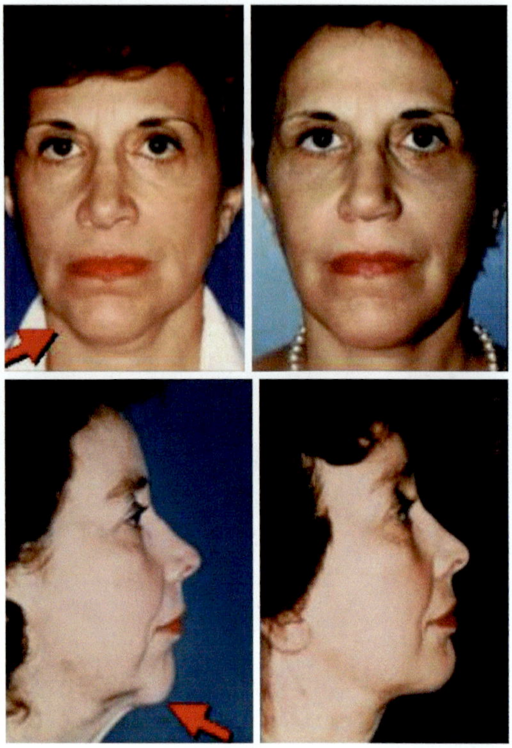

Fig. 20.12 Examples of "witches chin" deformity and pre-jowl sulcus accentuated by central traditional implants. Right photos show preoperative improvement by anatomic design implants

20.3.4 Preoperative Planning

The key to successful facial contouring is determined completely by effective communication with the patient. A surgeon must completely duplicate and understand a patient's desired contour changes. Facial implant patients have specific perceptions about their midface, cheek, and jawline contours. They are meticulous in their observation of details. Facial images from fashion magazines or other sources, as well as photographs of the patient, perhaps modified by them, are extremely useful and necessary to understand a patient's specific expectations (Fig. 20.19). At the present time, magnetic resonance imaging (MRI) and other diagnostic tools such as cephalometrics do not provide sufficient data to assist the surgeon in achieving a predictable outcome. 3D CAT SCAN provides the necessary technology for individual customization of facial con-

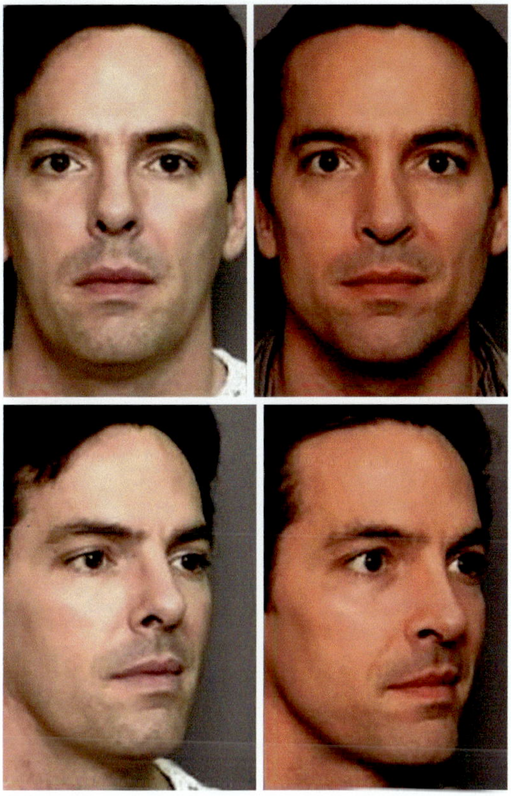

Fig. 20.13 A strong square posterior jawline is created by inserting mandibular angle implants. Post-operative views are seen on the right square style implants are often used for more anterior projection and shape

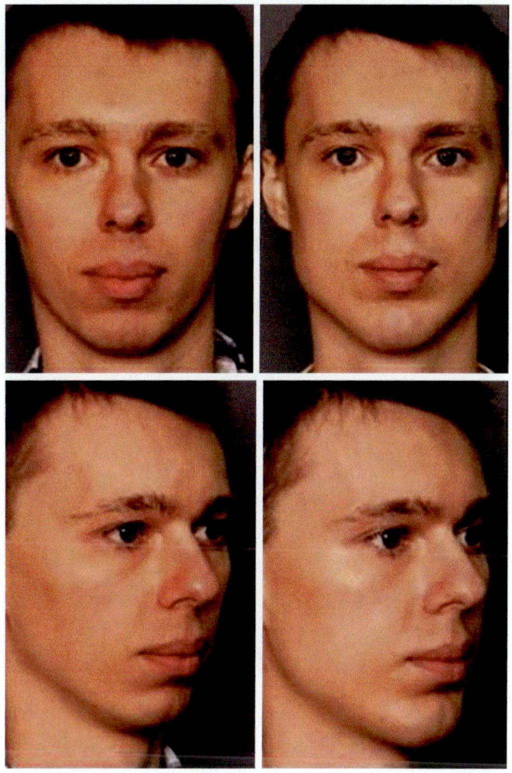

Fig. 20.14 A strong square posterior jawline is created by inserting mandibular angle implants. Post-operative views are seen on the right square style implants are often used for more anterior projection and shape

tour. However, the author first in consultation uses computer imaging technology indispensable in learning what a patient desires and showing them with a high degree of accuracy and success what they can realistically expect.

Preoperative planning must include evaluation of the patient's zonal anatomy to determine the specific implant location, as well as to determine the extent of volume enhancement to be achieved. Multiple consultations may be necessary. The author spends a great deal of time on the morning of surgery marking, measuring, and discussing details with the patient. By directly drawing the midfacial anatomic zones on the patient's facial skin, the patient and the surgeon can more accurately choose implants together that will produce the desired result (Fig. 20.20).

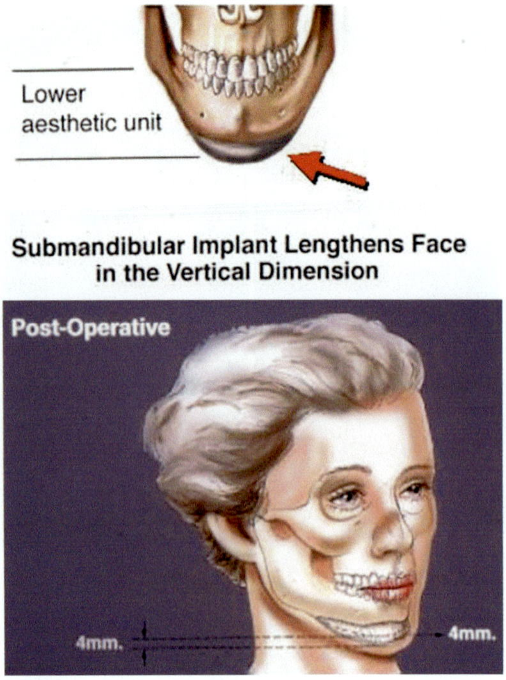

Fig. 20.15 Illustration of "vertical extension" implant designed by the author in 1978 and which extends the length of the face by 4 mm as well as adding 4 mm of projection

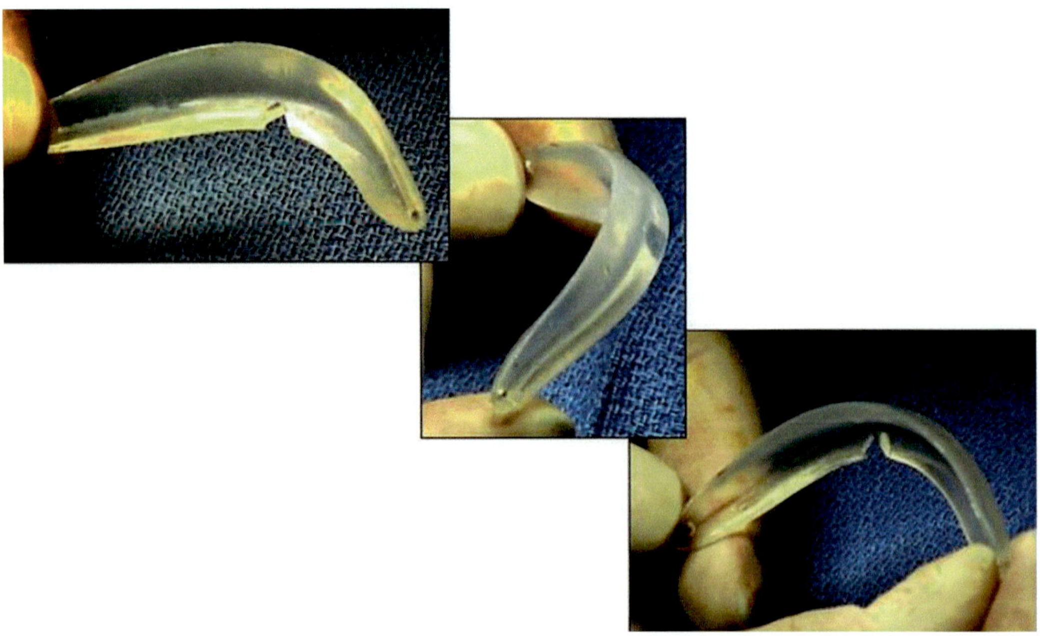

Fig. 20.16 A "vertical extension" wrap-around implant can extend the length of the lower 1/3 aesthetic facial segment by 4 mm

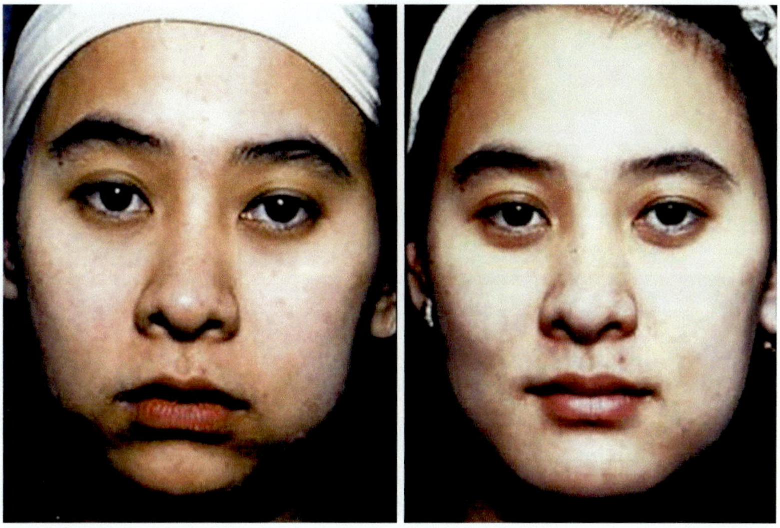

Fig. 20.17 22-year-old Asian female whose hereditary microgenia was corrected by a vertical extension implant

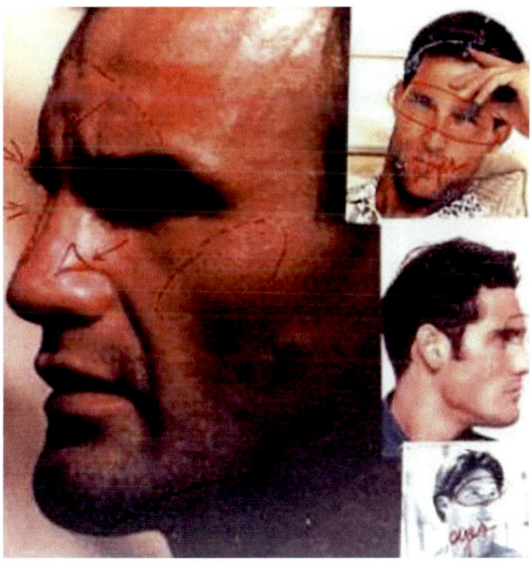

Fig. 20.18 Some patients bring extensive drawings of their own faces or magazine photos showing “dos and don’ts” of their desires

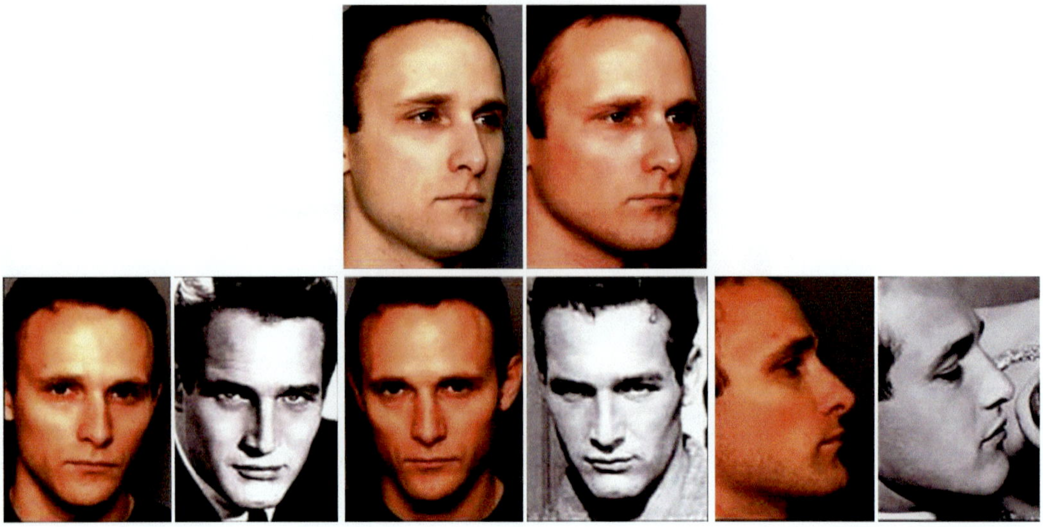

Fig. 20.19 A 30-year-old male aspiring actor desiring improved contours to help him appear more similar to his screen idol

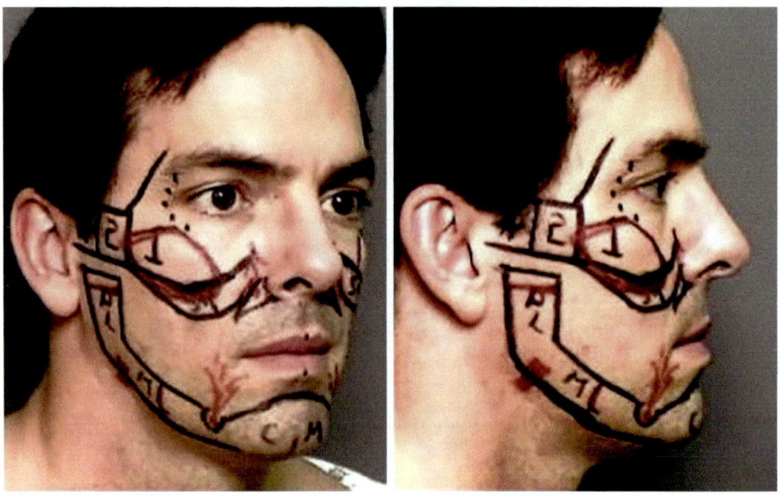

Fig. 20.20 Preoperative skeletal and anatomic zonal markings placed on the morning of surgery

20.4 Technique

Insertion of silastic facial implants into various subperiosteal locations is safe, easy, and essentially minimally invasive. The basic principles for augmenting the facial skeleton are identical to those for contouring both the malar/midface and the premandibular regions. These techniques result in successful procedures that have few serious or permanent complications.

It must be emphasized that there are three critical parameters: shape, size, and positioning. The degree to which these parameters are properly controlled determines the overall final facial contour and, in most cases, results in significant patient satisfaction.

20.5 Anesthesia

It has been learned from a large experience of several thousand facial implant procedures that anesthesia is a critical factor in determining the safety and precision with which facial contouring can be accomplished.

Two basic principles must be followed: First, the subperiosteal plane, as well as the subcutaneous layers, must be infiltrated generously. A solution of dilute lidocaine and epinephrine is used. The epinephrine concentration is 1/800,000, and the lidocaine—Marcaine concentration is 0.125%. This is prepared by mixing 250 mls of 0.5% lidocaine cntaining 1/200,000 adrenaline with 500 mls of sterile saline and 250 mls of 0.5% Marcaiine (total volume 1000 mls).

Generous tumescent infiltration of up to 30 or 40 mls of this dilute lidocaine/epinephrine solution appears to create an increased interstitial pressure at the capillary level, which contributes to optimum hemostasis.

Secondly, all procedures are performed under general anesthesia, making certain that the blood pressure is maintained at a systolic level of 90 to 110 mms of mercury. It can be consistently and predictably demonstrated that elevation of the blood pressure over this limit results in significant troublesome oozing and bleeding.

20.6 Operative Technique

1. Stay on the bone. When implants are placed directly over bone, a firm and secure attachment is formed. Symptomatic capsular contracture has not been seen with these implants.
2. Avoid trauma to the soft tissue, which could produce mental nerve injury.
3. Expand the pocket adequately to accommodate the chosen prosthesis comfortably.
4. Minimize bleeding by keeping the dissection immediately on the bone and by using both local and general anesthesia.

Once the basic principles of dissection are understood, the technical aspects of implant insertion are straightforward. It is advisable to visualize the mental nerves and their foramina because in rare instances there may be more than 1 or both [6]. Frequent irrigation using Bacitracin solution is performed.

To extend a centrally placed implant into the midlateral or posterolateral zones, dissection is performed along the inferior border of the mandible in the "safe zone" posterior to the mental nerve.

The premandible space can be accessed with the standard intraoral route or the submental route (Fig. 20.21). If the author is performing a procedure that requires a submental approach, e.g., submental liposuction and subplatysmal fat removal or platysma plication, then the submental approach is used.

In either case, the incision may be made posterior to the mental nerve to accurately place lateral bar mandibular implants, which extend back to the midlateral and posterolateral zones. A one-centimeter vertical mucosal incision made medial to the first molar allows access to the premandi-

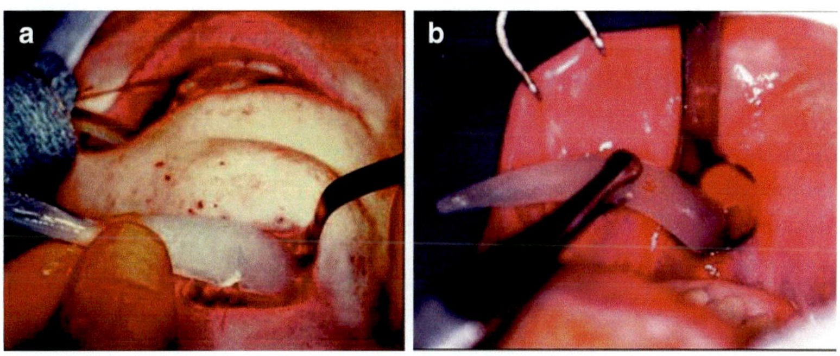

Fig. 20.21 Central chin implants can be placed by either (**a**) a submental or (**b**) an intraoral approach

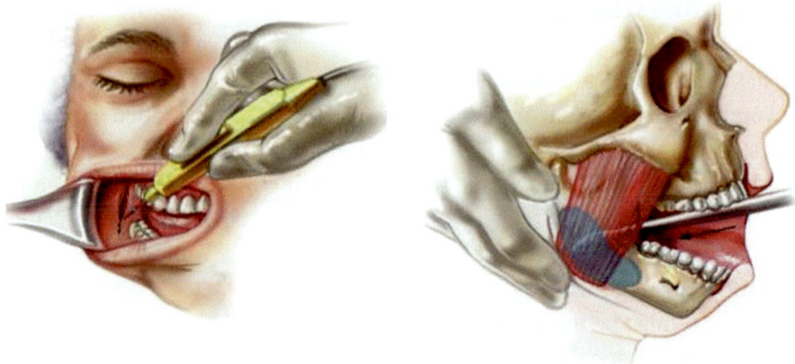

Fig. 20.22 Intraoral dissection is performed subperiorsteally beneath the masseter muscle along the posterior and inferior border of the mandible

ble space. This incision allows accurate placement of the posterior lateral mandibular implant.

To position an implant with long tail extensions, a tunnel or space must be created. The dissection must extend further than necessary, especially to one side. The implant can then be inserted from the central incision far into one side, folded upon itself, and introduced into the opposite mandibular tunnel.

Posterior mandible angle of jaw implants are intraorally placed through an intraoral posterolateral incision. This incision is 3 cm transverse and is located anterior and 1.5 cm adjacent to the buccal sulcus above the angle of the mandible and the posterior 3 molar teeth (Fig. 20.22). This leaves a strong adequate cuff of mucosa and buccinator muscle to strengthen the closure.

A curved elevator is used to dissect subperiosteally around the inferior and posterior aspects of the angle and the ascending ramus. Mandibular angle implants are designed to fit securely around the angle of the mandible once the bony margins have been "de-gloved." A secure closure of muscle and mucosa is optimum for all facial implant incisions.

20.7 Complications

Although placement of lower face implants is technically not difficult, occasional problems can develop. The author's series of over 8000 facial implants since 1971 is as follows [7].

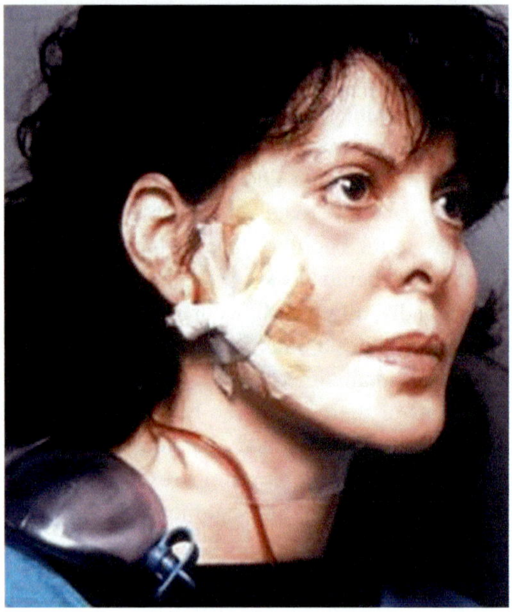

Fig. 20.23 Silicone rubber facial implant infections can usually be resolved by using antibiotics and occasionally drainage techniques as shown here

In order of importance and frequency: (1) patient and/or doctor dissatisfaction 15%; (2) minor asymmetries 10%; (3) malposition requiring correction 4%; (4) hematoma, seroma 5%; (5) (Fig. 20.23) infection and removal 0.1%. Detailed discussion and treatment of these complications are beyond the scope of this chapter but have been discussed extensively elsewhere (Fig. 20.24).

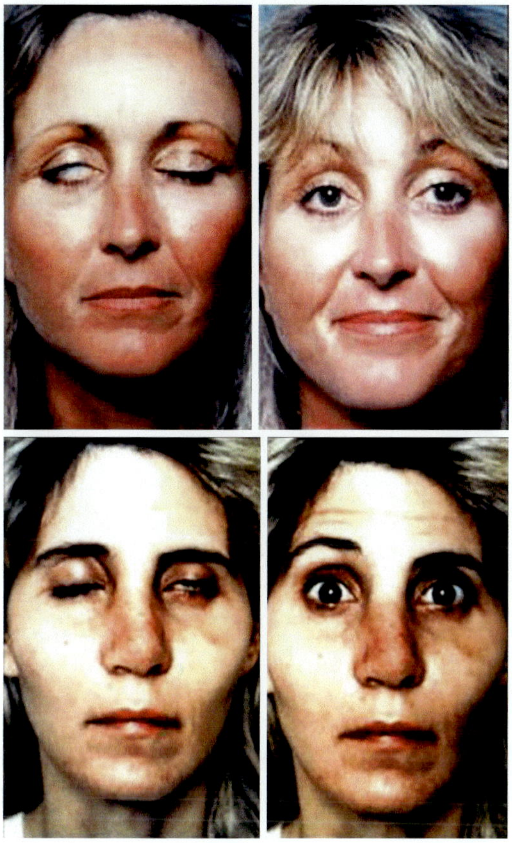

Fig. 20.24 Two examples of patients who, due to excessive traction trauma, developed temporary paresis of facial movement. TOP: Weakness of orbicularis oculi function, right eye. Right photo: Complete return of function after 6 weeks. BOTTOM: Weakness of the function of both the left frontalis and orbicularis muscles. This completely recovered in 1 month

20.8 Conclusions

Plastic surgeons are now better prepared to fulfill the primary goal of facial cosmetic surgery. By manipulating and combining various new alloplastic techniques, they can restore, rejuvenate, and enhance hereditary facial forms and improve aging changes.

Whereas soft tissue plane tightening and lifting techniques are essentially two-dimensional, skeletal augmentation represents surgery on the deepest plane and is three-dimensional in nature. The use of implants on the facial skeleton represents volume, mass augmentation, and alteration of facial form. Manipulations of the other three planes (i.e., skin, subcutaneous fat, and SMAS) are attempts to reverse aging qualities of loosening, sagging, and drooping in a two-dimensional fashion, which are limited by the bioplastic dynamics of aging tissues.

Skeletal augmentation now represents a final phase for facial plastic surgery. Three-dimensional volume-mass modifications of the fourth plane skeletal framework enable surgeons to dramatically or subtly alter inherited facial images, as well as compensate for the deterioration, sagging, and atrophy of facial tissue mass that comes with age.

Now, virtually all aspects of the facial skeleton can be augmented satisfactorily. It can truthfully be said that alloplastic implants may become the "open sesame" of aesthetic surgery, the door by which facial changes can be made that are almost "magical" and heavily rely on the imagination and the skill of the surgeon.

References

1. Guerrerosantos J. The role of the platysma muscle in rhytidoplasty. Chin Plast Surg. 1978;5:29.
2. Millard RD. Chin implants. Plast Reconstr Surg. 1953;13:70.
3. Pitanguy I. Augmentation mentoplasty. Plast Reconstr Surg. 1968;42:441.
4. Terino EO. The art of alloplastic facial contouring, "alloplastic contouring in the Premandible—jawline lower third facial aesthetic unit", 10:153–65, Mosby, 2000.
5. Terino EO. Unique mandibular implants including lateral and posterior angle implants. Facial Plast Surg Clin North Am. 1994;2(3):311–28.
6. Serman NJ. Differentiations of double mental foramina mandibular nerve: anatomic study. Dental Med. 1987;5(3):20–1.
7. Terino EO. Complications of chin and malar augmentations. In: Peck G, editor. Complications and problems in aesthetic plastic surgery. New York: Gower Medical Publishers; 1991.

Part IV

Body

21 Adolescent Gynecomastia

Joshua T. Henderson and Aaron C. Mason

21.1 Introduction

Gynecomastia was first described by Paulus Aegineta (625–690 AD), and removal of the excess "formation of fat" through submammary lunar incisions was recommended [1]. It is very common and demonstrates a trimodal age distribution in the neonatal period, during adolescence, and in the elderly. This chapter focuses on the adolescent population, wherein up to 60% of males are affected [2–4]. While observation is often the initial treatment strategy once young men come to medical attention, those who do not resolve may be candidates for either pharmacologic treatment or surgical intervention.

21.2 The Development of Adolescent Gynecomastia

Gynecomastia is the benign proliferation of glandular tissue in the male breast. Though multiple etiologies exist, the common pathophysiology involves an imbalance of estrogen and androgen, where estrogen effects dominate and lead to ductal hyperplasia [5, 6]. Pathologic origins for the hormonal imbalance must be considered in each patient and include endocrinological and exogenous etiologies. Tumors secreting estrogen or its precursors and, more commonly, increased extragonadal conversion of androgens to estrogens by tissue aromatase, lead to a sex-hormonal imbalance stimulating breast glandular development. Androgen resistance syndromes may also produce the same effect. Additionally, conditions like hyperthyroidism and liver disease, and certain medications may alter sex hormone-binding globulin levels, thereby shifting the balance between free testosterone and estrogen. All these must be excluded. Exogenous medications, including antacids, antimicrobials, hormones, chemotherapeutic agents, psychotropics, and antiretroviral therapies (Table 21.1), are all associated with the development of gynecomastia. Most commonly, no pathology is identified as the reason for breast glandular development. This typically results in a diagnosis of benign adolescent gynecomastia. Even if the majority of sex hormone levels are normal, free testosterone levels are lower than those of controls without gynecomastia.

J. T. Henderson · A. C. Mason (✉)
Department of Surgery, Division of Plastic Surgery, University of Arizona, Tucson, AZ, USA

K. Jeffords et al. (eds.), *Aesthetic Surgery for Men*, https://doi.org/10.1007/978-3-032-03840-1_21

Table 21.1 Medications associated with gynecomastia

Antacids	Cimetidine, ranitidine, omeprazole
Antibiotics	Metronidazole, ketaconazole, minocycline, isoniazid
Cardiovascular drugs	Captopril, digoxin, enalapril, diltiazem, nifedipine, verapamil, amiodarone, spironolactone, minoxidil
Chemotherapeutics	Methotrexate, vinca agents, alkylating agents
Hormones	Androgens, anabolic steroids, estrogens, hCG
Psychoactive drugs	Diazepam, tricyclics, haloperidol, phenothiazines
Miscellaneous	Antiretroviral drugs for HIV, metoclopramide, penicillamine, phenytoin

Table 21.2 History and physical examination of the gynecomastia patient

History	Physical examination
Change in weight; obesity (former or current)	BMI
Inciting medications (Table 21.1)	Chest contour, inframammary fold
Illicit drug use (marijuana, methadone, amphetamines)	NAC position, size
Hormone supplements	Palpable glandular breast mass
Family history of gynecomastia	Diffuse and subareolar fat
Infertility	Genital exam (varicocele, microorchidism)

21.3 Assessment and Medical Management of Adolescent Gynecomastia

As treatable etiologies of breast glandular hyperplasia must be excluded, a careful history and physical examination must be performed on each male patient presenting with breast hyperplasia (Table 21.2). History should include any change in weight, identification of inciting medications, illicit drug use (marijuana, methadone, and amphetamines), and family history of gynecomastia. Up to 58% of males with persistent adolescent gynecomastia will have a positive family history. As obesity is associated with a higher prevalence of gynecomastia, body mass index (BMI) and change over time should be evaluated.

Careful assessment of the chest should include evaluation for tissue make-up, masses, and skin changes. Gynecomastia typically affects both breasts but may also be unilateral or asymmetric. A tender, firm, and mobile mass is usually palpable beneath the nipple-areolar complex (NAC). An exam may also reveal diffuse breast enlargement and subareolar fat without a palpable glandular mass, also known as pseudogynecomastia. Patients with the above findings generally do not need further workup. In contrast, patients with excess tissue peripheral to the NAC, unilateral masses that are hard or fixed, or those with associated nipple discharge, skin changes, or lymphadenopathy warrant further evaluation prior to consideration of surgery. A genital examination should be performed to exclude masses and document the presence of any varicoceles, which have a strong association with gynecomastia. Rare instances may necessitate mammography or alternative breast imaging.

Adolescent gynecomastia is most often benign in nature and is usually self-limited. Reassurance, observation, and appropriate follow-up are the typical initial management, and most cases regress within 12 months. When it persists beyond a year, is associated with persistent pain, and/or if psychological distress evolves, pharmacologic or surgical options are available. Medical therapies seek to intervene before the hyperplastic glandular tissue is replaced with more fibrous tissue. Estrogen receptor modulators (tamoxifen and raloxifine) appear to be safe and beneficial in patients whose glandular tissue is in active proliferation. These patients report a reduction in pain and mass size. Dihydrotestosterone, danazol, clomiphene, and testolactone may also have benefits but have been less studied to date.

If symptoms persist despite observation and medical management, surgical intervention is indicated.

Adolescent gynecomastia that is present for greater than 12 months rarely regresses because of stromal hyalinization and fibrous replacement of glandular tissue [7–9]. Further, the psychosocial consequences of persistent gynecomastia in the adolescent male should not be underestimated. The condition is frequently painful and causes social embarrassment and emotional discomfort. Thus, the intent of surgery is not only to restore normal contour to the male chest but to rebalance the psychological discomfort caused by the condition.

21.4 Classification

Several classification systems have been proposed for gynecomastia. As the condition progresses, the enlarged male breast undergoes increased stromal hyalinization [7, 8]. An appreciation of the degree of transformation is essential in consideration of a proper surgical technique. Additionally, the degree of skin redundancy around the nipple and along the inferior border of the breast influences the operative decision. Classification systems that take these factors into consideration may assist in categorizing patients for whom specific surgical interventions will yield optimal results.

21.4.1 Webster Classification

Webster proposed a classification system based on tissue composition alone [1] (Table 21.3).

Type III is now commonly referred to as pseudogynecomastia and is less common in the adolescent population [10].

21.4.2 Simon Classification

Simon et al. classified gynecomastia based on the degree of hypertrophic tissue and skin redundancy (Table 21.4) [11].

Table 21.3 Webster classification

Type I	Predominantly glandular
Type II	Combination of fatty and glandular tissue
Type III	Adipose tissue hypertrophy alone

Table 21.4 Simon classification

Type I	Minor breast enlargement without skin excess
Type II	Moderate breast enlargement
II a	Without skin excess
II b	With minor skin redundancy
Type III	Gross breast enlargement with skin excess; pendulous breast

Table 21.5 Rohrich classification

Grade I	Minimal hypertrophy (<250 g) with no ptosis
I a	Primary glandular
I b	Primary fibrous
Grade II	Moderate hypertrophy (250–500 g) with no ptosis
II a	Primary glandular
II b	Primary fibrous
Grade III	Severe hypertrophy (>500 g) with grade I ptosis
Grade IV	Severe hypertrophy with grade II or grade III ptosis

21.4.3 ROHRICH Classification

Rohrich et al. created a staging system that incorporated ptosis, advocating for ultrasound- or suction-assisted lipectomy in all stages, with higher grades necessitating additional open excision (Table 21.5) [12].

21.5 Surgical Intervention

Many techniques exist for the correction of gynecomastia. It is important to first make an accurate assessment of what needs to be targeted in recontouring the patient's chest. One or multiple findings may be present, including excess glandular tissue, excess adipose tissue, excess skin, ptosis, or any combination thereof. Identifying and understanding how each contributes to the deformity allow the surgeon to generate the best surgical plan.

21.5.1 Excess Glandular Tissue: The Role of Open Excision

Open excision addresses the removal of symptomatic, firm, and often tender sub-areolar glandular tissue. Webster's inferior semicircular intra-areolar approach has been the pillar of open excision for gynecomastia [1]. A semicircular incision made along the inferior margin of the areola allows access to the underlying tissue and conceals the scar in the areola. Importantly, at least 1 cm of tissue should remain beneath the NAC to give normal bulk to the areola [13]. The Webster technique falls short when confronted with significant breast enlargement, ptotic breasts requiring skin reduction, and enlarged NACs for which reduction is needed [9]. For glandular excess with additional volume effect from adipose tissue, lipoaspiration techniques with and without ultrasound energy are adjuncts that may be considered. While significant glandular and fibrotic tissue excess are often found in bodybuilders (and thus renders liposuction insufficient for adequate correction), liposuction can be a noteworthy adjunct to overall chest contouring and can assist with glandular excision in indicated cases [14, 15]. In severe cases of glandular hypertrophy, a subcutaneous mastectomy via a periareolar approach with or without liposuction is warranted.

21.5.2 Excess Adipose Tissue: The Role of Liposuction

The advent of suction-assisted lipectomy (SAL) in the 1970s ushered in a new era of aesthetic breast surgery, and it has become a powerful technique for the management of gynecomastia (both alone and in combination with excision techniques) [16]. For many, liposuction has become the primary first-stage surgical treatment for gynecomastia [17, 18]. An advantage of liposuction is minimal scarring. The ideal patient has pathology that involves excess adipose tissue, limited or easily excised fibrous tissue, and skin redundancy/ptosis that does not require more extensive techniques [12]. Via strategically placed small stab incisions, the excess volume of the breast is evacuated, and the chest wall is recontoured. The placement of infiltration and suction cannula may be along the lateral inframammary crease, at the superior aspect of the anterior axillary fold, or transareolar, depending upon the specific contouring plan for the individual [13]. These locations reliably camouflage access sites. The tumescent solution most commonly used includes lactated Ringer's solution with lidocaine and epinephrine. Tranexamic acid has recently also been added to the tumescent infiltrate. The infiltration incisions are the same locations for the suction cannula access as well. During liposuction, changes in contour should be assessed frequently, as should the color of the aspirate. To achieve the desired contour, it is recommended that the liposuction cannula extend past the boundaries of the breast to ensure a new normal male chest wall aesthetic [18–20]. Unique in the treatment of gynecomastia, it is very important to eliminate any semblance of an inframammary fold. Failure to do so will lead to a more feminine breast appearance.

Popularized by Zocchi, ultrasound-assisted liposuction (UAL) is considered a less-invasive measure for the treatment of male gynecomastia with greater proportions of fibrous tissue [12, 17, 21, 22]. While incision sites remain the same, ultrasound energy is delivered to the tissues prior to aspiration, improving extraction and contouring. Wong and Malata found that patients treated with UAL were 8.5 times less likely to require subsequent revision surgery and 1.5 times less likely to require conversion to open excision when compared to patients who underwent SAL. [17] UAL can also promote better skin contraction than SAL, potentially eliminating the need for open excision and skin reduction [13, 23]. Both may be used in a single case wherein SAL is used for final aspiration and contouring after UAL. [13]

As it is difficult for liposuction alone to adequately correct excessive subareolar tissue, direct excision is often included in the treatment strategy. Fruhstorfer and Malata's series of 48 patients supports this strategy [13]. They found the most common complication in those treated with liposuction alone was a residual lump [13]. As a result, they advocate for conversion and/or incorporation of open excision into the operative planning, regardless of preoperative assessment [13]. Wong reported intraoperative conversion of liposuction to open excision in 39% of cases involving significant proportions of subareolar fibrous tissue [17]. Thus, combining liposuction with a transareolar incision for glandular excision is commonly performed [24, 25]. Further, liposuction facilitates open excision more seamlessly after conversion, as it reduces bleeding and creates tunnels to ease resection of the residual glandular tissue [10]. It is important to re-evaluate the chest contour frequently intraoperatively to optimize outcomes in chest wall recontouring.

21.5.3 Skin Excess/Redundancy

Skin reduction is necessary in patients with significantly enlarged breasts and in those who possess a notable component of breast ptosis. In these patients, not only is there excess skin, but the NAC is translocated from its normal anatomic lie. Both deformities must therefore be addressed. The first determination is the degree of excess skin. In addition, one must assess the contractile capacity of the skin for the individual patient. Younger patients will generally have a much greater ability for skin to contract and recontour than older males. Small amounts of skin redundancy can be managed locally with circumareolar approaches, some of which incorporate a purse-string suture of the NAC. [26–29] Other approaches remove the excess tissue within an elliptical incision and then transpose the nipple on a developed pedicle [30, 31]. A concentric circle operation with the nipple supplied by a superior pedicle has also been described [9, 32].

More notable volumes of redundant skin around the nipple can be excised with a concentric mastopexy reduction or with an elliptical LeJour pattern [32, 33]. The advantage of the concentric mastopexy reduction is its ability to hide the scars at the periphery of the NAC. While the LeJour excision creates a noticeable vertical scar, it is more reliable in patients with large breasts and severe ptosis. This excision pattern decreases periareolar skin puckering [13, 33].

By contrast, large, ptotic breasts require more extensive open excisions with significant skin resection. These techniques targeting excess skin escalate in complexity as the area/volume of skin excess increases; however, they are also more likely to result in adverse scarring and potentially undesirable chest contour [34, 35]. While there is no consensus on the ideal method for skin reduction, the timing of the skin resection is usually easiest immediately following open excision. If the glandular excision and skin reduction are planned as a two-stage procedure, it is recommended that the skin excision be performed a minimum of 4–6 months following open glandular excision [36].

Normalization of the NAC position must also be addressed in cases where the patient demonstrates excess skin and breast ptosis. Relocation of the nipple can be accomplished in several ways. When positional changes are more finite, they can be transposed on a de-epithelialized pedicle [25, 37, 38]. In cases where a concentric mastopexy reduction or an elliptical LeJour pattern is used, it is an inherent consideration of the planned reconstruction. Finally, the NAC may be repositioned as a full-thickness graft [39, 40]. The goal of each technique is to achieve masculinization of the shape, diameter, and position of the NAC upon the recontoured chest wall.

21.5.4 Nipple-Areolar Complex Distortion

The diameter of the typical male NAC is 25–30 mm [41]. Breast hypertrophy distorts the normal male NAC, often yielding an abnormally wide areola. Reduction of the areolar diameter needs to be addressed in reconstructive endeavors. These techniques can be included in most incisions. Assuring NAC viability and sensibility, as well as concealing scars, are paramount in successfully addressing the male gynecomastia deformity. Saad proposed a circumareolar incision for reducing the diameter of the enlarged nipple [42]. This is particularly valuable in unilateral cases where one breast and nipple are enlarged relative to a contralateral normal-sized chest/nipple.

21.6 Masculinization of the Chest

Although many of the minimally invasive and excisional techniques share similarities with operative reduction and reconstruction of female breasts, it is vital that the result of gynecomastia surgery not resemble female breasts. Obliteration of the inframammary fold is important to restore the normal male chest aesthetic. Similarly, one must reduce the fullness of the superior and inferior poles. Extending liposuction and open excision past the normal confines of the breast aids in achieving this goal. Reduction of areolar diameter consistent with male proportions is also important in restoring the male aesthetic.

21.7 Conclusion

No single minimally invasive or open technique is suitable for every case of gynecomastia, and individualization is the rule. The truest assessment of tissue hypertrophy and skin redundancy is often made intraoperatively, and the surgeon must be knowledgeable of the available techniques and willing to change plans to best fit the patient's needs. Fortunately, the wide range of approaches affords the surgeon an opportunity to meet an ideal result. No algorithm or specific instruction is superior to expert technique. The surgeon must maintain an intent of perfection with each challenge.

References

1. Webster JP. Mastectomy for gynecomastia through a semicircular intra-areolar incision. Ann Surg. 1946;124(3):557–75.
2. Nydick M, Bustos J, Dale JH, Rawson RW. Gynecomastia in adolescent boys. JAMA. 19 61;178:449–54.
3. Nuttall FQ. Gynecomastia as a physical finding in normal men. J Clin Endocrinol Metab. 1979;48(2):338–40. https://doi.org/10.1210/jcem-48-2-338.
4. Johnson RE, Murad MH. Gynecomastia: pathophysiology, evaluation, and management. Mayo Clin Proc. 2009;84(11):1010–5. https://doi.org/10.1016/S0025-6196(11)60671-X.
5. Braunstein GD. Aromatase and gynecomastia. Endocr Relat Cancer. 1999;6(2):315–24.
6. Rochefort H, Garcia M. The estrogenic and antiestrogenic activities of androgens in female target tissues. Pharmacol Ther. 1983;23(2):193–216.
7. Nicolis GL, Modlinger RS, Gabrilove JL. A study of the histopathology of human gynecomastia. J Clin Endocrinol Metab. 1971;32:2173–8. https://doi.org/10.1210/jcem-32-2-173.
8. Willams MJ. Gynecomastia. Its incidence, recognition and host characterization in 447 autopsy cases. Am J Med. 1963;34:103–12.
9. Persichetti P, Berloco M, Casadei RM, Marangi GF, Di Lella F, Nobili AM. Gynecomastia and the complete circumareolar approach in the surgical management of skin redundancy. Plast Reconstr Surg. 2001;107(4):948–54.
10. Samdal F, Kleppe G, Amland PF, Abyholm F. Surgical treatment of gynaecomastia. Five years' experience with liposuction. Scand J Plast Reconstr Surg Hand Surg. 1994;28(2):123–30.
11. Simon BE, Hoffman S, Kahn S. Classification and surgical correction of gynecomastia. Plast Reconstr Surg. 1973;51(1):48–52.
12. Rohrich RJ, Ha RY, Kenkel JM, Adams WP. Classification and management of gynecomastia: defining the role of ultrasound-assisted liposuction. Plast Reconstr Surg. 2003;111(2):909–23; discussion 924–5. https://doi.org/10.1097/01.PRS.0000042146.40379.25.
13. Fruhstorfer BH, Malata CM. A systematic approach to the surgical treatment of gynaecomastia. Br J Plast Surg. 2003;56(3):237–46.
14. Aiache AE. Surgical treatment of gynecomastia in the body builder. Plast Reconstr Surg. 1989;83(1):61–6.
15. Blau M, Hazani R. Correction of gynecomastia in body builders and patients with good physique. Plast Reconstr Surg. 2015;135(2):425–32. https://doi.org/10.1097/PRS.0000000000000887.
16. Illouz YG. Body contouring by lipolysis: a 5-year experience with over 3000 cases. Plast Reconstr Surg. 1983;72(5):591–7.
17. Wong KY, Malata CM. Conventional versus ultrasound-assisted liposuction in gynaecomastia surgery: a 13-year review. J Plast Reconstr Aesthet Surg. 2014;67(7):921–6. https://doi.org/10.1016/j.bjps.2014.03.004.
18. RosenbergGJ. Gynecomastia: suction lipectomy as a contemporary solution. Plast Reconstr Surg. 1987;80(3):379–86.
19. Rosenberg GJ. A new cannula for suction removal of parenchymal tissue of gynecomastia. Plast Reconstr Surg. 1994;94(3):548–51.

20. Mladick RA. Gynecomastia. Liposuction and excision. Clin Plast Surg. 1991;18(4):815–22.
21. Zocchi M. Ultrasonic liposculpturing. Aesth Plast Surg. 1992;16(4):287–98.
22. Hodgson EL, Fruhstorfer BH, Malata CM. Ultrasonic liposuction in the treatment of gynecomastia. Plast Reconstr Surg. 2005;116(2):646–53; discussion 654–5.
23. Rohrich RJ, Beran SJ, Kenkel JM, Adams WP, DiSpaltro F. Extending the role of liposuction in body contouring with ultrasound-assisted liposuction. Plast Reconstr Surg. 1998;101(4):1090–102; discussion 1117–9.
24. Scuderi N, Dessy LA, Tempesta M, Bistoni G, Mazzocchi M. Combined use of power-assisted liposuction and trans-areolar incision for gynaecomastia treatment. J Plast Reconstr Aesthet Surg. 2010;63(1):e93–5. https://doi.org/10.1016/j.bjps.2009.01.025.
25. Teimourian B, Perlman R. Surgery for gynecomastia. Aesth Plast Surg. 1983;7(3):155–7.
26. Peled IJ. The concentric mastopexy and the purse-string suture. Plast Reconstr Surg. 1991;87(2):385.
27. Smoot EC. Eccentric skin resection and purse-string closure for skin reduction with mastectomy for gynecomastia. Ann Plast Surg. 1998;41(4):378–83.
28. Huang TT, Hidalgo JE, Lewis SR. A circumareolar approach in surgical management of gynecomastia. Plast Reconstr Surg. 1982;69(1):35–40.
29. Peters MH, Vastine V, Knox L, Morgan RF. Treatment of adolescent gynecomastia using a bipedicle technique. Ann Plast Surg. 1998;40(3):241–5.
30. Letterman G, Schurter M. Surgical correction of massive gynecomastia. Plast Reconstr Surg. 1972;49(3):259–62.
31. Coskun A, Duzgun SA, Bozer M, Akinci OF, Uzunkoy A. Modified technique for correction of gynaecomastia. Eur J Surg. 2001;167(11):822–4. https://doi.org/10.1080/11024150152717643.
32. Davidson BA. Concentric circle operation for massive gynecomastia to excise the redundant skin. Plast Reconstr Surg. 1979;3(3):350–4.
33. Lejour M. Vertical mammaplasty and liposuction of the breast. Plast Reconstr Surg. 1994;94(1):100–14.
34. Courtiss EH. Gynecomastia: analysis of 159 patients and current recommendations for treatment. Plast Reconstr Surg. 1987;79(5):740–53.
35. Steele SR, Martin MJ, Place RJ. Gynecomastia: complications of the subcutaneous mastectomy. Am Surg. 2002;68(2):210–3.
36. Malata CM, Wong KY. Gynecomastia surgery. In: Neligan PC, Nahabedian MY, editors. Plastic surgery: volume 5: breast. Elsevier; 2018. p. 174–95.
37. Brenner P, Berger A, Schneider W, Axmann HD. Male reduction mammoplasty in serious gynecomastias. Aesth Plast Surg. 1992;16(4):325–30.
38. Kornstein AN, Cinelli PB. Inferior pedicle reduction technique for larger forms of gynecomastia. Aesth Plast Surg. 1992;16(4):331–5.
39. Murphy TP, Ehrlichman RJ, Seckel BR. Nipple placement in simple mastectomy with free nipple grafting for severe gynecomastia. Plast Reconstr Surg. 1994;94(6):818–23.
40. Wray RC, Hoopes JE, Davis GM. Correction of extreme gynaecomastia. Br J Plast Surg. 1974;27(1):39–41.
41. Beckenstein MS, Windle BH, Stroup RT. Anatomical parameters for nipple position and areolar diameter in males. Ann Plast Surg. 1996;36(1):33–6.
42. Saad MN, Kay S. The circumareolar incision: a useful incision for gynaecomastia. Ann R Coll Surg Engl. 1984;66(2):121–2.

Gynecomastia

22

Edward H. Davidson and Brandon J. De Ruiter

22.1 Introduction

The word gynecomastia is derived from the Greek *gunḗ* meaning female and *mastós* meaning breast. The term was first described by Galen in the second century, though there are gynecomastia-like depictions dating as far back as King Tutankhamun in ancient Egypt [1].

Gynecomastia is defined as a benign proliferation of glandular breast tissue in men. It is highly prevalent, and studies have estimated as many as 41–65% of males are affected [2–4]. Gynecomastia displays a trimodal age distribution most commonly affecting infants, adolescents, and older men.

Management of gynecomastia varies depending on etiology, disease severity, and duration of symptoms. Some cases majority of cases may be treated by observation, medical therapy, or addressing the underlying cause. Selection of surgical candidates involves identifying those with persistent symptoms or high-grade disease.

22.2 Pathophysiology

The mechanism underlying gynecomastia is thought to involve local imbalances of androgens and estrogens. While numerous physiologic, pathologic, and iatrogenic entities may contribute to such an imbalance, a majority of cases are idiopathic [5].

Histologically, gynecomastia progresses from an initial florid state of glandular proliferation within the first four months, to an intermediate phase, to a predominantly fibrous state after approximately a year. Gynecomastia is a histologically distinct entity from pseudogynecomastia, which involves excess adiposity *without* glandular proliferation.

Physiologic gynecomastia refers to that which commonly is seen with obesity as well as that which predictably occurs in newborns, adolescents, and older adults. In neonates, gynecomastia is transiently caused by in-utero exposure to maternal estrogens. The majority of these cases

E. H. Davidson (✉)
Department of Plastic Surgery, Case Western Reserve University/University Hospitals Cleveland, Cleveland, OH, USA
e-mail: Edward.davidson@case.edu

B. J. De Ruiter
University of Washington, Seattle, WA, USA

K. Jeffords et al. (eds.), *Aesthetic Surgery for Men*, https://doi.org/10.1007/978-3-032-03840-1_22

are self-resolving and asymptomatic though transient galactorrhea and indurated breast swelling have been described [6, 7]. The cause of adolescent gynecomastia is thought to be a delay in endogenous androgen production relative to estrogen production [4, 8–12]. Pubertal gynecomastia classically begins around age 10–12 years and peaks around ages 13–14 [13]. Most adolescent patients experience resolution of their symptoms within a year or two of symptomatic onset as they achieve adult ratios of sex hormones [4, 14, 15]. Gynecomastia in older adults may result from increases in adiposity, medication use, or age-related decreases in endogenous testosterone production [16].

Pathologic gynecomastia may result from a number of disease processes [16, 17]. Testicular tumors can cause gynecomastia through the secretion of β-hCG, direct secretion of estrogens, or increased peripheral aromatization. Adrenal tumors may directly secrete estrogen or, alternatively, secrete weak androgens that are aromatized. Patients with liver disease display imbalances in hormonal levels due to decreased hepatic metabolism of estrogens and altered levels of sex-hormone binding globulin. Hyperthyroidism has been postulated to cause gynecomastia through increased aromatase activity and altered levels of sex hormone binding globulin. Patients with renal failure may have gynecomastia due to decreased renal clearance of luteinizing hormone and prolactin or due to uremic injury of the testes.

Numerous medications, supplements, and recreational drugs have been linked with gynecomastia. Common examples are listed in Table 22.1.

Table 22.1 Medications and recreational drugs associated with gynecomastia

Class	Agent
Anti-androgens	Finasteride Flutamide
Cardiovascular agents	Amiodarone
	Digoxin
	Diltiazem/verapamil
	Spironolactone
Gastrointestinal agents	Cimetidine Metoclopramide Proton pump inhibitors
Cardiovascular agents	Amiodarone
	Digoxin
	Diltiazem/verapamil
	Methyldopa
	Spironolactone
HIV medications	Efavirenz
	Protease inhibitors
	Reverse transcriptase inhibitors
Psychoactive agents	Diazepam
	Fluoxetine
	Haloperidol
Recreational drugs	Alcohol
	Anabolic steroids
	Opioids
	Marijuana

22.3 Evaluation

A thorough clinical history is foundational in the evaluation of patients with gynecomastia. Information on onset, timing, laterality, pain or tenderness, presence of discharge, and associated symptoms should be obtained along with a thorough list of medications and substance use history.

Physical examination should evaluate the distribution of the tissue, presence of ptosis, size of the breast, skin redundancy, skin elasticity, and distinguish between a fatty or glandular tissue predominance. Examination findings are important to planning management and distinguishing gynecomastia from pseudogynecomastia or breast cancer.

True gynecomastia classically presents as a firm rubbery mass that is concentrically positioned deep to the nipple-areola complex (NAC) [16]. Pseudogynecomastia and breast carcinoma may be distinguished from this on exam as adipose tissue in pseudogynecomastia provides less tactile resistance when pinched and as breast carcinoma tends to present as a hard, unilateral mass located away from the NAC [16]. Stigmata from liver, kidney, or thyroid disease should be assessed. A thorough testicular examination is *required* as testicular cancer is the most common cancer in young adult men and has an excellent prognosis if caught early. Gynecomastia, in some cases, may be the initial presenting symptom of testicular cancer [18, 19].

The need for an endocrine evaluation has long been controversial. Hormonal studies, including β-hCG, LH, FSH, testosterone, estradiol, T4, TSH, prolactin, GH, and a metabolic panel, have been considered. However, recent evidence suggests an endocrine workup is unnecessary in a majority of cases as it rarely identifies the underlying abnormality, subjects the patient to unnecessary invasive testing, and costs the medical system additional monetary expenditures [20]. Testicular ultrasound, chest x-ray, computed tomography, sellar MRI, or diagnostic mammography may be ordered if clinical or laboratory findings dictate.

22.4 Management

Management of gynecomastia varies depending on etiology. Many cases can initially be managed with observation or by treatment of the underlying cause (i.e., removing inciting medications, weight loss, etc.). More intensive interventions may be required for patients with persistent or disfiguring symptoms.

Medical management options for gynecomastia have been described but demonstrate mixed efficacy. Selective estrogen receptor modulators, including Tamoxifen and Raloxifene, have shown an effect improving symptoms, and a short course of therapy may be appropriate for those with mild gynecomastia of recent onset [16, 21–23]. Androgenic therapy may be effective for patients with primary hypogonadism, however may exacerbate gynecomastia in other patients due to peripheral aromatization [16]. Aromatase inhibitors have shown limited benefit in the management of gynecomastia and are not recommended for use [16]. All medical therapy is prone to undercorrection, cannot address skin laxity, may be prone to relapse, and is ineffective after approximately a year of symptoms due to fibrosis of the affected tissue [16].

Surgical management options offer definitive therapy for patients with persistent or disfiguring symptoms. Numerous options exist, including open excision, liposuction, or some combination or modification of the above approaches [16].

The selection of technique must balance the need for adequate resection and the desire to minimize scarring. The authors here propose a management algorithm based upon the grade of disease as described by Simon et al. [24] (Table 22.2). While other grading classification systems for gynecomastia have been proposed, the authors here prefer this system as it provides simple guidelines for management.

Ultrasound-assisted liposuction (UAL) is an effective modality for managing low-grade disease as it minimizes scar burden and may cause some degree of skin retraction. Open excision is required for those with high-grade disease. For

Table 22.2 Surgical management of gynecomastia [24]

Classification	Presentation	Management
Grade I	Minor enlargement, no skin excess	UAL
Grade IIA	Moderate enlargement, no skin excess	UAL +/– secondary skin resection
Grade IIB	Moderate enlargement, skin excess	UAL
Grade III	Marked enlargement, skin excess	Open excision

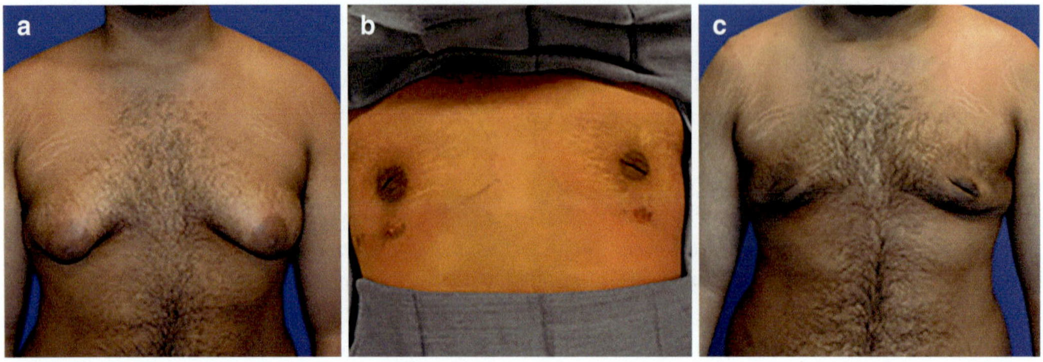

Fig. 22.1 Patient with Grade IIB gynecomastia (**a**). Immediate post-operative results following VASER liposuction (**b**). At 6-month follow-up, the patient has persistent skin excess and is a candidate for a secondary skin-resection procedure (**c**)

patients with intermediate disease severity (Grade IIB), a more nuanced approach is required. Liposuction techniques can be used; however, secondary skin resection procedures may be required (Fig. 22.1). Alternatively, patients may opt to immediately undergo open excision and trade the possibility of a second procedure for a single operation that is associated with a larger scar. Thorough pre-operative counseling on potential risks and benefits of each option is crucial to facilitating a shared decision-making process and guiding patient expectations.

22.5 Techniques

22.5.1 Liposuction

Patients with good skin elasticity, minimal skin redundancy, fatty predominant tissue, and relatively small breast size are ideal candidates for liposuction. Advantages of liposuction are its ability to remove large amounts of fatty tissue while minimizing overall scar burden (Fig. 22.2). Disadvantages include difficulty addressing skin redundancy and difficulty removing fibrotic or glandular tissue. Modifications to the traditional suction-lipectomy technique have been developed to help bypass these limitations.

Ultrasound-assisted liposuction (UAL) is one such modification that utilizes high-frequency sound waves to emulsify adipose tissue and thus facilitate removal of tissue from fibrotic areas that are otherwise challenging to reach with traditional suction-lipectomy [25, 26]. Studies have found better overall outcomes with UAL demonstrating better skin retraction and lower rates of post-operative revision and intraoperative conversion to open excision when compared with conventional liposuction techniques [26, 27]. VASER (vibration amplification of sound energy with resonance) liposuction is a form of UAL that utilizes *pulsed* ultrasonic energy and smaller, more efficient cannulas. When compared with prior generations of UAL devices, VASER devices have been shown to yield lower rates of complications, including internal burns, seroma, skin necrosis, rippling, and painful dysesthesias, while simultaneously cutting procedure time and using smaller instruments that are easier to use [28, 29]. Together, UAL techniques are important modalities for the surgical management of gynecomastia.

The technique:

1. Stab incision is made at the lateral inframammary fold.
2. Tumescent solution is infiltrated.
3. After a 15-min delay to allow for the tumescent effect, UAL probe is utilized for 8–15 min per quadrant (typically 1 min per 100 cc of tumescence infiltrated) with care to protect skin from thermal injury.

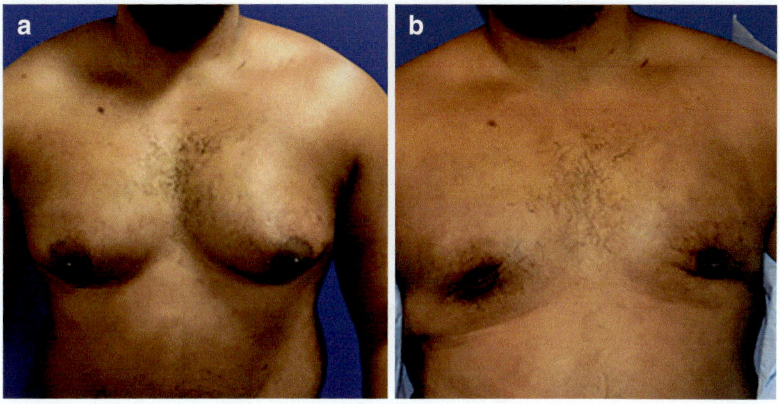

Fig. 22.2 Grade I gynecomastia (**a**). 6 month post-operative results following VASER liposuction (**b**)

4. Suction-assisted liposuction (SAL) is performed until a uniform pinch test of ~¼ inch throughout is achieved.
5. Residual retroareolar fibrous breast tissue is mechanically removed by avulsion technique with Kelly clamp.
6. A drain can be placed if there is significant skin redundancy and dead space.
7. Compression dressings for 4 weeks post-operatively.

22.5.2 Open Excision

Excisional techniques are required for high-grade gynecomastia with significant skin redundancy. Advantages of excisional techniques include their ability to easily address skin excess, eliminate large amounts of fatty and glandular tissue, and reposition the nipple-areolar complex. Disadvantages include a larger scar burden and potentially higher rates of operative complications, including nerve injury, fat necrosis, skin necrosis, seromas, and hematomas.

The specific approach and incisional pattern may be customized based on patient presentation. Peri-areolar incisions, crescent-shaped incisions on the superior pole of the nipple-areolar complex (NAC), and larger "donut-shaped" peri-areolar incisions may be used depending on the need for NAC repositioning.

For patients with severe disease and significant NAC displacement, the authors here advocate the use of an inferiorly based dermoglandular flap as it permits maximal tissue resection and NAC mobility while maintaining aesthetic results [30] (Fig. 22.3).

The technique:

1. Markings
   (a) Mark the new NAC position at the intersection of the lateral border of the pectoralis major muscle and the fifth rib.
   (b) The lower border of the elliptical excision is marked in the existing IMF.
   (c) The upper border of the elliptical excision is provisionally marked ~4 cm inferior to the planned nipple position and continued medially and laterally to meet the inframammary fold.
   (d) An inferiorly based pedicle of ≥10 cm width is marked.
2. A NAC of diameter 2 cm is marked utilizing a guide. The pedicle is then de-epithelialized and elevated maintaining a thickness of 1 cm.
3. The deep dissection of the superior flap is made along the pectoralis fascia up to the level of the clavicle.
4. The superficial dissection of the superior flap is performed in the mastectomy plane between the breast capsule and the subcutaneous fat. The resultant isolated breast tissue is then removed.
5. Closure is "tailor tacked" based on the marked superior excision to ensure tension-free closure as well as to confirm the correct position of the marked nipple position. The superior excision is then made, and the deep layer is

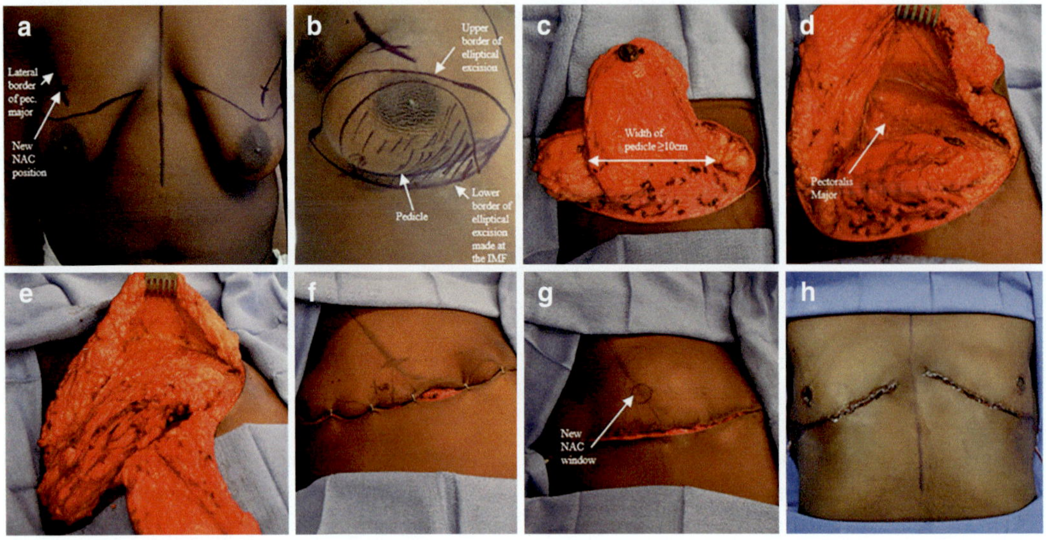

Fig. 22.3 Excision of gynecomastia. NAC repositioning markings (**a**). Pre-operative markings delineate the margins of excision (**b**). A thin dermoglandular pedicle is isolated (**c**). Deep dissection of the superior flap is made along the pectoralis fascia up to the clavicle (**d**). The superficial dissection of the superior flap is carried between the breast capsule and subcutaneous fat (**e**). Closure is "tailor tacked" (**f**). Location of new NAC window (**g**). Immediate post-operative results (**h**)

closed with absorbable sutures once meticulous hemostasis has been achieved and a drain has been placed.

6. A new NAC window is created using a 1 cm guide centered on the position marked in step 1a. The NAC is delivered, and closure is completed.

References

1. Paulshock BZ. Tutankhamun and his brothers. Familial gynecomastia in the eighteenth dynasty. JAMA. 1980;244(2):160–4.
2. Niewoehner CB, Nuttal FQ. Gynecomastia in a hospitalized male population. Am J Med. 1984;77:633–8.
3. Georgiadis E, Papandreou L, Evangelopoulou C, Aliferis C, Lymberis C, Panitsa C, Batrinos M. Incidence of gynaecomastia in 954 young males and its relationship to somatometric parameters. Ann Hum Biol. 1994;21(6):579–87.
4. Biro FM, Lucky AW, Huster GA, Morrison JA. Hormonal studies and physical maturation in adolescent gynecomastia. J Pediatr. 1990;116(3):450–5.
5. Rahmani S, Turton P, Shaaban A, Dall B. Overview of gynecomastia in the modern era and the Leeds Gynaecomastia investigation algorithm. Breast J. 2011;17(3):246–55.
6. Madlon-Kay DJ. 'Witch's milk'. Galactorrhea in the newborn. Am J Dis Child. 1986;140(3):252–3.
7. Raveenthiran V. Neonatal Mastauxe (breast enlargement of the newborn). J Neonatal Surg. 2013;2(3):31.
8. Moore DC, Schlaepfer LV, Paunier L, Sizonenko PC. Hormonal changes during puberty: V. Transient pubertal gynecomastia: abnormal androgen-estrogen ratios. J Clin Endocrinol Metab. 1984;58(3):492–9.
9. Ersöz H, Onde ME, Terekeci H, Kurtoglu S, Tor H. Causes of gynaecomastia in young adult males and factors associated with idiopathic gynaecomastia. Int J Androl. 2002;25(5):312–6.
10. Johnson RE, Murad MH. Gynecomastia: pathophysiology, evaluation, and management. Mayo Clin Proc. 2009;84(11):1010–5.
11. Daniels IR, Layer GT. Gynaecomastia. Eur J Surg. 2001;167:885–92.
12. Bhasin S. Testicular disorders. In: Kronenberg HM, Melmed S, Polonsky KS, Larsen PR, editors. Williams textbook of endocrinology. 11th ed. Philadelphia: Saunders Elsevier; 2008. p. 669–74.
13. Gikas P, Mokbel K. Management of gynaecomastia: an update. Int J Clin Pract. 2007;61:1209–15.
14. Lemaine V, Cayci, Simmons PS, Petty P. Gynecomastia in adolescent males. Semin Plast Surg. 2013;27(1):56–61.
15. Lazala C, Saenger P. Pubertal gynecomastia. J Pediatr Endocrinol Metab. 2002;15(5):553–60.
16. Braunstein GD. Gynecomastia. N Engl J Med. 2007;357(12):1229–37.

17. Braunstein GD. Gynecomastia. N Engl J Med. 1993;328(7):490–5.
18. Harris M, Rizvi S, Hindmarsh J, Bryan R. Testicular tumor presenting as gynaecomastia. BMJ. 2006;332(7545):837.
19. Hassan HC, Cullen IM, Casey RG, Rogers E. Gynaecomastia: an endocrine manifestation of testicular cancer. Andrologia. 2008;40(3):152–7.
20. Malhotra AK, Amed S, Bucevska M, Bush KL, Arneja JS. Do adolescents with gynecomastia require routine evaluation by endocrinology? Plast Reconstr Surg. 2018;142(1):9e–16e.
21. Lawrence SE, Faught KA, Vethamuthu J, Lawson ML. Beneficial effects of raloxifene and tamoxifen in the treatment of pubertal gynecomastia. J Pediatr. 2004;45(1):71–6.
22. Parker LN, Gray DR, Lai MK, Levin ER. Treatment of gynecomastia with tamoxifen: a double-blind crossover study. Metabolism. 1986;35(8):705.
23. Ting AC, Chow LW, Leung YF. Comparison of tamoxifen with danazol in the management of idiopathic gynecomastia. Am Surg. 2000;66(1):38–40.
24. Simon BE, Hoffman S, Kahn S. Classification and surgical correction of gynecomastia. Plast Reconstr Surg. 1973;51(1):48–52.
25. Rohrich RJ, Ha RY, Kenkel JM, Adams WP Jr. Classification and management of gynecomastia: defining the role of ultrasound-assisted liposuction. Plast Reconstr Surg. 2003;111(2):909–23.
26. Wong KY, Malata CM. Conventional versus ultrasound-assisted liposuction in gynaecomastia surgery: a 13-year review. J Plast Reconstr Aesthet Surg. 2014;67(7):921–6.
27. Zocchi ML. Ultrasonic-assisted lipoplasty: technical refinements and clinical evaluations. Clin Plast Surg. 1996;23(4):575–98.
28. Jewell ML, Fodor PB, de Souza Pinto EB, Al Shammari MA. Clinical application of VASER—assisted lipoplasty: a pilot clinical study. Aesthet Surg J. 2002;22(2):131–46.
29. de Souza Pinto EB, Abdala PC, Maciel CM, dos Santos FP, de Souza RP. Liposuction and VASER. Clin Plast Surg. 2006;33(1):107–15, vii
30. Toy JW, Rubin JP. Contouring of the arms, breast, upper trunk, and male chest in the massive weight loss patient. In: Warren R, Neligan P, editors. Plastic surgery, 3e. Vancouver: Saunders; 2012. p. 575–8.

The Athletes' Gynecomastia

23

Jaime R. Garza and Victor E. Stams

23.1 Etiology

In the general male population, gynecomastia is relatively common occurring in 36–70% of male subjects [1]. Gynecomastia often appears transiently at birth. The process is thought to be related to an increased level of circulating maternal estrogens. After birth, the estrogen level decreases, the gynecomastia resolves, and treatment is rarely necessary. Many cases are typically related to hormone variation during the neonatal period, puberty, or advanced age.

Gynecomastia is also a common adverse effect associated with anabolic steroid use. Research has demonstrated a prevalence rate of 37% in anabolic steroid users [2]. It is a benign enlargement of the male breast resulting from an altered estrogen-androgen balance, or increased breast sensitivity to a circulating estrogen level. Increases in estrogen production in men are seen primarily through the aromatization of circulating testosterone [3]. It develops in a minority of men who use anabolic steroids because a small amount of the androgens is metabolized to estrogens in fat cells, and hepatic function may be altered [4]. The overwhelming majority of these cases spontaneously resolve without intervention. In addition to performance-enhancing drugs and steroids, other medications can also induce gynecomastia. Anti-anxiety medications, such as diazepam, tricyclic antidepressants, ulcer medications, such as cimetidine, and cannabis have all been linked to gynecomastia development.

Anabolic steroids are the most common cause of gynecomastia development in athletes and continue to be abused by a variety of athletes, including bodybuilders, baseball players, football players, cyclists, and strength and conditioning athletes. Some of the more common offending steroid preparations include nandrolone deconate, trenbolone acetate, human chorionic gonadotropin, and testosterone.

Anabolic steroids can promote an increase in muscular size and strength when combined with supervised training programs and diet. Athletes will administer the drugs in a pyramid (step-up) pattern in which dosages are steadily increased over several weeks. Toward the end of the cycle, the athlete will "step down" to reduce the likelihood of negative side effects. At this point, some athletes will discontinue drug use or perhaps initiate another cycle of different drugs that may increase endogenous testosterone production to prevent the undesirable drop in testosterone concentrations that follows the removal of the pharmaceutical agents [3]. Due to the many anatomical, physiological, and psychological

J. R. Garza
UT Health-San Antonio, San Antonio, TX, USA

V. E. Stams (✉)
Department of Plastic and Reconstructive Surgery, UT Health-San Antonio, San Antonio, TX, USA

K. Jeffords et al. (eds.), *Aesthetic Surgery for Men*, https://doi.org/10.1007/978-3-032-03840-1_23

adverse effects of steroids, medical professionals have discouraged their use.

The first systematic use of anabolic steroids in sports has been attributed to a successful Soviet weightlifting team in the 1950s. Use of these drugs spread to other countries and, during the early 1960s, to other strength-intensive sports, from field events to football [5]. Thereafter, the use of steroids diffused to endurance sports such as long-distance running and swimming, as well as to recreational users attempting to "look good" or more muscular. Regardless, athletes seeking a competitive edge persist in their use. Previous studies have demonstrated that significant use of anabolic steroids has been reported among professional, collegiate, and even high-school athletes [6]. In recent studies of high-school seniors, 6.6% of males [7] and 1.3% of females [8] acknowledged prior use of anabolic steroids. Anabolic steroids are generally used in "cycles"—that is, taken for a period such as 8 weeks and then not used for several weeks or months or taken in lower doses. Several types of anabolic steroids may be used simultaneously, a method called "stacking."

After steroids are stopped, the breast tissue can become less prominent but does not disappear entirely. Many anabolic steroid users will use anti-estrogens (selective estrogen receptor modulators) such as tamoxifen and clomiphene or anastrozole (which is a non-steroidal aromatase inhibitor) to minimize the side effects of estrogen and stimulate testosterone production [3].

23.2 Diagnosis

A careful history and physical examination is paramount in the workup of gynecomastia, including assessment of age, duration and onset of breast enlargement, symptoms of pain or tenderness, medications, recreational drug use, and psychological and social effects. A review of systems should involve signs/symptoms of hepatic disease, hyperthyroidism or hypothyroidism, recent weight gain or loss, adrenal disease, alcoholism, renal failure, and malignancies. Physical examination includes assessment of the breast gland and includes the nature of the tissue (glandular versus fat), isolated masses, and tenderness. The thyroid is evaluated for enlargement. The testes are examined for asymmetry, masses, enlargement, or atrophy. Laboratory evaluation is based on the findings of the history and physical examination. Healthy adults with a normal physical examination (other than gynecomastia) and longstanding gynecomastia do not require further workup. Patients with feminizing characteristics should undergo endocrine testing. In addition, if a marfanoid body habitus is associated with feminization, Klinefelter syndrome must be ruled out [9]. Any other new positive findings on physical examination should be evaluated in an appropriate manner.

23.3 Classification of Gynecomastia

Gynecomastia has several classification schemes [10]. Originally classified in 1973, the initial scheme classified gynecomastia based on the physical appearance of the breast. Grades I and IIa include small-to-moderate breast enlargement without skin redundancy. Grade IIb and III include enlargement with skin redundancy. Later revision by Rohrich [9] includes tissue type, glandular vs fibrous, ptosis, and weight of breast tissue in its classification (Table 23.1). Ultimately, all classifications are designed with treatment in mind.

Table 23.1 Classification and management of gynecomastia

Classification	Treatment
Grade I: -Mminimal hypertrophy (<250 g of breast tissue) without ptosis	
I A. Primarily glandular[a]	Ultrasound-assisted liposuction or suction-assisted lipectomy
I B. Primarily fibrous[a]	Ultrasound-assisted liposuction
Grade II: Moderate hypertrophy (250–500 g of breast tissue) without ptosis	
II A. Primarily glandular[a]	Ultrasound-assisted liposuction or suction-assisted lipectomy
II B. Primarily fibrous[a]	Ultrasound-assisted liposuction
Grade III: Severe hypertrophy (>500 g of breast tissue) with grade 1 ptosis	
Glandular or fibrous[a]	Ultrasound-assisted liposuction with or without staged excision[b]
Grade IV: Severe hypertrophy with grade II or III ptosis	
Glandular or fibrous[a]	Ultrasound-assisted liposuction with or without staged excision[b]

From: Rohrich et al. [9]

[a]Fatty and glandular tissue is determined by a pinch test medially, laterally, and beneath the nipple-areola complex

[b]Delayed excision of remaining ptotic breast skin and/or breast parenchyma is performed 6–9 months after ultrasound-assisted liposuction to allow maximal skin retraction

23.4 Technique for Treatment of Gynecomastia

In patients with gynecomastia for more than 1 year and with a normal history and physical examination, surgery may be indicated. If there is a possible etiology noted in the patient's history, then an attempt should be made to either discontinue the drug believed to be causing the gynecomastia or correct the systemic condition. If an abnormality is found on physical examination, workup is indicated prior to surgical intervention for the gynecomastia. If the underlying condition is medically treated and the gynecomastia persists beyond a year, surgical correction is indicated [9]. The two key elements in treating gynecomastia are to remove the excess volume of glandular and/or fatty tissues and to decide if and how to best remove any excess skin [11]. Most fibrous lesions are treated with surgical excision or, in select cases, liposuction when there is only diffuse fibro-fatty tissue [12]. This surgical approach is most commonly a combination of liposuction and direct excision of retro-areolar glandular tissue.

Patients with lesions of fatty tissue located just beneath the areolae may be treated with just liposuction. Conventional approaches to liposuction of gynecomastia with standard cannulas, power-assisted liposuction, or ultrasound-assisted liposuction have been used successfully.

If surgical excision is chosen as the treatment, a periareolar incision is key. The skin incision is a half-moon incision from the 3 o'clock to 9 o'clock position marked in a wavy pattern just at the junction of the areolar skin and chest wall skin. If placed within the pigmented area, the scar may appear as a white line. If placed outside the areola, it may become hypertrophic. In both cases, the scar would be visible. The site of the incision should be marked prior to the distortion caused by injection of a lidocaine-epinephrine-containing solution to prevent distortion of the area to be marked. The patient is marked in the upright position. All areas of tissue excess are marked, including the inframammary fold and the periareolar incision. Sedation or general anesthesia is necessary. The area is infiltrated with a tumescent solution containing 1 cc of 1:1000 epinephrine solution and 50 cc of 1% lidocaine. The infiltration volume is about 2:1 with the expected aspiration volume and covers a wide area of the chest from the clavicle to below the inframammary fold. Liposuction is performed in radial directions and the inframammary fold is disrupted. It is important to perform liposuction of a wide area surrounding the gynecomastia deformity to obtain the maximal amount of skin shrinkage possible. In cases of pure fatty gynecomastia, no further surgery is necessary. After the periareolar incision is made, a cuff of subcutaneous and glandular tissue, 1–1.5 centimeters in thickness, is preserved directly under the nipple-areola complex to prevent postoperative nipple-areola distortion or adherence of the nipple/areola to the chest wall, resulting in a visible depression. The glandular tissue is dissected with electrocautery under direct vision, leaving the pectoralis fascia intact deep to the gland. The tissue is pulled out through the wound and removed with electrocautery. Drains can be placed if the dead space is large. We use a #10 Blake drain and leave it in place for 5–6 days. All patients are treated with compression garments for 8 weeks.

23.5 Complications

The most common early complication after gynecomastia surgery is hematoma. In an open case, the hematoma should be evacuated [13]. This prevents excessive scarring and distortion of the breast. Postoperative closed suction drainage decreases the incidence of this complication. In liposuction cases, evacuation may not be possible. Under-resection of tissue is the most common long-term complication of gynecomastia surgery. This is particularly common in liposuction cases when a residual mass of glandular tissue is not resected. This can usually be avoided using the pull-through technique. Under-resection at the periphery of the breast can result from poor tapering and cause a noticeable deformity. Over-resection of the nipple-areola can result in a saucer-type deformity that is difficult to correct. Loose skin is usually not considered a complication if it is part of the operative plan. Occasionally, loose skin occurs unexpectedly, and surgical excision is required [13].

23.6 Conclusion

Gynecomastia is an increasingly common condition that can be attributed to a hormonal imbalance caused by several factors. The purpose of gynecomastia assessment should be the detection of underlying pathological conditions, including reversible causes, and the discernment from other more serious pathologies, particularly breast cancer. After confirming the diagnosis, identifying the underlying etiology, and classifying the grade according to severity grade, therapy should be personalized. Lifestyle guidance, reassurance, medical treatment, and surgical correction are valid tailored therapeutic options.

References

1. Neuman JF. Evaluation and treatment of gynecomastia. Am Fam Physician. 1997;55(5):1835–50.
2. O'Sullivan AJ, Kennedy MC, Casey JH, Day RO, Corrigan B, Wodak AD. Anabolic-androgenic steroids: medical assessment of present, past and potential users. Med J Aust. 2000;173(6):323–7. https://doi.org/10.5694/j.1326-5377.2000.tb125667.x.
3. Hoffman JR, Ratamess NA. Medical issues associated with anabolic steroid use: are they exaggerated? J Sports Sci Med. 2006;5(2):182–93. Published 2006 Jun 1
4. Strauss RH, Yesalis CE. Anabolic steroids in the athlete. Annu Rev Med. 1991;42:449–57. https://doi.org/10.1146/annurev.me.42.020191.002313.
5. Yesalis CE, Wright JE, Lombardo JA. Anabolic-androgen steroids: a synthesis of existing data and recommendations for future research. Clin Sports Med. 1989;1(3):109–34.
6. Anderson WA, Albrecht RR, McKeag DB, Hough DO, McGrew CA. A national survey of alcohol and drug use by college athletes. Phys Sportsmed. 1991;19(2):91–104.
7. Buckley WE, Yesalis CE 3rd, Friedl KE, Anderson WA, Streit AL, Wright JE. Estimated prevalence of anabolic steroid use among male high school seniors. JAMA. 1988;260(23):3441–5.
8. Bachman JG, Johnston LD, O'Malley PM. Monitoring the future: a continuing study of the lifestyles and values of youth, 1990. Inter-university Consortium for Political and Social Research [distributor]; 2011. Available from: https://doi.org/10.3886/ICPSR09745.v2.
9. Rohrich RJ, Ha RY, Kenkel JM, Adams WP Jr. Classification and management of gynecomastia: defining the role of ultrasound-assisted liposuction. Plast Reconstr Surg. 2003;111(2):909–25. https://doi.org/10.1097/01.PRS.0000042146.40379.25.
10. Waltho D, Hatchell A, Thoma A. Gynecomastia classification for surgical management: a systematic review and novel classification system. Plast Reconstr Surg. 2017;139(3):638e–48e. https://doi.org/10.1097/PRS.0000000000003059.
11. Hammond DC. Surgical correction of gynecomastia. Plast Reconstr Surg. 2009;124(1 Suppl):61e–8e. https://doi.org/10.1097/PRS.0b013e3181aa2dc7.
12. Monarca C, Rizzo MI. Gynecomastia: tips and tricks-classification and surgical approach. Plast Reconstr Surg. 2013;131(5):863e–5e. https://doi.org/10.1097/PRS.0b013e318287a18f.
13. Petty PM, Solomon M, Buchel EW, Tran NV. Gynecomastia: evolving paradigm of management and comparison of techniques. Plast Reconstr Surg. 2010;125(5):1301–8. https://doi.org/10.1097/PRS.0b013e3181d62962.

Ptotic Male Chest

24

Keith Jeffords and Mitchell Lyons

Gynecomastia is problematic in the world with at least 1/3 of the male population with a disproportionate chest-to-waist ratio. A large subset of these men also have sagging breasts with areola that is below the inframammary fold. Plastic surgery statistics worldwide demonstrate the lack of male awareness of surgical solutions [1–5].

The initial advancement in gynecomastia surgery was made by Ivo Pitanguy in 1966 reporting a "Transareolar Incision for Gynecomastia." With advances in liposuction and reporting of combination liposuction, liposuction with glandular excision and inclusion skin excision techniques, gynecomastia surgery has advanced. The question remains, "How do I perform a minimal incision technique to acquire a flat and aesthetic chest?" [6, 7].

The goal of any aesthetic procedure is to look natural. The male ptotic chest goals should also consider this natural goal with minimal visible scars. The nomenclature for men is similar to women [8–10].

Class l: areola is above the inframammary fold
Class ll: areola is at or slightly below the inframammary fold
Class lll: areola is below the inframammary fold

The standard surgical treatment plan for Class l gynecomastia has been liposuction +/− -excision of glandular tissue. This is ALSO true for Class ll gynecomastia cases. Rarely, it is necessary to excise skin for Class ll cases. The liposuction should always extend from the clavicle past the inframammary fold and laterally into the axillary region. This is necessary to "redrape" the skin and allow the skin to contract onto the chest wall.

The standard technique for removing glandular tissue is making an incision from the 3 o'clock to the 9 o'clock position of the areola skin interface. Then the full thickness incision can be dissected to lift the areola superiorly to excise the glandular tissue. The same techniques for Type ll and lll gynecomastia cases are the same.

Liposuction is always used on Class ll and lll cases unless involved in massive weight loss with only skin sag remaining. The best analogy for patients is the "cheese" comparison. The skin-fat-muscle analogy is a block of "cheddar cheese." Liposuction creates "swiss cheese." Post-op compression garments allow the "Swiss cheese" holes to be compressed, forming fibrous connective tissue. This tissue contracts the skin with compression garments, creating tighter skin.

When removing glandular tissue, it is necessary to undermine the skin to alleviate depression deformities. It is common to use 2.0 and 3.0 Vicryl sutures to fat under the areola to prevent

K. Jeffords (✉)
Private Practice, Paramount Plastic Surgery, Smyrna, GA, USA
e-mail: kjeffords@paramountplasticsurgery.com

M. Lyons
Paramount Plastic Surgery, Smyrna, GA, USA

K. Jeffords et al. (eds.), *Aesthetic Surgery for Men*, https://doi.org/10.1007/978-3-032-03840-1_24

these depression deformities. Use the undermining of the skin to redrape the chest wall skin and create bilateral symmetry.

Class lll cases can be difficult. If it is a milder case with the areola just slightly below the inferior mammary fold, the treatment can be the same. If it is a significant sag, the nipple-areola complex may point vertically toward the man's toes.

In this case, the chest might require a traditional chest lift—the most aesthetic procedure. The midclavicular line is measured and marked. The areola size is spread under tension. Then, a smaller areola is marked with a round device with a marking pen. The areola is incised, and the new areola circulation is preserved on an inferior pedicle. The excessive skin is amputated with a full-thickness horizontal incision at the inferior mammary fold. The is sutured in multiple layers as a horizontal scar.

Before the surgery, a new position of the smaller areola is marked from the mid-clavicular marking with a tape measure. The new smaller areola is raised in a new position using the smaller areola sizer. The new areola position is excised, the pedicle is raised, and the smaller areola is sutured in the new position.

Gynecomastia is life-changing surgery for men. Complex cases can be routine and worthwhile to both the patient and the surgeon. Techniques are simple but very life changing. This population is underserved in the plastic surgery community.

Case 24.1 Combination of glandular excision plus liposuction (extending the liposuction past the inferior mammary fold)

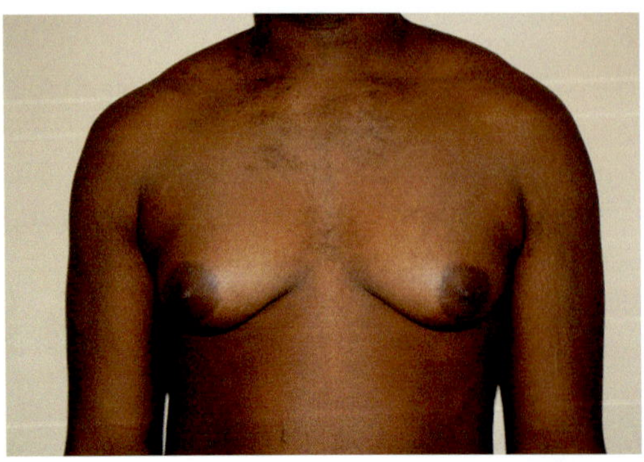

Postop 2 months

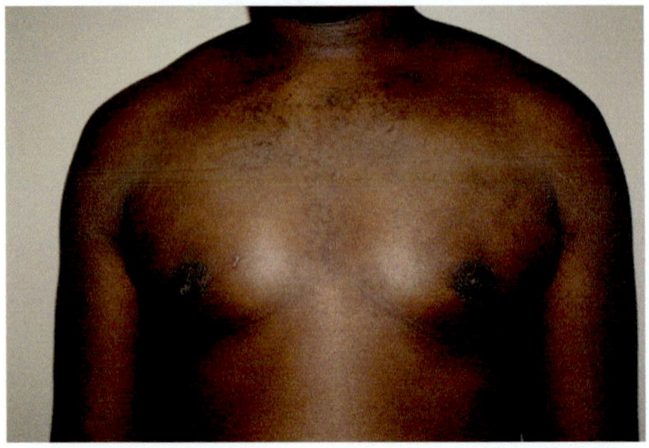

Case 24.2 Chest Liposuction with glandular excision. The liposuction extended past the inframammary fold

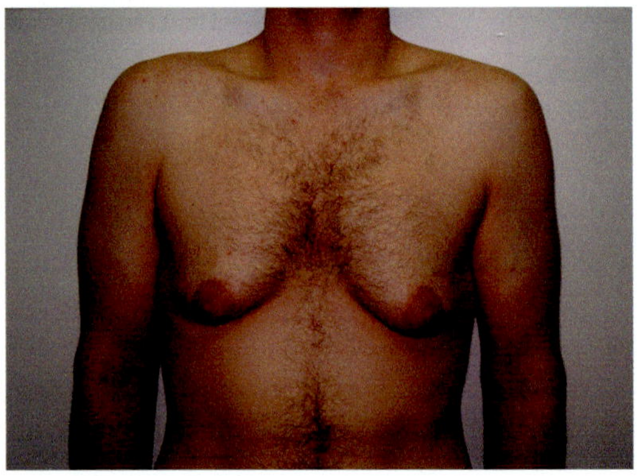

Postop 1 year

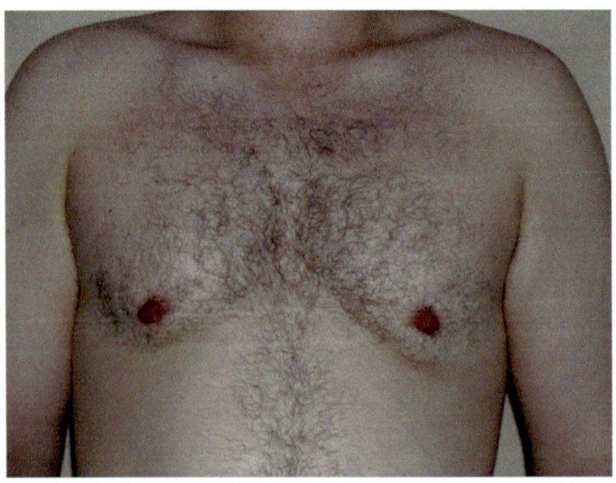

Case 24.3 Chest liposuction with glandular excision. Abdominal liposuction also. Liposuction extending past the inframammary fold

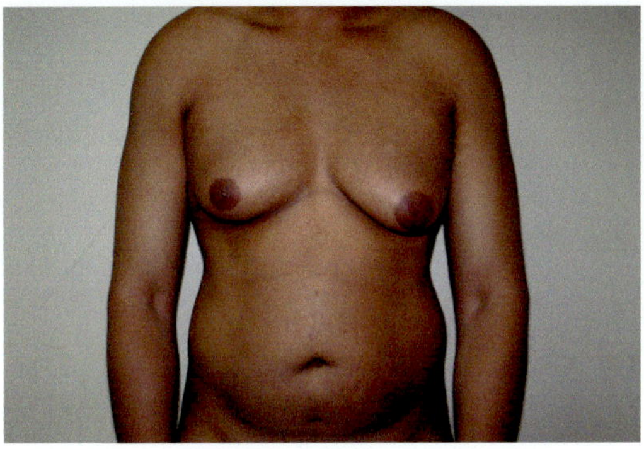

Postop 1 year after exercise

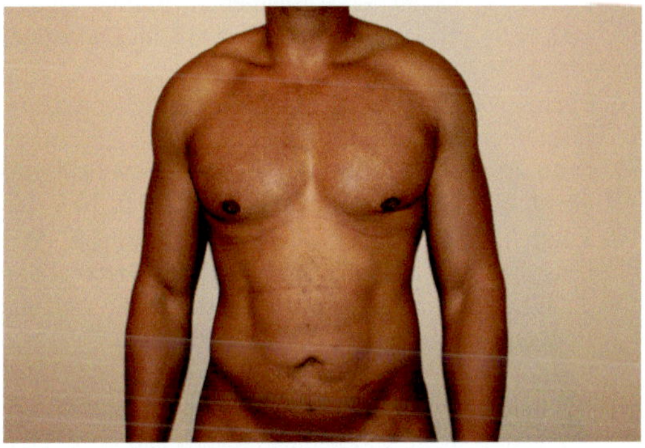

Case 24.4 Chest asymmetry with Grade III ptosis. Perioareolar excision with pedicle flap, excision of chest skin at inframammary fold, and insertion of reduced pedicle nipple/areola complex in new anatomic position

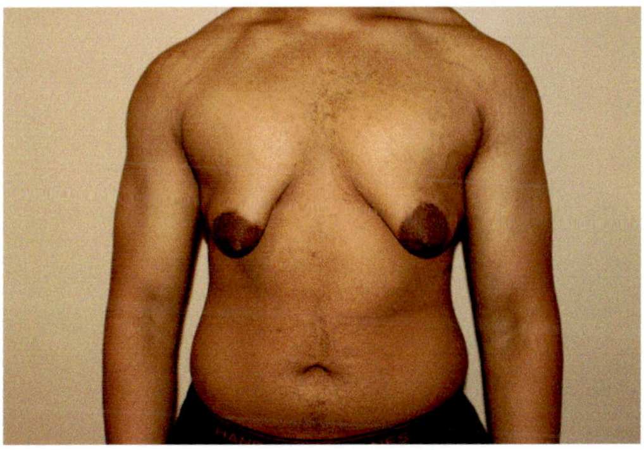

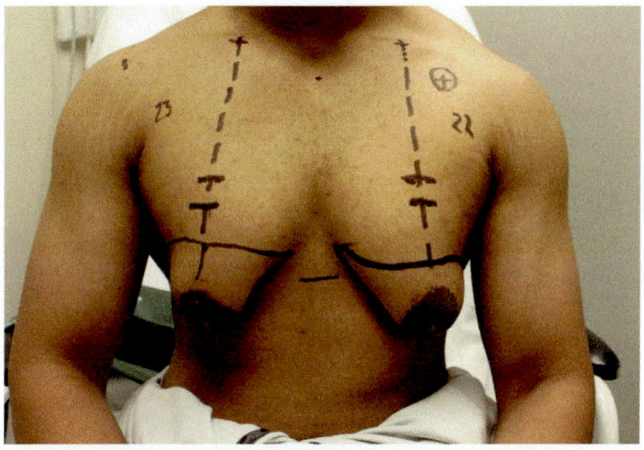

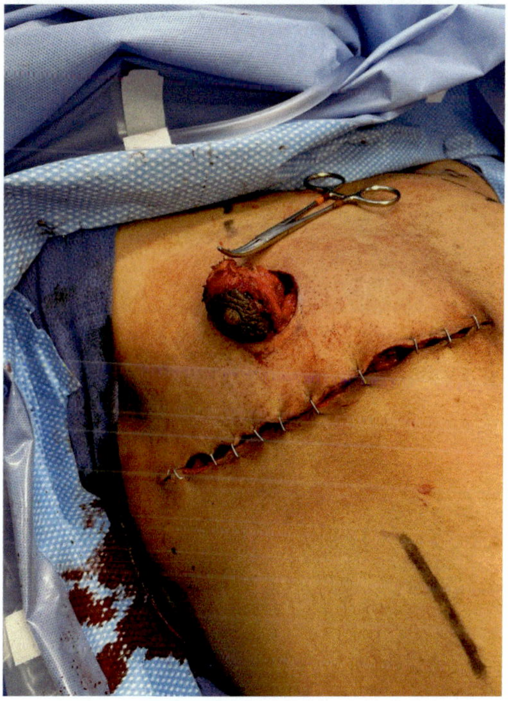

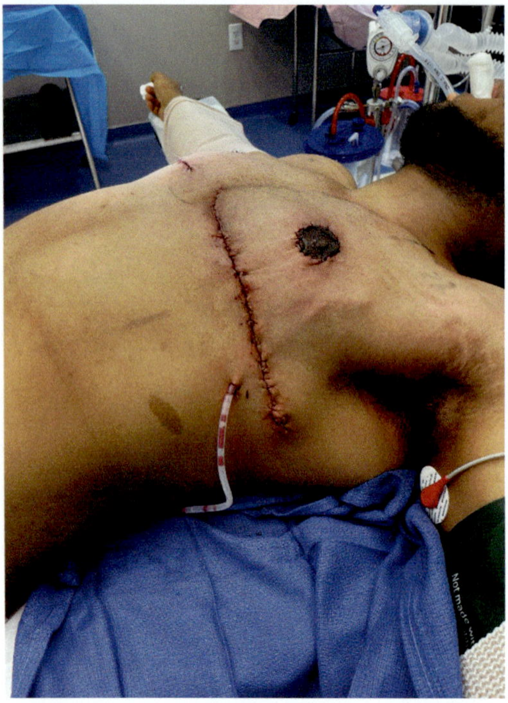

Postop 1 week

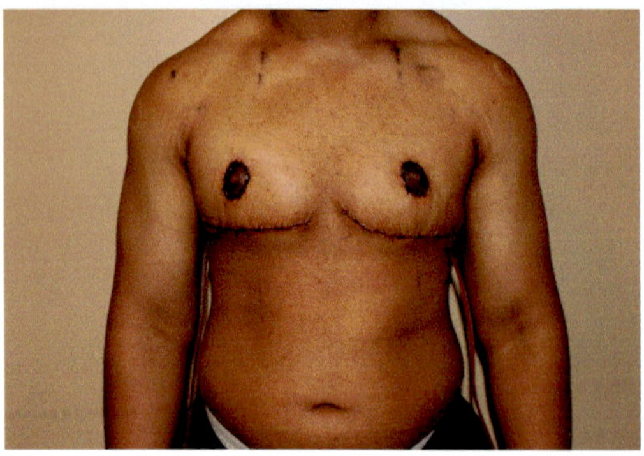

References

1. Nuttall FQ. Gynecomastia as a physical finding in normal men. J Clin Endocrinol Metab. 1979;48(2):338–40. https://doi.org/10.1210/jcem-48-2-338.
2. Carlson HE. Gynecomastia. N Engl J Med. 1980;303(14):795–9. https://doi.org/10.1056/NEJM198010023031405. https://doi.org/10.1210/jcem-48-2-338.
3. Williams MJ. Gynecomastia: its incidence, recognition and host characterization in 447 autopsy cases. Am J Med. 1963;34:103–12.
4. Nydick M, Bustos J, Dale JH Jr, Rawson RW. Gynecomastia in adolescent boys. JAMA. 1961;178:449–54.
5. Rubens R, Dhont M, Vermeulen A. Further studies on Leydig cell function in old age. J Clin Endocrinol Metab. 1974;39:40–5.
6. Pitanguy I. Transareolar incision for gynecomastia. Plast Reconstr Surg. 1966;38(5):414–9.
7. Dufourmentel CI. L'incision aréolaire dans la chirurgie du sein. Bull Mem Soc Chir Paris. 1928;20:9–14.
8. Rohrich RJ, Ha RY, Kenkel JM, Adams WP. Classification and management of gynecomastia: defining the role of ultrasound-assisted liposuction. Plast Reconstr Surg. 2003;111(2):909–23; Discussion 924.
9. Waltho D, et al. Gynecomastia classification for surgical management: a systematic review and novel classification system. Plast Reconstr Surg. 2017;139(3): 638e-648e.
10. Innocenti A, et al. Management of gynecomastia of patients with different body types: Considerations in 312 consecutive treated cases. Ann Plast Surg. 2017; 78:492–6.

The Male Chest After Massive Weight Loss

25

Michael S. Hu, Jonathan Brower, Walter J. Joseph, and J. Peter Rubin

25.1 Introduction

Obesity is a global pandemic. Progressing unabated, 2.7 billion adults are projected to be overweight or obese by 2025 [1]. The negative sequelae of obesity are well known, but no country has yet reversed its obesity epidemic [2]. Bariatric surgery can produce remarkable and sustained weight loss, improving health and reducing mortality for patients with severe obesity [3, 4]. Consequently, the number of patients with a history of severe obesity and MWL has significantly increased. The resulting contour deformities and surplus skin cause both functional and aesthetic impairment [5]. Thus, patients frequently desire body contouring surgery after MWL [6]. Moreover, the number of cosmetic surgical procedures in men continues to increase, with surgery of the male chest among the top five most common procedures [7].

Massive weight loss is defined by a deliberate loss of 100 pounds or more to treat morbid obesity. Most commonly, MWL is a result of bariatric surgery, but it can also be achieved by diet and exercise alone. Patients who have undergone gastric bypass (GBP) in particular require special consideration due to surgical manipulation of the gastrointestinal tract, placing these patients at risk for metabolic complications. Distinguishing among these causes of MWL is important for patient selection and preoperative nutritional considerations [8].

M. S. Hu · J. Brower · W. J. Joseph
Pittsburgh, PA, USA

J. P. Rubin (✉)
Department of Plastic Surgery, University of Pittsburgh, Pittsburgh, PA, USA
e-mail: rubinjp@upmc.edu

25.1.1 Patient Selection

Careful consideration must be taken in patient selection for male chest surgery after MWL. Nutritional derangements—particularly after GBP—are common, psychosocial issues occur frequently, and sequelae of past and present medical problems can affect both surgical planning and outcomes [9]. On initial patient consultation, the surgeon should obtain the following information: weight loss method, bariatric procedure type/date, bariatric surgeon, maximum weight/body mass index (BMI), current weight/BMI, goal weight, and last appointment with bariatric surgeon/nutritionist [10, 11]. Weight fluctuations over 1- and 3-month intervals should be assessed to determine recent weight loss/gain and evaluate whether the patient has reached a plateau near his goal weight [12]. Constitutional symptoms, such as nausea, vomiting, constipation, or diarrhea, should be considered and may require follow-up with the bariatric surgeon [9]. A list of medications and nutritional supplements should be obtained. Protein intake

K. Jeffords et al. (eds.), *Aesthetic Surgery for Men*, https://doi.org/10.1007/978-3-032-03840-1_25

should be evaluated with a goal of 70–100 grams per day. Patients who have undergone GBP often have deficiencies of protein, iron, vitamin B12, folate, calcium, and fat-soluble vitamins (A, D, E, K) [13]. Utilization of an on-site or referred nutritionist may be useful to provide a detailed assessment and recommendations. Preoperative laboratory assessment should include metabolic and nutritional tests (e.g., hemoglobin, hematocrit, basic metabolic panel, albumin, prealbumin).

Body contouring surgery after MWL should be performed when weight is stable for at least 6 months and no sooner than 12 months following bariatric surgery [14]. BMI at the time of surgery has been shown to predict outcome, with lower values associated with better cosmetic results and higher values portending increased complications [8]. Other medical and psychosocial problems should be addressed prior to surgery with appropriate consultations as needed. Body dysmorphic disorder exists among MWL patients and must be identified and addressed. Smoking cessation for at least 1 month should be confirmed with urine cotinine testing, as possible, to prevent wound healing complications [15].

25.1.2 Managing Expectations

Management of expectations is essential for providing patient satisfaction. The patient will benefit from careful elucidation of these expectations in the initial consultation. As with all surgeries, patients should be counseled on the risks, benefits, and alternatives. Potential results and complications, such as wound healing issues, scarring (asymmetry, prominent, hypertrophic/keloid, etc.), seroma, and contour deformity, should be discussed. It is important to note that body contouring procedures can improve body image but produce dissatisfaction with new deformities not previously appreciated [16]. Lastly, informed consent should include a statement that no guarantees are made regarding outcomes of surgery. Adhering to these patient selection guidelines will optimize patient satisfaction.

25.2 Diagnosis

Pseudogynecomastia, the term used to describe the male chest after MWL, is characterized by an excess of redundant skin with increased subareolar fat, typically without enlargement of glandular breast tissue [17]. In contrast to asymptomatic gynecomastia, in which there is enlargement of glandular breast tissue, pseudogynecomastia lacks the firm mound of tissue under the nipple-areola complex (NAC) [18]. Our group developed a classification scheme to grade pseudogynecomastia as a means to standardize diagnosis and direct management. The grading system is based on the degree of ptosis, the presence of a lateral chest roll, and inframammary fold (IMF) stability/upper abdominal laxity (Table 25.1) [19].

Grade 1 pseudogynecomastia is defined as a minimal excess of skin and fat without alteration of the NAC. Grade 1 is further subdivided based on the absence (grade 1a) or presence (grade 1b) of lateral skin roll extension (Fig. 25.1). Grade 2 is defined by NAC and IMF below the ideal position of the IMF (the inferior border of the pectoralis major muscle), presence of lateral chest roll,

Table 25.1 Classification and treatment algorithm for pseudogynecomastica after massive weight loss

Grade	Description	Treatment
1	Minimal excess skin and fat, minimal alteration of NAC, normal IMF	
1a	No lateral skin roll	Liposuction[a]
1b	Lateral skin roll	Liposuction[a] and direct excision of roll
2	NAC and IMF below the ideal IMF[b], lateral chest roll, minimal upper abdominal laxity	Pedicled nipple reconstruction
3	NAC and IMF below the ideal IMF[b], lateral chest roll, significant upper abdominal laxity	Free-nipple graft reconstruction

NAC nipple-areola complex, *IMF* inframammary fold
Reprinted with permission from Gusenoff et al. [19]
[a]Ultrasonic liposuction was followed by suction-assisted lipectomy
[b]Ideal inframammary fold was defined as the inferior border of the pectoralis major

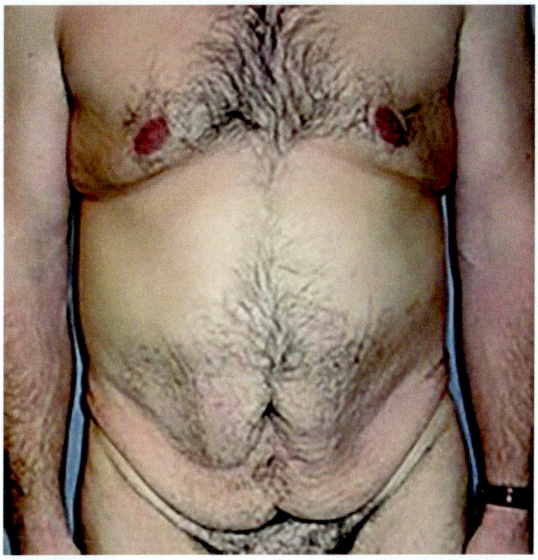

Fig. 25.1 Grade 1b pseudogynecomastia: minimally displaced NAC, normal IMF, and lateral chest skin roll. (Reprinted with permission from Gusenoff et al. [19])

and minimal upper abdominal laxity (Fig. 25.2). Grade 3 is defined as NAC and IMF below the ideal IMF, presence of lateral chest roll extension, and IMF instability/significant upper abdominal laxity (Fig. 25.3) [19].

25.2.1 Techniques

Treatment of pseudogynecomastia after MWL depends on grade (Table 25.1). Grade 1a is treated with liposuction. We recommend ultrasonic liposuction followed by suction-assisted lipectomy for these patients, who benefit from a minimally invasive procedure and maximal skin retraction. Secondary excision may be employed if results are inadequate. Grade 1b is similarly treated with ultrasonic liposuction with the addition of direct excision of the lateral chest roll. Any patient treated with liposuction as a primary

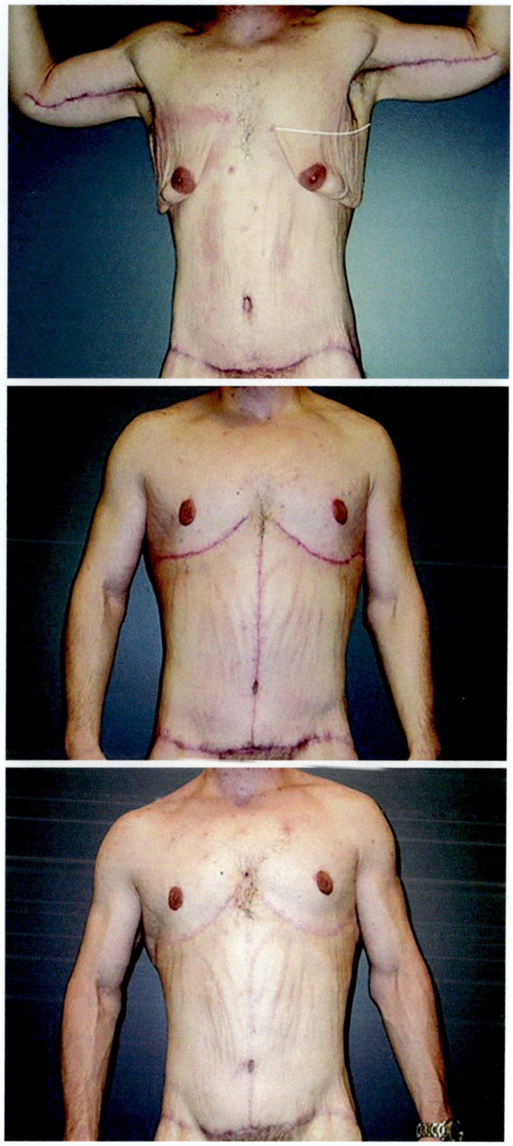

Fig. 25.2 Grade 2 pseudogynecomastia, characterized by NAC and IMF below ideal IMF, lateral chest skin rolls, and minimal abdominal laxity (**top**), treated with pedicled nipple reconstruction at 3- (**middle**) and 10-month (**bottom**) follow-up. (Reprinted with permission from Gusenoff et al. [19])

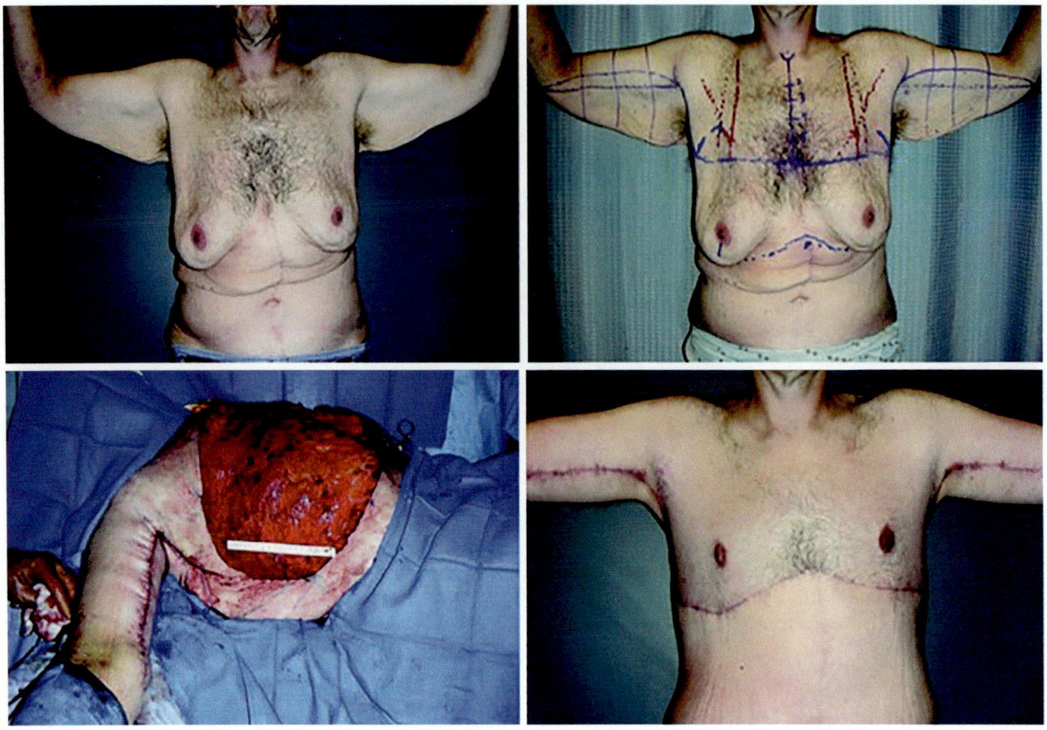

Fig. 25.3 Grade 3 pseudogynecomastia, defined by NAC and IMF below ideal IMF, lateral chest skin roll, and significant upper abdominal laxity (**top left**). Preoperative markings (**top right**) estimate new NAC above upper incision (**bottom left**). Appearance at 3-month follow-up (**bottom right**). (Reprinted with permission from Gusenoff et al. [19])

modality should be advised of the risk of loose skin and possible need for secondary excision.

Grade 2 pseudogynecomastia may be treated with either a nipple preservation technique (Fig. 25.2) or with free nipple grafting. Grade 3 deformities are best addressed with free nipple grafting (Fig. 25.3). In both techniques, preoperative markings begin with an elliptical excision of chest skin. To determine the superior edge of the resection, downward traction is manually applied to the chest skin. The skin is marked where the chest skin meets the location of the intended IMF scar. The inferior margin is determined by pinch test and extended as far laterally as necessary to include the lateral chest roll and provide the desired contour. If nipple preservation is planned, a broad-based dermal pedicle is fashioned extending from the IMF to the superior border of the NAC (Fig. 25.4) [19].

The anticipated new NAC position is marked on the patient preoperatively to involve him in decision making, though it is confirmed on the operating table once the resection is complete. Authors have proposed various anatomic landmarks for relocation of the medialized NAC characteristic of pseudogynecomastia [20]. We now prefer to center the nipple at the intersection of the lateral border of the pectoralis muscle and the fifth intercostal space. Additionally, we aim to leave 3–4 cm of skin between the inferior border of the NAC and the IMF scar. The new position is confirmed by visual inspection with the patient sitting upright on the operating table before any incisions are made, committing to the new location.

Perioperative antibiotics are administered, and spontaneous compression devices are applied prior to induction of general anesthesia. The

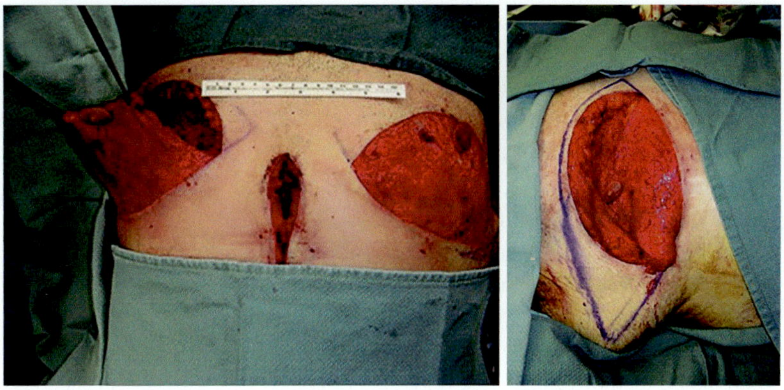

Fig. 25.4 Thinned dermoglandular pedicle (**left**) and area of excision extending to lateral skin roll (**right**). (Reprinted with permission from Gusenoff et al. [19])

patient is positioned supine on the operating table with the shoulders abducted 90 degrees. In the nipple preservation technique, the NAC is marked on the table to have a diameter of 2.8 cm before it is incised to the mid-dermis. The excess areola and skin within the area of the marked pedicle are de-epithelialized. The thin, broad-based dermoglandular pedicle (Fig. 25.4) is then raised as the mastectomy proceeds as usual. Superior undermining is carried as far as necessary to deliver the NAC to the determined new nipple position.

Closure is estimated with towel clips, and the superior wound edge is secured to the deep fascia as described by Lockwood [21]. The patient is positioned sitting on the operating table, and the position of the new NAC is confirmed before a 2 cm circle is marked at the site. We find the back of a 10-cc syringe plunger is a useful template for this marking. Incision is carried full thickness through the skin. Tension of the surrounding skin will stretch the 2 cm opening to approximately 2.5 cm in diameter, permitting delivery of the underlying NAC. A closed suction drain is placed before final skin closure is completed.

If the NAC is to be replaced as a graft, the operation begins with the same NAC marking 2.8 cm in diameter before it is sharply lifted as a graft. The mastectomy proceeds as usual with an elliptical resection. Drain placement and incision closure are completed as above before the patient is sat up on the operating table to confirm NAC position. A 2.8 cm circular marking is made centered at this position and de-epithelialized in preparation for placement of the nipple graft. The NAC graft is secured with a xeroform tie-over bolster.

25.2.2 Postoperative Dressings

Upon completion of surgery, closed chest incisions are covered with gauze fluff dressings and abdominal pads. Firm compression is applied with circumferential elastic wrap or compressive garment. Dressings are taken down for evaluation at postoperative check 4–6 h following surgery and daily beginning on postoperative day 1. Gentle compression of the chest is maintained, and physical activity is limited for 4–6 weeks.

25.3 Managing Complications

Common complications after body contouring surgery include wound dehiscence, seroma, tissue loss, infection, and hematoma. In particular, men who undergo body contouring surgery are at increased risk of hematoma and seroma formation [22]. Other postoperative issues include problems with scarring (asymmetry, prominent, hypertrophic/keloid, etc.) and contour deformities. Managing patient expectations prior to surgery can alleviate patient dissatisfaction postoperatively. Complications are typically amenable to outpatient management and rarely require return to the operating room for treatment.

25.4 Options

We describe the classification scheme and treatment protocol based on our patient series [19]. However, a modified treatment algorithm has been described, whereby grade 1a is treated with liposuction with NAC minimizing, grade 1b is treated with liposuction and NAC transposition with horizontal IMF scar run, and grades 2 and 3 are treated with modified mastectomy with free nipple transplantation [23]. Others have approached high-grade pseudogynecomastia with an inferior dermoglandular pedicle approach [24, 25]. Grade 2 pseudogynecomastia utilizing posterolateral torsoplasty with nipple translocation has been demonstrated to minimize visible scarring from the frontal view [26]. Aesthetically pleasing results have been obtained using obliquely oriented closures over the anterior chest [27], as well as boomerang pattern correction of pseudogynecomastia [28].

References

1. SwinburnB,DietzW,KleinertS.Alancetcommissionon obesity. Lancet (London, England) [Internet]. Lancet; 2015 [cited 2020 Apr 11];386. Available from: https://pubmed.ncbi.nlm.nih.gov/26545418/?from_single_result=26545418&expanded_search_query=26545418
2. Roberto CA, Swinburn B, Hawkes C, Huang TT-K, Costa SA, Ashe M, et al. Patchy progress on obesity prevention: emerging examples, entrenched barriers, and new thinking. Lancet (London, England) [Internet]. Lancet; 2015 [cited 2020 Apr 11];385:2400–9. Available from: http://www.ncbi.nlm.nih.gov/pubmed/25703111.
3. Chang S-H, Stoll CRT, Song J, Varela JE, Eagon CJ, Colditz GA. The effectiveness and risks of bariatric surgery: an updated systematic review and meta-analysis, 2003–2012. JAMA Surgery [Internet]. JAMA Surg; 2014 [cited 2020 Apr 11];149:275–87. Available from: http://www.ncbi.nlm.nih.gov/pubmed/24352617.
4. Bray GA, Frühbeck G, Ryan DH, Wilding JPH. Management of obesity. Lancet (London, England) [Internet]. Lancet; 2016 [cited 2020 Apr 11];387:1947–56. Available from: http://www.ncbi.nlm.nih.gov/pubmed/26868660.
5. Song AY, Jean RD, Hurwitz DJ, Fernstrom MH, Scott JA, Rubin JP A classification of contour deformities after bariatric weight loss: the Pittsburgh rating scale. Plastic and Reconstructive Surgery [internet]. Plast Reconstr Surg; 2005 [cited 2020 Apr 11];116. Available from: https://pubmed.ncbi.nlm.nih.gov/16217505/?from_term=A+Classification+of+Contour+Deformities+after+Bariatric+Weight+Loss%3A+The+Pittsburgh+Rating+Scale
6. Kitzinger HB, Abayev S, Pittermann A, Karle B, Bohdjalian A, Langer FB, et al. After massive weight loss: patients' expectations of body contouring surgery. Obesity Surgery [Internet]. Obes Surg; 2012 [cited 2020 Apr 11];22:544–8. Available from: http://www.ncbi.nlm.nih.gov/pubmed/22101887.
7. American Society of Plastic Surgeons (ASPS). 2018 Plastic Surgery Statistics Report.
8. Gusenoff JA, Rubin JP. Plastic surgery after weight loss: current concepts in massive weight loss surgery. Aesthetic Surgery journal [Internet]. Aesthet Surg J; 2008 [cited 2020 Apr 11];28:452–5. Available from: http://www.ncbi.nlm.nih.gov/pubmed/19083561.
9. Naghshineh N, Rubin JP. Preoperative evaluation of the body contouring patient: the cornerstone of patient safety. Clinics in Plastic Surgery [Internet]. Clin Plast Surg; 2014 [cited 2020 Apr 11];41:637–43. Available from: http://www.ncbi.nlm.nih.gov/pubmed/25283451.
10. Bossert RP, Rubin JP. Evaluation of the weight loss patient presenting for plastic surgery consultation. Plastic and Reconstructive Surgery [Internet]. 2012 [cited 2020 Apr 11];130:1361–9. Available from: http://content.wkhealth.com/linkback/openurl?sid=WKPTLP:landingpage&an=00006534-201212000-00034
11. O'Toole J, Rubin J. Evaluation of the massive weight loss patient who presents for body-contouring surgery. In: Rubin J, Matarasso A, editors. Aesthetic surgery after massive weight loss. New York: Elsevier Health Sciences; 2008. p. 13–20.
12. Rubin JP, Nguyen V, Schwentker A. Perioperative management of the post-gastric-bypass patient presenting for body contour surgery. Clinics in Plastic Surgery [Internet]. Clin Plast Surg; 2004 [cited 2020 Apr 11];31:601–10, vi. Available from: http://www.ncbi.nlm.nih.gov/pubmed/15363913.
13. Bloomberg RD, Fleishman A, Nalle JE, Herron DM, Kini S. Nutritional deficiencies following bariatric surgery: what have we learned? Obesity Surgery [Internet]. Obes Surg; 2005 [cited 2020 Apr 11];15. Available from: https://pubmed.ncbi.nlm.nih.gov/15802055/?from_single_result=15802055&expanded_search_query=15802055
14. Amy S Colwell. Current concepts in post-bariatric body contouring. Obesity Surgery [Internet]. Obes Surg; 2010 [cited 2020 Apr 16];20. Available from: https://pubmed.ncbi.nlm.nih.gov/20349284/?from_term=Current+concepts+in+post-bariatric+body+contouring
15. Gravante G, Araco A, Sorge R, Araco F, Delogu D, Cervelli V. Wound infections in post-bariatric patients undergoing body contouring abdominoplasty: the role of smoking. Obesity Surgery [Internet]. Obes Surg;

2007 [cited 2020 Apr 11];17:1325–31. Available from: http://www.ncbi.nlm.nih.gov/pubmed/18000726.

16. Song AY, Rubin JP, Thomas V, Dudas JR, Marra KG, Fernstrom MH. Body image and quality of life in post massive weight loss body contouring patients. Obesity (Silver Spring, Md) [Internet]. Obesity (Silver Spring); 2006 [cited 2020 Apr 11];14:1626–36. Available from: http://www.ncbi.nlm.nih.gov/pubmed/17030974.
17. Waltho D, Hatchell A, Thoma A. Gynecomastia classification for surgical management. Plast Reconstr Surg [Internet]. 2017 [cited 2020 Apr 11];139:638e–48e. Available from: http://journals.lww.com/00006534-201703000-00019
18. Braunstein GD. Gynecomastia. The New England Journal of Medicine [Internet]. N Engl J Med; 1993 [cited 2020 Apr 11];328. Available from: https://pubmed.ncbi.nlm.nih.gov/8421478/?from_single_result=8421478&expanded_search_query=8421478
19. Gusenoff JA, Coon D, Rubin JP. Pseudogynecomastia after massive weight loss: detectability of technique, patient satisfaction, and classification. Plast Reconstr Surg [Internet]. 2008 [cited 2020 Apr 11];122:1301–11. Available from: http://www.ncbi.nlm.nih.gov/pubmed/18971712.
20. Beer GM, Budi S, Seifert B, Morgenthaler W, Infanger M, Meyer VE. Configuration and localization of the nipple-areola complex in men. Plastic and Reconstructive Surgery [Internet]. Plast Reconstr Surg; 2001 [cited 2020 Apr 11];108:1947–52; discussion 1953. Available from: http://www.ncbi.nlm.nih.gov/pubmed/11743381.
21. Lockwood T. Reduction mammaplasty and mastopexy with superficial fascial system suspension. Plastic and Reconstructive Surgery [Internet]. Plast Reconstr Surg; 1999 [cited 2020 Apr 11];103:1411–20. Available from: http://www.ncbi.nlm.nih.gov/pubmed/10190437
22. Chong T, Coon D, Toy J, Purnell C, Michaels J, Rubin JP. Body contouring in the male weight loss population: assessing gender as a factor in outcomes. Plastic and Reconstructive Surgery [Internet]. Plast Reconstr Surg; 2012 [cited 2020 Apr 11];130:325e–30e. Available from: http://www.ncbi.nlm.nih.gov/pubmed/22495205.
23. Ziegler UE, Lorenz U, Daigeler A, Ziegler SN, Zeplin PH. Modified treatment algorithm for pseudogynecomastia after massive weight loss. Annals of Plastic Surgery [Internet]. Ann Plast Surg; 2018 [cited 2020 Apr 11];81:290–4. Available from: http://www.ncbi.nlm.nih.gov/pubmed/29916894.
24. Murat Diyarbakirlioglu, Alp Ercan, Yunus Dogan. Correction of high-grade pseudogynecomastia after massive weight loss: modified inferior dermoglandular pedicled transverse scar reduction. Aesthetic Plastic Surgery [internet]. Aesth Plast Surg; 2020 [cited 2020 Apr 11];44. Available from: https://pubmed.ncbi.nlm.nih.gov/31451852/?from_term=Correction+of+High-Grade+Pseudogynecomastia+After+Massive+Weight+Loss%3A+Modified+Inferior+Dermoglandular+Pedicled+Transverse+Scar+Reduction&from_pos=2
25. Brower JP, Rubin JP. Invited discussion on: correction of high-grade pseudogynecomastia after massive weight loss: modified inferior dermoglandular pedicled transverse scar reduction. Aesthetic Plastic Surgery [Internet]. Aesthetic Plast Surg; 2020 [cited 2020 Apr 11];44:442–4. Available from: http://www.ncbi.nlm.nih.gov/pubmed/31834521.
26. Atiyeh BS, Dibo SA, Hayek SN. Contouring of the male anterior chest following bariatric surgery and massive weight loss. Aesthetic Surgery Journal [Internet]. Aesthet Surg J; 2008 [cited 2020 Apr 11];28:688–96. Available from: http://www.ncbi.nlm nih.gov/pubmed/19083600.
27. Letterman G, Schurter M. Surgical correction of massive gynecomastia. Plastic and Reconstructive Surgery [Internet]. Plast Reconstr Surg; 1972 [cited 2020 Apr 11];49:259–62. Available from: http://www.ncbi.nlm.nih.gov/pubmed/5060315.
28. Hurwitz D. Enhancing masculine features after massive weight loss. Aesthetic Plastic Surgery [Internet]. Aesthetic Plast Surg; 2016 [cited 2020 Apr 11];40:245–55. Available from: http://www.ncbi.nlm.nih.gov/pubmed/26893282.

26 Medium Definition Abdominal Etching: Looking Natural

Giuliano Borille

Improvement of abdominal muscle details is noticeable at 10–15% of Body Fat Index (BFI) in individuals under intense exercise (muscular hypertrophy) and a strict dieting routine. Even so, most people will never achieve that much muscular definition.

The concept of Medium Definition Abdominal Etching is to achieve a fit and natural look in select patients with a committed and consistent exercise routine. The thing is not to look like an athlete, but rather, to create an athletic aesthetic in patients who lack abdominal definition even following a regular exercise routine.

Medium Definition Liposuction is an alternative liposuction technique that prevents the eventual stigmata of the current procedure of High Definition liposuction. It's not about shaping the six packs in the subcutaneous fat, a superficial, artificial, and non-pre-existing anatomy.

Medium Definition liposuction uncovers the abdominal musculature outlines by showing and enhancing the deep anatomy and muscular topography [1].

G. Borille (✉)
Clinica Borille, Porto Alegre, RS, Brazil

26.1 Patient Selection

The main limitation of the Medium Definition technique is patient selection. The ideal patient should follow a consistent workout program and a dieting routine. The patient has to have an overall athletic look, even though he does not look ripped or shredded.

The best overall patient, in my opinion, would benefit from a holistic approach with proportionality of their abdomen in relation to their whole body.

26.2 Anatomic Criteria

1. No saggy skin.
2. Abdominal muscle hypertrophy, but not necessarily any visible outline of the muscles (intersections should be palpable).
3. Limited areas in Patients up to approximately 15% overall Body Fat Index.

26.3 Technique

26.3.1 Skin Markings

Skin markings are guided by palpation of muscular tendinous intersections—the rectus abdominis muscle, linea alba, and linea semi-lunaris. The patient's individual and singular anatomy

K. Jeffords et al. (eds.), *Aesthetic Surgery for Men*, https://doi.org/10.1007/978-3-032-03840-1_26

must be taken into account, because there are several different tendinous intersections between the abdominal muscles among patients. That is fundamental to prevent an artificial disconnection between the subcutaneous etched shape and the muscle layer in the deeper plane [1, 2]. Any artificial disconnection between the skin and the abdominal muscle can potentially be seen during a sit-up, rising from a chair to standing, or other torso movements (Fig. 26.1).

26.3.2 Pre-liposuction Subcutaneous Solution Infiltration

Usually, we perform liposuction under general or regional anesthesia. In both situations, we infiltrate less volume than in the regular wet or tumescent liposuction approach. This way we can prevent distortions, intense postoperative swelling, and still manage bleeding. 250 cc tumescent solution, 1–250,000 (0.9% concentration of 250 cc saline + adrenaline/epinephrine, 0.5 cc) is usually enough to reach adequate and well-controlled vasoconstriction in the average procedure for the abdomen.

Whenever under general anesthesia, we add 20 cc of ropivacaine 7.5 mg and 40 cc of lidocaine 20 mg to the tumescent solution for post-surgery pain control.

26.3.3 Access Site for Liposuction

In order to get the right angle, safely access all the subcutaneous fat layers, and avoid symmetrical and visible access sites, we use a liposuction cannula access site systematic plan (guided by the skin marks) (Fig. 26.2).

26.3.4 Cannulas

There is no need for a VASER or LASER approach. We only use 3, in-line, perforated cannulas (3 mm, 3.5 mm, 4 mm caliber) to perform the liposuction according to the location of the superficial abdominal fat levels (Fig. 26.3).

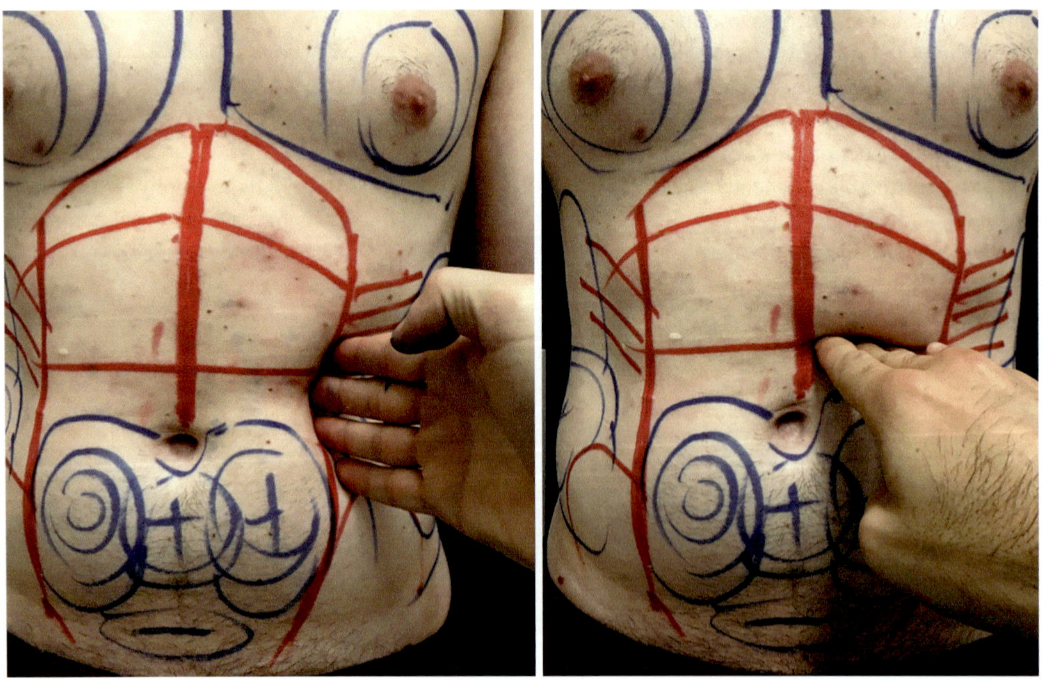

Fig. 26.1 Skin markings based on muscle intersections

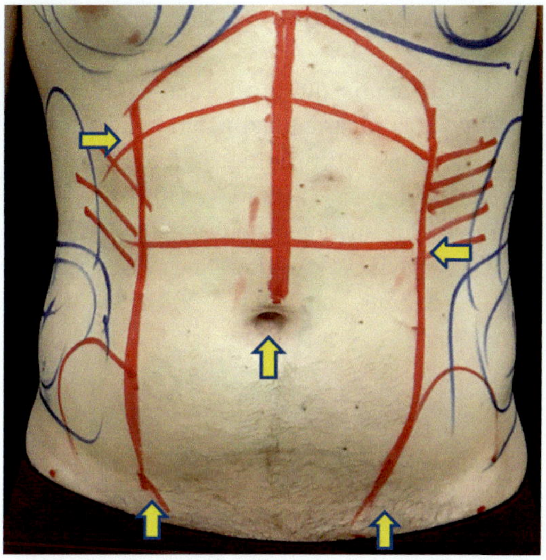

Fig. 26.2 Liposuction access sites

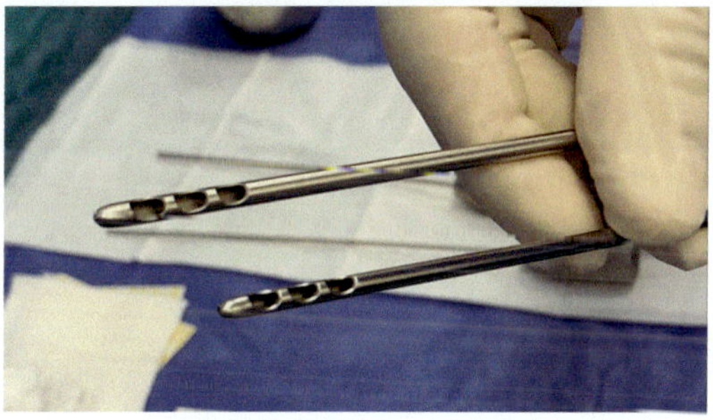

Fig. 26.3 Liposuction cannulas (3 and 3.5 mm)

26.3.5 3D Sculpting

The abdominal musculature is topographically visualized according to the skin markings guided by the palpation of the linea alba, linea semilunaris, and the tendinous intersections of rectus abdominis muscle. These landmarks are enhanced with localized superficial liposuction to deepen the natural grooves or furrows, creating curves, light, and shadow effects on the skin [3, 4].

We start debulking the deep layers with 4 mm cannulas and continue to the mid-lamellar layer and between muscle groups with 3.5 mm cannulas.

Superficial liposuction, in the muscle outline áreas, is performed to define the relevant anatomy for the muscle groups in each treatment area by using a 3 mm cannula.

To induce extra skin tightening at intersection areas, we do a subdermal pass with the cannula with the cannula holes facing up towards the skin.

It's important to create a delicate transition zone between the abdominal muscular intersections to define the superficial anatomy landmarks, smoothing the surfaces and eventual sharp edges. At this time, we can remove some of the remaining fat over the muscles to finish the transition between the muscles with a 3.5 mm cannula [5–7].

26.3.6 Handcrafted Abdominal Pads

The key step to creating Medium Definition abdominal muscle outlines is the proper use of localized and continuous compression, mainly in the transition zones between individual abdominal groups. This way, we can create a guided and well-controlled fibrosis in specific, predetermined areas.

Generally, the more local compression is made, the deeper the outline of the abdominal muscle and the more etched the área will be long term. Customized hand crafted cotton and gauze pads are used to produce diverse pressure points. These handcrafted pads create the desired shape of the abdominal muscles (Fig. 26.4). These pads should be used for at least 1 month (Fig. 26.5).

These pads are positioned at the end of the surgery, covered by a semi-rigid cardboard plaque placed over the anterior abdomen and a compression garment (Fig. 26.5).

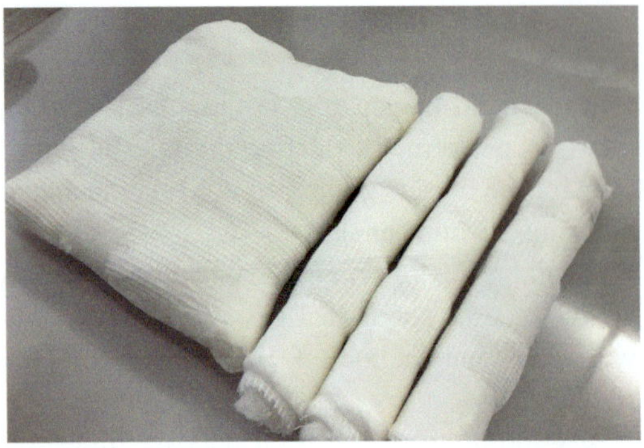

Fig. 26.4 Gauze and cotton customized handcrafted pads

26.4 Advantages

This approach is quite safe and reproducible, resulting in a pleasant and natural athletic look, with low risk of distortions, retractions, and undesirable fibrosis (Fig. 26.6). This method uses traditional liposuction cannulas without the need for such devices as Laser and Vaser devices [8–10]. Drains are not needed with this technique.

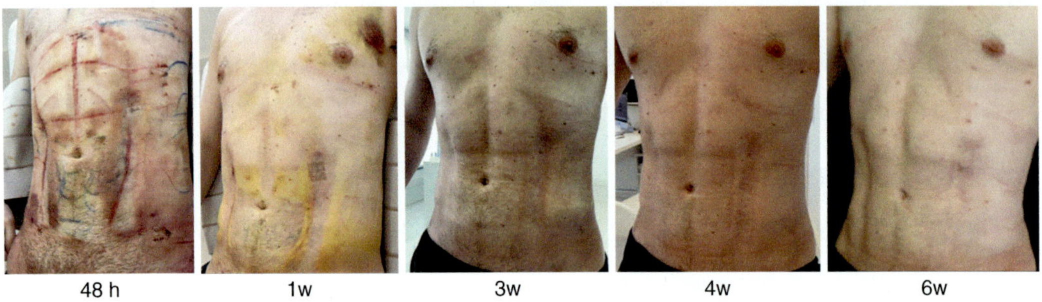

Fig. 26.5 Evolution during the abdominal pads utilization (48 h to 6 weeks)

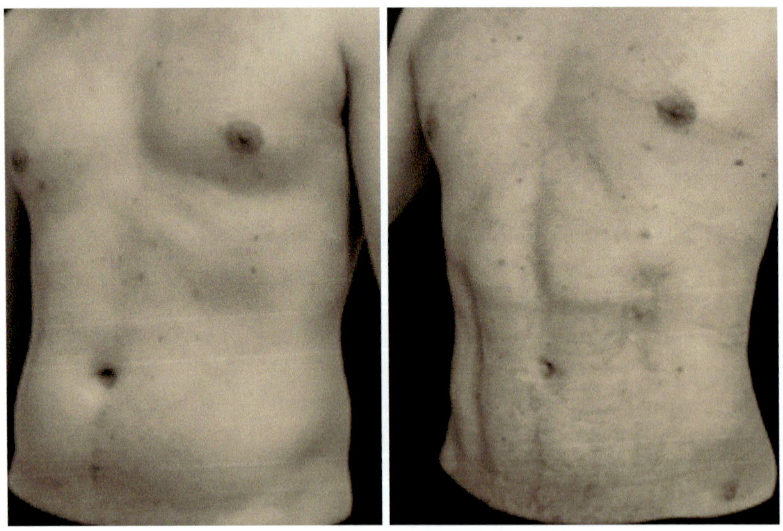

Fig. 26.6 Pre and post op (8 weeks)

References

1. Hoyos A, Perez ME, Guarin DE, Montenegro A. A report of 736 high-definition lipoabdominoplasties performed in conjunction with circumferential VASER liposuction. Plast Reconstr Surg. 2018;142(3):662–75.
2. Danilla S. Rectus abdominis fat transfer (RAFT) in lipoabdominoplasty: a new technique to achieve fitness body contour in patients that require tummy tuck. Aesth Plast Surg. 2017;41(6):1389–99.
3. Hoyos AE, Perez ME, Castillo L. Dynamic definition mini-lipoabdominoplasty combining multilayer liposculpture, fat grafting, and muscular plication. Aesthet Surg J. 2013;33(4):545–60.
4. Zhang YX, Lazzeri D, Grassetti L, Silvestri A, Trisliana Perdanasari A, Han S, Torresetti M, di Benedetto G, Castello MF. Three-dimensional superficial liposculpture of the hips, flank, and thighs. Plast Reconstr Surg Glob Open. 2015;3(1):e291.
5. Mentz HA 3rd, Gilliland MD, Patronella CK. Abdominal etching: differential liposuction to detail abdominal musculature. Aesth Plast Surg. 1993;17(4):287–90.
6. Ersek RA, Salisbury AV. Abdominal etching. Aesth Plast Surg. 1997;21(5):328–31.
7. Singh B, Keaney T, Rossi AM. Male body contouring. J Drugs Dermatol. 2015;14(9):1052–9.
8. Hoyos AE, Millard JA. VASER-assisted high-definition liposculpture. Aesthet Surg J. 2007;27(6):594–604.
9. Nagy MW, Vanek PF Jr. A multicenter, prospective, randomized, single-blind, controlled clinical trial comparing VASER-assisted Lipoplasty and suction-assisted Lipoplasty. Plast Reconstr Surg. 2012;129(4):681.
10. de Souza Pinto EB, Abdala PC, Maciel CM, dos Santos FP, de Souza RP. Liposuction and VASER. Clin Plast Surg. 2006;33(1):107–15.

27 High Definition Liposuction: Tumescent Technique

David Mattos and Daniel Del Vecchio

27.1 Introduction

27.1.1 History

Liposuction is a widespread procedure undergone by nearly 250,000 US patients in 2017 [1]. It is more common in women, but as the stigma of undergoing plastic surgery continues to diminish in men, men are increasingly likely to consider surgery. A survey in 2007 showed that 17% of men think they may be interested in cosmetic surgery in the future, and 14% are currently interested in liposuction, with or without an additional procedure [2]. This compares to 23% and 33% in women, respectively. High Definition Liposuction (HDL), which accentuates the male muscular anatomy and form, is not a new piece of technology, but a concept of creating irregularities in the subcutaneous fat that create an illusion of aesthetically pleasing muscular definition. In studies, evolutionary biologists have found that secondary sexual characteristics, such as muscular form, can act as cues for offspring viability and reproductive success [3]. Along similar lines, studies show that women rate muscular men as sexier and more dominant, which is part of the fitness indicator hypothesis [4]. For these reasons, HDL has the potential to increase in popularity in the years to come, and understanding how we got here and how to deliver successful outcomes will be crucial for any plastic surgeon interested in taking care of this patient population.

Liposuction, also known as suction-assisted lipectomy or lipoplasty, was popularized by Ives-Gerard Illouz in Paris in the early 1980s [5]. He originally called the technique lipolysis aspiration and used it to treat lipodystrophies throughout the body. His technique was based on four premises: (1) Each person has a fixed number of adipocytes, (2) Lipodystrophy can be hereditary, (3) Localized lipodystrophy remains after dieting, and (4) Lipodystrophy is affected by dietary habits, hormones, genes, and body type. His pioneering technique used a slightly hypotonic solution containing hyaluronidase, which he infiltrated into the tissues to facilitate the aspiration of fat. Early adopters of the technique were appropriately focused on patient safety, minimizing blood loss, and preventing irregularities. The cannulas were large, up to 1 cm in diameter, and required focusing on patients with deep fat layers, where early instrumentation could still produce an improved appearance. As such, further pivotal advances were necessary before HDL could be conceived.

The following decades led to refinements in liposuction that moved away from its usual constraints and better defined its safety thresholds.

D. Mattos
Massachusetts General Hospital, Boston, MA, USA

D. Del Vecchio (✉)
Back Bay Plastic Surgery, Boston, MA, USA

K. Jeffords et al. (eds.), *Aesthetic Surgery for Men*, https://doi.org/10.1007/978-3-032-03840-1_27

Pivotal to these changes were the studies by Jeffrey Klein in 1987 and 1990, where he first described his tumescent technique using large volumes of fluid with dilute lidocaine and epinephrine, and then further set a safe threshold of lidocaine in this solution to be 35 mg/kg [6, 7]. In further study, almost a decade later, data suggested 55 mg/kg to also be safe, but the American Society of Plastic Surgeons (ASPS) recommends 35 mg/kg as the limit [8]. This development overcame limitations originally set by prior infiltrative local anesthesia techniques. It made liposuction easier, helped prevent contour irregularities, and minimized blood loss significantly. The years following witnessed a rapid development of techniques. While early liposuction was limited to the deep layer of fat for safety and prevention of irregularities, multiple surgeons in the early 1990s began experimenting with superficial (also referred to as subdermal) liposuction, including Gasparotti, Gasperoni, and Souza Pinto [9–11]. Different cannulas were developed during that time to facilitate liposuction. Typically, smaller cannulas were used for more superficial layers of fat. Although superficial liposuction increased the risk of contour irregularities, early adopters noted its increased ability to cause skin contraction over the treated region, allowing some areas to be treated with liposuction alone that would have previously also required a surgical excision. For example, in 1997, Mark Gilliland noted he was able to treat upper arms with circumferential superficial liposuction alone using the tumescent technique that previously would have also required a brachioplasty. Other advances in superficial liposuction included abdominal etching, first described by Mentz in 1993, and then by Ersek in 1997, where the abdomen underwent liposuction to differing degrees throughout to better detail the abdominal musculature underneath [12, 13]. Mentz would also go on to describe his pectoral etching technique in men using similar concepts [14].

The following decade saw the advent of Power-Assisted Liposuction (PAL), Ultrasound-Assisted Liposuction (UAL), and VASER (vibration amplification of sound energy at resonance) Liposuction techniques as ways to remove tissue less traumatically and without as much force. UAL technology caused lipolysis to produce a fat emulsion that could be more easily aspirated with a cannula [15, 16]. Unfortunately, the energy generated sometimes burned the skin. VASER technology, first reported by Jewell in 2002, used a pulsed, low-power ultrasound that only applied about a quarter of the energy typically applied by UAL [17]. This lower energy application, combined with its ability to treat fibrous areas of the body, such as the trunk and back, to facilitate aspiration, made it a promising tool to treat superficial fat. More selective areas of fat were now being treated as a result of these advancements.

27.1.2 High Definition Liposuction

HDL was first presented in Colombia by Alfredo Hoyos in 2003, with the first publication describing his technique being published in 2007 [18, 19]. As Hoyos described, HDL combines the study of art and anatomy to perform, as an "artistic treatment of the human form to create not only a slim figure, but also the appearance of a highly developed musculature" [19]. The technique requires greater attention to detail and is more time consuming, as superficial fat removal requires an additional step over the traditional deep layer of fat removal. More importantly, fat has to be removed very selectively, from both layers, to create a natural 3D result that accentuates the muscular anatomy underneath. In the past, we were only able to focus on feathering techniques to keep an even layer of thickness in all of the areas treated. This method stymied our ability to emphasize the muscular form underneath. HDL focuses on understanding how the manipulation of subcutaneous layer thickness, both acutely and gradually throughout the body, can naturally enhance the muscular form underneath. It requires a thorough appreciation of the underlying muscles and their attachments. HDL creates irregularities and depressions that are beautiful through acute planar changes along curves, such as the tendinous intersections and the semilunar lines of the abdomen. These planar changes can be achieved by selectively removing fat in one area or, conversely, inserting fat in another. In males, these procedures can be especially useful along the chest, abdomen, back, and upper arms.

27.1.3 Patient Selection

To some degree, the concept of HDL can be applied to every patient that is a liposuction candidate. The most important aspect of the preoperative visit is the surgeon and patient interaction, as it is critical to fully understand the patient's goals and expectations. Then, after an assessment of body type and skin quality, one can have a frank discussion with the patient about whether his goals and expectations can be met. Just as the male facelift is a very different operation from the female facelift, HDL in men is also very different than it is in women. It requires more fat removal and muscular definition than in women, and less fat transfer. The first important step is selecting healthy patients who can safely undergo this procedure. This procedure should be avoided in patients with significant medical comorbidities or abdominal procedures and hernias that may increase the risk of injury to the abdominal wall or viscera. Caution should be taken with smokers, as superficial liposuction increases the risk of ischemia to the skin. Perhaps most importantly, patients chosen for the procedure should have good skin quality and tone to allow redraping and contraction of the skin to the underlying anatomy.

There are three broad patient presentations that are amenable to improvement. They range from the muscular to the slightly overweight man (BMI < 30). First, a muscular patient with normal BMI may have difficulty defining a particular aspect of his body, such as the abdominal wall muscles, despite diet and exercise. Second, a normal weight male without easily visible muscular tone may benefit from HDL to seek more tone and muscular definition, though his result will not be as defined on a muscular level as that of a patient who already has an athletic form preoperatively. Third, a slightly overweight male (BMI between 25 and 30) who may have one or more areas of his body that are more prominent and benefit from the reduction of lipodystrophy to give him the gradual curves of a normal weight male, perhaps with some mild muscular form. In effect, this last patient benefits more from debulking than from reshaping.

Patients who have had prior abdominoplasty or liposuction may fall into any of the categories above, and are perhaps the best patients, as they are often dissatisfied with their lack of definition, still have residual fat to remove, and can get amazing results. However, patients with moderate to severe skin laxity should be cautioned, because they will require staged procedures to address the contour and skin laxity, such as an abdominoplasty. For these patients, expectations must be set that the outcome cannot be satisfactorily achieved in one procedure, and should be staged with the liposuction first. This will both delay the abdominoplasty flap and allow aggressive liposuction that would not be safe to do at the time of abdominoplasty. Conversely, patients with none to mild skin laxity, especially in areas where there is superficial and circumferential liposuction, such as the upper arm or the abdomen and back, do not need a skin resection procedure.

27.2 Technique

27.2.1 Markings-Arms

The inferior edge of the deltoid muscle delineates the most prominent planar change of the arm, following the convexity created by the deltoid muscle itself [20]. The muscle inserts on the most lateral aspect of the arm when the arm is at the patient's side, and gradually curves up from there anteriorly and superiorly, and is most easily noted with the arms abducted 90 degrees and the elbows flexed 90 degrees. Anteriorly, this curve reaches the anterior axillary fold, where it ends underneath it, and posteriorly, it ends a couple of centimeters above the posterior axillary fold, as the long head of the triceps reaches more proximally in this region. Asking the patient to contract their muscle helps define these planar changes more easily. The biceps and triceps can be enhanced by marking the medial bicipital groove and the lateral intermuscular septum. Finally, the depression just distal to the deltoid between the long and lateral head, which is triangular with the point aiming proximally, is marked, and the distal posterior aspect of the arm over the triceps tendon is also marked for further thinning to enhance the insertion of the muscle. Typically, most of the fat for deep extraction lies posteriorly in the arm, assessed with a pinch test.

27.2.2 Markings-Chest

Start anteriorly with the pectoralis major and mark the patient standing and with his arms adducted [21]. Mark areas with deep fat, such as around the areola in patients with gynecomastia. Depressions can be noted to treat with fat grafting. Have the patient push down with one arm on a table or your shoulder to contract the latissimus. The anterior edge of the latissimus in the posterior chest can be palpated and marked, as can the serratus anterior. Next, delineate the curve where acute planar changes need to be defined: the inferior and lateral edges of the pectoralis. For this portion, it is especially important to have the arms at the patient's side. Then mark areas that need further liposuction to highlight the pectoralis prominence. These are (1) the superolateral portion of pectoralis, limited by the clavicle, (2) the area between the inferomedial attachments of the pectoralis major muscles, and limited by the rectus abdominus inferiorly, (3) the triangle between the lateal pectoral edge, the latissimus, and the costal margin, and (4) the small area just lateral to the semilunar line and medial to the triangle over serratus.

27.2.3 Markings-Abdomen

Delineate the areas where there is excessive fat that would benefit from traditional liposuction, typically in the lower abdominal region and flanks [22]. Carefully mark the curves and areas where acute planar changes need to be made for added definition: areas that will get superficial liposuction. Ask the patient to hold an inspiration to define the costal margin. Have the patient contract abdominal muscles and mark out the semilunar lines bilaterally. If the patient is thin enough to feel the horizontal tendinous intersections during muscle contraction, mark them also. Next, mark the borders of the external oblique. In patients with higher BMI, whose rectus abdominis muscles are harder to define, have the patient do an abdominal crunch and elevate the legs off the table to further contract the rectus and improve palpability. Any areas between the excessive fat and the superficial areas of liposuction should be treated as transition zones.

27.2.4 Markings-Back

These markings are a continuation of the abdominal markings [23]. Start by marking out areas that have lipodystrophy and need additional deep extraction to even the overlying skin contour. Then mark out the regions of deep and added superficial liposuction. From the midline of the back, focused on the lower back, a line is drawn from the midline that curves gently out superiorly, and ultimately follows the anterior edge of the latissimus muscle as it continues into the external oblique zone anteriorly, both along the superior margin and the inferior margin of the external oblique zone. Focus on the two most important areas of acute planar changes in the back. First is the triangle delineated by the beginning of the intergluteal cleft inferiorly (where the gluteus maximus muscles first almost come together) and the two posterior superior iliac spines (PSIS) points superiorly. The second area of the triangle is bordered by the paraspinous muscle medially, the edge of the latissimus dorsi laterally, and the inferior costal margin superiorly. The bottom of the triangle comes to the point at approximately the PSIS. These latter two triangles will require both deep and superficial liposuction, as they form the indentations necessary to emphasize the shape of the back. Finally, the paralumbar lines and median line are marked for superficial definition.

27.2.5 Anesthesia

This technique can be done with tumescent anesthesia and sedation or general anesthesia, and the anesthesia chosen largely depends on the patient and the area to be treated. In order for tumescent anesthesia with sedation to be effective, the tumescent must be infiltrated slowly and given enough time for its anesthetic effect to take hold. Smaller areas, such as the arms, could potentially be done under tumescent local anesthesia alone, similar to the technique described for autologous fat transfer to the buttocks [24]. One potential benefit of doing cases under tumescent local anesthesia, when the patient can tolerate it, is that the awake patient himself acts as a physiologic monitor and should respond to painful stimuli if the cannula hits the muscle layer, protecting the surgeon from surgical misadventure.

27.2.6 Incision Placement

Incision placement for men is particularly important, as they are typically more conscious of hiding any evidence of surgery. Incisions must balance the surgeon's need to perform the procedure effectively with the goal of hiding the scars successfully, such as in areas covered by underwear, as some patients will avoid showing off their results if any scars are visible. To minimize incisions, use of long 5 mm × 50 cm liposuction cannulas is essential to reach more areas from each incision.

In the anterior torso, incisions can be placed in the areolas, pubis, umbilicus, and anterior axillary fold. For the creation of horizontal tendinous intersections, asymmetric incisions may be placed along the abdomen that can be more easily camouflaged into its surroundings [25]. However, using curved cannulas, one should be able to access the horizontal tendinous intersections using a combination of the pubic, umbilical, and areolar incisions. The areolar incisions provide access to the pectoral region, flanks, upper abdomen, and axillary region. The pubis region should have two incisions, both placed within the hair-bearing region, and ideally at the level of the semilunar lines. These provide access to most of the abdomen. The umbilical incision can be hidden well and give access to the linea alba superiorly, as well as the upper half of the abdomen. Finally, the anterior axillary incisions provide access to the arm, pectoral region, and lateral chest. In addition, focused liposuction of the arms also requires incisions in the posterior axillary fold and at the elbow near the olecranon. The back also benefits from the posterior axillary fold incisions, but requires a cannula long enough to reach the lower aspects of the back needed for contouring. Additionally, an intergluteal cleft incision is done for patients undergoing HDL of the back. This incision should be placed at the highest point possible in the midline that can be hidden by the buttocks, and high enough to make sure you can reach over the buttocks and to the side of the body from the incision. For patients undergoing liposuction or fat grafting from this incision, it is beneficial from an infectious standpoint to cover the anus with a betadine-soaked gauze, which should be sutured in place around the anus with a nylon running suture to prevent contamination. Gloves should be changed, and the needle driver should be set aside.

27.2.7 Tumescent

Simultaneous separation and tumescence (SST) is used for infiltration of tumescence in the desired areas efficiently. This technique involves the use of a basket tip, or "exploded tip" cannula, to tumesce and separate, or mechanically emulsify, the fat [26]. The basket cannula is 4 mm in diameter, 30 cm long. Tumescence is done with a solution containing dilute lidocaine, epinephrine, and bicarbonate mixed in normal saline. The ultimate concentration of lidocaine depends on the volume to be infiltrated, but should range from 0.05% to 0.1% and remain under the ASPS guidelines of 35 mg/kg of lidocaine. Of note, the peak plasma concentration of lidocaine occurs 12–18 h after administration, but residual lidocaine lingers for over 24 h, providing useful analgesia [8]. One ampule (1 mL) of 1 mg/mL epinephrine should be placed in each liter of saline, for a final concentration of 1:1,000,000. Both the superficial and deep layers to be treated need infiltration, and typically, the deep layer is infiltrated first, particularly if an energy probe is to be used, to make sure some solution remains in the superficial layer at the time of liposuction to prevent thermal injury and abnormal contours. Having tumescence in the superficial layer also makes liposuction easier in the superficial plane.

27.2.8 Liposuction

For the best result, liposuction should be done in three stages: deep, superficial, and intermediate liposuction. Following the markings done preoperatively, the liposuction follows the same principles in all areas to be treated.

Start with deep liposuction using a PAL handpiece to facilitate the removal of fat, using a 5 mm multihole cannula (Wells Johnson 5 mm × 50 cm Delvecchio Cannula) for deep extraction and for improved efficiency. The senior author (D.D.V.) prefers to use the MicroAire™ handpiece (MicroAire Surgical Instruments; Charlottesville, VA) for this portion. Cannulas should be curved so that the tips point up toward the ceiling, minimizing the risk of penetrating a body cavity. This procedure does not require the use of VASER or UAL, but simply the ability to create beautiful contours that enhance the body's underlying definition. Create even thickness flaps of tissue, first focusing on the areas of particular adiposity, to even them out with the surrounding skin. In the abdomen, this is typically about 1 cm thickness over the rectus abdominus muscles first, and thinner, but with even flaps of tissue laterally over the external obliques. Similar depths hold true for the torso, but should be slightly thinner for the arms. Some surgeons believe that additional thinning of subcutaneous fat, such as over the rectus abdominis, creates additional definition, but we caution against that attempt, as completely evacuating the abdominal area could result in undesirable skin laxity. Of note, any liposuction close to the costal margin should be done through the areolar or axillary fold incisions, to avoid intra-abdominal or intrathoracic injury if doing liposuction from below.

The superficial liposuction will now begin to better define the underlying muscles with a 4 mm cannula (Wells Johnson 4 mm × 40 cm Delvecchio Cannula) for finer control, focusing on their tendinous connections and the transitions between the muscles. To create abrupt depressions in the linea semilunaris and the linea alba, a basket cannula can also be used very carefully. The basket cannula also works well for the deltoid grooves and paraspinous muscle depressions. To thin the flaps, pinch the skin with your fingers and pass the cannula through the guided skin flap until it is thin exactly where you want it. Remember, the muscle edges, such as the semilunar line, are not straight lines, so the natural curvature of the muscles should be followed as closely as possible for a more natural result. To minimize the incisions needed, curved liposuction cannulas can be used to follow the curves of the muscles in all body regions without unnecessary incisions. For example, the rectus abdominis horizontal tendinous intersections can be done through the umbilical incision, the areolar incisions, and the pubic incisions. If absolutely necessary for better contour, alternating lateral incisions along the horizontal incisions can be done. Superficial liposuction of the upper abdomen should be done from the areolar incisions to avoid inadvertent puncture underneath the costal margin. Suctioning should start superficially and proceed to the deeper layer until the required definition is achieved. Depressions should have a gradual definition of the grooves for a natural appearance.

Always remember that preoperative markings done in the standing position can shift when supine, such as the costal margin, so the preoperative markings are more accurate predictors of what is needed. The same principle of defining structure using superficial liposuction in selected locations is followed in all HDL cases, regardless of where in the body it is done. The preoperative markings do most of the work for you.

Intermediate liposuction provides the finishing touch and transitions between the superficial and deep liposuction regions. This is mostly done adjacent to the superficial liposuction curves in areas of acute planar changes. For example, for the rectus abdominis, begin with the area just lateral to the semilunar line definition, and do not do any further liposuction underneath the high definition curves. Areas to refine include the semilunar line laterally, the line along the external oblique fascia inferiorly, and the triangle between the pectoralis major, the latissimus dorsi, and the costal margin. The same differential liposuction principles are applied in the arms and back. As a last step, the basket cannula is used for the equalization technique, as described by Wall, to smooth surface irregularities and transitions [26]. An example of a patient's preoperative and postoperative photos is presented in Fig. 27.1.

27.2.9 Patient Safety

To maximize patient safety at all times, fat should only be injected into the subcutaneous layer, with few exceptions. Given the deaths that have resulted from autologous fat transfer to the buttocks, recent studies have found that intramuscular injection of fat can lead to migration of fat and ultimately venous fat emboli, which can be fatal [27, 28]. Through the Venous Traction Theory, fat may enter a nearby vein without direct cannula injury to the vessel, simply by causing stretch on the muscle, which can lead the vessels to fail, becoming a portal of entry for fat. This theory is particularly concerning for truncal muscles (latissimus dorsi, rectus abdominis, gluteus maximus, etc.) that do not have a posterior fascia, unlike extremity muscles that are typically enclosed circumferentially by a fascial membrane. In addition, lack of a posterior fascia allows fat to dissect through muscle fibers into the retro-muscular space, negative the desired effects. For these reasons, while some authors previously injected into the rectus abdominis muscle for augmentation or added definition of the "six pack," we do not currently recommend augmenting the muscle with intramuscular injection [29]. However, in the deltoid, there does appear to be a role in inserting small amounts of fat within the muscle to increase volume and definition of the upper arm, consistent with a high testosterone state and fitness level.

27.2.10 Postop and Recovery

Any area treated needs compression for 6 weeks. The chest is compressed with a vest, and the abdomen/back with a garment. Foam under the garments can be used for further compression and to minimize ecchymoses. The arms should also ideally be compressed with a garment, though an elastic bandage wrap may also be used. The disadvantage of the latter is that it is harder

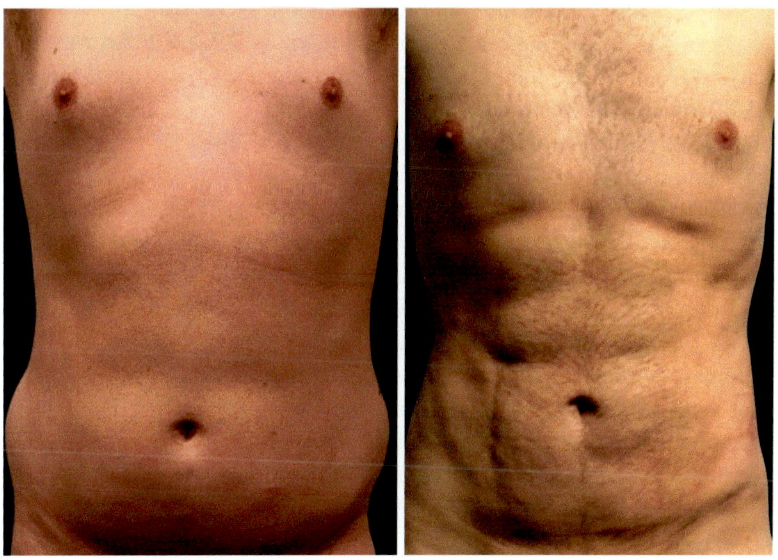

Fig. 27.1 Side-by-side comparison of the anterior view of a male abdomen before (left) and after (right) surgery. The preoperative photo shows lateral abdominal adiposity with negligible abdominal definition. The postoperative photo shows the newly defined form, with visible tendinous intersections of the abdominal wall, no fat in the lateral flanks of the abdomen, and an improved contour

to put on and may have a higher profile, which is harder to conceal under clothing, making the patients less likely to follow strict postoperative instructions. Patients should be cautioned against buying other compression garments, as the patients are often drawn to expensive garments with to define patient shape more effectively, yet may provide inappropriately high compression and place the skin at risk secondary to the transient numbness that patients may have after surgery. In addition to continuous compression, patients benefit from manual lymphatic massage to improve pain, swelling, and minimize fibrosis. The massages can help patients in their healing process and begin 3 days after surgery for 2–3 weeks. Drains can be beneficial for the dependent aspect of the abdomen and back, as fluid is more likely to accumulate there, though this is a balance each surgeon must define for himself. If your seroma rate is 25%, you may choose to aspirate those who develop them instead of prophylactically draining all patients. If placed, they should be placed through the pubic or intergluteal incisions.

27.2.11 Complications

While safe, HDL also has possible complications that need to be managed appropriately. There is a rare risk of serious complications, such as infection, deep venous thrombosis, fat emboli (especially if fat grafting is done), lidocaine toxicity, abdominal or thoracic perforation, and death, which may occur but should be preventable if safe principles of liposuction are followed. In addition, there are more relevant and more common complications, which, although not as severe, can demolish the aesthetic outcome if they occur. These include contour irregularities, skin patterns or necrosis, skin laxity, access site burns, unfavorable scarring, and seromas. Seromas, common to other surgical procedures that involve large areas of dissection, are most common in the dependent areas of the torso, and for this reason, some practices choose to drain these dependent areas.

Contour irregularities are most common, resulting from too much superficial tissue in one area, leading to an unexpected amount of contraction, or too little, which may lead to inappropriate redraping of the skin in some areas. Skin contraction may also occur unpredictably if compression is not applied evenly postoperatively. These defects can be treated with a revision to remove insufficiently removed fat, or to smooth the contour with the surrounding, more prominent area. Some defects will require fat transfer into the deficiency to improve it.

Skin changes range from changes in the appearance of the skin to increased laxity. Aggressive subdermal liposuction, especially with ultrasound or other energy-producing instruments, can damage the subdermal plexus and cause ischemia or burn the overlying skin and cause necrosis. In rare scenarios, patients may not develop necrosis but may still develop a marbled appearance with purple and red hues that may be permanent [30]. Protection of the entry sites for the cannulas is also important to minimize friction and prevent a burn at the incision site that could potentially leave a hypertrophic scar. Finally, another possible skin change is increased laxity, which may occur in patients with limited skin tone that undergo removal of too significant a volume of fat, not allowing the skin to contract back down appropriately.

27.2.12 Advantages and Disadvantages

The HDL technique that the senior author (D.D.V.) uses in his practice, with tumescent and without additional energy sources (e.g., UAL), has multiple advantages that should be reviewed, but the final choice of instrumentation is ultimately based on physician preference. Use of a PAL handpiece helps to minimize surgeon fatigue and facilitates longer procedures. Additionally, by making the pushing and pulling of the cannula smoother and by reducing risk of abrupt movements, it may minimize the risk of inadvertent injury of the viscera caused by overpowering of the liposuction cannulas. While some prefer to use VASER, given its additional energy source and its diminished need for physical effort, certain additional precautions need to be taken with VASER to avoid "end hits" that can result in subdermal burns, including around the port sites. Additionally, the price point of the VASER technology may be cost-prohibitive for some in practice. Nonetheless, VASER can be very useful for HDL once the learning curve has been overcome and the surgeon knows how to use it safely.

Additionally, given the recent findings of increased risk of fat emboli with intramuscular injection, by avoiding intramuscular injection with the exception of the deltoid, risk of fat emboli and other serious complications is minimized. Nonetheless, with the varying locations of superficial liposuction, the aesthetic results possible with this technique are capable of significantly increasing a male patient's muscular appearance and accentuating his anatomy.

Disadvantages of the technique may mostly be minimized and improved as one becomes more proficient in HDL. One argument against doing the procedure this way is that while safer without the use of VASER or UAL, the skin retraction that occurs may be less, and more likely to leave some skin laxity. However, as the patients who most benefit from this procedure are normal weight men, the skin laxity is less often a problem. The other main disadvantages of the technique are that the level of technical difficulty in performing HDL successfully is higher, as there is very little margin for error, and it's the difference between unsuccessful and overdone is very slim. However, after one overcomes the steep learning curve and pays close attention to detail, the benefits of this advance in liposuction become obvious, and the disadvantages are less likely to cause problems.

References

1. ASPS 2017 Plastic Surgery Statistics Report 2018 [updated 03–31–2019. Available from: https://www.plasticsurgery.org/documents/News/Statistics/2017/plastic-surgery-statistics-report-2017.pdf.
2. Frederick DA, Lever J, Peplau LA. Interest in cosmetic surgery and body image: views of men and women across the lifespan. Plast Reconstr Surg. 2007;120(5):1407–15.
3. Kokko H, Brooks R, Jennions MD, Morley J. The evolution of mate choice and mating biases. Proc Biol Sci. 2003;270(1515):653–64.
4. Frederick DA, Haselton MG. Why is muscularity sexy? Tests of the fitness indicator hypothesis. Personal Soc Psychol Bull. 2007;33(8):1167–83.
5. Illouz YG. Surgical remodeling of the silhouette by aspiration lipolysis or selective lipectomy. Aesth Plast Surg. 1985;9(1):7–21.
6. Klein JA. Tumescent technique for regional anesthesia permits lidocaine doses of 35 mg/kg for liposuction. J Dermatol Surg Oncol. 1990;16(3):248–63.
7. Klein JA. The tumescent technique for lipo-suction surgery. Am J Cosmet Surg. 1987;4(4):263–7.
8. Ostad A, Kageyama N, Moy RL. Tumescent anesthesia with a lidocaine dose of 55 mg/kg is safe for liposuction. Dermatologic Surg. 1996;22(11):921–7.
9. Gasperoni C, Salgarello M, Emiliozzi P, Gargani G. Subdermal liposuction. Aesth Plast Surg. 1990;14(2):137–42.
10. Gasparotti M. Superficial liposuction: a new application of the technique for aged and flaccid skin. Aesth Plast Surg. 1992;16(2):141–53.
11. Pinto EB, Indaburo PE, Muniz Ada C, Martinez YP, Gerent KM, Iwamoto H, et al. Superficial liposuction. Body contouring. Clin Plast Surg. 1996;23(4):529–48; discussion 49.
12. Mentz HA 3rd, Gilliland MD, Patronella CK. Abdominal etching: differential liposuction to detail abdominal musculature. Aesth Plast Surg. 1993;17(4):287–90.
13. Ersek RA, Salisbury AV. Abdominal etching. Aesth Plast Surg. 1997;21(5):328–31.
14. Mentz HA, Ruiz-Razura A, Newall G, Patronella CK, Miniel LA. Pectoral etching: a method for augmentation, delineation, and contouring the thoracic musculature in men. Plast Reconstr Surg. 2007;120(7):2051–5.
15. Scuderi N, Paolini G, Grippaudo FR, Tenna S. Comparative evaluation of traditional, ultrasonic, and pneumatic assisted lipoplasty: analysis of local and systemic effects, efficacy, and costs of these methods. Aesth Plast Surg. 2000;24(6):395–400.
16. Zocchi ML. Ultrasonic assisted lipoplasty. Technical refinements and clinical evaluations. Clin Plast Surg. 1996;23(4):575–98.
17. Jewell ML, Fodor PB, de Souza Pinto EB, Al Shammari MA. Clinical application of VASER—assisted lipoplasty: a pilot clinical study. Aesthet Surg J. 2002;22(2):131–46.
18. Hoyos A. High definition liposculpture. Bucaramanga, Colombia: XIII International Course of Plastic Surgery; 2003.
19. Hoyos AE, Millard JA. VASER-assisted high-definition liposculpture. Aesthet Surg J. 2007;27(6):594–604.
20. Hoyos A. Chapter 10: male arms. In: High definition body sculpting: art and advanced lipoplasty techniques. Springer; 2014.

21. Hoyos A. Chapter 9: male chest. In: High definition body sculpting: art and advanced lipoplasty techniques. Springer; 2014.
22. Hoyos A. Chapter 8: male abdomen and torso. In: High definition body sculpting: art and advanced lipoplasty techniques. Springer; 2014.
23. Hoyos A. Chapter 11: male torso and back. In: High definition body sculpting: art and advanced lipoplasty techniques. Springer; 2014.
24. Chia CT, Theodorou SJ, Dayan E, Tabbal G, Del Vecchio D. "Brazilian butt lift" under local anesthesia: a novel technique addressing safety concerns. Plast Reconstr Surg. 2018;142(6):1468–75.
25. Hoyos A. High definition body sculpting: art and advanced lipoplasty techniques. Springer; 2014. 244 p
26. Wall SH Jr, Lee MR. Separation, aspiration, and fat equalization: SAFE liposuction concepts for comprehensive body contouring. Plast Reconstr Surg. 2016;138(6):1192–201.
27. Del Vecchio DA, Villanueva NL, Mohan R, Johnson B, Wan D, Venkataram A, et al. Clinical implications of gluteal fat graft migration: a dynamic anatomical study. Plast Reconstr Surg. 2018;142(5):1180–92.
28. Del Vecchio D. Common sense for the common good: staying subcutaneous during fat transplantation to the gluteal region. Plast Reconstr Surg. 2018;142(1):286–8.
29. Danilla S. Rectus abdominis fat transfer (RAFT) in lipoabdominoplasty: a new technique to achieve fitness body contour in patients that require tummy tuck. Aesth Plast Surg. 2017;41(6):1389–99.
30. Porto da Rocha R, Porto da Rocha EL, de Souza Pinto EB, Sementilli A, Nakanishi CP. Cutis marmorata resemblance after liposuction. Aesth Plast Surg. 2005;29(4):310–2.

Aesthetic Surgery for Men: Ultrasound High-Definition Liposuction

28

Alfredo Ernesto Hoyos Ariza
and Mauricio Ernesto Perez Pachon

28.1 Introduction

Since the first description of Liposuction surgery [1] and the first large case report of lipoplasty [2], many authors and surgeons have come up with new improvements to the original technique. In fact, the original procedure was just focused on removing adipose tissue from undesirable zones in order to reduce the metabolic risk and also improve the human figure, but then it became very popular among women who desired more defined buttocks and thighs. Many improvements like the "wet technique" were developed later, and also to limit the use of possibly harmful instruments in the abdomen [3]. With this premise, Ultrasound lipoplasty was first designed [4] and became very popular since it was reported to decrease bleeding, ameliorate recovery, and ease the procedure itself. After that, many publications [5] and papers reported the great benefits of ultrasound technologies on liposculpture techniques and established new standards regarding body contour surgery. Consequently, we based our techniques in lipoplasty and improved the concepts of ultrasound-assisted liposuction by creating High Definition Liposculpture (HDL) [6], which introduced a new approach to understand the difference between a natural, slim, and athletic appearance above a plastic or irregular one.

In recent years, people's concern about fat and diet, exercise, and healthy living, as well as slim body shape, has been geometrically increasing; however, fitness lifestyle is still challenging for most individuals, and moreover, getting those desired six-pack bellies is almost reserved for a few. Social media and networks share a common economic interest in different markets: gym centers publicity, protein shakes and supplements, garments, and clothes, etc., but few of them really care about health and well-being according to each patient type. That's why we continuously take care of patients at our office, asking for advice not only on lipoplasty surgery but also on exercise and healthy living. Our purpose with HDL was to create a new standard for body sculpting surgery and improve healthy habits in our patients, helping them to achieve their own goals in addition to preventing weight gain.

The advent of new medical devices and technologies has allowed aesthetic surgeons to enhance results and perform an easier and safer liposuction with better outcomes. Although each surgeon has his/her own technique and preferred device(s) to achieve his/her own results, there are some premises and features that need to be followed in order to get optimal postoperative effects. Henceforth, patients search for aesthetic surgeons according to their results and constantly

A. E. H. Ariza (✉)
Private Practice, Bogota, Colombia

M. E. P. Pachon
Bogota, Colombia

K. Jeffords et al. (eds.), *Aesthetic Surgery for Men*, https://doi.org/10.1007/978-3-032-03840-1_28

compare technologies and ask for multiple procedures to improve their appearance, but the real contradiction lies in the type of procedure the female or the male patient asks for. Men prefer a more muscular and athletic appearance, as compared to the slim and natural buttock enhancement that women like.

Artistic Anatomy Throughout history, men have been associated with leadership, power, and reproduction. Almost all human cultures around the world share evolutionary concepts about natural selection between male and female mates for species preservation. So, the "best" male partners would be those with strength, intelligence, energy, and some other specific characteristics according to their customs that will evince a healthy optimum mate for reproductive purposes. Those features have shown us that the definition of the male figure has really different aspects compared to the female.

First of all, the male musculature has been designed to run, climb, jump, and finally hunt. The main anatomic differences regarding the more powerful quadriceps and hamstrings muscles, the bigger latissimus dorsi and pectoral muscles, the longer arm/body ratio, and other aerodynamics will help males in these labors as compared to females. In general, the male shape is defined by sharp angular edges rather than round ones (Fig. 28.1): e.g., the V-shape of the male posterior torso, the rectangular pectoral and gluteal areas, and the rhomboid thighs and legs [7]. These unique male features are crucial as we define and enhance muscles and the underlying anatomy through HDL. On the other hand, fat deposits are located predominantly over the abdominal area in a 360-degree fashion on the male patient (Fig. 28.2).

Another crucial concept that we have elucidated over the years is the Dynamic component of several muscles in the resting position vs. contraction. This concept is critical for making decisions in the preoperative period, since there are some different spaces and shapes defined by muscles that have a determinant active component while they move the anatomic structures they are aimed at. We will explain the Dynamic concept further in the markings section.

Although surgery is performed in the resting position, we need to be aware that the muscular definition perception has to be adapted, not only by how the appearance must be in rest but also in harmony with the natural movement of the underlying muscles. We have taken advantage of third-generation ultrasound technology to improve the liposculpture technique in the superficial and deep layers by easing the extraction of the adipose tissue, while diminishing the blood loss and improving the graft harvesting for ulterior injection.

As a further premise, HDL must be performed in as much muscle groups as possible. Regional or partial interventions are prohibited since an unnatural and asymmetric appearance is very

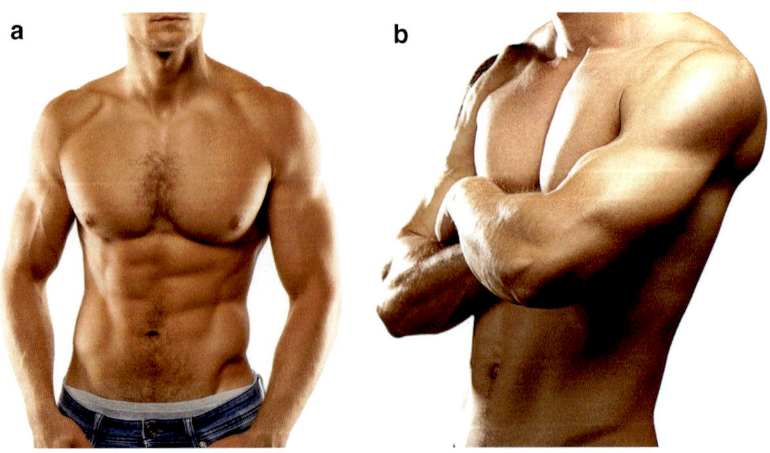

Fig. 28.1 Male shape: Notice the rectangular shape of the pectoral area and the well-defined abdominis muscle (**a**). Sharp ends and prominent muscles distinguish the male from the female. Arms and posterior torso (**b**) are harshly outlined by muscle bounds with prominent grooves. (Copyright Dr. Alfredo Hoyos and Total Definer)

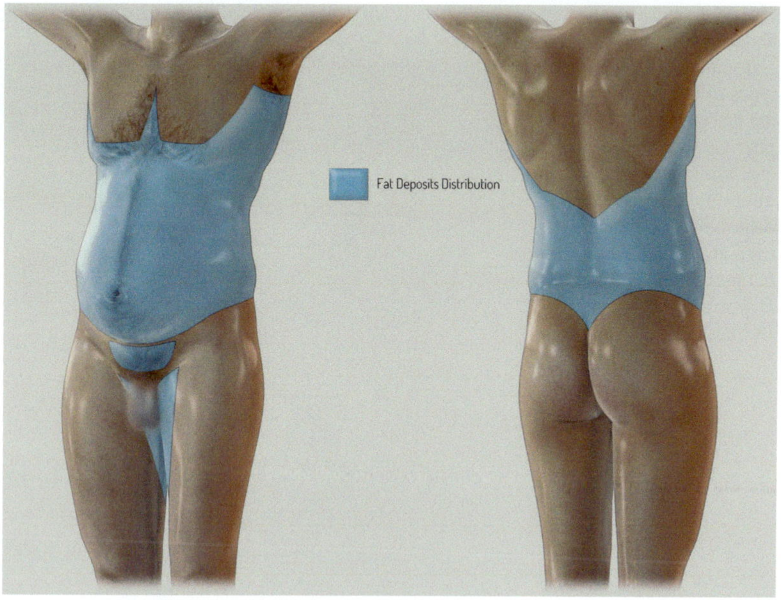

Fig. 28.2 Male fat deposits: Notice the predominant anterior and lateral disposition of fat pads. Also, the inner thighs are prone to adipose tissue accumulation. (Copyright Dr. Alfredo Hoyos and Total Definer)

likely to result. For instance, contour surgery performed only or limited to the anterior abdomen will end up with a fat chest over a defined belly ("Fit Fat Man," "Ninja Turtle" Belly). As a result, HDL needs to be performed as a whole-body contour surgery, rather than a localized one.

28.2 Patient Selection

The surgeon needs to prepare their patients from the first appointment at the office by making a meticulous physical exam, as well as a deep history of the patient, in order to support including criteria but more importantly excluding criteria for a major surgery as HDL. As a general consideration, we decided to base our patient selection according to the American Heart Association (AHA) guidelines for preoperative assessment and risk calculation. Patients who meet the exclusion criteria are rescheduled for an appointment with their attending physician or redirected to another type of procedure. Exclusion criteria are:

- Patients with Body Mass Index (BMI) 34 kg/m^2 or above
- Massive weight loss patients
- Patients who had previous bariatric surgery
- Patients with second or third-time liposuction or severe underlying scarring and fibrosis
- Patients with biopolymers or other substances previously injected in the surgical zone
- Patients with high cardiovascular risk

Note: The obese patient (BMI between 30 and 34 kg/m^2) might be a good candidate for HDL. However, it is important to address how much of fat in the anterior abdomen belongs to the intra-abdominal area (Fig. 28.3). Patients with massive intra-abdominal fat accumulation would benefit from dietary counseling before surgery and may be rescheduled within 3–6 months.

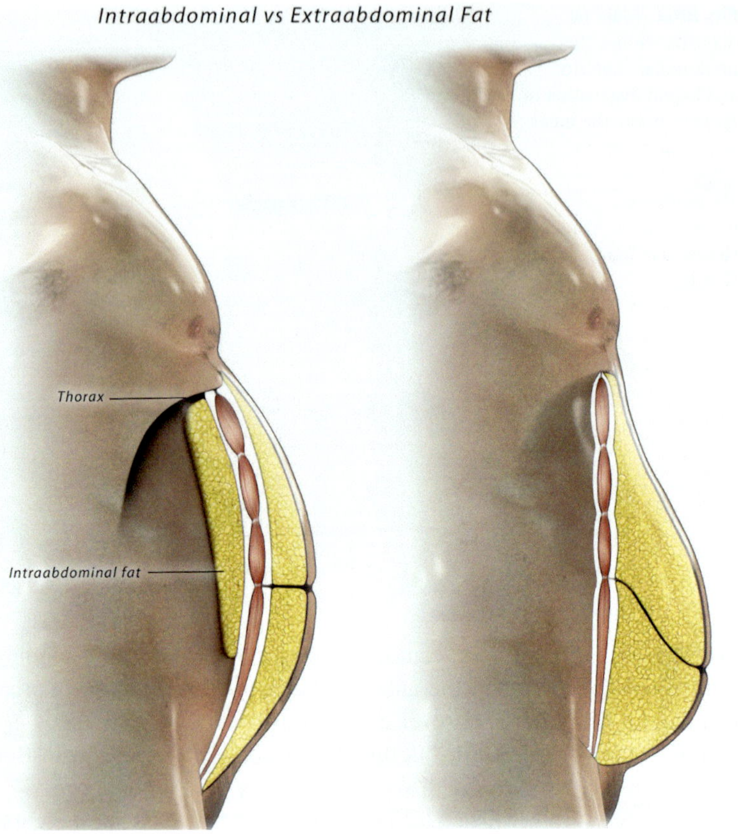

Fig. 28.3 Intra-abdominal vs. extra-abdominal fat: Both types of fat distribution are recognizable in the physical exam. Also, we can take advantage of ultrasonography to determine the amount of intra-abdominal pad. (Copyright Dr. Alfredo Hoyos and Total Definer)

Remember that on physical exam, it is important to detail the presence of:

- Hernias
- Irregularities due to trauma
- Asymmetries due to bone structure (scoliosis, rib cage asymmetries, previous fractures)
- Muscular deformities or asymmetries due to training, complexion, or overtraining (a tennis player, for example)
- Gynecomastia

28.3 High Definition Lipoplasty Technique

We perform HDL following the basic three-step process for ultrasound-assisted liposuction: (1) Infiltration, (2) Emulsification, and (3) Extraction. But before we start the surgery itself, we must perform specific markings that will portray the landmarks and zones that need to be treated according to the type of concavity or convexity, as well as the smooth or thorough definition.

28.3.1 Markings

We draw preoperative markings with the patient in the standing position with the arms in a resting state and then in 90-degree shoulder abduction. We mark the different zones with distinctive color markers in order to safely guide our performance in the surgery room.

28.3.1.1 Deep Markings

These are general markings, just focusing our attention to those classic fat deposits, usually over the central infraumbilical area, the "love-handles," the flanks, the pectoral area, and the lateral upper chest toward the axilla (Fig. 28.4).

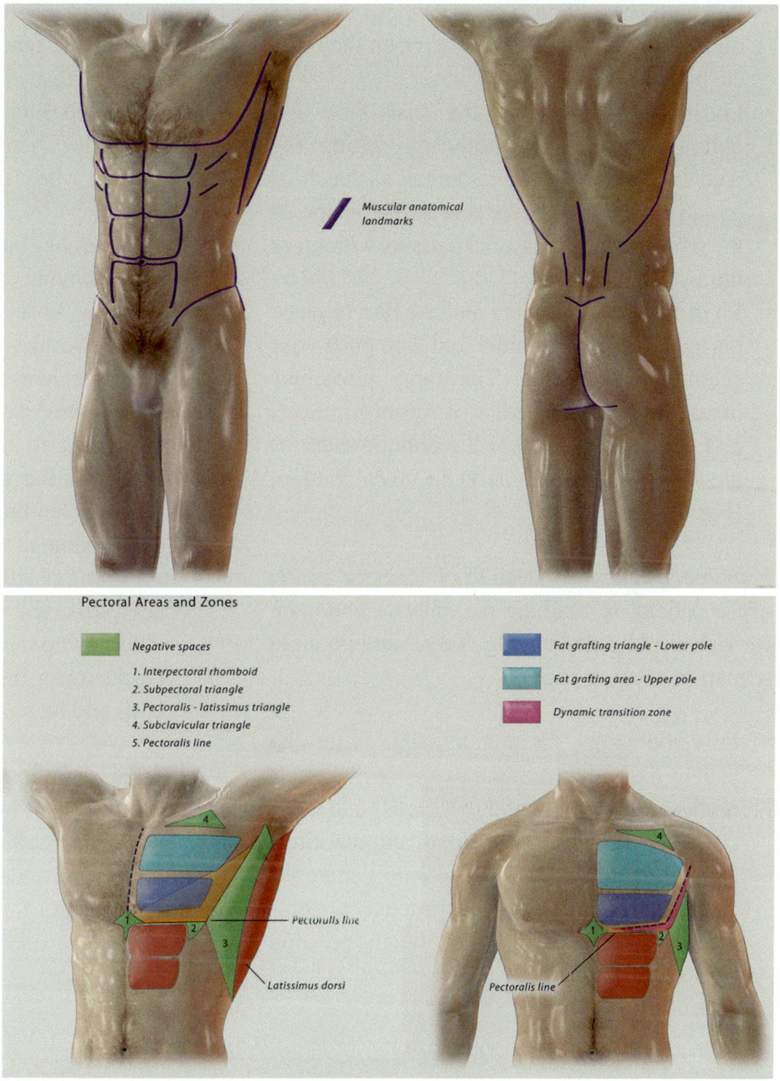

Fig. 28.4 Male markings: Main anatomical landmarks (**a**). Different zones for definition and fat grafting are marked following a code of colors (**b**). The importance of negative spaces and dynamic zones is going to be explained further in the text. *See also* Figs. 28.7 and 28.8. (Copyright Dr. Alfredo Hoyos and Total Definer)

28.3.1.2 Muscularization

First, we need to outline the underlying muscle anatomy by drawing the actual position of the muscles and other superficial anatomical landmarks. It might be done by palpation with the patient in the resting position and may require the patient to contract the muscles in specific areas and positions to determine the Dynamic zones. Ultrasonography guidance is particularly useful in the obese patient, not just to make out the muscle structure but also to evaluate the amount of intra-abdominal fat, which is crucial to avoid unnatural results, as we mentioned before.

Patient in the standing position:

- Ask the patient to inhale deeply until the costal margin is visible. Mark the costal margin bilaterally to define the thoracic arch.
- Mark the Linea Alba in the midline from the supraumbilical area to just below the xiphoid process. Remember that no midline should be marked below the umbilicus.
- Draw the lateral borders of rectus abdominis. If possible, try also to locate the transverse tendinous intersections by carefully palpating with the tips of the fingers. Ask the patient in

the standing position to contract the abdominal muscles to find the grooves between the muscle bellies (Fig. 28.5).
- Locate the borders of the transverse and oblique muscles bilaterally by asking the patient to push out the abdomen as much as possible. This maneuver reveals the shape of the muscles, particularly in patients with more intra-abdominal fat.
- Sit in front of the patient and ask him to place his hand on your shoulder and then push your shoulder downwards. The large latissimus dorsi, the anterior bundles of serratus muscle, and the upper portion of the oblique muscles are easily visible and marked as they contract (Fig. 28.4).

Some special facts need to be assessed in the obese patient, as marking the anterior abdomen for HDL can be challenging. There are two main scenarios in obese patients:

- Intra-abdominal fat predominant: After the patient has reduced this fat content by means of diet (high protein and low carbs) and exercise, then surgery is scheduled, and markings are performed. The rectus abdominis anatomical arrangement might be distorted by abdominal contents (rectus diastasis), but the position of the muscular bellies should be easy to pinpoint, as with other patients. Fat resection should be exhaustively performed over the central area in order to diminish the curvature of the anterior abdomen. The intra-abdominal fat cannot be reached by liposuction (Fig. 28.6).
- Extra-abdominal fat predominant: This is the most challenging patient to deal with, as excessive fat obscures the rectus abdominis landmarks. So, the following additional positions must be demarcated:
  - In the supine position, ask the patient to perform a partial sit-up and mark the lateral borders of the rectus during contraction. The upper tendinous intersections are often also palpable in this position.
  - In a sitting position, ask the patient to lean backwards and hold a 45-degree angle while raising the legs. During this maneuver, the lower insertions of rectus abdominis should be palpable or even visible.

As a rule, resection should be focused on the lower abdomen, and retraction is highly encouraged by performing thorough superficial fat resection to achieve definition of the underlying muscle landmarks.

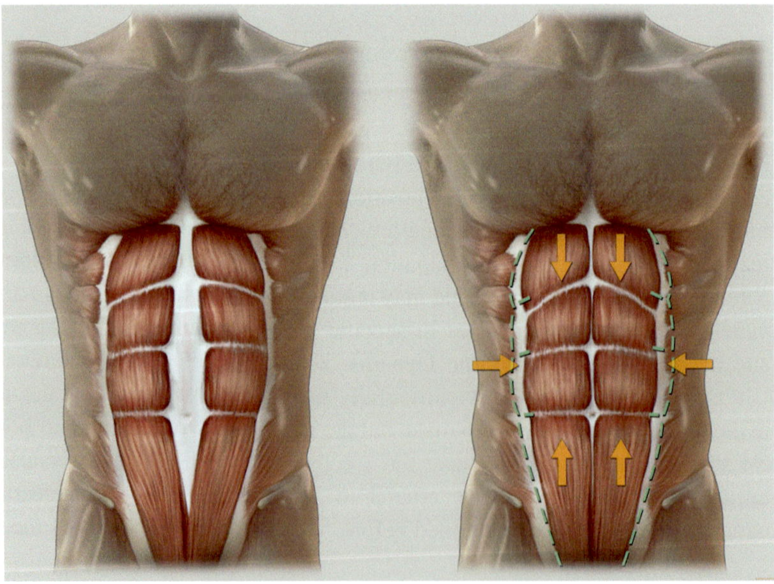

Fig. 28.5 Marking the rectus abdominis muscle: In the standing position (left), ask the patients to contract the abdomen and mark the lateral borders of the muscle (right). (Copyright Dr. Alfredo Hoyos and Total Definer)

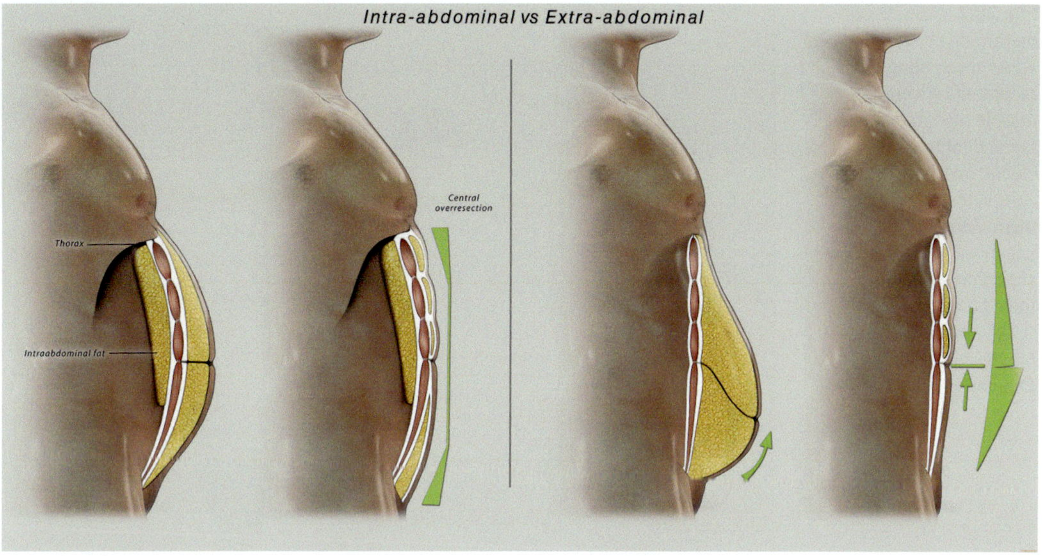

Fig. 28.6 Intra-abdominal vs. extra-abdominal fat resection: Over-resection must be performed in the patient with intra-abdominal fat deposits in order to correct the excessive curvature, but also leaving a little pad over and under the central region. (Copyright Dr. Alfredo Hoyos and Total Definer)

28.3.1.3 The Negative Spaces

They represent the transitional areas formed by the shadows of the already marked underlying anatomy, where superficial and deep lipoplasty is going to be performed. By combining these two layers, an intermediate zone for markings will result. Superficial liposuction, where controlled skin adhesions are desired, will make this surgery a unique one [8].

Another special consideration must be made regarding zones of high mobility and definition. They are called Dynamic Zones and are specific for each muscle, but most predominant for muscles in the arms and pectorals, where the dynamic concept takes place (Figs. 28.4, 28.5, 28.6, and 28.7). So, the negative spaces should resemble concavities and convexities with the aim to reveal the volume of the underlying muscular anatomy as follows (Fig. 28.8):

- A large triangular area between the lateral border of pectoralis major and the lateral aspect of latissimus dorsi (pectoral-latissimus dorsi triangle).
- A triangular-shaped area between the superior-lateral border of rectus abdominis and the lower border of pectoralis major (pectoral-rectus triangle).
- Areas between the transverse inscriptions of the rectus muscle, small triangles following the lateral border of the indentations (subcostal and semilunaris triangle).
- Area below the external oblique and transverse muscles (sub-oblique triangle).
- Posterior Area below the rib cage (paravertebral triangle).
- Area between sacral depressions and the intergluteal crease (sacral triangle).
- Dynamic Zones are marked depending on each patient's muscle features.

28.3.2 Stealth Incisions

As surgeons, we need to find a balance between operating comfortably from easy access sites that leave visible scars and hidden incisions over anatomic folds or creases, but at the cost of working from awkward positions that may require specially designed tools to reach all the areas to be contoured.

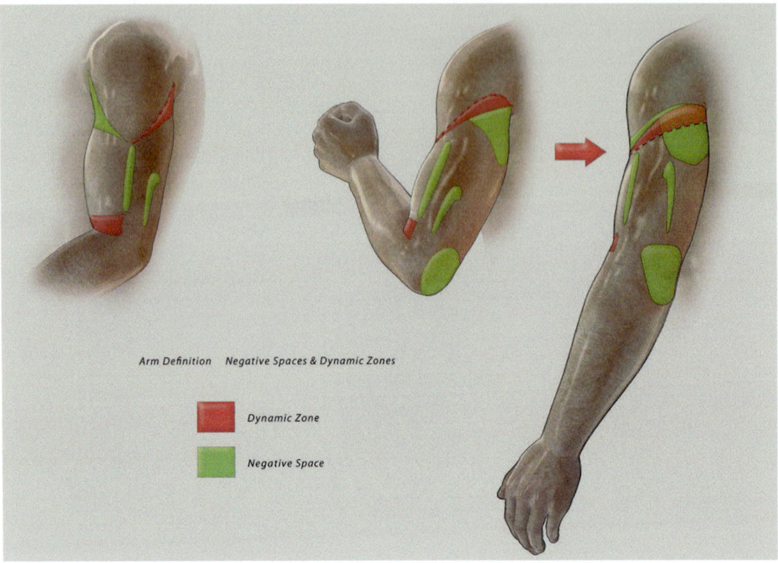

Fig. 28.7 Arm markings: Dynamic zones resembling the biceps and triceps muscle movement. Ask the patient to gently extend and flex the arm completely to mark them. Also see the negative spaces where superficial definition must be made. (Copyright Dr. Alfredo Hoyos and Total Definer)

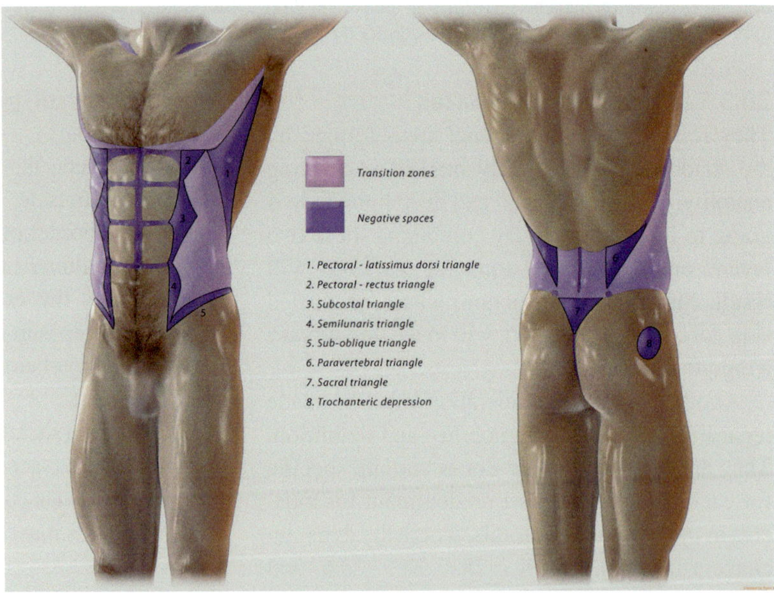

Fig. 28.8 Negative spaces: Triangles defined by zones where careful liposuction must be done to improve shadows (purple). Remember that the male muscular appearance requires sharp muscle borders but also smooth definition to achieve natural athletic results. (Copyright Dr. Alfredo Hoyos and Total Definer)

Even small incisions can leave conspicuous scars, particularly in patients with skin types V and VI or those with medical history of hypertrophic scars or Keloids. The ideal access points should not leave visible scars over the abdomen or the back and should be hidden in the underwear or in the natural folds of the skin. Even with good contouring results, some patients are reluctant to wear a bikini or sunbathe if noticeable scars are present. As a consequence, we have mastered the use of hidden or "stealth" incisions in HDL and also designed special cannulas to easily access the entire anatomy. In men, the ideal incision points should be (Fig. 28.9):

- Pubis: Below the hairline, two parallel incisions are made over the boundary of the semilunaris lines (lateral rectus abdominis). They will provide access to most of the abdominal area, including the flanks, waistline, and the rectus abdominis bellies.

- Umbilical: Provides access to the inferior abdominal area, vertical midline above the umbilicus, and central supra-umbilical abdomen.
- Nipple crease: It will provide access to the pectoral area, the upper abdomen, and the superior flank and axillary areas. In men, this incision is clearly concealed.
- Anterior axillary fold: Placed in the internal border of the crease, they will provide access to the arm, pectoral area, and lateral chest. This site is essential for fat grafting in pectoralis major and minor, also helps for mammary tissue removal in gynecomastia.
- Posterior axillary fold: Located in the internal border of the crease, they will provide access to the upper back, the posterior deltoid area, and the triceps muscles.
- Intergluteal crease: Placed just at the top of the intergluteal groove, it will provide access to the gluteal area, the lower back, and the posterior flanks. It will also provide access for fat grafting in the gluteal area.

In the abdominal area, stealth incisions are always preferable. But sometimes, for men it is often difficult to avoid additional ones. If additional access sites are necessary to define the horizontal tendinous intersections of rectus abdominis, asymmetric incisions can be placed along the abdomen, ideally mimicking cholecystectomy incisions. They will be done according to the anatomical configuration of the rectus abdominis muscle (four-, six-, or eight-pack). Other additional incisions can be made depending on the muscular groups to treat, but also when excess fat is located in some segments that are not safely reached by the previously described incisions: They include the elbow incision, the inferior gluteal crease, and the popliteal zones (Fig. 28.9). For most incisions, we recommend primary closure with subdermal continuous sutures; some others will remain open for drainage (intergluteal and pubic).

28.3.3 Procedure

With the patient under general anesthesia and placed in the supine position, we start our three-step process.

28.3.3.1 Infiltration

We use the standard tumescent solution consisting of: 1000 cc Ringer's lactate and 1:100,000 epinephrine, in addition to lidocaine 20 cc of 1%. Following a 2:1 ratio, half of the volume is infiltrated in the superficial layer and the other half in the deep layer. Infiltration should begin in the deep layer and then proceed to the superficial layer. The reason for infiltrating the superficial layer at last is to ensure that there will be tumescent solution in this layer during ultrasound delivery. If the superficial layer were infiltrated first, migration into deeper layers as time elapses could leave the skin unprotected from the VASER probe energy.

28.3.3.2 Emulsification

We begin in the superficial layer and later move to the deep layer. Although it is important to wait at least 5–10 min for the epinephrine to cause adequate vasoconstriction, prolonged delay should be avoided to prevent the migration of fluid to the inferior layers. The probe movement should be gentle, and the VASER system is tuned to pulsed mode to prevent excessive heat generation. Additional VASER time may be applied to zones for sharp definition and the negative spaces.

Once the superficial layer has been fully treated, proceed to the deep layer. Begin with the deepest areas by rubbing the probe against the muscular layer; this will ensure emulsification over almost all of the fat. Once there is loss of resistance in the deeper layers, the probe moves again toward the superficial layer until all layers are treated symmetrically and uniformly.

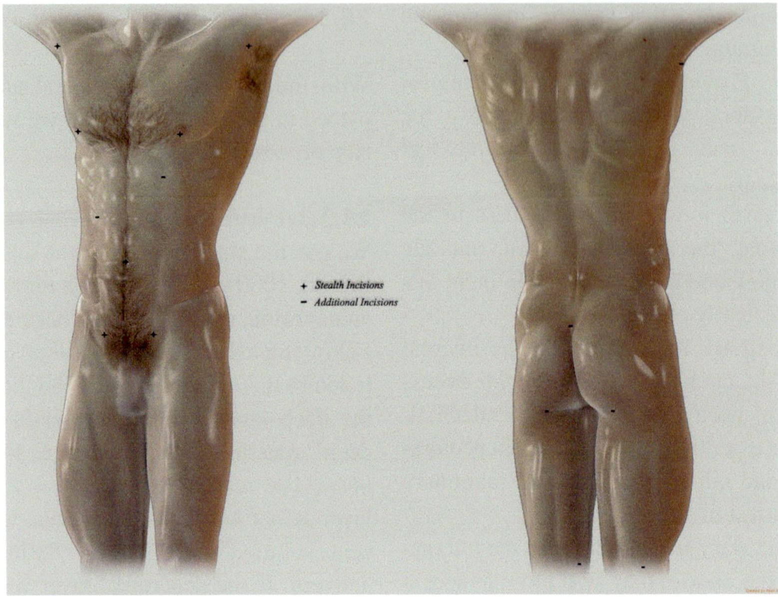

Fig. 28.9 Stealth incisions: Pubis (2), umbilicus (1), anterior axillary fold (2), and nipple crease (2). Additional ones could be done for horizontal demarcation of the rectus bellies. Note the asymmetrical fashion to avoid scar stigma. Other additional can be made in the posterior axillary fold and the intergluteal crease to reach the posterior abdomen and torso. The others can be made in the inferior gluteal crease and the popliteal region to achieve lower limb definition. (Copyright Dr. Alfredo Hoyos and Total Definer)

28.3.4 Extraction

28.3.4.1 Deep Extraction

We start with the deep layer, especially focusing on the infra-umbilical area and the flanks. Once this area is complete, start with the deep layer in the supra-umbilical anterior abdomen. Remember that most of the thickness in the upper abdomen is superficial fat (extra-abdominal), so the extraction should be performed using small cannulas. We use a 3.0-mm or 4.0-mm cannula in the deep layer. Do not over-extract in this area, as deformities can result. When suctioning the central abdomen, use smooth, non-forced crisscrossing movements and do not try to use the pinch maneuver; just feel the tip of the cannula the whole time. A 1-cm flap should remain.

Then, proceed to the pectoral area: Remove the deep fat over the pectoral muscles, including glandular tissue when gynecomastia is present. However, the upper poles should not be over-resected, as they will help with chest volume and projection. Then empty the deep fat of the pectoralis–lattisimus triangle from the nipple and axillary fold incisions. For safety reasons, try to avoid resecting the upper abdominal fat from the lower incisions. When working in the upper abdomen, the upper flanks, and the rib cage, use the incisions placed in the nipple crease.

Note: Once the anterior zone is completed (superficial and deep), the patient is placed in prone position and the posterior torso is treated. We use the posterior axillary folds to perform deep and superficial liposculpture over the latissimus dorsi muscles and the upper arms, including the deltoid muscle. Smooth definition must be done over the triceps muscle and the deltoid crease, taking special care of the dynamic zones, to avoid unnatural results. Afterwards, the posterior flanks and the gluteal areas also need to be treated with superficial and deep lipoplasty. Definition of the gluteus maximus and gluteus medius must be done thoroughly as sharp ends are critical for a masculine appearance, but not too much or a fake-looking can result. The posterior torso, the gluteal area, and the posterior thighs are zones that may need specific treatments regarding fat grafting and muscular definition, but they overcome the purpose of this chapter.

28.3.4.2 Superficial Liposuction

As mentioned before, once a 1 cm flap is achieved in the superficial layer, we proceed with the deep area of the flanks. This time, you should leave a flap of just 0.5 cm thickness. Later, we begin the sculpting process of superficial extraction by defining rectus abdominis in the lower abdomen and the transverse and oblique definition laterally. In this stage, you can take advantage of the pinch maneuver to place cannula between your fingers to thin the flap and obtain a ridge or indentation over the skin. Use a 3.0 mm cannula for this purpose.

After that, superficial etching continues from the nipple incisions: Using a 4.0-mm cannula, the lateral border of rectus abdominis is defined by suctioning superficially just below the preoperative markings. This area is critical for HDL; it is important to pause and check the appearance and symmetry of the tissues once in a while, in order to avoid over-resection. Remember that Linea semilunaris (lateral lines of the rectus abdominis muscle) follow the curvature of each muscle indentation (especially on the upper abdomen); hence, it should not be a straight line but rather would reveal the anatomical curvature of the rectus to ensure a natural result.

Hereafter, we start the definition of the pectoralis major and latissimus dorsi by emptying the triangular space between the two muscles (Figs 28.4, 28.5, 28.6, 28.7, and 28.8). The inferior and lateral borders of pectoralis major are defined by suctioning the superficial layer starting with a 4.0-mm cannula from the anterior axillary fold incision, followed by a 3.0-mm cannula to soften the contour. Use the same incision to sculpt the anterior border of the latissimus dorsi muscle by smoothly emptying the triangle. The nipple access is also used to further define the pectoralis line between the inferior margin of pectoralis major and rectus abdominis.

28.3.4.3 Defining the Rectus Abdominis Muscle

This is the most rewarding, but also the most challenging area to work in. The horizontal inscriptions are created to define the horizontal tendinous intersections of rectus abdominis muscle. There are three main ways to create the horizontal inscriptions:

- Directly, parallel to the incision point. This will require an intercalated incision at every level in line with the horizontal inscription (*see* stealth incisions section).
- Directly, using curved cannula. This obviates the need for additional incisions at every level of inscription (Fig. 28.9).
- Indirectly, by creating the inscription perpendicular to the incision point. Using compression over the marked tendinous intersections, the linear depressions are gradually formed by repeatedly passing the 3.0-mm cannula below the focally compressed tissue. This is more difficult than the other techniques and may be used alone or as an adjunct to the other methods.

Always start with a small cannula (3.0 mm), either straight or curved. Begin from the umbilical incision in the very superficial layer from the lower zone to the upper one, and later proceed deeper, until the groove is formed. You can take advantage of the nipple incisions to complete this task in the upper abdomen. Crisscrossing from three access sites produces a natural, rounded tonal progression from the grooves to the convex surfaces of the rectus abdominis bellies.

The midline Always leave the midline last. The horizontal inscriptions should be completed before defining the Linea alba. Starting from the umbilical incision, a 3.0 mm cannula is used to define the midline. The groove is then deepened using the 4–0 mm cannula and rounded by further suctioning and crisscrossing from the superior access incisions.

28.3.4.4 The Intermediate Layer

The secret of an exceptional result in HDL belongs to this step. The surgical art of transforming carved fat into shapes that look and feel natural takes its origins from the interaction of lights and shadows over the underlying anatomy (Figs. 28.10 and 28.11).

We start carving the lower negative space with a full extraction just below the oblique-transversalis muscle line, but also making it smoother as we go further distal. Then, we proceed with the semilunar lines and access through the upper incisions to meet the lower semilunar lines. Remember that the lateral borders of rectus abdominis form curves, not straight lines along the way. Suctioning below the costal margin from the sub-nipple incisions creates the negative space in the subcostal region. Always guide yourself by markings, as this zone changes considerably from the standing to supine positions. From the nipple and anterior axillary incisions, proceed to the space below the pectoralis major. Depending on the anatomy, this space may appear as a linear groove or as a broader triangle between the upper bellies of rectus abdominis and pectoralis major.

Finally, we sculpt the triangular negative space between pectoralis major and the anterior border of latissimus dorsi with a strong shadow; this sharp end will help to create the masculine appearance of the thorax (Fig. 28.11).

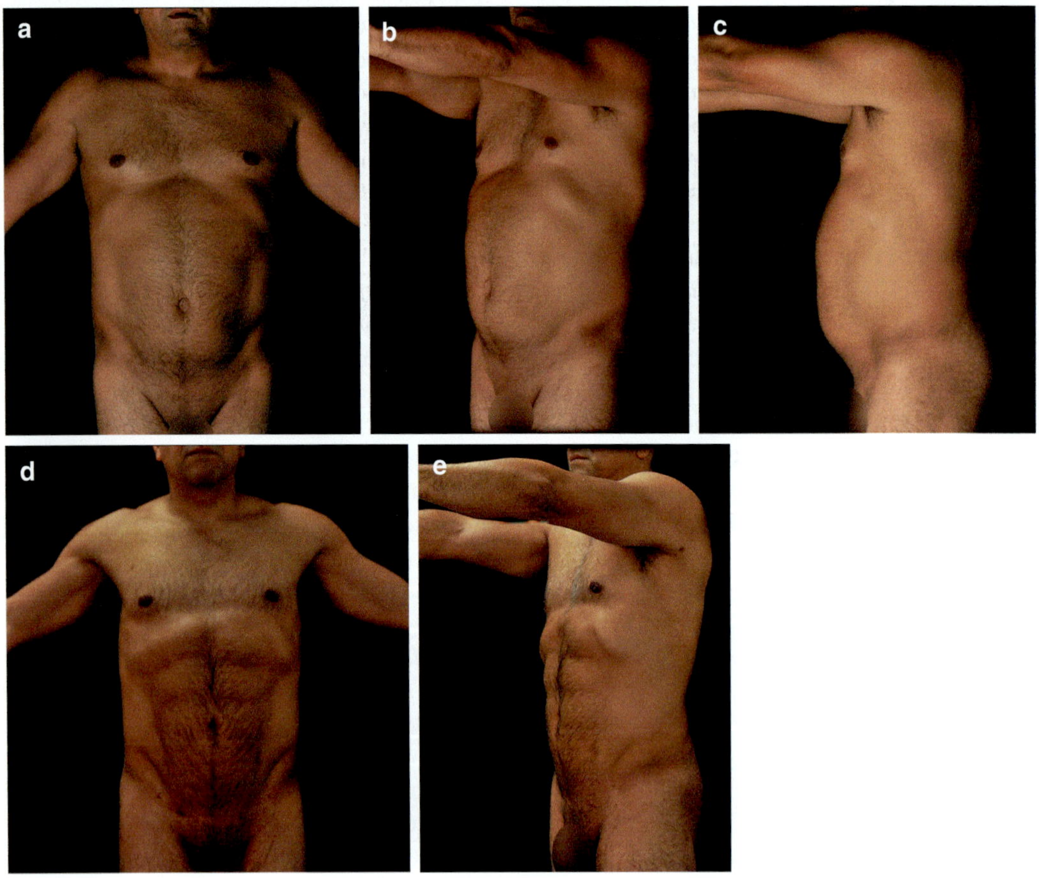

Fig. 28.10 A 51-year-old male patient: High Definition Lipoplasty was performed in the torso, arms, legs, and gluteal area. Note the difference in the preoperative pictures (**a**–**c**), where a large amount of fat pad is noticeable in the central abdomen, compared to the new athletic and muscular appearance in the 6-month post-operative pictures (**d**–**e**). (Copyright Dr. Alfredo Hoyos and Total Definer)

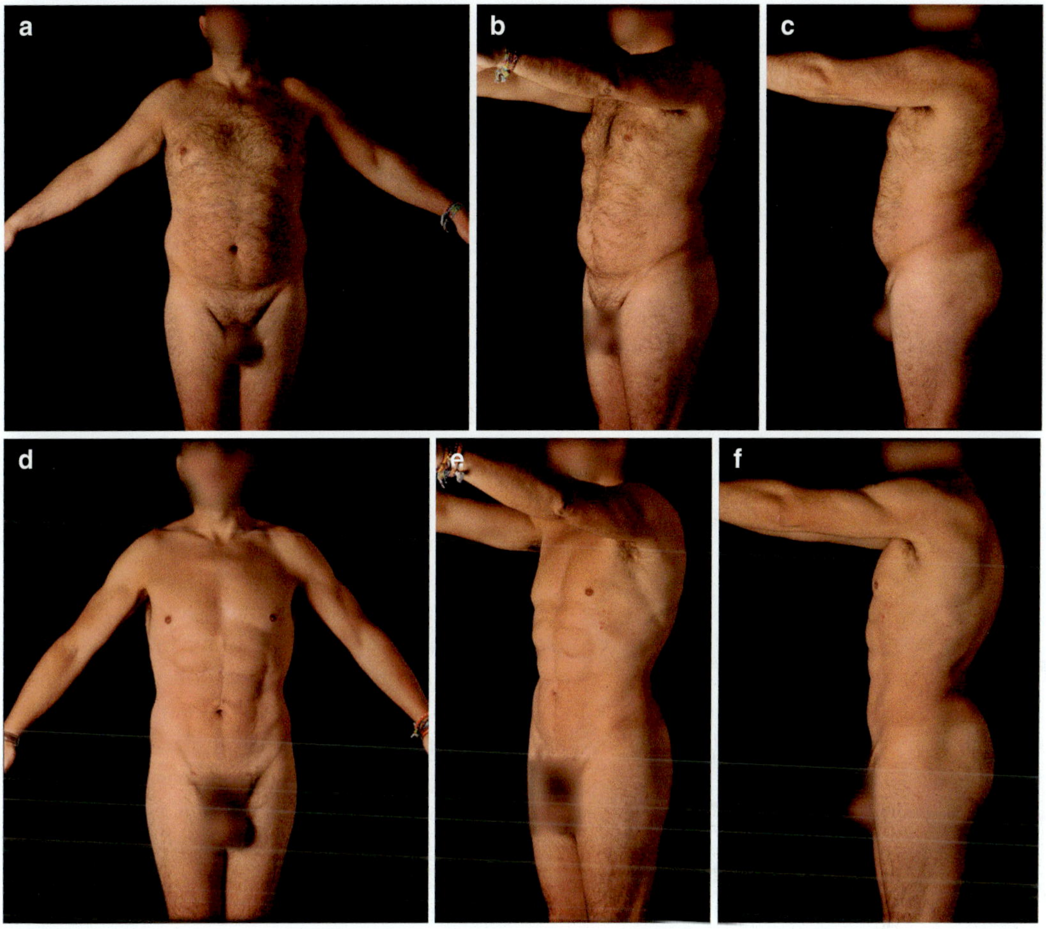

Fig. 28.11 A 39-year-old male patient: High Definition Lipoplasty was performed in the torso, arms, legs, and gluteal area, including fat grafting over the gluteus medius. Note the fat and overweight appearance in the preoperative pictures (**a**–**c**), compared to the new muscular and lean appearance in the 2-month post-operative pictures (**d**–**f**). Also, the contrasting contour over the gluteal area and the inter-trochanteric depression are evident. (Copyright Dr. Alfredo Hoyos and Total Definer)

The posterior torso HDL is performed through the intergluteal crease for the gluteal area, posterior flanks, and lumbar region. If needed, infragluteal fold incisions can be accessed to perform liposuction over the lateral gluteus and thighs. We need to be careful with the intertrochanteric depression and the popliteal region when performing gluteal and thigh HDL, since these zones are forbidden for superficial liposuction. The male gluteal region also differs from the female counterpart, as it tends to be sharper and rectangular-shaped, rather than round. We start the gluteus maximus and medius definition with a 4.0-mm curved cannula in order to reach the flanks and the lateral border of the gluteus medius. Then, smooth definition is made in the lumbar triangle, but defining the erector spinae thoroughly to enhance the muscular appearance. Pinch maneuver could be difficult to define its borders, but a 3.0-mm cannula could help you achieve this task. Finally, we sculpt the lower gluteus and thighs with smooth definition guided by markings to avoid excess roundness over the inferior gluteal crease.

The last step in male HDL is assessed by careful inspection: Negative spaces and controlled irregularities can be deepened at this stage using a 3.0-mm cannula if more definition is considered. Always be aware of the subdermal vascular plexus to avoid bleeding complications and flap suffering.

28.4 Fat Grafting

Some zones may need special enhancement in the male HDL, and fat grafting is the best choice for natural and long-lasting outcomes [9–12]. We focus especially on those areas that lack projection or not have enough volume to harmony with their surrounding anatomy. Virtually, any muscle might be subject to fat grafting; we have developed five essential premises for a safe fat grafting approach:

1. The access should be as far from the pedicle as possible.
2. The tip of the cannula should be directed in a perpendicular fashion in relation to the anatomical axis of the pedicle.
3. Place the graft at the superficial layer of the muscle.
4. Fat grafting is done in a retrograde fashion.
5. Use 3.0-mm to 4.0-mm diameter cannulas for fat grafting (Bigger than the diameter of the pedicle).

Most common areas are: the Deltoid m., the Biceps brachii m., the Triceps brachii m., the Latissimus dorsi m., the Trapezius m., the Rectus abdominis bellies, the Obliques m., the Serratus m., the Pectoralis major m., the Gluteus medius m. and the buttocks, the Vastus lateralis and Vastus medialis m., the Rectus femoris m., the hamstrings, the Biceps femoris m., and the Gastrocnemius m. (Figs. 28.4b, 28.5, 28.6, 28.7, 28.8, 28.9, 28.10, 28.11, and 28.12). Selective fat grafting can be performed on these muscles by accessing through the hidden incisions and staying as far from the main vascular pedicles as possible, using a muscle pinch technique, a 3.0-mm blunt tip curved cannula, and injecting intramuscular fat graft by delicate retrograde lipoinjection (Fig. 28.13). We use intraoperative ultrasound imaging to ensure the proper placement of the graft for those small and/or thin muscles (e.g., Latissimus dorsi, Serratus, Rectus Abdominis, Obliques, etc.). Remember that subcutaneous fat grafting is mandatory at the gluteal region, due to the increased risk of embolic complications. The technique for fat grafting of the muscles relies on the principles we have described before; however, describing each one of them will overcome the purpose of this chapter. Each zone for fat grafting must be carefully compared and assessed by ways of several angle views in the surgery room. This will decrease the chance of unnatural results and/or irregularities.

Lastly, as mentioned before, upper incisions may be closed using subdermal rapid absorbable sutures. Drains are placed in the lower declining incisions. We prefer not to fix them but rather place an absorbable pad until the postoperative control visit. Finally, the patient is dressed in compression foam vest and garments.

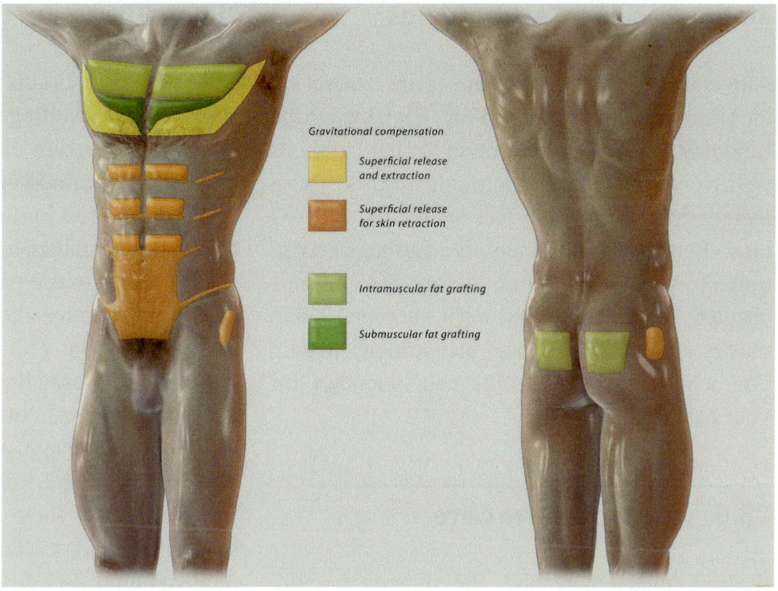

Fig. 28.12 Body sculpting summary: Areas for superficial release and grooves where fat extraction must be made in the superficial layer to improve skin adhesions (gravitational compensation), and zones that usually require Fat grafting. Note the difference between intramuscular vs. submuscular fat grafting in the upper pole vs. the lower pole, respectively. (Copyright Dr. Alfredo Hoyos and Total Definer)

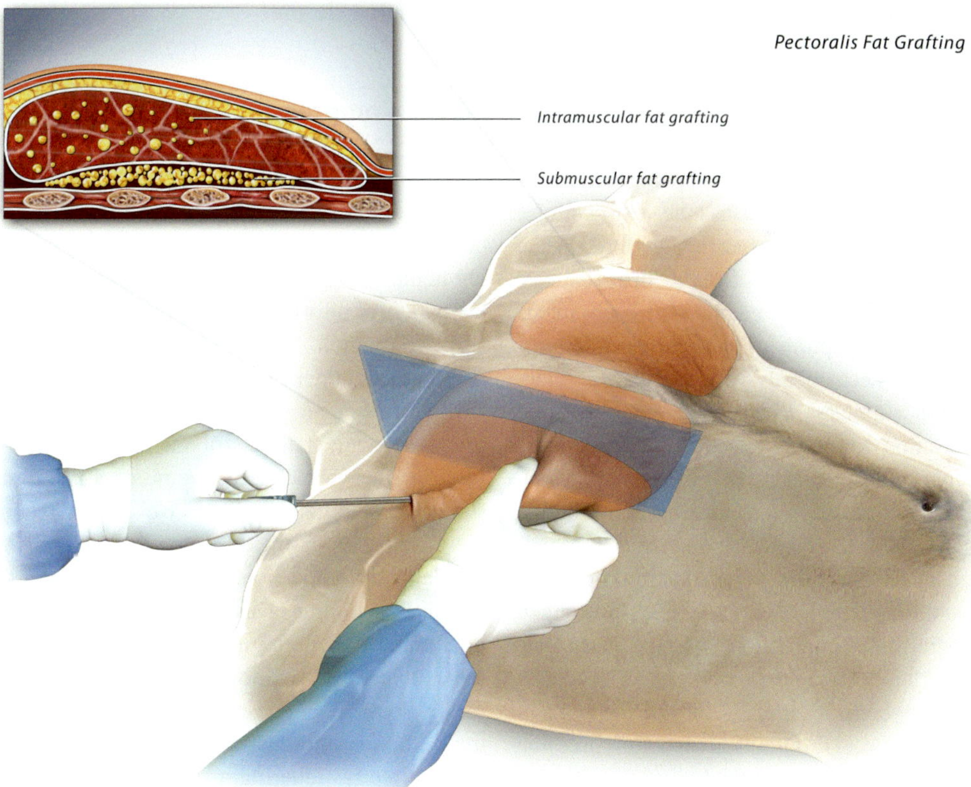

Fig. 28.13 Pectoral fat grafting: Accessing from the anterior axillary fold incisions, the graft is placed submuscular in the lower pole and intramuscular in the upper pole on the pectoralis major. (Copyright Dr. Alfredo Hoyos and Total Definer)

28.5 Ancillary Technologies

Although we have focused the entire chapter on the Ultrasound-assisted (VASER) High Definition Lipoplasty, we use some other technologies as well to help us achieve optimum results. These include Microaire, BodyTite technologies, YAG laser, PureGraft, and others, the further description of which overcomes the purpose of this chapter. We do agree that each surgeon should master some techniques and technologies to help you achieve the best results and outcomes for your patients.

28.6 Postoperative Care

It starts immediately after the surgeon has finished the procedure and the patient is dressed up with the foams and garments. Compression of the superficial layer toward the underlying newly defined anatomy is the main purpose of HDL. Most common relatively minor complications of lipoplasty procedures include prolonged swelling, bruising, and persistent pain. Tumescent technique abruptly increases the extracellular fluid fraction and creates an acute third space, which may lead to electrolyte disturbances. Moreover, liposculpture edema and ecchymosis occur when disruption of capillaries and lymphatics is mechanically produced; by then, increased capillary hydrostatic pressure and extravasation of blood, water, and large molecular-weight substances into the interstitium result in an increase in the extravascular osmotic pressure [10]. Closing incisions and trapping pooled interstitial fluid, injudicious intravenous fluid administration, and excessive, prolonged postoperative compression could exacerbate these pathophysiologic processes. As a consequence, we consider three pillars of the postoperative care: (1) Drains, (2) Compression garments, and (3) Lymphatic drainage.

28.6.1 The Use of Drains

Open or closed drains are encouraged to reduce postoperative swelling and pain and to reduce the systemic absorption of lidocaine where the concentration in tumescent fluid is high. Silicone drains are placed in dependent sites, such as the pubic and sacral incisions, so as to keep them patent during the entire postoperative drainage therapy. In the anterior abdomen, the drain tubes are placed along the groove that defines the Linea semilunaris. Closed drains get large drainage volumes that require frequent emptying. On the contrary, open drainage plus super-absorbent pads are placed over the drain to improve patient comfort and protect them against messy leakage of blood-tinged tumescent fluid. They are usually removed after 3–7 days, depending on the fluid production rate. The incision is left open for second intention closure.

28.6.2 Compression Garments

At the end of surgery, the patient is dressed up with a compression garment with the immediate purpose of reducing liposuction edema, providing hemostasis, closing potential spaces, providing patient comfort, and facilitating skin adhesion and retraction. Coated foam dressings (Epifoam—Biodermis® 2022, Henderson, NV—USA) have been used extensively under the compression garment to distribute the compressive force of the garment, overcome capillary pressure, and stabilize the skin. We do not recommend adhesion garments/taping since significant problems have arisen as a result of crimping the dermis, including avascular bullae and post-inflammatory hyperpigmentation. Silicone foams are specifically designed for patients after lipoplasty, so as to ameliorate excessive pressure on the dermal capillaries. Problems resulting from foam directly adhering to the skin have been overcome by incorporating foam into material vests.

The compression garments and vests are removed after 24 h to change the dressings, check the condition of the skin, and gently massage the trapped subcutaneous fluid toward the drains or opened incisions. The patient is allowed a sponge bath as well, and then the garments are worn again. Drain production is assessed daily until production is almost zero to be removed.

28.6.3 Lymphatic Drainage Massage

The CARE system (cosmetic active recovery) is designed to accelerate tissue healing and reduce recovery time. Several treatments have been studied separately, but the combination of them in a specific sequence is considered superior. This therapeutic method is commonly used after surgery, but can also be used sometimes before surgery to prepare the tissue for intervention. We use a standard protocol achieved by highly trained personnel in this specific assignment, as follows:

1. Lymphatic drainage
2. External ultrasound
3. Pressotherapy
4. Diathermy
5. Radiofrequency
6. Wet heat

Massages that promote lymphatic drainage can be performed long time after surgery. Some patients feel very comfortable with this therapy even 6 months after surgery and continue it for long periods of time.

28.7 Complications

Effective high-definition body sculpting employs advanced techniques and extensive superficial lipoplasty; hence need a long learning curve and specific training to achieve optimum results.

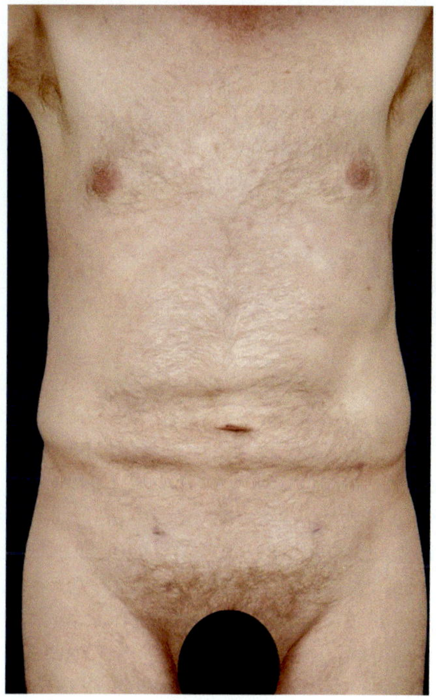

Fig. 28.14 HDL pitfall: Note the Seroma in the Lower abdomen associated with the lack of Garment use. The patient also looks fat and without muscular definition. (Copyright Dr. Alfredo Hoyos and Total Definer)

Patients should be aware during informed consent that HDL is different from conventional lipoplasty, and prolonged bruising, pain, and swelling might be expected, although ultrasound technologies have considerably reduced these effects. Patients who may not be motivated to attend frequent postoperative visits should be excluded since postoperative therapies play an important role in optimizing results and minimizing complications (Fig. 28.14). The patient must also understand the importance of constant compression with foam vests and garments in the postoperative period.

Common minor complications include:

- Prolonged bruising and swelling
- Seroma
- Fluid overload
- Polyuria
- Decreased sensitivity

Major complications include:

- Hematoma
- Infection
- Asymmetries
- Irregularities
- Aberrant skin adhesions
- Flap suffering and/or necrosis
- Burns
- Peritoneal injury

Many other complications derived from conventional lipoplasty, and HDL has been decreasing in recent decades, since new technologies and safer procedures can be performed. However, we have to mention that advanced lipoplasty techniques and fat grafting for HDL must be preceded by adequate training and hands-on experiences before starting in your own practice, as we have noticed that non-trained and/or junior surgeons sometimes try to recreate just muscular lines and surface details without addressing the anatomic features of the patient properly (Fig. 28.15).

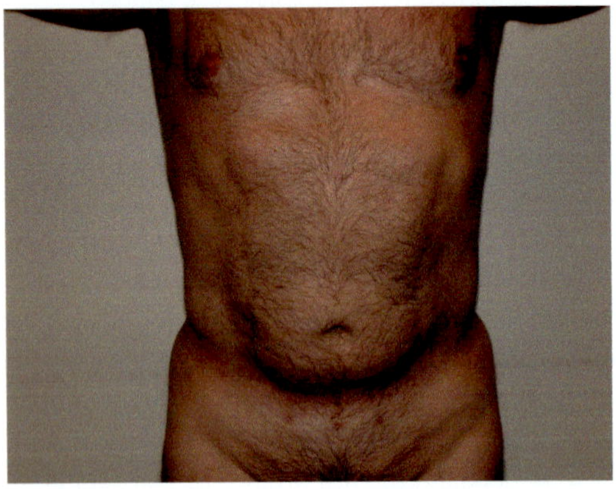

Fig. 28.15 "Fat Fit Man": Note the residual fat pad on the middle and lower abdomen. The patient looks athletic but fat at the same time. (Copyright Dr. Alfredo Hoyos and Total Definer)

References

1. Liposculpture: the "correct" history of liposuction - Giorgio fisher. Elsevier Science Publishing; 1990.
2. Illouz YG. Body contouring by lipolysis: a 5-year experience with over 3000 cases. Plast Reconstr Surg. 1983;72:591–7.
3. Illouz YG. History and current concepts of lipoplasty. Clin Plast Surg. 1996;23:721–30.
4. Zocchi ML. Ultrasonic assisted lipoplasty. Technical refinements and clinical evaluations. Clin Plast Surg. 1996;23:575–98.
5. Rochrich RJ, Beran SJ, Di Spaltro F, et al. Extending the role of liposuction in body contouring with ultrasound assisted liposuction. Plast Reconstr Surg. 1998;101:1090–102.
6. Hoyos AE, Millard JA. Vaser-assisted high definition lipoplasty. Aesthetic Surg J. 2007;27:594–604.
7. Hoyos AE, Pendergast PM. High definition body sculpting: art and advanced lipoplasty techniques. 1st ed. Springer; 2014.
8. De Souza Pinto EB, Indaburo PE, Da Costa MA, Martinez YP, Gerent KMM, Iwamoto H, Marão Miziara AC. Superficial liposuction: body contouring. Clin Plast Surg. 1996;23(4):529–48.
9. Toledo L, Mauad R. Fat injection: a 20-year revision. Clin Plast Surg. 2006;33:47–53.
10. Hoyos A, Perez M. Arm dynamic definition by liposculpture and fat grafting. Aesthet Surg J. 2012;32(8):974–87. https://doi.org/10.1177/1090820X12461498.
11. Hoyos AE, Perez ME, Domínguez-Millán R. Variable sculpting in dynamic definition body contouring: procedure selection and management algorithm. Aesthet Surg J. 2021;41(3):318–32. https://doi.org/10.1093/asj/sjaa133.
12. Hoyos AE, Perez ME, Domínguez-Millán R. Gynecomastia treatment through open resection and pectoral high-definition liposculpture. Plast Reconstr Surg. 2021;147(5):1072–83.

The Applied Science of Fat Grafting

29

Donald T. Browne, Marion W. Tapp, Adam J. Katz, and Ramon Llull

29.1 Introduction

The first adipose tissue transfer was performed and described 120 years ago by Gustav Neuber. He relocated adipose tissue from the upper extremity to the peri-orbital area to correct a contour abnormality and adherent scar after osteomyelitis [1]. The promise of successful autologous tissue transfers to correct soft tissue deficits has transfixed plastic surgeons since the origins of the profession. In so many ways, a technique originally described over 100 years ago remains at the cutting edge of restorative and regenerative medicine.

For much of the twentieth century, fat grafting struggled to take hold as a viable reconstructive option. The major criticisms included non-standardized graft harvest, variable processing techniques, inconsistent injection strategies, and graft "take," which was different for each surgeon [2]. A number of significant innovations during the twentieth and twenty-first centuries have increased the basic understanding of autolo gous fat grafting [3]. Major advancements were made in graft harvest and quantity with the development and refinement of vacuum-assisted liposuction. Now numerous variations and techniques exist to harvest viable adipose tissue [4]. The first effort at practice standardization for harvest, processing, and grafting was described by Sydney Coleman [5–7]. Lastly, the door to the regenerative potential of fat was opened in 2001 when Zuk et al. conceived and demonstrated adipose tissue as host to a large population of multipotent stromal cells [8, 9]. These discoveries among numerous others have built the foundation for the clinical practice of autologous fat grafting.

Understanding how to achieve sustainable results becomes all the more important as autologous fat grafting continues to grow in popularity. Long-term success will come from key comprehension of how the science relates to the patient. Fat grafting can be broken down into five crucial areas necessary to successful fat grafting: (1) the graft itself, (2) graft procurement, (3) graft processing, (4) the recipient bed, and (5) the engraftment process. Each of these areas will be explored in this chapter. To date, the science of fat grafting has been female focused. The fat graft and regenerative potential of fat have largely been studied in female fat. Yet the techniques and core principles are easily generalizable to the growing male plastic surgery population.

D. T. Browne · M. W. Tapp · A. J. Katz
Winston-Salem, NC, USA

R. Llull (✉)
Department of Plastic and Reconstructive Surgery,
Wake Forest School of Medicine,
Winston-Salem, NC, USA
e-mail: rllull@wakehealth.edu

K. Jeffords et al. (eds.), *Aesthetic Surgery for Men*, https://doi.org/10.1007/978-3-032-03840-1_29

29.2 The Graft

A graft is a segment of tissue transferred from one site of the body to another, in which its survival is completely reliant on the recipient bed. Fat grafting utilizes the malleable and supple composition of adipocytes and its surrounding environment in order to augment perceived deficits of the body. At surface level, the plastic surgeon may feel they have a good grasp on the fundamentals of fat grafting with approximately 80% of plastic surgeons utilizing the procedure in their practice as of 2013 [10, 11]. Nevertheless "take" rates are highly variable with observations of 25–70% [12]. Low graft survival rates, in addition to a lack of a universally adopted standard, require the surgeon to re-analyze their individual technique. This must begin with an understanding of the composition of the lipoaspirate and its donor site.

29.2.1 Physical Composition of Lipoaspirate

Adipose tissue consists of mature adipocytes and a surrounding heterogeneous mixture of stromal vascular cells (fibroblasts, immune cells, pericytes, and endothelial cells) in addition to blood vessels, lymph nodes, and nerves [13]. Adipose-derived stromal cells, first discussed by Zuk et al. in 2001, are prevalent within adipose tissue and comprise a large portion of the stromal vascular fraction [14]. They are of particular interest in therapeutic medicine and resemble mesenchymal stem cells. Additionally, they are capable of releasing numerous growth factors to trigger blood vessel formation, and their activation allows replacement of degenerative adipocytes [13, 15]. The presence of adipose-derived stromal cells is the basis of the graft replacement theory of successful fat transfer, while the preservation of viable adipocytes, along with a healthy vascular bed, is the basis of the graft survival theory, which we will discuss later.

The composition of adipose tissue is best understood by the practicing surgeon when considering the intraoperative lipoaspirate and its components. After centrifugation or simply after gravity separation, the lipoaspirate will begin to settle into three distinct layers based on density: oil on the top, fatty tissue in the middle layer, and serosanguinous fluid in the bottom (Fig. 29.1). The oil is routinely removed and the serosanguinous fluid, comprised of tumescent solution and cellular debris, is decanted [11]. The remaining injectable tissue layer contains viable cells with a cellular gradient. The top layer is composed primarily of loose adipocytes. As the density gradient increases toward the water layer, tissue fragments are of heavier density, larger in vol-

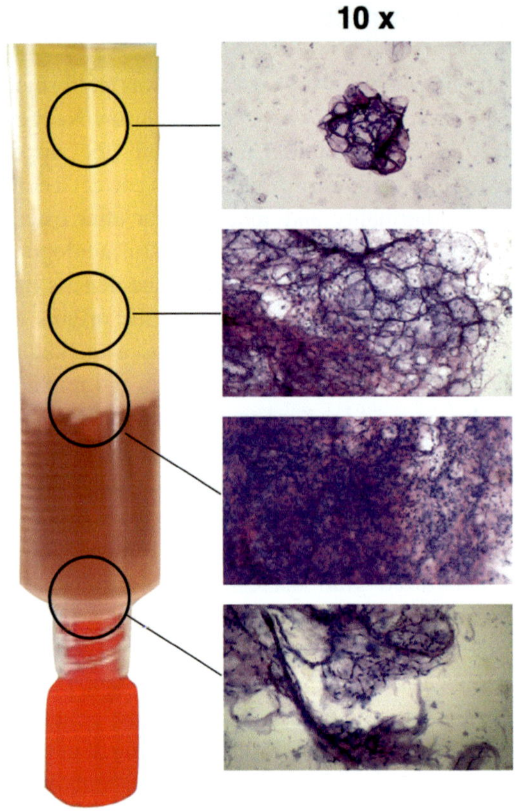

Fig. 29.1 Fat graft composition and cell density. This 10 cc syringe contains a typical lipoaspirate sample after centrifugation. The components separate based on density: a top oil, a middle tissue, and a bottom water layer. As illustrated by the right microphotographs, tissue layers display different cell composition. Loose adipocytes in the top layer and denser layers with decreasing adipocytes and increasing stromal cells. At the syringe tip, the pellet is constituted by heavy, small, adipocyte-free, fibrous fragments with vascular structures surrounded by a plethora of stromal cells

ume, and populated with decreasing adipocytes and increasing stromal cells [16]. These higher-density cells are of clinical importance as histologic assessment of fat grafts from these lower (more dense) layers demonstrates increased numbers of stromal progenitor cells and high prevalence of angiogenic factors [11, 16].

29.2.2 Liposuction and the "Ideal Donor Site"

Harvesting of adipose tissue may be performed at several locations on the body. Some authors suggest dividing fat compartments into three layers (superficial, intermediate, and deep) with judicious harvesting of the superficial sublayer due to vascular compromise and contour deformities. Additionally, fat composition varies by region; for example, the adipose tissue of the back is more fibrous than the inner thigh [17, 18]. Zones of adherence to be aware of when harvesting in both men and women include the lateral gluteal depression, gluteal crease, mid-medial thigh, distal posterior thigh, and infero-lateral iliotibial tract, to name a few [17, 19]. Numerous studies have looked at identifying the "ideal donor site." An ideal donor site should allow the surgeon easy access to areas of high-density adipose tissue without causing donor site morbidity, including trauma or unwanted contour deformities. Such sites may include the abdomen, thigh, flank, and breast. Kaufman et al. reported that the preferred site among surgeons for fat harvest is the abdomen (89%) followed by the thighs [20, 21] (Fig. 29.2). Several authors have studied the ideal donor site; however, current literature has found no significant difference in terms of cell viability or volume of grafted fat from various donor sites [11, 22, 23]. Rohrich et al. observed no difference in adipocyte viability when comparing four different donor sites, and this was further supported by Ullman et al. when comparing fat viability in a nude mouse model [22–24]. A caveat to this is literature describing adipose-derived stromal cell function, and suggests that stromal cells obtained from superficial depots in the abdomen may permit better graft survival [24, 25]. The increased potential of adipose-derived stromal cells in these superficial depots has also been supported in other studies [26].

29.2.3 Gender Differences

Anecdotally, fat grafting is more commonly performed on women, and based on literature review, gender has rarely been considered in the analysis of fat grafting [20]. Two things a surgeon may question, when approaching the male patient for fat grafting, are differences in adipose tissue quality and distribution. A lower level of evidence study by Ogawa et al. showed higher markers of adipogenesis in adipose-derived stromal cells harvested from female mice compared to male mice; however, high levels of evidence in in vitro human studies have not replicated these results [27–30]. When considering male patients, it is important to understand that male fat distribution differs from females. Age and sex hormones are known to play a role in fat distribution. Whole body imaging has shown men have less subcutaneous adipose tissue in the abdominal and gluteo-femoral areas when compared with pre-menopausal women [31, 32] (Fig. 29.2). Additionally, men are found to have higher levels of visceral adipose tissue compared to females. When performing liposuction, it is important to keep in mind different aesthetic qualities in men versus women so as to not inappropriately masculinize or feminize the patient's physique [17]. Sivak and Rubin suggest harvesting from the medial thigh in thinner patients, especially males, as this yields adequate harvest and an otherwise overlooked area [24].

Key Point: Gender-specific fat distribution affects both harvesting and grafting.

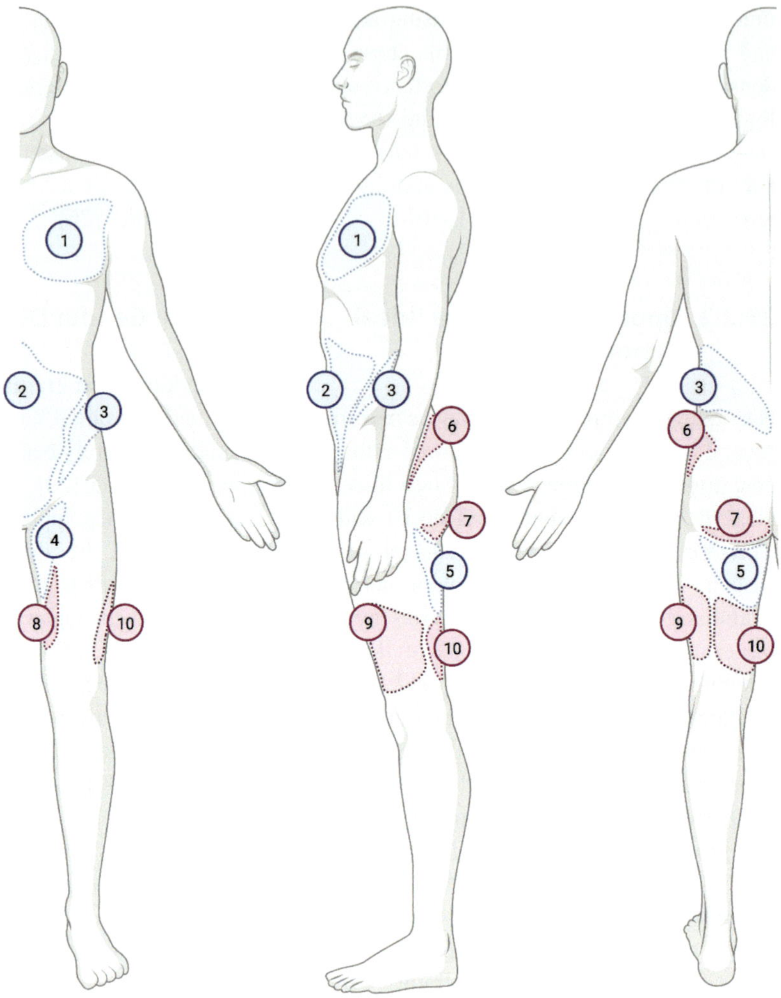

Fig. 29.2 Male fat deposits and adherence zones in men. (Created with biorender.com). *Zones of fat deposit and procurement*. Fat harvest may improve contour and mitigate donor site morbidity. (**1**) Pectoral regions, (**2**) abdominal and pubic regions, (**3**) lateral abdominal regions, (**4**) superior medial thigh, (**5**) superior posterior thigh. *Zones of adherence*, susceptible to contour depressions and deformities if violated. (**6**) Lateral gluteal depression (gluteo-trochanteric), (**7**) gluteal sulcus, (**8**) middle medial thigh, (**9**) inferior lateral thigh, (**10**) inferior posterior thigh

29.3 The Graft Procurement

The goal during each step of the fat grafting process is to protect the viability of the graft. The first potential for graft to be adversely affected is during the harvest and procurement phase. In order to achieve predictable and standardized results, the viability of adipocytes and adipose-derived stromal cells must be maintained. When viable adipocytes are harvested, viable adipocytes can then be transferred. Numerous techniques exist for the harvest of adipose tissue. It is unlikely that one harvesting method can apply to all autologous fat transfer procedures as donor site, recipient site, and desired outcome all need to be considered pre-operatively.

Liposuction provides superior access to large amounts of adipose tissue with minimal donor morbidity. As opposed to the dermal-fat grafts, fat grafts obtained by suction-assisted lipectomy are significantly fragmented and dispersed in a liquid phase. The small size of lipoaspirated grafts confers the ability of implanting grafts via percutaneous injection, thus mitigating the recipient injury.

Prior to fat aspiration, the donor site is typically infused with tumescent solution, usually consisting of a local anesthetic for pain relief and epinephrine for hemostasis in a crystalloid solution. Several studies have examined the effect of the local anesthetic and epinephrine on fat viability. The design of in vitro studies seems to be flawed, with many inconsistencies, though in summary, there is no strong evidence that suggests the use of local anesthetics or epinephrine adversely affects fat graft survival [33, 34].

Currently available liposuction methods are all relatively adipocyte-friendly harvesting techniques [35]. Although there is no clear evidence for the superiority of any one type of harvesting technique, a survey of members of the American Society of Plastic Surgeons revealed that handheld manual suction appears to be the preferred technique [10].

In addition to the method of liposuction, other variables such as suction pressure and cannula size could also impact on adipocyte viability. Irrespective of the method of liposuction, a blunt-tip harvesting cannula is utilized to withdraw the lipoaspirate from the donor site. Several studies have also concluded that the use of large-bore cannulas (4 mm in cannula diameter) yields a greater number of viable adipocytes in the lipoaspirate [36–38]. With regards to suction pressure, the literature concurs that the use of low harvest pressure (−250 mmHg) is preferable to that of high harvest pressure (−760 mmHg) [39].

The authors have previously provided comprehensive reviews of graft procurement, and though literature supports superiority in certain aspects, they have yet to be translated into a universal protocol for fat grafting [11, 40–42]. Previous results and comparisons between methods tend to vary according to the outcome measured, thus posing a restriction to determine the most competent techniques to affect fat grafting procedures. Additional human studies are necessary to aid in the development of a universal protocol for clinical practice in order to settle differences between existing harvesting techniques, recommended harvesting cannula diameters, pressure application, and composition of tumescent solution [43]. Additionally, the lack of a standard assay to determine graft viability or simply volumetric changes at the recipient site remains another limitation to obtain universally accepted grafting procedures and protocols.

Key point: Harvest at low pressure with large bore cannulas to maintain the graft's vascular structure, cell density, and viability.

29.4 The Graft Processing

During liposuction, the lipoaspirate harvested is a slurry of numerous components, irrespective of being manual, ultrasound, mechanical, or water-jet assisted. We conceive a lipoaspirated sample as a complex suspension in which solid tissue remains temporarily suspended in a liquid phase [44]. The liquid phase is an emulsion of two heterogenous fluids, including aqueous and lipid components.

In addition to adipocytes, the solid component of a graft contains other cellular elements including preadipocytes, endothelial cells, and adipose-derived stromal cells [45]. The goal of processing lipoaspirate suspension is to obtain an adipose graft nearly free of the liquid phase while simultaneously maintaining the integrity of adipocytes and stromal cells. Conceivably, both number and quality of grafted cells determine the potential of clinical benefit.

Various processing methods take advantage of the different particle densities of the material harvested from lipoaspirate. The most popular techniques for fat processing are centrifugation, gauze rolling, gravity separation, decantation and sedimentation, and washing and filtration [46]. Each processing method effectively removes the heterogenous liquid phase from the adipose tissue. The goal is to achieve consistent volumes of high-quality fat for injection.

In the coarse dispersion model, it is of paramount importance to remove excess liquid phase, rendering solid adipose tissue phase. The goal is to keep the graft in near physiologic conditions by removing excess oil and red blood cell breakdown products as well as returning the graft to physiologic osmolarity [47, 48]. Some data suggests, the aqueous fluid fraction can be reduced to a known and reproducible volume or percentage (about 16%) via fat washing systems. Consistent aqueous volume in graft tissue to be injected allows fluidity, facilitating ease of injection, and minimization of shear stress while balancing a predictable post-implantation volume resorption. Excess aqueous fluid fraction will be promptly absorbed after implantation [47, 48]. Removal of oil is also necessary for consistent clinical outcomes. The free oil content of a graft is variable among aspirates. Salinas et al. demonstrated that grafts containing excess oil, when compared to all residual lipoaspirate products, most closely resemble control fat graft in terms of degree of cellular injury and overall adipocyte health [49]. However, the oil layer adds no appreciable volume, is acellular, and may result in increased inflammation [50, 51]. Additionally, blood products such as erythrocytes, platelets, free hemoglobin, and leukocytes are found in lipoaspirate and are generally accepted as proinflammatory mediators [51–53].

Cotton gauze rolling has the benefits of being low trauma to the adipose tissue as well as low cost. Gravity separation, decantation, and sedimentation are also low trauma, low cost, and effectively separate tissue components [46]. Graft consistency may be lost if adequate time is not allowed for components to separate. The complete separation of components via gravity is reached when the system is in equilibrium; however, adipocyte viability begins to decline after 30 min, thus an upper limit exists on how long components should be allowed to separate [54].

Centrifugation, most commonly used with the Coleman Technique, adequately separates suspension into viable adipose graft at 3000 rpm for 3 min [5]. Other studies have attempted to further define centrifugation parameters; however, there remains significant variability in methods and little clinical difference in results [46].

Washing and filtration methods are now available through a number of commercial systems. These systems are best suited for larger processing volumes. Some studies suggest the washing and filtration systems may be less traumatic than centrifugation while also maintaining a greater number of adipose-derived stromal cells [12, 55]. At this stage, no studies have been able to demonstrate superior take with the above processing techniques [46, 55–57]. The authors advocate for the consistent use of processing platforms and understanding the benefits and drawbacks of various methods. Conceptual understanding of how a given technique may influence both the desirable portion of lipoaspirate (i.e., tissue fragments) and the undesirable components (i.e., free oil, blood, water) will likely result in superior volume retention.

Key point: Standardize your graft: Know your graft's physical composition, keep it oil-free and under physiological conditions.

Key point: Maximizing the graft's cell constitutive density. Minimize graft's cellular damage.

29.4.1 Stromal Vascular Fraction and Cellular Supplementation

The stromal vascular fraction is generated after enzymatic processing and centrifugation of lipoaspirate, which is a source of adipose-derived stromal cells, hematopoietic stem and progenitor cells, endothelial cells, and other stromal cellular components [45, 58, 59].

Much focus remains on increasing cellular density of fat grafting via the addition of stromal vascular fraction cells and/or culture-expanded adipose-derived stromal cells [48, 60, 61]. Animal models suggest concentrated adipose-derived stromal cells carry a graft volume retention benefit [45]. Of note, supportive studies to date are associated with the use of exceptionally high cell doses for positive effect—doses that are not readily obtained using non-enzymatic methods of cell isolation. Due to current FDA regulations, enzyme-mediated cellular supplementation to fat grafting remains available only in research settings [62, 63].

With extensive efforts aimed at proving clinical benefit, adipose-derived stromal cells containing both reparative and regenerative subsets continue to be the object and subject of multiple publications and engage the attention of researchers and clinicians alike.

Key point: Adipose-derived stromal cells may help grafts as a filler, but also may turn the graft into a healer. Much more research is required on these matters.

29.4.2 The Graft Mechanically Disaggregated

Another area of research on fat processing is focused on reduction of graft particle size. Smaller grafts are likely to be easier to inject through narrower needle bores; in shallow implantation sites for small volume requirements (i.e., face); while increasing the graft-recipient surface contact to further secure engraftment. The question remains, what is the smallest functional graft unit?

Further fragmentation of lipoaspirated fat grafts has given rise to a sequential list of other inoculants such as milligrafts, micrografts, nanofat, gel, and others. Extensive research continues to histologically and functionally characterize these inoculants and their efficacy [64–68]. Many of these "preparations" involve the injection of tissue particles suspended within an emulsion of oil and water, the benefits/activity of which, if any, remain unknown.

29.4.3 Adipose-Derived Subcellular Elements

Currently, further fragmentation of adipose-derived cells has evolved from disaggregating tissues into fragmenting cells, thus generating subcellular elements like micro-vesicles, exosomes, or even membrane rafts, all cytosolic or cell membrane portions with biological properties still to be unveiled, but heavily investigated for angiogenesis, wound healing, and tissue regeneration, among others [69–72].

Key Point: Subcellular elements exert in vitro biological functions with yet unknown impact in clinical fat grafting.

29.5 The Recipient Bed

While the donor site for fat grafting may allow the surgeon some choice, the recipient bed is often pre-determined based on the patient's goals. Ultimately, the role of the recipient bed is to provide an environment that allows maximal viability of the fat graft. In 2009, the ASPS Fat Graft Task Force found that there is no evidence whether the injection site significantly affects graft viability [73]. Nevertheless, we know that without a suitable recipient bed, we are destined for an unsuccessful graft, and thus, we must be able to identify an adequate recipient site and optimize it to the best of our ability.

29.5.1 The Ideal Recipient Bed

Definitions may vary, but it is our belief that several critical requirements must be met for a healthy recipient bed, whether that applies to fat, skin, or any other graft. The bed must be compatible, adjacent, perfused, and competent. As a general rule, the closer the two tissues are genetically, the more likely engraftment will occur. The bed must be compliant to the volume of graft placed [41]. It should have a supple behavior supported by visco-elastic properties that allow both distention and accommodation of the graft. The bed must have adequate perfusion with a reliable vascular supply and avoid areas with precarious flow [74]. Finally, the bed must have the capacity for wound healing. A healthy extracellular matrix is essential to a competent bed that allows synthesis, lysis, and remodeling processes to occur while effectively supplying gas and nutrients to support healing processes [75].

It is important to recognize the compromised vascular bed. This entails a thorough evaluation of the patient history as well as physical exam and identification of patient-specific factors. Be wary of the following compromised scenarios: radiation, diabetes, vasculopathic, post-traumatic scarring, infection, aging, and post-oncological recipient beds.

29.5.2 Optimizing the Recipient Site

Systemic and local factors must be accounted for when considering fat grafting. On a systemic level, we must consider modifiable risks and comorbidities. The issue is that sometimes the inherent characteristics of the patient that caused them to seek an augmentation may be deleterious to the grafting process. This requires some finesse on the part of the physician to give the patient a desirable result. Patients with severe scarring, fibrosis, and even hemi-facial atrophy prove to be very difficult. Oftentimes, these patients require serial injections to reach the desired volume [11, 75–77]. While serial injections are always an option, others have considered prophylactic intervention. Surgeons may choose to prepare the recipient site and precondition it to optimize their outcome. Examples of this include the external, sub-atmospheric expansion techniques. Studies regarding this device suggest some benefit based on increased parenchymal space and reduced interstitial pressure resulting in higher graft survival rates [11, 78]. Optimization of the recipient bed requires modifying it to meet as many of the "ideal recipient" requirements as possible.

29.5.3 Optimizing Injections and Anatomic Considerations

Re-injection of the fat graft and its recipient bed are not mutually exclusive. Vascularization of the graft while dependent on the injection site must be optimized by the manner in which it is injected.

Historically, the Coleman technique has been championed as the standard of care. The ASPS task force determined that the key characteristics of injection technique are centered on minimizing damage to the tissue of both the graft and the recipient site. Small, 2 or 2.5 mm blunt-tipped cannulas are to be used with small deposits of fat in each pass in order to optimize the surface area between graft and recipient bed [73]. Coleman uses a 17-gauge (~ 1.5 mm OD) cannula. Additionally, Coleman recommends an incision of approximately 2 mm, just large enough for the cannula to be inserted through, and that fat should only be injected upon withdrawal of the cannula so that it may fall into the newly created tissue planes [79]. Digital manipulation may be used to flatten minor contour deformities due to larger fat deposits; however, one should not rely on this and care be taken to place small amounts of fat in several planes as the basis of the contouring. Additionally, slower injection speeds have indicated improved results due to the decrease in shear stress [11, 80].

The levels in which the fat is injected can dictate different effects on the recipient site. Superficial grafting directly beneath the dermis may improve the quality of the skin through decreased wrinkling, pore size, and scarring [24]. The surgeon must be judicious as this plane has the drawback of potential contour irregularities and de-vascularization. Additionally, modifications to the bony skeleton can be simulated by placement of fat just above the periosteum [24]. If the goal is bulk, fat may even be placed intramuscularly although deep muscle injection especially in the gluteal region is now discouraged following the 2017 review by The Aesthetic Surgery Education and Research Foundation Task Force [24, 81].

While the general principles of the Coleman technique apply to the entire body, various recipient sites have intricacies worth noting. Corporal regions have greater volumetric requirements to make notable differences, but they often have more precarious vascular supply compared to the face and are subject to greater tension. The face meanwhile is only able to handle relatively smaller volumetric requirements. The trade-off is that it has well-vascularized territories and is subject to less tension.

Fat grafting of the face offers the benefits of restoring a youthful appearance in older patients and may restore a more natural form in patients with hemi-facial atrophy among numerous other scenarios. Prior studies have found that the success of fat grafting in the face depends on the aesthetic subunit targeted. Malar regions have favorable outcomes; however, areas such as the upper and lower lip as well as the temporal region and glabella have less success potentially due to being overall more highly mobile regions [75, 82].

Key point: The ideal recipient bed should be compatible, adjacent, perfused, and competent, but this is not always possible. The surgeon must know how to optimize the graft and recipient bed based on the anatomy and patient-specific factors.

29.6 The Engraftment Process

Engraftment is the reconstitution of the vascular and structural continuity between implanted living cells or tissues and their recipient bed, leading to graft homeostasis. As mentioned in the previous section, there are certain requirements that must be met for a fruitful engraftment process. There must be compatibility, vascular alignment, and competence between both the graft and the recipient bed. The success of a graft depends primarily on the extent and speed at which vascular perfusion is restored to this parasitic, ischemic tissue [83]. Given equal clinical and technical conditions, two qualities of a fat graft influence its fate: the intrinsic blood supply of the graft from which the graft was obtained and its metabolic activity at the time of implantation. Both will dictate its inherent tolerance to the period of ischemia [83]. When a graft fails, it is presumed that there was a lack of perfusion, excessive inflammation, or mechanical trauma resulting in loss of adipocytes and histological conversion to fibrous tissue and cysts [13, 84]. The mechanism by which the fat graft survives after injection is a point of contention among two different theories alluded to earlier, "graft replacement" and "graft survival."

29.6.1 Graft Replacement Versus Graft Survival Theories

Studies on cell viability have shown adipocytes to be extremely fragile compared to preadipocytes and adipose-derived stromal cells due to their low metabolic activity, allowing them to survive an ischemic environment much longer [12, 85–87]. The increased resistance of these cells gave rise to the thought that graft survival may be based on the adipose-derived stromal cells via the graft replacement theory [12, 79]. The cell survival theory was first touted by Peer et al. in the 1950s when they attempted to study how adipocytes survive after transplant. He stated that grafts survive through imbibition until revascularization occurs. He deduced that adipocytes must remain viable after being harvested and that mechanical trauma is likely to lead to degeneration, and therefore, proponents of his theory advocate for atraumatic processing [13, 15, 88]. We find ourselves biased toward the graft survival theory, as it appears engraftment differs little from one kind of tissue to another. Much can be learned from the elements of the skin engraftment process, and while elements of this process occur in a continuous, integrated manner, it is convenient to divide the overall process into four overlapping phases: implantation, imbibition, revascularization, and integration.

29.6.2 Implantation

When a fat graft is placed in a subcutaneous adipose tissue bed, its homeostasis is altered. Such changes brought about by the implantation intervention can also be described as a general adaptation of connective tissue to a diminished blood supply. The healing response is initiated at the moment of injury. Surgical wounds disrupt the tissue architecture and cause hemorrhage. The blood itself stimulates a number of amplification systems which result in accumulation of chemoattractant at the site of the wound [89]. This results in clinical findings such as edema due to vasodilation.

29.6.3 Imbibition

The graft is ischemic for an undetermined period of time that varies according to the wound bed, which in skin grafts ranges from 24 to 48 h [83]. The exact significance of plasmatic imbibition to healing of a graft is not clear. It may range from the supplying of essential nutrients to merely preventing it from drying out, yet it is clear that the imbibition process is crucial. Plasmatic imbibition allows a graft to survive the immediate post-graft ischemic period until such a time as graft vasculature is reestablished [83, 90].

29.6.4 Revascularization

At the end of the imbibition phase, capillary buds from blood vessels in the recipient bed contact vessels of the graft (i.e., inosculation). From there follows the process of revascularization, although the specifics of which are unclear. Three mechanisms have been theorized. The first asserts that the definitive vasculature of the graft consists of blood vessels originally present within the graft, the second that the graft is perfused from new vessels originating from the recipient bed, and the third is a combination of the two [83].

29.6.5 Integration

The final phase takes place over several months. It involves vascular remodeling, some degree of wound contraction, in-growth of surrounding extracellular matrix, and cell turnover.

Key Point: Engraftment is a continuous process that must ultimately result in transformation of temporarily ischemic graft into a well-vascularized, integrated tissue. There must be compatibility, vascular alignment, and competence between both the graft and the recipient bed. Selection of the proper sites is key.

29.7 Indications and Techniques

As discussed earlier, we believe fat grafting can be broken down into five crucial areas necessary for successful fat grafting: the graft itself, the graft procurement, the graft processing, the recipient bed, and the engraftment process. A foundation in these areas outlined above equips the surgeon to utilize the full potential of fat grafting with reproducible results. The utility of fat grafting can be generalized to the correction of both volumetric and regenerative deficits.

29.7.1 Volumetric Applications

Volumetric deficits address those needs in both reconstructive and aesthetic surgery. As Coleman indicated, grafted fat is the ideal filler. It is autologous, biocompatible, readily available, naturally integrated, and long-lasting [79]. In reconstructive surgery, fat grafting offers numerous beneficial characteristics with a low side effect profile and low cost. These applications include breast reconstruction, scar revisions, burns, HIV-associated lipodystrophy, and congenital anomalies [24, 82]. In aesthetic surgery, we see the utility of fat grafting in facial rejuvenation, hand rejuvenation, rhinoplasty, breast augmentation/asymmetry, and gluteal augmentation [82]. A male patient may present to your office looking for surgical correction including any of these above indications. Additionally, there are numerous male-specific fat grafting applications found in literature including, but not limited to, penile augmentation, facial feminization, and pectoral shaping and enhancement [91–93].

29.7.2 Regenerative Applications

The aim of regenerative medicine is to repair damaged tissues and restore functionality by stimulating the body's own regenerative capacity [94]. Adipose-derived stromal cells have proven to be an ideal candidate for this field. It seems that some of the unexplainable improvements in skin quality secondary to fat grafting noted early on by Dr. Coleman were only the beginning [79]. As of 2016, there were approximately 130 active clinical trials investigating the potential of adipose-derived stromal cells ranging from soft tissue regeneration to immune disorders [94]. Examples include the use of adipose-derived stromal cells in bone regeneration, myocardium regeneration, and even neo-vascularization in the setting of radiation treatment [94–98]. A comprehensive list of regenerative applications is beyond the scope of this chapter.

Key point: The regenerative potential of adipose-derived stromal cells is vast. While most surgeons will focus solely on the volumetric applications of fat grafting, we believe a better understanding of the potential found within the graft benefits everyone and may lead to a greater respect for what we thought was once just fat.

29.8 Summary/Conclusions

It is crucial to keep in mind the male-specific fat distribution which will affect both harvesting and grafting. When harvesting, low-pressure liposuction and large-bore cannulas will help maintain adipose structure and viability. Processing the graft should result in minimal trauma to adipose tissue while reliably separating the liquid phase of lipoaspirate. Aqueous fluid, oil, cellular debris, and other tissue should be removed from the graft that is to be implanted. Know your graft and its components! By remaining true to these principles, you will maximize the cellular component of your graft. Consistent high-quality graft is the goal. Optimizing the recipient bed is essential for graft take and integration of graft and recipient bed. Continued advances in fat grafting science will analyze the effects of stromal vascular fraction and expanded adipose-derived stromal cells in conjunction with standard fat grafting. Additionally, many around the globe continue to work to unlock and refine the regenerative properties hidden in adipose tissue.

References

1. Mazzola RF, Mazzola IC. History of fat grafting: from ram fat to stem cells. Clin Plast Surg. 2015;42:147–53.
2. Sinno S, Wilson S, Brownstone N, Levine SM. Current thoughts on fat grafting: using the evidence to determine fact or fiction. Plast Reconstr Surg. 2016;137:818–24.
3. Flynn TC. The history of liposuction. Liposuction Princ Pract. 2006:3–6.
4. Chia CT, Neinstein RM, Theodorou SJ. Evidence-based medicine: liposuction. Plast Reconstr Surg. 2017;139:267e–74e.
5. Coleman SR. Structural fat grafting. Aesthetic Surg J. 1998; https://doi.org/10.1016/S1090-820X(98)70098-6.
6. Coleman SR. The technique of periorbital lipoinfiltration. Oper Tech Plast Reconstr Surg. 1994; https://doi.org/10.1016/S1071-0949(10)80002-2.
7. Coleman SR, Saboeiro AP. Structural fat grafting. In: Neligan PC, Rubin JP, editors. Plastic surgery, Aesthetic, vol. 2. 4th ed. Elsevier; 2018. p. 390–401.
8. Mayer R. University of Pittsburgh of Commonwealth System of Higher Education v. Hedrick.
9. Zuk PA, Zhu M, Mizuno H, Huang J, Futrell JW, Katz AJ, Benhaim P, Lorenz HP, Hedrick MH. Multilineage cells from human adipose tissue: implications for cell-based therapies. Tissue Eng. 2001; https://doi.org/10.1089/107632701300062859.
10. Kling RE, Mehrara BJ, Pusic AL, Young VL, Hume KM, Crotty CA, Rubin JP. Trends in autologous fat grafting to the breast: a national survey of the american society of plastic surgeons. Plast Reconstr Surg. 2013; https://doi.org/10.1097/PRS.0b013e318290fad1.
11. Strong AL, Cederna PS, Rubin JP, Coleman SR, Levi B. The current state of fat grafting: a review of harvesting, processing, and injection techniques. Plast Reconstr Surg. 2015;136:897–912.
12. Bellini E, Grieco MP, Raposio E. The science behind autologous fat grafting. Ann Med Surg. 2017; https://doi.org/10.1016/j.amsu.2017.11.001.
13. Doornaert M, Colle J, De Maere E, Declercq H, Blondeel P. Autologous fat grafting: latest insights. Ann Med Surg. 2019; https://doi.org/10.1016/j.amsu.2018.10.016.
14. Zuk PA, Zhu M, Ashjian P, De Ugarte DA, Huang JI, Mizuno H, Alfonso ZC, Fraser JK, Benhaim P, Hedrick MH. Human adipose tissue is a source of multipotent stem cells. Mol Biol Cell. 2002; https://doi.org/10.1091/mbc.E02-02-0105.
15. Gal S, Xue Y, Pu LLQ. What do we know now about autologous fat grafting? Ann Plast Surg. 2019;83:S17–20.
16. Allen RJ, Canizares O, Scharf C, Nguyen PD, Thanik V, Saadeh PB, Coleman SR, Hazen A. Grading lipoaspirate: is there an optimal density for fat grafting? Plast Reconstr Surg. 2013; https://doi.org/10.1097/PRS.0b013e3182729cc6.
17. Stephan PJ, Dauwe P, Kenkel JM. Plastic surgery. In: Neligan PC, Rubin JP, editors. Plastic surgery, Aesthetic, vol. 2. 4th ed. Elsevier; 2018. p. 545–67.
18. Lockwood TE. Superficial fascial system (SFS) of the trunk and extremities: a new concept. Plast Reconstr Surg. 1991; https://doi.org/10.1097/00006534-199106000-00001.
19. Rohrich RJ, Smith PD, Marcantonio DR, Kenkel JM. The zones of adherence: role in minimizing and preventing contour deformities in liposuction. Plast Reconstr Surg. 2001; https://doi.org/10.1097/00006534-200105000-00043.
20. Varghese J, Griffin M, Mosahebi A, Butler P. Systematic review of patient factors affecting adipose stem cell viability and function: implications for regenerative therapy. Stem Cell Res Ther. 2017;8:45.
21. Kaufman MR, Miller TA, Huang C, Roostaien J, Wasson KL, Ashley RK, Bradley JP. Autologous fat transfer for facial recontouring: is there science

behind the art? Plast Reconstr Surg. 2007; https://doi.org/10.1097/01.prs.0000260712.44089.e7.
22. Rohrich RJ, Sorokin ES, Brown SA. In search of improved fat transfer viability: a quantitative analysis of the role of centrifugation and harvest site. Plast Reconstr Surg. 2004; https://doi.org/10.1097/01.PRS.0000097293.56504.00.
23. Ullmann Y, Shoshani O, Fodor A, Ramon Y, Carmi N, Eldor L, Gilhar A. Searching for the favorable donor site for fat injection: in vivo study using the nude mice model. Dermatologic Surg. 2005; https://doi.org/10.1097/00042728-200510000-00007.
24. Sivak WN, Rubin JP. Plastic surgery. In: Neligan PC, Gurtner GC, editors. Plastic surgery, Princ, vol. 1. 4th ed. Elsevier; 2018. p. 327–39.
25. Schipper BM, Marra KG, Zhang W, Donnenberg AD, Rubin JP. Regional anatomic and age effects on cell function of human adipose-derived stem cells. Ann Plast Surg. 2008; https://doi.org/10.1097/SAP.0b013e3181723bbe.
26. Aksu AE, Rubin JP, Dudas JR, Marra KG. Role of gender and anatomical region on induction of osteogenic differentiation of human adipose-derived stem cells. Ann Plast Surg. 2008;60:306–22.
27. Faustini M, Bucco M, Chlapanidas T, et al. Nonexpanded mesenchymal stem cells for regenerative medicine: yield in stromal vascular fraction from adipose tissues. Tissue Eng Part C Methods. 2010; https://doi.org/10.1089/ten.tec.2010.0214.
28. Harris LJ, Zhang P, Abdollahi H, Tarola NA, Dimatteo C, McIlhenny SE, Tulenko TN, Dimuzio PJ. Availability of adipose-derived stem cells in patients undergoing vascular surgical procedures. J Surg Res. 2010; https://doi.org/10.1016/j.jss.2010.04.025.
29. Ogawa R, Mizuno H, Watanabe A, Migita M, Shimada T, Hyakusoku H. Osteogenic and chondrogenic differentiation by adipose-derived stem cells harvested from GFP transgenic mice. Biochem Biophys Res Commun. 2004; https://doi.org/10.1016/j.bbrc.2003.12.017.
30. Van Harmelen V, Röhrig K, Hauner H. Comparison of proliferation and differentiation capacity of human adipocyte precursor cells from the omental and subcutaneous adipose tissue depot of obese subjects. Metabolism. 2004; https://doi.org/10.1016/j.metabol.2003.11.012.
31. Frank AP, De Souza SR, Palmer BF, Clegg DJ. Determinants of body fat distribution in humans may provide insight about obesity-related health risks. J Lipid Res. 2019; https://doi.org/10.1194/jlr.R086975.
32. Karastergiou K, Smith SR, Greenberg AS, Fried SK. Sex differences in human adipose tissues – the biology of pear shape. Biol Sex Differ. 2012; https://doi.org/10.1186/2042-6410-3-13.
33. Moore JH, Kolaczynski JW, Morales LM, Considine RV, Pietrzkowski Z, Noto PF, Caro JF. Viability of fat obtained by syringe suction lipectomy: effects of local anesthesia with lidocaine. Aesth Plast Surg. 1995; https://doi.org/10.1007/BF00451659.
34. Kim IH, Yang JD, Lee DG, Chung HY, Cho BC. Evaluation of centrifugation technique and effect of epinephrine on fat cell viability in autologous fat injection. Aesthetic Surg J. 2009; https://doi.org/10.1016/j.asj.2008.09.004.
35. Fisher C, Grahovac TL, Schafer ME, Shippert RD, Marra KG, Peter Rubin J. Comparison of harvest and processing techniques for fat grafting and adipose stem cell isolation. Plast Reconstr Surg. 2013;132:351–61.
36. Özsoy Z, Kul Z, Bilir A. The role of cannula diameter in improved adipocyte viability: a quantitative analysis. Aesthetic Surg J. 2006; https://doi.org/10.1016/j.asj.2006.04.003.
37. Erdim M, Tezel E, Numanoglu A, Sav A. The effects of the size of liposuction cannula on adipocyte survival and the optimum temperature for fat graft storage: an experimental study. J Plast Reconstr Aesthetic Surg. 2009; https://doi.org/10.1016/j.bjps.2008.03.016.
38. Gause TM, Kling RE, Sivak WN, Marra KG, Rubin JP, Kokai LE. Particle size in fat graft retention: a review on the impact of harvesting technique in lipofilling surgical outcomes. Adipocytes. 2014; https://doi.org/10.4161/21623945.2014.957987.
39. Cheriyan T, Kao HK, Qiao X, Guo L. Low harvest pressure enhances autologous fat graft viability. Plast Reconstr Surg. 2014; https://doi.org/10.1097/PRS.0000000000000185.
40. Gabriel A, Champaneria MC, Maxwell GP. Fat grafting and breast reconstruction: tips for ensuring predictability. Gland Surg. 2015; https://doi.org/10.3978/j.issn.2227-684X.2015.04.18.
41. Zielins ER, Brett EA, Longaker MT, Wan DC. Autologous fat grafting: the science behind the surgery. Aesthetic Surg J. 2016;36:488–96.
42. Ross RJ, Shayan R, Mutimer KL, Ashton MW. Autologous fat grafting: current state of the art and critical review. Ann Plast Surg. 2014; https://doi.org/10.1097/SAP.0b013e31827aeb51.
43. Fontes T, Brandão I, Negrão R, Martins MJ, Monteiro R. Autologous fat grafting: harvesting techniques. Ann Med Surg. 2018; https://doi.org/10.1016/j.amsu.2018.11.005.
44. Everett DH. Manual of symbols and terminology for physicochemical quantities and units, appendix II: definitions, terminology and symbols in colloid and surface chemistry. Pure Appl Chem. 2008; https://doi.org/10.1351/pac197231040577.
45. Moustaki M, Papadopoulos O, Verikokos C, Karypidis D, Masud D, Kostakis A, Papastefanaki F, Roubelakis MG, Perrea D. Application of adipose-derived stromal cells in fat grafting: basic science and literature review. Exp Ther Med. 2017;14:2415–23.
46. Xue EY, Narvaez L, Chu CK, Hanson SE. Fat processing techniques. Semin Plast Surg. 2020;34:011–6.
47. Vilaboa SDA, Llull R, Mendel TA. Returning fat grafts to physiologic conditions using washing. Plast Reconstr Surg. 2013;132:1–10.

48. Dos Anjos S, Matas-Palau A, Mercader J, Katz AJ, Llull R. Reproducible volume restoration and efficient long-term volume retention after point-of-care standardized cell-enhanced fat grafting in breast surgery. Plast Reconstr Surg Glob Open. 2015; https://doi.org/10.1097/GOX.0000000000000511.
49. Salinas HM, Broelsch GF, Fernandes JR, McCormack MC, Meppelink AM, Randolph MA, Colwell AS, Austen WG. Comparative analysis of processing methods in fat grafting. Plast Reconstr Surg. 2014;134:675–83.
50. Ørholt M, Larsen A, Hemmingsen MN, Mirian C, Zocchi ML, Vester-Glowinski PV, Herly M. Complications after breast augmentation with fat grafting: a systematic review. Plast Reconstr Surg. 2020:530E–7E.
51. Ansorge H, Garza JR, McCormack MC, Leamy P, Roesch S, Barere A, Connor J. Autologous fat processing via the revolve system: quality and quantity of fat retention evaluated in an animal model. Aesthetic Surg J. 2014;34:438–47.
52. Sommer B, Sattler G. Current concepts of fat graft survival: histology of aspirated adipose tissue and review of the literature. Dermatologic Surg. 2000;26:1159–66.
53. Kato GJ, Taylor VIJG. Pleiotropic effects of intravascular haemolysis on vascular homeostasis. Br J Haematol. 2010;148:690–701.
54. Mecott GA, Cueto-Ramos RG, González-Martinez A, Perez-Trujillo JJ, Chacon-Martinez H, De Oca RM, Garcia-Perez MM. Determination of the ratio of the decantation time and the separation of components in lipoaspirate. Ann Plast Surg. 2020;85:e7–e11.
55. Condé-Green A, Gontijo De Amorim NF, Pitanguy I. Influence of decantation, washing and centrifugation on adipocyte and mesenchymal stem cell content of aspirated adipose tissue: a comparative study. J Plast Reconstr Aesthetic Surg. 2010;63:1375–81.
56. Cleveland EC, Albano NJ, Hazen A. Roll, spin, wash, or filter? Processing of lipoaspirate for autologous fat grafting: an updated, evidence-based review of the literature. Plast Reconstr Surg. 2015;136:706–13.
57. Gir P, Brown SA, Oni G, Kashefi N, Mojallal A, Rohrich RJ. Fat grafting: evidence-based review on autologous fat harvesting, processing, reinjection, and storage. Plast Reconstr Surg. 2012;130:249–58.
58. Han J, Koh YJ, Moon HR, Ryoo HG, Cho CH, Kim I, Koh GY. Adipose tissue is an extramedullary reservoir for functional hematopoietic stem and progenitor cells. Blood. 2010;115:957–64.
59. Bourin P, Bunnell BA, Casteilla L, Dominici M, Katz AJ, March KL, Redl H, Rubin JP, Yoshimura K, Gimble JM. Stromal cells from the adipose tissue-derived stromal vascular fraction and culture expanded adipose tissue-derived stromal/stem cells: a joint statement of the International Federation for Adipose Therapeutics and Science (IFATS) and the International So. Cytotherapy. 2013;15:641–8.
60. Kølle SFT, Fischer-Nielsen A, Mathiasen AB, et al. Enrichment of autologous fat grafts with ex-vivo expanded adipose tissue-derived stem cells for graft survival: a randomised placebo-controlled trial. Lancet. 2013; https://doi.org/10.1016/S0140-6736(13)61410-5.
61. Kølle SFT, Duscher D, Taudorf M, Fischer-Nielsen A, Svalgaard JD, Munthe-Fog L, Jønsson B, Selvig PB, Mamsen FP, Katz AJ. Ex vivo-expanded autologous adipose tissue-derived stromal cells ensure enhanced fat graft retention in breast augmentation: a randomized controlled clinical trial. Stem Cells Transl Med. 2020; https://doi.org/10.1002/sctm.20-0081.
62. Gottlieb S. Statement from FDA Commissioner Scott Gottlieb, M.D. on the FDA'S new policy steps and enforcement efforts to ensure proper oversight of stem cell therapies and regenerative medicine. In: U.S. Food Drug Adm; 2017.
63. Sharpless N. Statement on stem cell clinic permanent injunction and FDA'S ongoing efforts to protect patients from risks of unapproved products. In: U.S. Food Drug Adm; 2019. https://www.fda.gov/news-events/press-announcements/statement-stem-cell-clinic-permanent-injunction-and-fdas-ongoing-efforts-protect-patients-risks. Accessed 29 Mar 2021.
64. Svolacchia F, Svolacchia L. Dermal regeneration with MilliGraft® Kit of nanofat: the micrograft of adipose tissue: a clinical assessment study. Scr Med (Brno). 2019; https://doi.org/10.5937/scriptamed50-21881.
65. Onur Erol O, Rohrich R, Reagan B. Facial autologous soft-tissue contouring by adjunction of tissue cocktail injection (micrograft and minigraft mixture of dermis, fascia, and fat). Plast Reconstr Surg. 2000; https://doi.org/10.1097/00006534-200011000-00027.
66. Kaufman MR, Bradley JP, Dickinson B, Heller JB, Wasson K, O'Hara C, Huang C, Gabbay J, Ghadjar K, Miller TA. Autologous fat transfer national consensus survey: trends in techniques for harvest, preparation, and application, and perception of short- and long-term results. Plast Reconstr Surg. 2007;119:323–31.
67. Zeltzer AA, Tonnard PL, Verpaele AM. Sharp-needle intradermal fat grafting (SNIF). Aesthetic Surg J. 2012; https://doi.org/10.1177/1090820X12445082.
68. Yao Y, Dong Z, Liao Y, Zhang P, Ma J, Gao J, Lu F. Adipose extracellular matrix/stromal vascular fraction gel: a novel adipose tissue-derived injectable for stem cell therapy. Plast Reconstr Surg. 2017; https://doi.org/10.1097/PRS.0000000000003214.
69. Krawczenko A, Bielawska-Pohl A, Paprocka M, Kraskiewicz H, Szyposzynska A, Wojdat E, Klimczak A. Microvesicles from human immortalized cell lines of endothelial progenitor cells and mesenchymal stem/stromal cells of adipose tissue origin as carriers of bioactive factors facilitating angiogenesis. Stem Cells Int. 2020; https://doi.org/10.1155/2020/1289380.
70. Huang B, Huang LF, Zhao L, et al. Microvesicles (MIVs) secreted from adipose-derived stem cells (ADSCs) contain multiple microRNAs and promote the migration and invasion of endothelial cells. Genes Dis. 2020; https://doi.org/10.1016/j.gendis.2019.04.005.

71. Ren S, Chen J, Duscher D, et al. Microvesicles from human adipose stem cells promote wound healing by optimizing cellular functions via AKT and ERK signaling pathways. Stem Cell Res Ther. 2019; https://doi.org/10.1186/s13287-019-1152-x.
72. Tsujimaru K, Takanashi M, Sudo K, Ishikawa A, Mineo S, Ueda S, Kumagai K, Kuroda M. Extracellular microvesicles that originated adipose tissue derived mesenchymal stem cells have the potential ability to improve rheumatoid arthritis on mice. Regen Ther. 2020; https://doi.org/10.1016/j.reth.2020.08.004.
73. Gutowski KA, Baker SB, Coleman SR, Khoobehi K, Lorenz HP, Massey MF, Pusic A, Rubin JP. Current applications and safety of autologous fat grafts: a report of the ASPS Fat Graft Task Force. Plast Reconstr Surg. 2009;124:272–80.
74. Karacaoglu E, Kizilkaya E, Cermik H, Zienowicz R, Bucky LP, Lee WPA. The role of recipient sites in fat-graft survival: experimental study. Ann Plast Surg. 2005;55:63–8.
75. Mojallal A, Shipkov C, Braye F, Breton P, Foyatier JL. Influence of the recipient site on the outcomes of fat grafting in facial reconstructive surgery. Plast Reconstr Surg. 2009; https://doi.org/10.1097/PRS.0b013e3181af023a.
76. Ranganathan K, Wong VC, Krebsbach PH, Wang SC, Cederna PS, Levi B. Fat grafting for thermal injury: current state and future directions. J Burn Care Res. 2013; https://doi.org/10.1097/BCR.0b013e318280e2dd.
77. Slack GC, Tabit CJ, Allam KA, Kawamoto HK, Bradley JP. Parry-Romberg reconstruction: beneficial results despite poorer fat take. Ann Plast Surg. 2014; https://doi.org/10.1097/SAP.0b013e31827aeb0d.
78. Khouri RK, Eisenmann-Klein M, Cardoso E, Cooley BC, Kacher D, Gombos E, Baker TJ. Brava and autologous fat transfer is a safe and effective breast augmentation alternative: results of a 6-year, 81-patient, prospective multicenter study. Plast Surg Complet Clin Masters PRS Breast Augment. 2015; https://doi.org/10.1097/PRS.0b013e31824a2db6.
79. Coleman SR. Structural fat grafting: more than a permanent filler. Plast Reconstr Surg. 2006;118:108–20.
80. Lee JH, Kirkham JC, McCormack MC, Nicholls AM, Randolph MA, Austen WG. The effect of pressure and shear on autologous fat grafting. Plast Reconstr Surg. 2013; https://doi.org/10.1097/PRS.0b013e3182879f4a.
81. Mofid MM, Teitelbaum S, Suissa D, Ramirez-Montañana A, Astarita DC, Mendieta C, Singer R. Report on mortality from gluteal fat grafting: recommendations from the ASERF task force. Aesthetic Surg J. 2017; https://doi.org/10.1093/asj/sjx004.
82. Simonacci F, Bertozzi N, Grieco MP, Grignaffini E, Raposio E. Procedure, applications, and outcomes of autologous fat grafting. Ann Med Surg. 2017;20:49–60.
83. Thornton J, Gosman A. Skin grafts and skin substitutes and principles of flaps. Sel Readings Plast Surg. 2004;
84. Niechajev I, Sevcuk O. Long-term results of fat transplantation: clinical and histologic studies. Plast Reconstr Surg. 1994; https://doi.org/10.1097/00006534-199409000-00012.
85. Raposio E, Bertozzi N. How to isolate a ready-to-use adipose-derived stem cells pellet for clinical application. Eur Rev Med Pharmacol Sci. 2017;
86. Von Heimburg D, Hemmrich K, Haydarlioglu S, Staiger H, Pallua N. Comparison of viable cell yield from excised versus aspirated adipose tissue. Cells Tissues Organs. 2004; https://doi.org/10.1159/000081719.
87. Wolter TP, Von Heimburg D, Stoffels I, Groeger A, Pallua N. Cryopreservation of mature human adipocytes: in vitro measurement of viability. Ann Plast Surg. 2005; https://doi.org/10.1097/01.sap.0000181345.56084.7d.
88. Peer LA. Cell survival theory versus replacement theory. Plast Reconstr Surg. 1955; https://doi.org/10.1097/00006534-195509000-00001.
89. Beldon P. Basic science of wound healing. Surgery. 2010; https://doi.org/10.1016/j.mpsur.2010.05.007.
90. Angrigiani C, Grilli D, Siebert J. Latissimus dorsi musculocutaneous flap without muscle. Plast Reconstr Surg. 1995;
91. Xu L, Zhao M, Chen W, Li Y, Yang Z, Ma N, Wang W, Feng J, Liu Q, Ma T. Augmentation phalloplasty with autologous dermal fat graft in the treatment of "small penis". Ann Plast Surg. 2016; https://doi.org/10.1097/SAP.0000000000000782.
92. Altman K. Facial feminization surgery: current state of the art. Int J Oral Maxillofac Surg. 2012; https://doi.org/10.1016/j.ijom.2012.04.024.
93. Hoyos A, Perez M. Dynamic-definition male pectoral reshaping and enhancement in slim, athletic, obese, and gynecomastic patients through selective fat removal and grafting. Aesth Plast Surg. 2012; https://doi.org/10.1007/s00266-012-9940-z.
94. Frese L, Dijkman PE, Hoerstrup SP. Adipose tissue-derived stem cells in regenerative medicine. Transfus Med Hemotherapy. 2016; https://doi.org/10.1159/000448180.
95. Lendeckel S, Jödicke A, Christophis P, Heidinger K, Wolff J, Fraser JK, Hedrick MH, Berthold L, Howaldt HP. Autologous stem cells (adipose) and fibrin glue used to treat widespread traumatic calvarial defects: case report. J Cranio-Maxillofacial Surg. 2004; https://doi.org/10.1016/j.jcms.2004.06.002.
96. Rigotti G, Marchi A, Galiè M, Baroni G, Benati D, Krampera M, Pasini A, Sbarbati A. Clinical treatment of radiotherapy tissue damage by lipoaspirate transplant: a healing process mediated by adipose-derived adult stem cells. Plast Reconstr Surg. 2007; https://doi.org/10.1097/01.prs.0000256047.47909.71.
97. Tsuji W. Adipose-derived stem cells: implications in tissue regeneration. World J Stem Cells. 2014; https://doi.org/10.4252/wjsc.v6.i3.312.
98. Nagata H, Ii M, Kohbayashi E, Hoshiga M, Hanafusa T, Asahi M. Cardiac adipose-derived stem cells exhibit high differentiation potential to cardiovascular cells in C57BL/6 mice. Stem Cells Transl Med. 2016; https://doi.org/10.5966/sctm.2015-0083.

Male Fat Grafting (Face/Body)

30

David M. Turer, Keith Jeffords,
and Jeffrey Gusenoff

30.1 Intramuscular Augmentation

Male aesthetic ideals are defined by the ability to visualize the musculature underlying the subcutaneous tissue. In previous chapters, liposuction has been demonstrated to be a powerful tool in providing definition to a variety of locations in the torso and extremities. Fat grafting can also be a useful adjunct to male body contouring procedures to augment muscular bulk and improve appearance.

The appearance of the male chest is dominated by the pectoralis major muscles [1]. A masculine appearance of the pectoralis major includes definition from the surrounding structures and more bulk in the superior portion of the muscle. Bulkiness of the inferior portion of the pectoralis major can give the male chest a glandular appearance. When augmenting the pectoralis major, most of the graft should be applied to the superior region and may be injected intramuscularly and submuscularly to avoid contour deformities. A blunt cannula should be used and always directed away from the chest to avoid inadvertent entry into the thoracic cavity [2].

D. M. Turer · J. Gusenoff (✉)
Department of Plastic Surgery, University of Pittsburgh, Pittsburgh, PA, USA
e-mail: gusenoffja@upmc.edu

K. Jeffords
Private Practice, Paramount Plastic Surgery, Smyrna, GA, USA

The muscles of the upper and lower extremities are other areas that can benefit from intramuscular fat grafting. In the upper extremity, often the deltoid and biceps brachii are augmented [3]. In the lower extremity, calf augmentation with injection of the gastrocnemius has been described [4].

While most regions of the body can be enhanced with intramuscular fat grafting, surgeons should be cautioned against intramuscular injection of the gluteal region. Multiple studies have demonstrated that intramuscular injection of fat can lead to fatal fat embolism as a result of injury to the gluteal veins [5–9]. As a result of this complication, any fat grafting to the gluteal region should be strictly limited to the subcutaneous plane [10]. So far, there have been no reports of fatal fat embolism from intramuscular fat grafting to other regions of the body; however, surgeons should still be aware of the possibility of intravascular injection with subsequent embolic complications.

30.2 Abdominal Fat Grafting

The aesthetic male torso includes well-defined and visible musculature of the abdomen and flanks. Specifically, the visible inscriptions and linea alba of the rectus abdominus give the abdomen its characteristic "six-pack" appearance. A visible serratus anterior can also be considered

K. Jeffords et al. (eds.), *Aesthetic Surgery for Men*, https://doi.org/10.1007/978-3-032-03840-1_30

part of the aesthetic ideal. As mentioned previously, abdominal liposuction has helped to provide definition to the muscles of the abdomen and flanks. However, in patients with minimal bulk of the rectus abdominus and serratus anterior, fat grafting can help to accentuate their abdominal contour [11]. The subcutaneous tissue overlying the space between each inscription is injected with fat to provide additional volume. Multiple lines of fat are then placed diagonally over the region of the serratus anterior to give additional definition to that area as well.

30.3 Gynecomastia

Correction of gynecomastia is a common operation performed to improve the appearance of the male chest, with roughly 26,000 operations performed in 2018 alone [12]. More severe cases often require excision of significant amounts of skin and subcutaneous tissue. However, less severe cases can often be treated by resecting a small amount of glandular tissue underlying the nipple with or without the use of liposuction [13]. A detailed discussion of the management of gynecomastia can be found in Chaps. 25, 26, and 27.

At the time of correction of gynecomastia, the contour of the chest may be improved using intramuscular fat grafting. A number of authors have described their techniques for intramuscular injection at the time of primary gynecomastia correction [2, 14]. Specifically, the superior portion of the pectoralis major is injected to avoid a glandular appearance of the chest. In thin and athletic patients, a small amount of subcutaneous fat grafting can also be used to smooth the transition from the subareolar region to the surrounding tissue.

Fat grafting can also be used to correct postoperative contour deformities after gynecomastia correction. A "crater deformity" results when glandular tissue is resected from the subareolar region without adequate contouring of the surrounding subcutaneous tissue. This can result in a sunken or retracted appearance of the nipple. A combination of liposuction and fat grafting can be used to reduce the surrounding tissue while elevating the nipple, providing for a more natural appearance. Fat grafting has also been used to correct contour abnormalities of the male chest after mastectomy for breast cancer [15].

30.4 Hand

Apart from the face, the hands are the most constantly exposed region of the body. While most surgeons are mainly concerned with the function of the hand, aging hands can be a major aesthetic concern. It can be difficult to define aesthetic ideals of the hand, but undoubtedly, there are significant changes to both the skin and soft tissues of the hand that occur with aging [16]. Atrophy of the fat and dermis produces lax skin that appears transparent with increased visibility of the underlying structures [16, 17]. Fat grafting has proven to be a reliable method to improve the appearance of the aging hand [17–19]. In general, fat is harvested from the torso and lower extremities and processed in a standard fashion. Generally, between 10 and 30 cc of injectable fat is required per hand. Procedures can be performed under regional blocks or general anesthesia.

Typically, fat grafting is performed to the dorsal surfaces of the hands and digits, with no grafting of the volar surfaces. Multiple access sites are used around the periphery of the dorsum of the hand and within the web spaces. Small blunt cannulas are typically used to perform fat grafting in small aliquots. It is critical to avoid injecting large volumes during each pass and to cross fields of injection to avoid contour irregularities and lumps. Massaging the fat can help to create an even and smooth layer. Patients are instructed to elevate their hands and avoid significant activity or heavy lifting for several days after the procedure.

Fat grafting to the hand is generally well tolerated with few complications [17, 18]. Some patients will experience temporary parasthesias and swelling that will resolve with time. There are reports of infections after fat grafting to the hand [18, 20, 21] but in general, infection is a rare complication. The majority of patients are

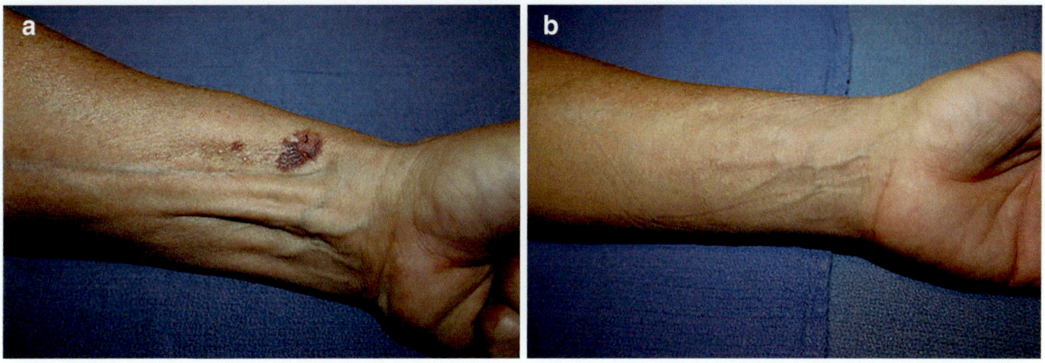

Fig. 30.1 A 51-year-old male who suffered a sports injury to the left wrist with resultant lipoatrophy (**a**). Results 3 months after fat grafting (**b**). Note the improved contour and less visibility of the underlying structures

satisfied with their results, but some may need additional rounds of fat grafting depending on the degree of atrophy and graft take (Fig. 30.1).

30.5 Foot

Fat pad atrophy of the forefoot or heel is the loss of fat on the bottom of the foot, characterized by pain that can be severe enough to have a significant effect on a patient's quality of life [22]. Patients may experience severe pain, which can lead to significant debilitation, including the inability to walk. Pedal fat pad atrophy is a diagnosis of exclusion without well-defined diagnostic criteria. This condition may be associated with advanced age, obesity, steroid injections, use of high-heeled shoes, iatrogenic surgical complications, or abnormal foot mechanics [23]. The current standard of care for treating pedal fat atrophy includes the use of external pressure offloading devices or augmentation with synthetic fillers or dermal substitutes. These strategies have not produced acceptable long-term results.

Autologous fat grafting has been proven to produce a significant improvement in pain in these patients [22, 23]. Patients underwent a thorough evaluation by a podiatrist, and then 4–6 mL of fat was injected into areas that demonstrated significant soft tissue atrophy. Although there was minimal long-term change to the thickness of the pedal fat pad, dermal thickness was significantly improved, and this correlated with long-term improvement in pain. Overall, pedal fat grafting has a significant positive impact on patients' quality of life. The combined expertise of plastic surgery and podiatry is important for optimizing the care of these patients.

30.6 Facial Fat Grafting

The characteristics that constitute an aesthetic male face are considerably different than those in women [24, 25]. In general, men have squarer faces with larger and wider jaws. These structural differences define the male facial aesthetic, and therefore the desired changes most male patients will request. The most common areas for augmentation in men include the jawline, chin, and malar region (Fig. 30.2). There is an increasing number of men requesting the use of facial fillers, and while fat grafting has been used extensively in the facelift [26] and reconstructive population [27], the use of facial fat grafting to replace fillers is still in its infancy.

There are several studies that demonstrate the safe and effective use of primary facial fat grafting, but none focus specifically on men [28–31]. Unlike hyaluronic acid fillers that will fade over time or can be dissolved, fat grafting is generally considered to be permanent. Additionally, as is often observed in the pediatric craniofacial population, grafted fat may hypertrophy with weight

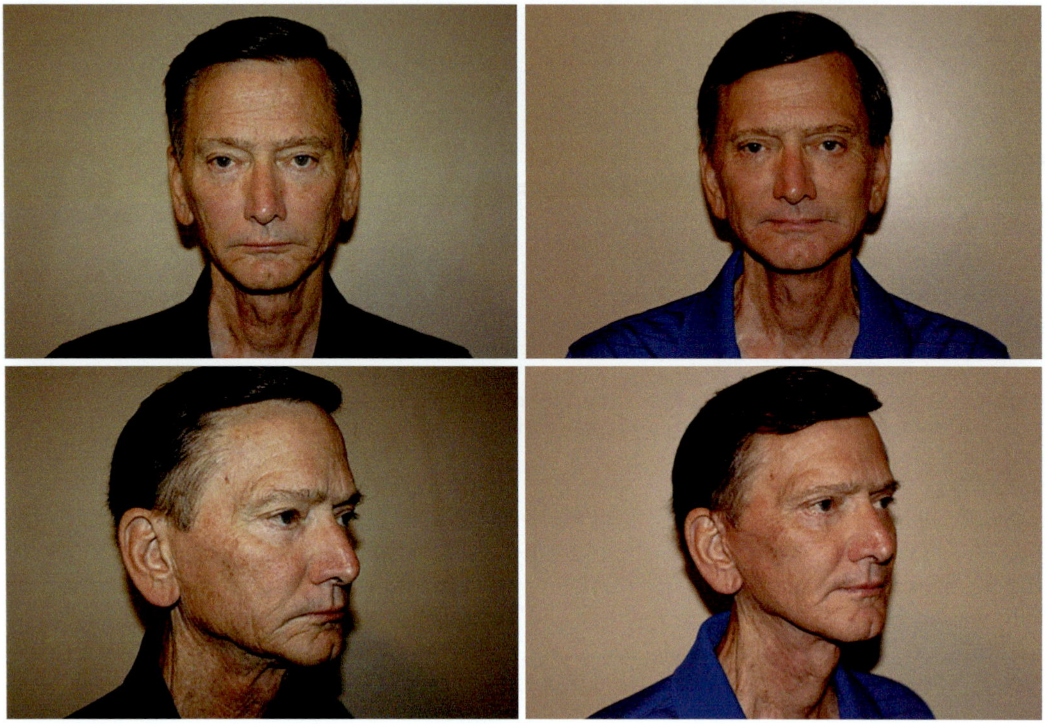

Fig. 30.2 A 65-year-old male with a history of head and neck cancer, right radical neck dissection, and radiation therapy. Patient is shown preop (**a**, **b**) and 4 months postop after fat grafting to bilateral cheeks, malar regions, and chin (**c**, **d**)

gain and may require secondary liposuction or direct excision.

One application of facial fat grafting that has been well reported is for treatment of HIV-associated lipodystrophy. This well-documented side effect of HAART therapy is characterized by lipoatrophy of the face, arms, and buttocks, as well as lipohypertrophy of the abdomen, breast, and dorsocervical region (known as the "buffalo hump") [32, 33]. These changes are potentially very stigmatizing for this population, and a number of treatments have been attempted [34]. In patients with truncal lipohypertrophy, these regions can be used as donor sites for facial fat grafting. Graft harvest is completed in a standard fashion and most commonly injected to correct temporal wasting, sunken cheeks, and a prominent nasolabial fold. There are reports of patients having unexpected lipohypertrophy [33]; however, most patients tolerate this well with a very low risk of complications [35].

References

1. Mentz HA, Ruiz-Razura A, Newall G, Patronella CK, Miniel LA. Pectoral etching: a method for augmentation, delineation, and contouring the thoracic musculature in men. Plast Reconstr Surg. 2007;120(7):2051–5. https://doi.org/10.1097/01.prs.0000287394.22375.2e.
2. Hoyos A, Perez M. Dynamic-definition male pectoral reshaping and enhancement in slim, athletic, obese, and gynecomastic patients through selective fat removal and grafting. Aesth Plast Surg. 2012;36(5):1066–77. https://doi.org/10.1007/s00266-012-9940-z.
3. Hoyos A, Perez M. Arm dynamic definition by liposculpture and fat grafting. Aesthetic Surg J. 2012;32(8):974–87. https://doi.org/10.1177/1090820X12461498.
4. Mundinger GS, Vogel JE. Calf augmentation and reshaping with autologous fat grafting. Aesthetic Surg J. 2016;36(2):211–20. https://doi.org/10.1093/asj/sjv166.
5. Mofid MM, Teitelbaum S, Suissa D, et al. Report on mortality from gluteal fat grafting: recommendations from the ASERF task force. Aesthetic Surg J.

2017;37(7):796–806. https://doi.org/10.1093/asj/sjx004.
6. Villanueva NL, Del Vecchio DA, Afrooz PN, Carboy JA, Rohrich RJ. Staying safe during gluteal fat transplantation. Plast Reconstr Surg. 2018;141(1):79–86. https://doi.org/10.1097/PRS.0000000000003934.
7. Cárdenas-Camarena L, Durán H, Robles-Cervantes JA, Bayter-Marin JE. Critical differences between Microscopic (mife) and Macroscopic (mafe) fat embolism during liposuction and gluteal lipoinjection. Plast Reconstr Surg. 2018;141(4):880–90. https://doi.org/10.1097/PRS.0000000000004219.
8. Vadseth L, Dreyer S, Jönsson V, Kalaaji A, Maric I, Haukebøe TH. Gluteal augmentation with fat: retrospective safety study and literature review. Aesthetic Surg J. 2018;39(3):292–305. https://doi.org/10.1093/asj/sjy153.
9. Condé-Green A, Kotamarti V, Nini KT, et al. Fat grafting for gluteal augmentation: a systematic review of the literature and meta-analysis. Plast Reconstr Surg. 2016;138(3):437e–46e. https://doi.org/10.1097/PRS.0000000000002435.
10. Mills D, Rubin JP, Saltz R. Multi-society gluteal fat grafting task force issues safety advisory urging practitioners to reevaluate technique. https://www.surgery.org/sites/default/files/Gluteal-Fat-Grafting-02-06-18_0.pdf. Published 2018.
11. Steinbrech DS, Sinno S. Utilizing the power of fat grafting to obtain a naturally-appearing muscular "6-pack" abdomen. Aesthetic Surg J. 2016;36(9):1085–8. https://doi.org/10.1093/asj/sjw072.
12. American Society of Plastic Surgeons. 2024 National Plastic Surgery Statistics. 2025. https://www.plasticsurgery.org/documents/News/Statistics/2018/plastic-surgery-statistics-report-2018.pdf. https://www.plasticsurgery.org/documents/news/statistics/2024/plastic-surgery-statistics-report-2024.pdf.
13. Brown RH, Chang DK, Siy R, Friedman J. Trends in the surgical correction of gynecomastia. Semin Plast Surg. 2015;29(2):122–30. https://doi.org/10.1055/s-0035-1549053.
14. Pilanci O, Basaran K, Aydin HU, Cortuk O, Kuvat SV. Autologous fat injec tion into the pectoralis major as an adjunct to surgical correction of gynecomastia. Aesthetic Surg J. 2015;35(3):NP54–61. https://doi.org/10.1093/asj/sju015.
15. Al-Kalla T, Komorowska-Timek E. Breast total male breast reconstruction with fat grafting. Plast Reconstr Surg Glob Open. 2014;2(11):e257. https://doi.org/10.1097/GOX.0000000000000221.
16. Jakubietz RG, Jakubietz MG, Kloss D, Gruenert JG. Defining the basic aesthetics of the hand. Aesth Plast Surg. 2005;29(6):546–51. https://doi.org/10.1007/s00266-005-0100-6.
17. Fantozzi F. Hand rejuvenation with fat grafting: a 12-year single-surgeon experience. Eur J Plast Surg. 2017;40(5):457–64. https://doi.org/10.1007/s00238-017-1337-4.
18. Coleman SR. Hand rejuvenation with structural fat grafting. Plast Reconstr Surg. 2002;110(7):1731–44; discussion 1745-7. https://doi.org/10.1097/01.PRS.0000033936.43357.08.
19. Weiss D, Carraway J. Hand rejuvenation. Aesthetic Surg J. 2004;24(6):567–73. https://doi.org/10.1016/j.asj.2004.08.002.
20. Galea LA, Nicklin S. Mycobacterium abscessus infection complicating hand rejuvenation with structural fat grafting. J Plast Reconstr Aesthetic Surg. 2009;62(2):e15–6. https://doi.org/10.1016/j.bjps.2007.12.035.
21. Vara AD, Miki RA, Alfonso DT, Cardoso R. Hand fat grafting complicated by abscess: a case of a bilateral hand abscess from bilateral hand fat grafting. Hand. 2013;8(3):348–51. https://doi.org/10.1007/s11552-013-9508-7.
22. Farber SE, Minteer D, Gusenoff BR, Gusenoff JA. The influence of fat grafting on skin quality in cosmetic foot grafting: a randomized, cross-over clinical trial. Aesthetic Surg J. 2018;39(4):405–12. https://doi.org/10.1093/asj/sjy168.
23. Gusenoff JA, Mitchell RT, Jeong K, Wukich DK, Gusenoff BR. Autologous fat grafting for pedal fat pad atrophy: a prospective randomized clinical trial. Plast Reconstr Surg. 2016;138(5):1099–108. https://doi.org/10.1097/PRS.0000000000002667.
24. Morrison SD, Vyas KS, Motakef S, et al. Facial feminizationn: systematic review of the literature. Plast Reconstr Surg. 2016;137(6):1759–70. https://doi.org/10.1097/PRS.0000000000002171.
25. Burgess C, Awosika O. Ethnic and gender considerations in the use of facial injectables: male patients. Plast Reconstr Surg. 2015;136:28S–31S. https://doi.org/10.1097/prs.0000000000001813.
26. Sinno S, Mehta K, Reavey PL, Simmons C, Stuzin JM. Current trends in facial rejuvenation: an assessment of ASPS members' use of fat grafting during face lifting. Plast Reconstr Surg. 2015;136(1):20e–30e. https://doi.org/10.1097/PRS.0000000000001329.
27. Strong AL, Cederna PS, Rubin JP, Coleman SR, Levi B. The current state of fat grafting: a review of harvesting, processing, and injection techniques. Plast Reconstr Surg. 2015;136(4):897–912. https://doi.org/10.1097/PRS.0000000000001590.
28. Pezeshk RA, Stark RY, Small KH, Unger JG, Rohrich RJ. Role of autologous fat transfer to the superficial fat compartments for perioral rejuvenation. Plast Reconstr Surg. 2015;136(3):301e–9e. https://doi.org/10.1097/PRS.0000000000001506.
29. Basile FV, Basile AR. Prospective controlled study of chin augmentation by means of fat grafting. Plast Reconstr Surg. 2017;140(6):1133–41. https://doi.org/10.1097/PRS.0000000000003895.
30. Marten TJ, Elyassnia D. Fat grafting in facial rejuvenation. Clin Plast Surg. 2015;42(2):219–52. https://doi.org/10.1016/j.cps.2014.12.003.
31. Coleman SR. Structural fat grafting: more than a permanent filler. Plast Reconstr Surg. 2006;118(3 SUPPL):108–20. https://doi.org/10.1097/01.prs.0000234610.81672.e7.

32. Mallewa JE, Wilkins E, Vilar J, et al. HIV-associated lipodystrophy: a review of underlying mechanisms and therapeutic options. J Antimicrob Chemother. 2008;62(4):648–60. https://doi.org/10.1093/jac/dkn251.
33. Guaraldi G, De Fazio D, Orlando G, et al. Facial Lipohypertrophy in HIV-infected subjects who underwent autologous fat tissue transplantation. Clin Infect Dis. 2004;40(2):e13–5. https://doi.org/10.1086/426686.
34. Davison SP, Timpone J, Hannan CM. Surgical algorithm for management of HIV lipodystrophy. Plast Reconstr Surg. 2007;120(7):1843–58. https://doi.org/10.1097/01.prs.0000267341.14550.a7.
35. Reilly MJ, Burke KM, Davison SP. Wound infection rates in elective plastic surgery for HIV-positive patients. Plast Reconstr Surg. 2009;123(1):106–11. https://doi.org/10.1097/PRS.0b013e3181904dd9.

31 Muscular Augmentation in Males with Implants and BodyBanking Composite Lipocell Transfer

Douglas S. Steinbrech and Eduardo Gonzalez

31.1 Introduction to Muscular Augmentation in Males

In males, a muscular build is the principal dimorphic characteristic, and perhaps the only one aside from facial features. A muscular physique is representative of health, capacity to perform tasks, ability to interact with a hostile environment, endurance, and capability of physically caring for others. Furthermore, it also gives the perception of youth and fertility, as it is a result of healthy development of the testosterone-dependent secondary sexual characteristics.

The surgeon must be cognizant that, unlike female body contouring, the classic approach of creating transitions between slenderness and fullness is not applicable to male plastic surgery. The ideal male physique must deliver a muscular appearance, which consequently will also provide some projection and contour; nevertheless, the targeted visual impression must be one of virility and health. The contemporary plastic surgeon must be well versed in managing a male patient consultation, understanding the male aesthetic ideal, selecting a male-specific surgical technique, and considering muscular augmentation, if indicated, as a tool to get their patients closer to the male aesthetic ideal.

Safe and excellent aesthetic outcomes in muscular augmentation with implants are achieved by abiding by the following surgical principles: precise implant pocket dissection, maintaining excellent hemostasis, and watertight closure of the fascia overlying the implant. Perhaps the most critical of these factors is good control of the implant pocket. The biggest pitfall for the surgeon is over-dissection of the pocket, which will lead to implant malposition and migration. The pocket should be snug and slightly smaller than the implant itself; keep in mind that when the implant is inserted, it will expand the pocket further. The surgeon will know when an implant pocket is too small if it causes the implant to bend or the edges to curl; the implant can be removed, and the pocket carefully dissected further. Graded expansion of the pocket is always preferred to over-dissection. A useful strategy to achieve precise implant pocket dissection is to draw the implant footprint on the skin overlying it and to keep the dissection one to two millimeters short of it. Maintaining a bloodless field helps the surgeon have full visibility of the pocket and avoids postoperative hematomas and seromas. Hemostasis must be maintained prospectively as dissection is ongoing and checked prior to insert-

D. S. Steinbrech (✉)
Gotham Plastic Surgery, New York, NY, USA
e-mail: dss@steinbrech.com

E. Gonzalez
Private Practice in Dnever, CO, USA

K. Jeffords et al. (eds.), *Aesthetic Surgery for Men*, https://doi.org/10.1007/978-3-032-03840-1_31

ing the implant. Local anesthetic (1% lidocaine, 1:100,000 epinephrine) is used at all incision sites and is a key step in achieving dry dissection in a bloodless field; at least 10 min of dwelling time is allowed after infiltration. Lastly, the skin incision must not lie directly above the fascial incision on the muscle and be kept as far away as possible by subcutaneous tunneling—this decreases the possibility of implant extrusion and/or implant contamination if a superficial surgical site infection occurs.

Muscular enhancement in males can be achieved with several plastic surgery techniques of augmentation and body contouring. Pertaining to this chapter, the authors will focus on muscular enhancement through silicone implant placement with adjunctive "fat grafting" in the way of BodyBanking as previously described by the senior author. This composite approach is very powerful: while implants provide volume and subsequent projection, BodyBanking allows for fine-tuning of aesthetic focal points and enhancement of light reflection transitions. For example, in chest augmentation with pectoral implants, the sought-after central pectoral inscription on the sternum can be enhanced with BodyBanking for a very dramatic result, which is difficult to achieve solely with implants. Of note, the senior author (D.S.) feels strongly that we as a medical aesthetic and reconstructive community need to move away from the term "fat grafting" as it connotes the transplantation of jelly-like globule parcels of gelatinous material into a new area, resulting in flabby contours. In contradistinction to this patient perception, we must educate the public that "lipocells" are isolated from undesired areas to be processed and transferred to new desired areas for structure and beefy volume. "Lipocell" is the preferred term, as lipocytes give the patient a fear that the cell is a type of foreign invader, such as a parasite.

In the following sections of this chapter, the authors describe the surgically relevant anatomy and preoperative considerations in males, followed by a "bullet-step" description of the surgical technique for each muscle group, as well as postoperative care and management of complications.

31.2 Surgical Anatomy

The plastic surgeon must have a thorough understanding of the skeletal, neurovascular, muscular, and fascial anatomy of the extremities and torso in order to achieve an optimal aesthetic result while avoiding complications. In this section, we will point out distinct anatomical features pertaining to males, as well as the surgical landmarks the senior author utilizes for staying safe.

31.2.1 Pectoral Anatomy

Male chest aesthetics are predominantly defined by the shape and development of the pectoralis major muscles. A muscular male chest exhibits superior fullness with a transition to a flat inferior chest at the level of the infra-pectoral fold and medially over the central sternum. The lateral edge of the pectoralis muscle extends upward from the linea semilunaris to the anterior axillary line. The pectoralis major is divided into clavicular and sternocostal heads. The clavicular head originates from the anterior border of the medial half of the clavicle, while the sternocostal head originates from the anterior surface of the sternum, the superior six costal cartilages, and the aponeurosis of the anterior rectus sheath and external oblique muscle. The fibers converge to insert on the anteromedial proximal humerus along the lateral lip of the bicipital groove. The pectoral branch of the thoracoacromial artery and perforating vessels from the internal mammary artery provide blood supply to the pectoralis major. The lower two-thirds of the pectoralis major muscle are innervated by the medial pectoral nerve, which is closely associated with the lateral thoracic vessels. The medial pectoral nerve is at risk for injury during lateral sub-pectoral dissection, as it passes through or around the pectoralis minor muscle to enter the pectoralis major along the inferolateral border. The lateral pectoral nerve travels more superiorly with the thoracoacromial vessels and innervates the upper third of the pectoralis major muscle. This nerve may also be damaged during more superior sub-pectoral dissection. The pectoralis minor is a thin triangular muscle beneath the pectoralis major. It arises from the superolateral surfaces of ribs 3 through 5 and inserts onto the medial border of the coracoid process of the scapula. Arterial supply is derived from the pectoral branch of the thoracoacromial artery, and the medial pectoral nerve provides innervation.

31.2.2 Biceps and Triceps Anatomy

The upper arm is conceptualized into anterior and posterior muscular compartments, which are separated by the medial and lateral intermuscular septa and humerus. The anterior compartment contains the biceps brachii, brachialis, and coracobrachialis. The posterior compartment contains the triceps brachii muscle. The deep fascia of the arm overlies the biceps and is a continuation of the fascia overlying the deltoid and pectoralis major muscles. Distally, the fascia becomes the strong intermuscular septa to the medial and lateral aspects that separate the anterior and posterior compartments of the arm. The biceps muscle is composed of two heads: short and long, which converge into a single unit. The short head of the biceps originates from the coracoid process at the superior aspect of the scapula. The long head originates from the supraglenoid tubercle. The long head has a tendon that courses up along the intertubercular groove of the humerus into the joint capsule of the shoulder. The tendon of the short head runs adjacent to the tendon of the coracobrachialis and attaches to the coracoid process. Both heads join in the middle of the humerus to form a single muscle mass near the insertion of the deltoid, forming a common muscle belly. Distally, the biceps ends in two tendons: the radial tuberosity on the radius and the bicipital aponeurosis, which radiates into the ulnar part of the antebrachial fascia. The distal biceps tendons are completely separated in 40% and bifurcated in 25% of cases. The brachial artery is the continuation of the axillary artery beyond the lower margin of the teres major muscle and provides the major blood supply to the biceps. The venous drainage of the upper extremity is provided by the cephalic vein along with the basilic vein. Fibers of the fifth and sixth cervical nerves make up the components of the musculocutaneous nerve, which supply motor innervation to the biceps. The lateral antebrachial cutaneous nerve is a continuation of the musculocutaneous nerve and runs in the submuscular region and providing sensory innervation to the skin overlying the lateral arm. This nerve is at risk for injury during submuscular implant biceps augmentation. The medial antebrachial cutaneous nerve is derived from the medial cord of the brachial plexus and provides sensory innervation to the skin overlying the medial arm. The ulnar nerve is located in the medial extra-compartmental location and runs along the posteromedial aspect of the humerus. Great care must be taken not to injure the ulnar nerve when performing submuscular dissection. The biceps work across three joints: the proximal radioulnar, the humeroulnar, and the glenohumeral joint. The most important of these functions is to flex the elbow and supinate the forearm. The triceps have three heads: long, lateral, and medial. The long head, the most superficial of the three, arises from the infraglenoid tubercle of the scapula. It extends distally and anteriorly to the teres minor and posteriorly to the teres major. The medial head arises distally from the groove of the radial nerve, from the dorsal surface of the humerus, and from the medial intermuscular septum; its distal part also arises from the lateral intermuscular septum. The medial head is mostly covered by the lateral and long heads and is only visible distally on the humerus. The lateral head arises from the dorsal surface of the humerus, lateral and proximal to the groove of the radial nerve, from the greater tubercle down to the region of the lateral intermuscular septum. The three heads of the triceps then converge into one tendon that begins and inserts into the posterior portion of the olecranon of the ulna. All three heads of the triceps brachii are innervated by the radial nerve, which arises from the seventh and eighth cranial nerves. In some cases, the long head of the triceps brachii is innervated by a branch of the axillary nerve. The radial nerve is located deep within the posterior compartment adjacent to the posterior aspect of the humerus and medial head of the triceps. The radial nerve and two of its smaller cutaneous branches, the posterior cutaneous nerve of the arm and the dorsal antebrachial cutaneous nerve, are at risk for injury. Great care should be taken not to injure the radial nerve and its branches when performing a submuscular dissection. The triceps is an extensor muscle of the elbow joint and an antagonist of the biceps and brachialis muscles. The lateral head is used for movements requiring occasional high-intensity force, while the medial fascicle enables more precise, low-force movements. The long head also acts on the shoulder joint and is involved in retroversion and adduction of the arm.

31.2.3 The Forearm Anatomy

The anatomy of the anterior (volar) forearm consists of muscles that are conceptualized into three planes: superficial, intermediate, and deep. These muscle groups are responsible for hand and finger flexion and pronation. Most of the topography of the anterior forearm is based on the superficial muscles. Specifically, these muscles include the pronator teres, the flexor carpi radialis, palmaris longus, and flexor carpi ulnaris. For medial forearm augmentation, this is the muscle group that the implant pocket is dissected into. In addition, the brachioradialis is a superficial muscle on the radial side of the forearm that acts as a flexor of the elbow. The brachioradialis gives definition to the radial aspect of the anterior forearm. Analogous to the anterior forearm, the anatomy of the posterior forearm consists of muscles that are conceptualized into three planes: superficial, middle, and deep. Again, the topography is based on the muscles of the superficial layer, including the digitorum communis, the extensor carpi ulnaris, and the extensor digiti minimi. For lateral forearm augmentation, this is the muscle group that the implant pocket is dissected into. With the exception of superficial veins and sensory nerves, the major neurovascular structures are found deep to the aforementioned superficial layer of the anterior and posterior muscle groups. In the superficial place between the subcutaneous tissue and the superficial fascial system, the cephalic vein and its tributaries lie radially, the basilic vein and its tributaries lie ulnar, while the lateral antebrachial cutaneous nerve lies radially following the cephalic nerve, and the medial antebrachial cutaneous nerve lies ulnar following the basilic vein. When performing subcutaneous dissection in the forearm, care must be taken not to injure the cephalic or basilic veins, as this results in significant venous bleeding, and not to injure the medial or lateral antebrachial cutaneous nerves, as this results in anesthesia of the medial and lateral aspect of the volar forearm, respectively.

31.2.4 The Abdominal Anatomy

The rectus abdominis is a paired muscle extending from the xiphoid and costal cartilages of the fifth to seventh ribs superiorly to the pubis inferiorly. The muscle is encased in an anterior sheath along its entire course, as well as posterior sheath superiorly to the level of the arcuate line. Its blood supply arises from the bilateral superior and inferior epigastric arteries, while it is innervated by segmental thoracolumbar spinal nerves meeting the muscle on its posterolateral surface. Three to four transverse tendinous inscriptions typically divide the muscle into three to four muscular sections on each side. These inscriptions are often present at the level of the xiphoid, the umbilicus, as well as at a level halfway between these two landmarks. The marked transition between these tendinous inscriptions and well-developed rectus muscle fibers results in the sought-after contoured and indented abdomen of young athletic males. Laterally, the rectus abdominis joins the oblique musculature at the linea semilunaris bilaterally. An aesthetic, concave gutter extends from the origin of the rectus abdominis on the pubis, extending toward the flanks, and may be accentuated using adjunctive liposuction. The natural shadows along the linea semilunaris offer an excellent site for a single, small access incision, allowing for upper implant placement. The umbilicus is preferred for lower abdominal implant placement given its inconspicuous scarring.

31.2.5 The Gluteal Anatomy

The buttocks region should be conceptualized as a frame of bony structures that support the gluteal musculature through ligaments and fascial planes, which ultimately attach to the skin, resulting in the characteristic aesthetic contours (Fig. 31.1). The external landmarks of this frame in a clock-wise orientation are: the sacral triangle at the midline which is defined by the paired posterior superior iliac spines (PSIS) cephalad (as the base of the inverted triangle) and the coccyx caudally (as the tip of the triangle); parting from the PSIS's, the iliac crests then continue as an arch in a cephalad, anterior (ventral), and lateral direction; the highest point of the iliac crest defines the cephalad limit of the bony frame of the buttocks which intersects the axis of the apex of the scapula; the most lateral aspect of the frame is marked by the greater trochanter of the femur to which tendinous muscular insertions define the distinctive lateral trochanteric depression desired in males; caudally, the ischial tuberosity defines the most inferior extent of the osseous frame of the buttocks. This bony frame not only provides sites of insertion for the important gluteal musculature but also connects with the skin of the buttocks through osteo-cutaneous ligaments. Two of these ligaments are noted, both of which originate at midline: the sacro-cutaneous ligament and the ischio-cutaneous ligament. The sacro-cutaneous ligament originates at the lateral border of the sacrum and is densely attached to the skin overlying it; it then extends as an arch superolaterally to interdigitate with the adhesions of the iliac crest periosteum to the dermis. Through descriptions of cadaveric studies, Lockwood reported that this sacro-cutaneous ligament is more adherent in males compared to females; this results in a pronounced transition between the sacral triangle and the gluteal upper pole that is characteristic of an aesthetic male physique. The ischio-cutaneous ligament is fan-shaped and originates from the ischial tuberosity to extend toward the dermis of the mid-buttocks. As it fans supero-medially, it merges with the fascio-cutaneous ligament of the natal cleft, and as it fans infero-laterally, it merges with the fascio-cutaneous ligament of the infra-gluteal crease. There are three aesthetic focal points of the buttocks that result from fascio-cutaneous adherences. The natal cleft medially, the trochanteric depression laterally, and the infra-gluteal crease caudally. In 1989, Illouz characterized

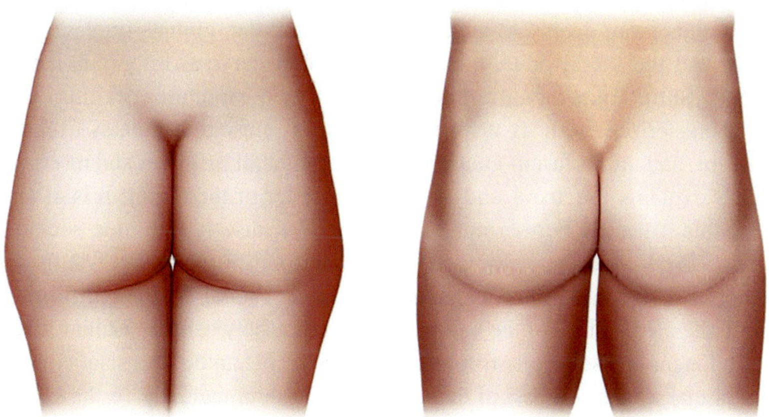

Fig. 31.1 Contrasting features of the buttocks relationships between females and males that lead to their dimorphic aesthetics. In females, the waist-to-hip ratio leads to the hourglass silhouette, while in males, the muscular projection and definition of the gluteus muscle result in an aesthetic appeal. In males, note the visible trochanteric depressions, the tall buttocks in which the projection of the upper pole of the gluteus musculature continues cephalad toward the lumbar region well beyond the beginning of the gluteal cleft. The gluteal cleft in males is shorter than in females, and the inferior gluteal crease in males is limited to the inner third of the breadth of the buttocks, while in females it occupies the inner half, approximating the meridian of the buttocks

these zones as "fixed points" that should not be surgically disrupted, as they cannot be recreated. Lockwood subsequently characterized them as "zones of adherence" of the superficial fascial system to the dermis. These fascio-cutaneous tissues take the form of septa that encase, support, and shape the adipose tissue, and can be used to the surgeon's advantage during liposculpting; parenthetically, they are thicker in males compared to females. At the midline, the natal cleft fascio-cutaneous adherence extends from the gluteal fascia (i.e., the deep fascial plane, which in this location corresponds to the aponeurosis of the gluteus maximus) to the dermis, merging cephalad with the sacro-cutaneous ligament and caudally with the ischio-cutaneous ligament. Laterally, the trochanteric depression is formed by the ligamentous and tendinous attachments of the gluteus medius, vastus lateralis, quadratus femoris, and gluteus maximus muscles to the greater trochanter of the femur as they approximate the superficial fascial system, with minimal adipose tissue in between these planes. The important infra-gluteal crease is a unique structure that, unlike prior assumptions, is distinct from the superficial fascial system. It originates from the dermis of the medial one-third of the lower buttocks, forming a heavy and thick septum that not only interdigitates with the gluteal fascia but also extends more deeply to attach to the ischial ramus and the sacral bone, taking a horizontal J-shaped form. Thus, the infra-gluteal crease can be characterized both as an osteo-cutaneous ligament and as a fascio-cutaneous adherence, which explains the fixed and well-defined nature of this structure. Furthermore, the infra-gluteal crease is a key aesthetic component of the male buttocks. The definition of its length should not exceed the medial third of the width of the buttocks, as a longer crease results from skin redundancy, lax fascial planes, and loss of muscle mass, suggesting a ptotic and aged buttocks. Once the reader can delineate the patient's bony frame, as well as the osteo-cutaneous and fascio-cutaneous planes, the musculature can be conceptualized as occurring within this scaffold. The most superficial muscle of this group is the gluteus maximus which is the body's thickest muscle (approximately 4–7 cm); it originates from the lateral coccyx, lateral sacrum, sacro-tuberous ligament, fascia of the erector spinae, posterior ilium, and the medial third of the posterior iliac crest; it runs a caudo-lateral course with its superficial fibers inserting to the ilio-tibial tract and the deeper fibers inserting to the gluteal tuberosity of the femur. The gluteus medius muscle originates from the lateral two-thirds of the iliac crest, inserting on the greater trochanter of the femur. It is immediately deep to the gluteus maximus, except for its origin at the iliac crest, where it resides uncovered by the gluteus maximus. Beyond this point, the two muscles interdigitate and can only be differentiated by the course of their fibers. The fibers of gluteus maximus are identified running obliquely, while the deeper fibers of the gluteus medius are identified running vertically. The gluteus minimus lies deep to the gluteus medius, and has a similar course originating from the gluteal surface of the ilium with vertically oriented fibers inserting to the hip joint capsule and greater trochanter of the femur. A group of smaller muscles deep to the gluteus minimus consists of the piriformis (most cephalad), followed by the gemellus superior, obturator internus, gemellus inferior, and quadratus femoris (most caudally). These muscles are not routinely encountered during dissection for intramuscular gluteal implant placement; however, they serve as important landmarks for neurovascular structures exiting the pelvis. The piriform muscle originates from the sacrum and sacro-tuberal ligament and inserts into the greater trochanter of the femur; it is of anatomic importance because it splits the sciatic foramen. The sciatic nerve exits the pelvis through the sciatic foramen caudal to the piriformis muscle, at a midpoint between the ischial tuberosity and the greater trochanter. The sciatic nerve then courses laterally and caudally to the pelvic acetabulum, which can be palpated intraoperatively for orientation. The superior gluteal artery exits in a cephalad direction to the piriformis muscle, dividing into a superficial and deep branch; the superficial branch courses along the deep surface of the gluteus maximus muscle, while the deep branch courses between the gluteus medius and minimus muscles. This trajectory of the superior gluteal artery can be traced along an axis from the PSIS to the greater trochanter of the femur. The inferior gluteal artery emerges caudally to the piriformis muscle, coursing along the deep aspect of the gluteus maximus, toward the posterior thigh. The superior and inferior gluteal veins follow the respective gluteal arteries into the pelvis, where they join the pelvic venous plexus. In addition to preoperative markings of the aesthetic focal points and the areas to be addressed with lipectomy, the surgeon must identify external landmarks that delineate a safety triangle on each buttock. The apex of each triangle is the PSIS, with the lateral point located at the greater trochanter, and the medial point at the ischial tuberosity. It is within this triangle that the gluteal vessels and the sciatic nerve course, with lipocell transfer needing to be superficial to the gluteal fascia in this safety zone. Buttocks augmentation should be framed within these anatomic landmarks, which not only assures safety but also enhances gluteal aesthetics. In males, augmenting beyond these aesthetic focal points, or blunting them, will result in an augmented, but less muscular, endomorphic appearance.

31.2.6 The Calf Anatomy

The lower leg musculature is conceptualized into four compartments divided by fascial septae: anterior compartment (tibialis anterior, extensor digitorum longus, peroneus brevis), lateral compartment (peroneus longus), posterior deep compartment (flexor digitorum longus, tibialis posterior, flexor hallucis longus), and posterior superficial compartment (soleus, gastrocnemius). The contour of the calf is the result of the volume provided mostly by the gastrocnemius and soleus muscles, which are the largest muscles of the lower leg. The gastrocnemius muscle lies superficial to the soleus muscle and has two muscle belly heads each of which has tendinous insertions into the medial and lateral condyles of the femur. The medial head of the gastrocnemius is larger than the lateral head. The medial and lateral head fibers converge at the midline and form a broad aponeurosis that merges with the soleus tendon, forming the Achilles tendon, which inserts into the calcaneus. The small saphenous vein courses at the midline between the two heads of the gastrocnemius and runs superficially in the superficial fascial system; injury during dissection is avoided by retracting this structure either medially or laterally. The medial and lateral sural cutaneous nerves can also be encountered in this plane and typically follow the course of the small saphenous vein.

31.3 Preoperative Considerations and Markings

Preoperative physical examination is key to achieving an ideal aesthetic outcome and precise implant selection. During the preoperative evaluation, the following is reviewed with the patient: the degree of desired augmentation, any asymmetries present at baseline, skin firmness and soft tissue laxity, adipose padding overlying muscle group to be augmented, and incision location. For patients undergoing "six pack" abdominal enhancement, the surgeon must perform a comprehensive abdominal exam, palpating for rectus diastasis, peri-umbilical hernias, ventral hernias, Spigelian hernias, as well as prior hernia repair scars and laparoscopy scars, as this can preclude safe and adequate implant pocket dissection.

Several key principles hold true for preoperative marking of patients undergoing muscular augmentation regardless of body location. The surgeon should be sitting down with the patient standing at arms-length from the surgeon in order to allow for appreciation of whole-body perspective, symmetry, and light reflection on aesthetic focal points.

The midline should always be marked as well as cardinal lines, such as the anterior axillary line. Condensations of the dermis to the superficial fascial system should also be marked, such as the infra-pectoral and infra-gluteal folds. The origin, insertion, and borders of the muscle groups to be augmented are then marked. Examination of the muscles to be augmented is done in both contraction and repose.

For the pectoralis muscle, its medial insertion to the sternum determines the most medial extent of the implant pocket and is identified and marked by asking the patient to flex the pectoralis with his hands on his hips. Note that the pectoralis muscle's origin at the sternum is not exactly at the midline but rather appx. 1.0 cm lateral to it. Defining this preoperatively is critical to achieve the sought-after central inscription at the sternum seen after a well-planned pectoral augmentation. The lateral border of the pectoralis major is identified and marked by abducting the patient's arm and then raising it over the head.

For upper arm muscular augmentation, the origin and insertions of the biceps and triceps muscle bellies are palpated, marked, and measured. These markings determine the maximum length of the implant pocket. Measure bilateral arm circumference at mid-portion of the arm in both flexion and repose in order to determine the degree of muscular hypoplasia.

For biceps, triceps, and forearm augmentation, the patient's skin and subcutaneous tissue must be examined for laxity and expected tolerance of the implant size. Compartment syndrome is a described complication of upper extremity muscle implant augmentation. Younger and more muscular patients have firmer skin and soft tissues. When both biceps and triceps augmentation is desired, if examination reveals firm dermis and soft tissues, staging is recommended. Likewise, when medial and lateral forearm augmentation is desired, staging is also recommended. For calf augmentation, the implant can be placed in either the lateral or medial head of the gastrocnemius. More commonly, the medial gastrocnemius is augmented, as its contour is more visible, leading to a more dramatic result. If desired, lateral augmentation can be performed at a second stage; this allows for greater augmentation while avoiding the risk of lower leg compartment syndrome. Staging is not only a safe approach, but also allows for greater augmentation, which patients appreciate as a trade-off for a second procedure. A useful strategy is to educate the patient on the value of placing multiple implants, which are not "competing for soft-tissue space." A typical scenario the senior author reviews with patients is as follows: stage 1: biceps, pectoral, medial forearm, medial calf; stage 2: triceps, lateral forearm, lateral calf. Furthermore, implantation of the extremities should be avoided in patients with a history or physical exam findings of venous insufficiency or peripheral artery disease.

When marking the abdomen for "six-pack" enhancement, the linea alba along the midline is marked, as well as the linea semilunaris and the transverse tendinous inscriptions of the rectus abdominis muscle. Note that significant asymmetry often exists among the native tendinous inscriptions of the rectus abdominis, and these may be exacerbated after implant placement and/or liposuction; such asymmetries must be brought to the attention of the patient and documented.

For gluteal augmentation, the following anatomical landmarks are marked: midline along the lumbar spinous processes, the sacral triangle, posterior superior iliac spines, iliac crests, infragluteal creases, and lateral trochanters.

After marking the midline, cardinal lines, superficial fascial and dermis condensations, tendinous inscriptions, bony landmarks, and muscle insertions, the planned implant pocket must be delineated over the muscle group to be augmented. Perhaps this is the most critical marking, as it determines the implant pocket, which controls projection and symmetry. Either an implant template or an implant sizer is placed on the skin overlying the muscle group to be augmented, and the footprint of the implant is then marked on the skin with a dotted line. The footprint of the implant pocket can then be adjusted to account for any asymmetry.

Preoperative photography is critical for surgical planning, educating the patient on expected results, for postoperative comparison, and for medico-legal documentation. Photographs should encompass 360-degree views, with arms up and arms down, and should be taken with the patient in flexed and repose positions in order to highlight the musculature and aesthetic focal points.

For pectoral and gluteal implants, general endotracheal anesthesia is preferred as paralysis allows for adequate retraction of the musculature, optimizing dissection of the pocket. For biceps, triceps, forearm, and calf implants, local anesthetic with or without sedation is adequate. Cefazolin, or clindamycin, is administered intravenously prior to induction as prophylaxis. In the operating room, the patient undergoes standing chlorhexidine prep. Stockinettes over venodynes are placed for venous thromboembolism prophylaxis. When performing gluteal augmentation and abdominal contouring, the patient lies down on sterile drapes. If the patient needs to be prone, a crossing sterile Mayo stand cover is used as a "draw sheet," and after induction and intubation by the anesthesiologist is then undertaken and airway is secured, and the patient is rotated onto a prone position using the sterile draw sheet. Safety while mobilizing anesthetized patients is approached as a "team effort" by verbalizing the specific role of each team member. Areas of potential pressure are padded and checked every time the patient is repositioned.

31.4 Chest Augmentation with Pectoral Implants

- A 3–4 cm incision is placed along a natural crease in the hair-bearing area of the axilla with the patient's arm abducted to 90°.
- Carry out a very superficial subcutaneous dissection using scissors and electrocautery directed to the lateral border of the pectoralis muscle, avoiding the axillary contents.
- Once the lateral border of the pectoralis major is defined, blunt finger dissection is performed under the muscle edge to develop an intermuscular plane between the pectoralis major and minor. A lighted retractor is inserted. Using an Agris–Dingman dissector, blunt submuscular dissection is performed to open the potential space under the pectoralis major.
- The Agris–Dingman dissector is then re-inserted to confirm that the dissected pocket matches the planned implant dimensions.
- It is preferable to have the implant higher rather than lower, and the pocket should be designed with that in mind.
- The inferior edge of the implant should lie immediately under the inferior aspect of the areola. In male aesthetics, the inferior pectoral fold, which lies immediately below the inferior border of the areola, corresponds with the inferior insertion of the pectoralis major, and augmentation below this point will result in a "high nipple" and in a full, but not muscular, appearance of the chest. The inferior pectoral fold in males and the inframammary fold in females are not analogous structures.
- An endoscope is then used to visualize the medial and inferior insertions of the pectoralis muscle, and these are selectively released with cautery under direct visualization.
- The implant pocket is irrigated with betadine, triple-antibiotic, and bupivacaine.
- Change gloves for a "no touch" technique.
- The Pectoral implant (AART, Carson City, NV) should be selected based on height and weight of patient and the desired projection. The implant may be custom trimmed for best fit and to accommodate anatomic asymmetries (Fig. 31.2).

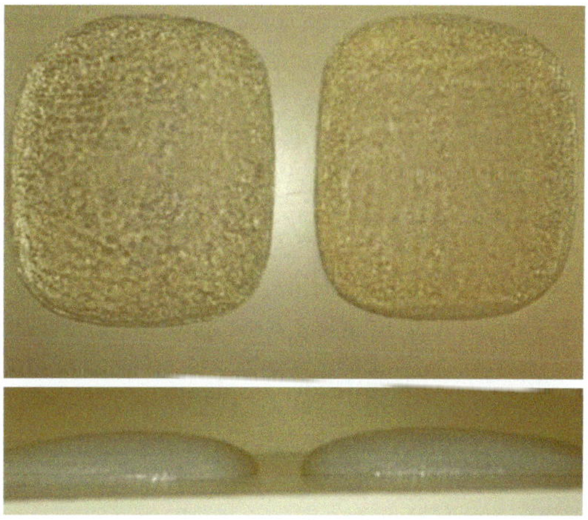

Fig. 31.2 Anterior and inferior view of a soft, solid pectoral implant (AART, Alpha Male Aesthetics, Carson City, NV). The square shape allows an appropriate fit for the intermuscular pocket between the pectoralis major and minor. The implant may be custom trimmed based on the unique anatomy of the patient

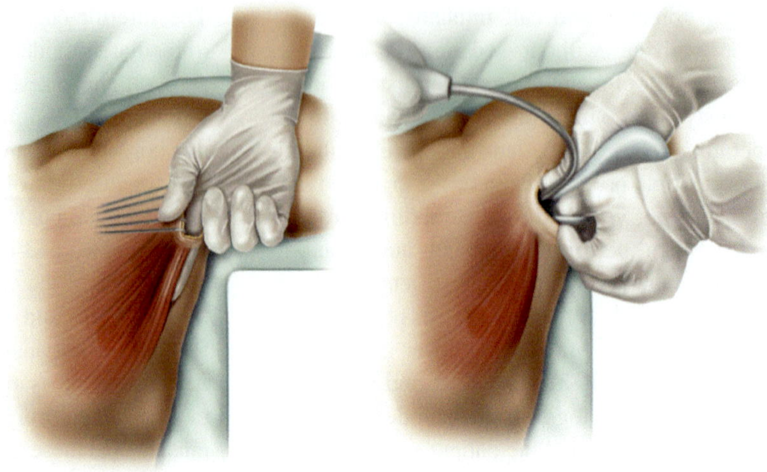

Fig. 31.3 With the assistant supplying retraction, gentle blunt finger dissection allows the surgeon to gain access to the intermuscular plane between the pectoralis major and minor (left panel). Insertion of gently folded silicone pectoral implant (right panel)

- An 8-mm notch is cut in the superolateral corner of the implant for orientation; the implant is folded like a "taco" and inserted carefully into the implant pocket; the Agris-Dingman dissector is re-inserted to correct any folds in the implant (Fig. 31.3).
- Once both sides of the chest have been implanted, the patient is seated upright to confirm adequate implant orientation and that the chest wall overall appears symmetric (Fig. 31.4).
- Although the senior author no longer utilizes drains, bilateral 10-mm drains may be placed directly superficial to the implant.
- Hemostasis within the subcutaneous tunnel must be assured using the lighted retractor prior to closure.
- The lateral pectoral border is reapproximated to the chest wall with interrupted 2–0 Vicryl (Johnson & Johnson, New Brunswick, NJ) to prevent lateral implant displacement. At this point, the senior author elects to take large bites in incorporating the corner of the implant with a loose tethering figure of eight to secure the implant into position.
- Reapproximate deep subcutaneous layer with a 3–0 Vicryl suture.

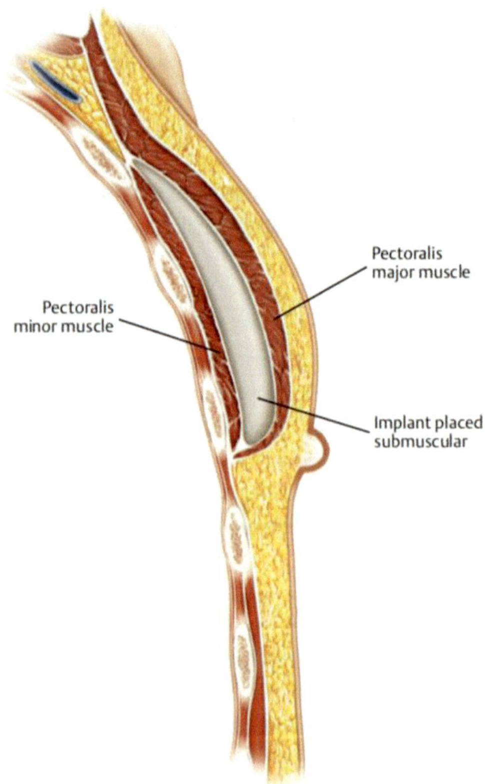

Fig. 31.4 Implant located at intermuscular plane between pectoralis major and pectoralis minor

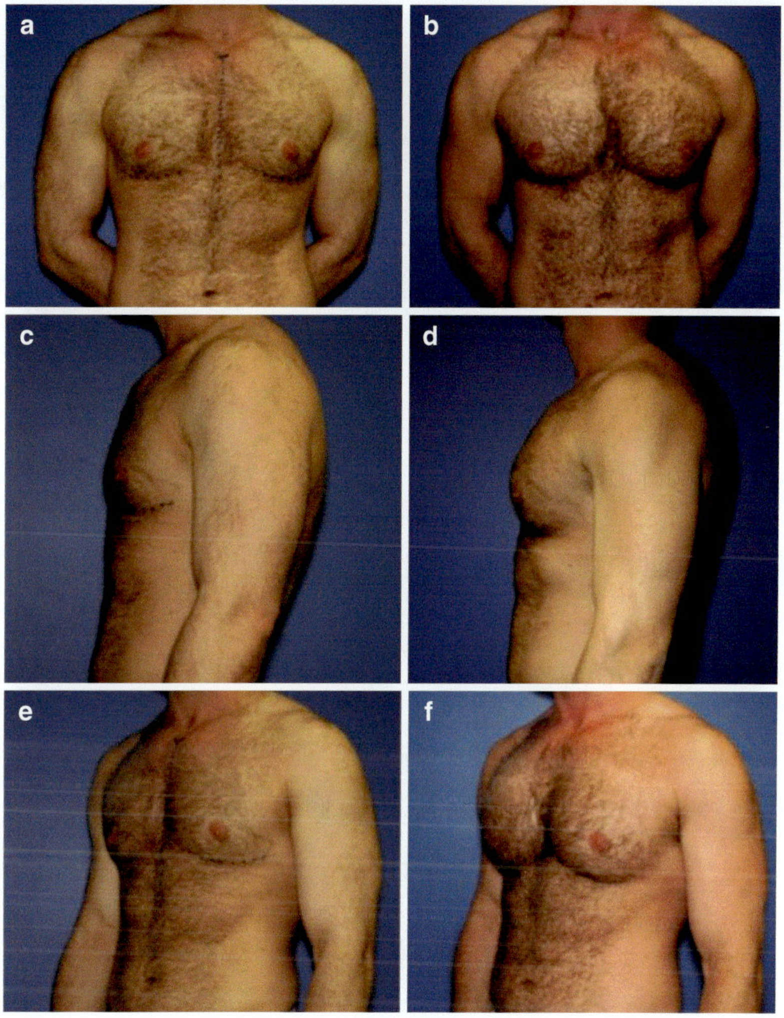

Fig. 31.5 A 36-year-old, 5 feet 10 inches, 215-pound, ecto-mesomorphic male who underwent endoscopic intermuscular pectoral implantation with a 385-cc silicone implant. Postoperative results at 16 months demonstrate increased volume with a natural contour and no visible incision

- Reapproximate skin with a running 3–0 Monocryl subcuticular suture.
- BodyBanking with lipocell transfer is then performed (see section below) at the recipient sites overlying the implanted muscles that were marked preoperatively (Fig. 31.5).

31.5 Upper Arm Augmentation with Bicep and Tricep Implants

- A 3–4 cm incision is placed along a natural crease in the hair-bearing area of the axilla with the patient's arm abducted to 90°.
- Carry out subcutaneous dissection using scissors and electrocautery, avoiding the axillary contents; when placing biceps implants, direct the subcutaneous tunnel toward the septum between the long and short head of the biceps muscle (Fig. 31.6); when placing triceps implants, direct the subcutaneous tunnel toward the long head of the triceps muscle (Fig. 31.7).
- Identify the glistening muscle fascia by sweeping areolar inter-fascial tissue with a peanut.
- Mark a 3-cm fascial incision and incise sharply with scalpel.

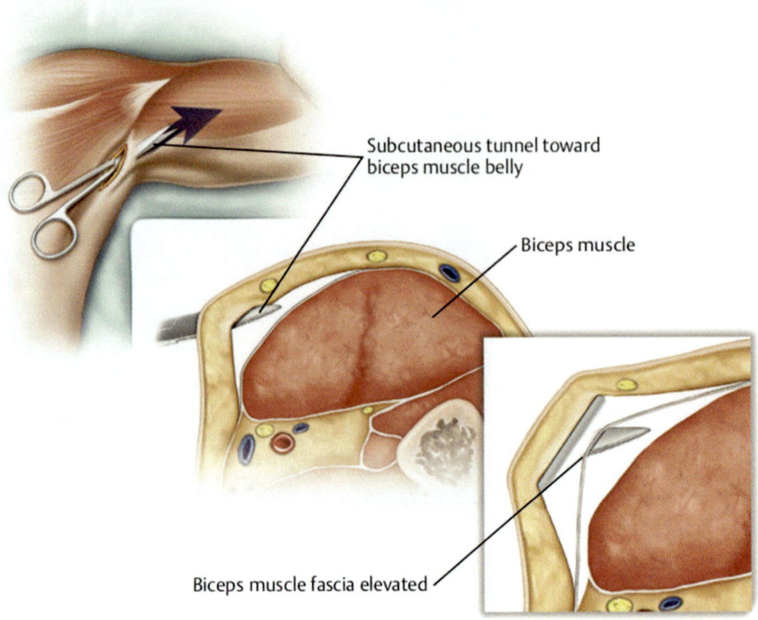

Fig. 31.6 While the assistant is retracting with an Army-Navy, the surgeon tunnels subcutaneously via areolar planes to the fascia of the biceps. A 2.5-cm longitudinal incision is made in the biceps fascia, and the fascia is gently teased away locally and minimally from the muscle with a tonsil clamp

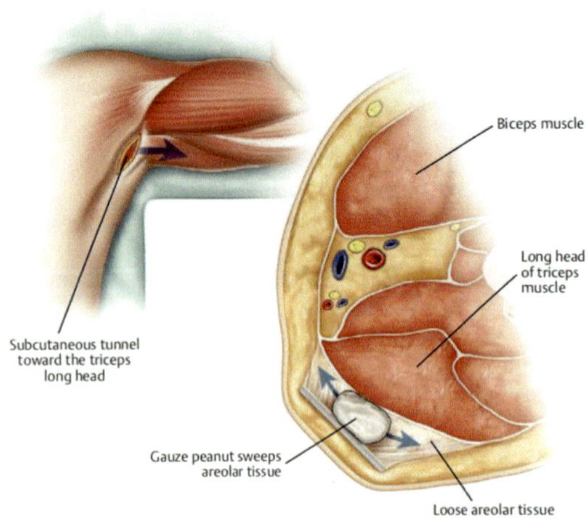

Fig. 31.7 After the standard axillary incision is made, subcutaneous dissection is carried out by sweeping the areolar tissue and then further sweeping with a gauze peanut to clean the glistening fascia off the long head of the triceps. A subsequent 3 cm axial incision is made on the fascia of the long head of the triceps, and the fascia is gently teased away locally from the underlying muscle

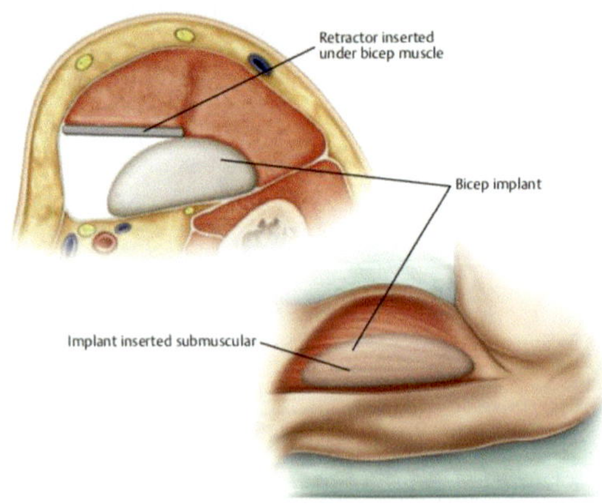

Fig. 31.8 As the assistant retracts with a narrow Deaver retractor, the surgeon folds the implant gently and maneuvers the "round bottom" (distal end) of the tear-shaped biceps implant first to result in the distal portion of the pocket

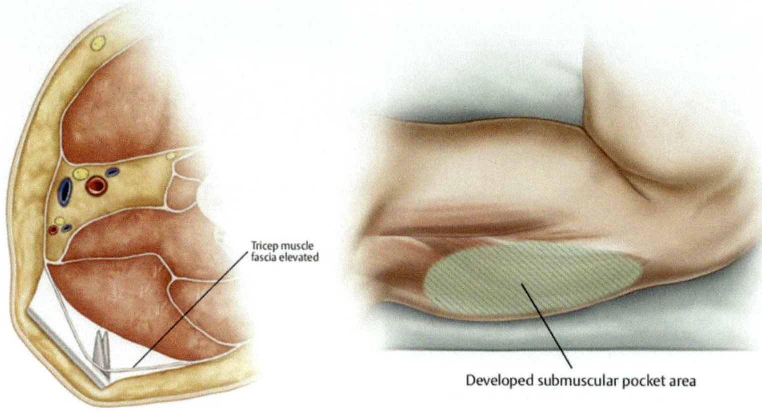

Fig. 31.9 While the assistant retracts with a lighted submental retractor, an S-retractor, or an Army-Navy, the surgeon progressively opens the sub-fascial pocket using blunt pocket dissection, implementing serial urethral sounds. A curved Deaver or a malleable ribbon retractor may be helpful in extending the sub-fascial pocket dissection. Principles of "precise pocket dissection" are employed

- Elevate the fascia and place 3–0 Vicryl stay sutures (Johnson & Johnson, New Brunswick, NJ) for subsequent closure.
- With a tonsil clamp, dissect a subfascial pocket for the triceps; for the biceps, gently tease between the muscle fibers for a submuscular pocket.
- Use progressive, judicial pocket expansion with urethral sounds.
- Do not over-dissect the respective pockets; with biceps implants, be mindful not to dissect the submuscular biceps pocket too anteriorly (Fig. 31.8); with triceps implants, be mindful not to dissect the subfascial pocket too distally (Fig. 31.9).
- Insert curved 2-cm-wide retractor.
- The implant pocket is irrigated with betadine, triple-antibiotic, and bupivacaine.
- Change gloves for a "no touch" technique.
- Implant (AART, Carson City, NV) may be custom carved as needed and is placed folded like a "taco," to avoid fracture of the implant (point of the tear-drop is proximal; fat belly distal).
- Manually range the elbow in order to ensure adequate dynamic implant position within the muscle complex.
- Tie the previously placed 3–0 Vicryl sutures (Johnson & Johnson, New Brunswick, NJ) on the muscle fascia.
- Hemostasis within the subcutaneous tunnel must be assured prior to closure.
- Reapproximate deep subcutaneous layer with a 3–0 Vicryl suture.
- Reapproximate skin with a running 3–0 Monocryl subcuticular suture (Figs. 31.10 and 31.11).

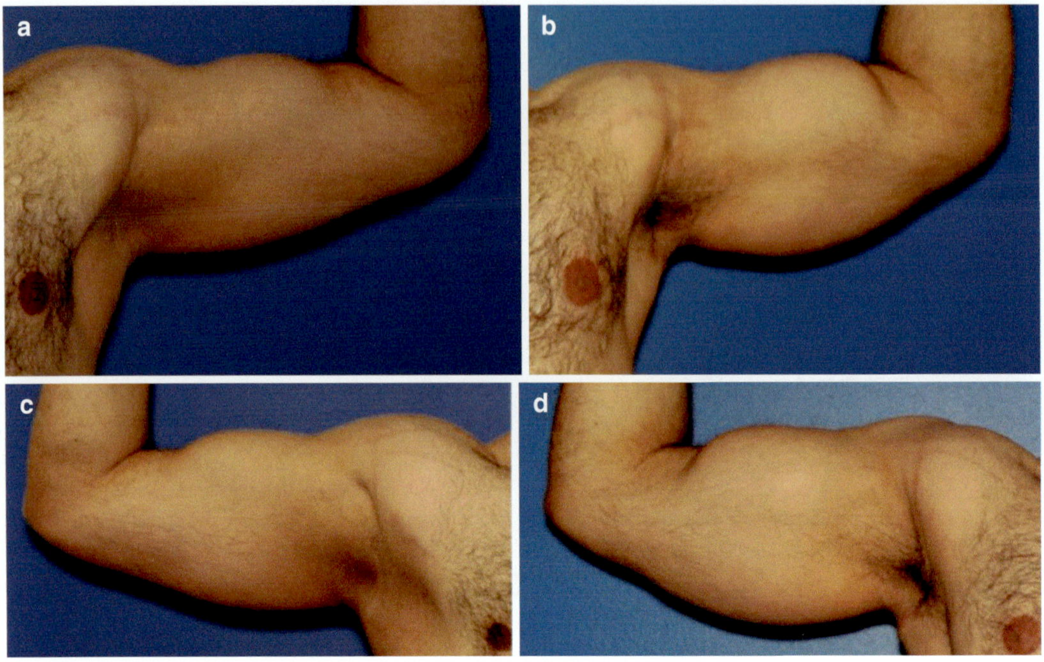

Fig. 31.10 A 43-year-old, 5 feet 10 inches, 205-pound, meso-endomorphic male underwent submuscular bicep implantation with a 146-cc custom-contoured, tear-shaped MuscleGel silicone implant

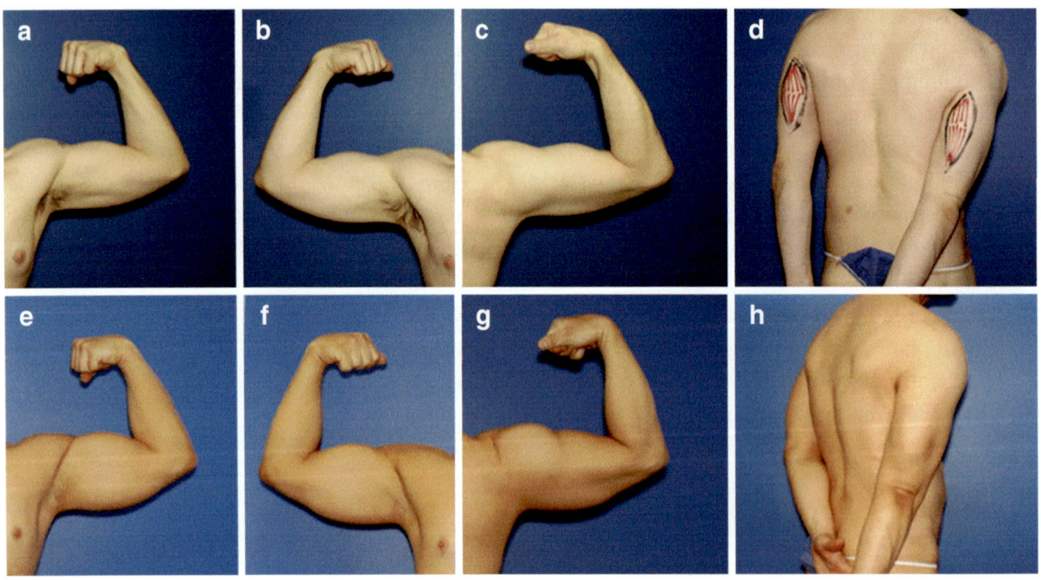

Fig. 31.11 A44-year-old, 5 feet 8 inch, 155pound, meso-ectomorphic male underwent sub-fascial tricep implantation with a 125 cc custom contoured, tear-shaped MuscleGel silicone implant. Note the natural contour with no visible incision, and no artificial step-off or visible implant-type look

31.6 Forearm Augmentation with Implants

- In the crease of the antecubital fossa of the forearm, a transverse 4 cm incision is made.
- The forearm can be augmented either medially (volarly, on the inner aspect of the arm) or laterally (dorsally, on the outer aspect of the arm). Carry out subcutaneous dissection using scissors and electrocautery, directing the subcutaneous tunnel medially toward the superficial flexor muscle bellies (pronator teres, flexor carpi radialis, palmaris longus, and flexor carpi ulnaris) or laterally toward the extensor muscle bellies digitorum, communis, extensor carpi ulnaris, and the extensor digiti minimi (Fig. 31.12).
- Carry out subcutaneous dissection using scissors and electrocautery directed either to the flexor or extensor muscle group, depending on whether medial or lateral forearm augmentation is desired.
- Identify the glistening muscle fascia by sweeping areolar inter-fascial tissue with a peanut.
- Mark a 3-cm longitudinal fascial incision along the intermuscular septum of the muscle bellies and incise sharply with scalpel.
- Elevate the fascia and place 3–0 Vicryl (Johnson & Johnson, New Brunswick, NJ) stay sutures for subsequent closure.
- With the tonsil clamp, tease in between fibers of the muscle belly to create a bloodless window into an intermuscular pocket just deep to the muscle bellies of the superficial group (Fig. 31.13).
- Use progressive, judicial pocket expansion with urethral sounds.

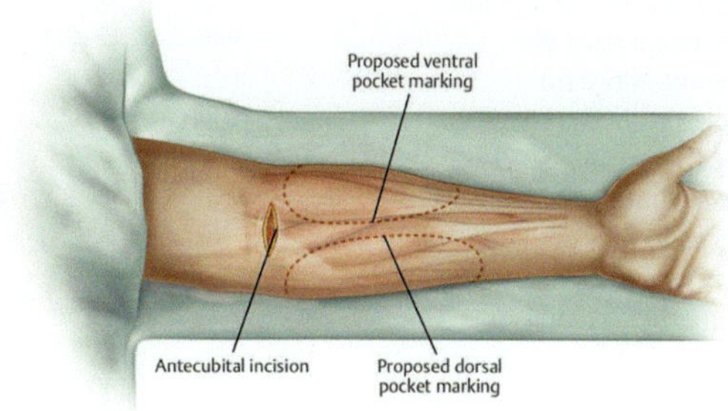

Fig. 31.12 A 4-cm incision is marked in the crease of the antecubital fossa. The proposed pocket is preoperatively determined by contraction of the dorsal extensor muscle groups. After incising the fascia, a tonsil clamp is employed to gently tease the fascia locally and conservatively to develop a pocket

- Do not over-dissect the submuscular pocket; be mindful not to dissect the pocket too distally.
- Insert curved 1-cm-wide retractor.
- The implant pocket is irrigated with betadine, triple-antibiotic, and bupivacaine.
- Change gloves for a "no touch" technique.
- Implant (AART, Carson City, NV) may be custom carved as needed, placed, and is folded like a "taco," to avoid fracture of the implant (wide belly is proximal) (Fig. 31.14).
- Manually range the wrist in order to ensure adequate dynamic implant position within the muscle complex; all muscle bellies must glide freely.
- Tie the previously placed 3–0 Vicryl sutures on the muscle fascia.
- Reapproximate deep subcutaneous layer with a 3–0 Vicryl suture.
- Reapproximate skin with a running 3–0 Monocryl subcuticular suture (Fig. 31.15).

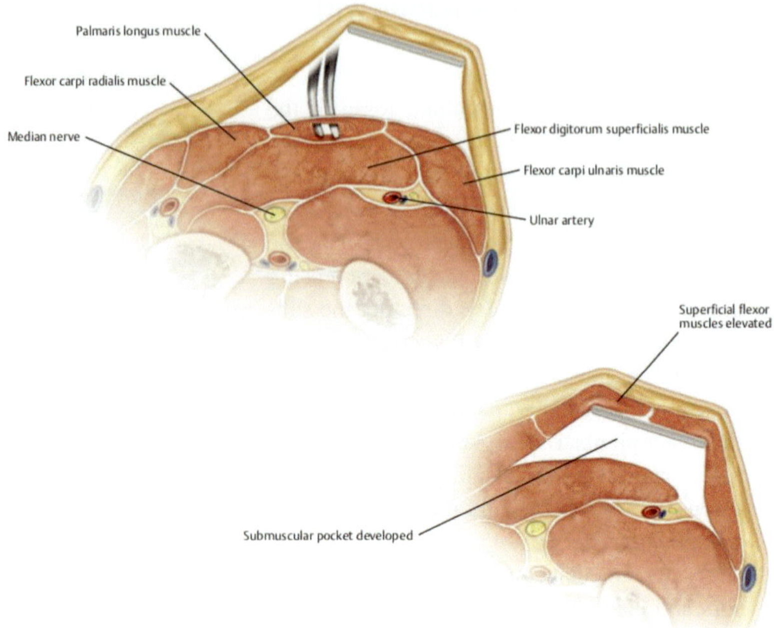

Fig. 31.13 While the assistant uses the Army-Navy for retraction, the surgeon gently progressively uses urethral sounds to expand the recipient pocket just below the superficial extensor group

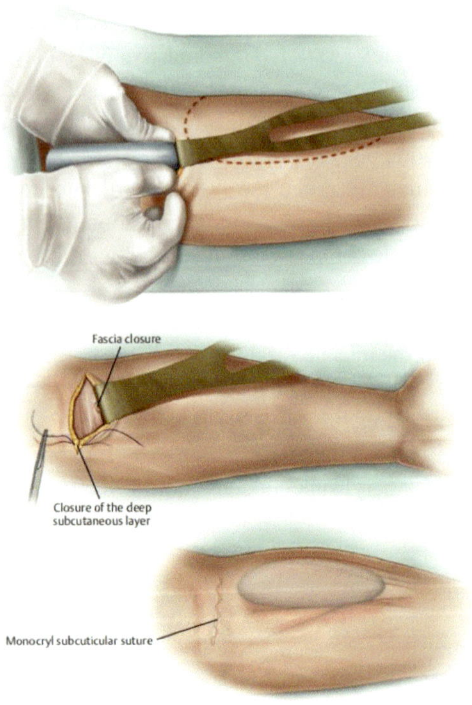

Fig. 31.14 While the assistant retracts with an Army-Navy, the surgeon gently maneuvers the "taco-folded" implant into the pocket. The fascial pocket of the superficial extensor group is loosely reapproximated with 4–0 Vicryl suture

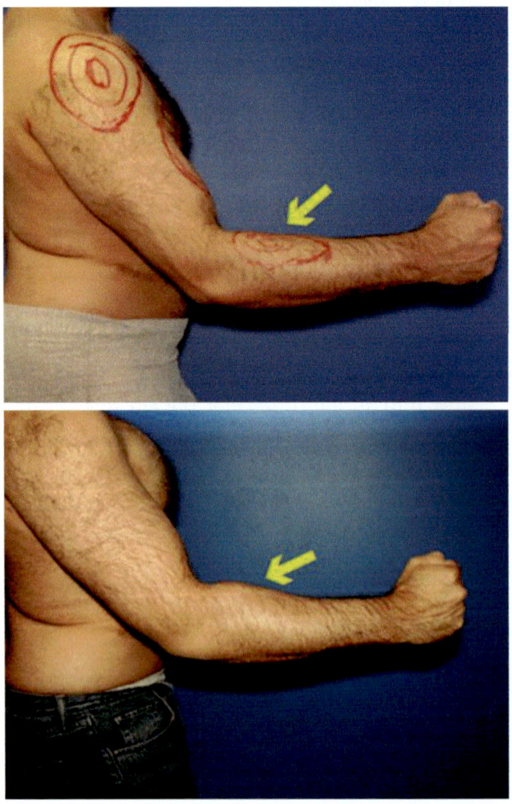

Fig. 31.15 A 42-year-old, 5 feet 10 inches, 205-pound, meso-endomorphic male underwent intermuscular forearm implantation with an 85-cc custom-contoured, tear-shaped MuscleGel silicone implant

31.7 Abdominal Muscular Definition with "Six-Pack" Implants

- A vertical 3.5 cm incision is placed in the natural crease of the linea alba centrally between the superior (first) and second set of muscular sections of the rectus abdominis. This incision gives access for implant augmentation of the supra-umbilical rectus abdominis (Fig. 31.16).
- A circumferential incision is placed around the umbilicus and hidden within the umbilical fold. This incision gives access for implant augmentation of the infra-umbilical rectus abdominis bilaterally.
- Carry out subcutaneous dissection using scissors and electrocautery, directed bilaterally to expose the medial edges of the rectus abdominis anterior fascia.
- A 1-cm vertical incision is marked on the anterior fascia at the medial edge of the first rectus abdominis muscle pocket and incised with a scalpel.
- The sub-fascial plane is entered through this incision, and the implant pocket is initially dissected gently with a tonsil clamp; any medial rectus abdominis perforators must be anticipated and cauterized to maintain a bloodless field.
- Use progressive, judicial pocket expansion with urethral sounds.
- Do not over-dissect the sub-fascial pocket; be mindful not to dissect the pocket too laterally off the rectus abdominis muscle.
- A lighted submental retractor is inserted for visualization of the implant pocket and for maintaining hemostasis.
- The implant pocket is irrigated with betadine, triple-antibiotic, and bupivacaine.
- Change gloves for the "no touch" technique.
- The implant (AART, Carson City, NV) may be custom-carved as needed in order to customize it to the profile, contour, or tapering of the native abdominal wall (Fig. 31.17).

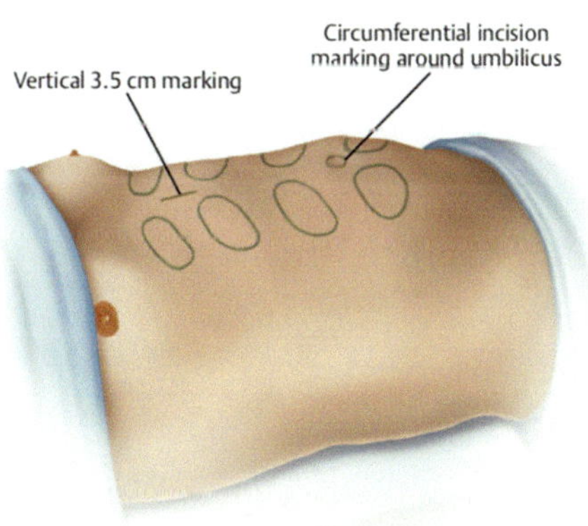

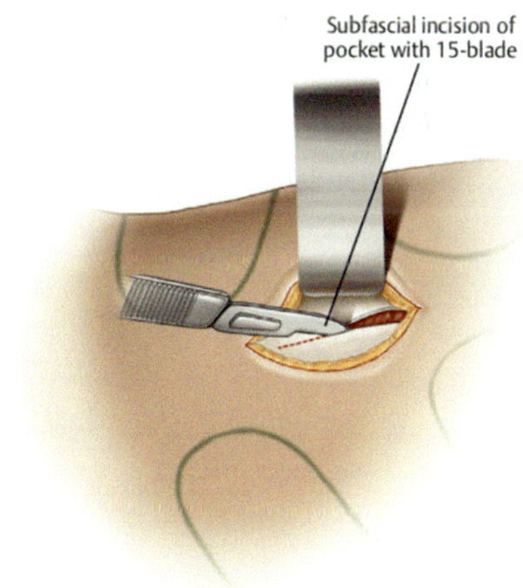

Fig. 31.16 An upper 3.5-cm incision and a lower circumferential incision are marked around the native umbilicus. Via the upper incisions, the superficial fascial system is incised, and the dissection is carried to the anterior fascia of the rectus pocket for placement of the upper two to four implants

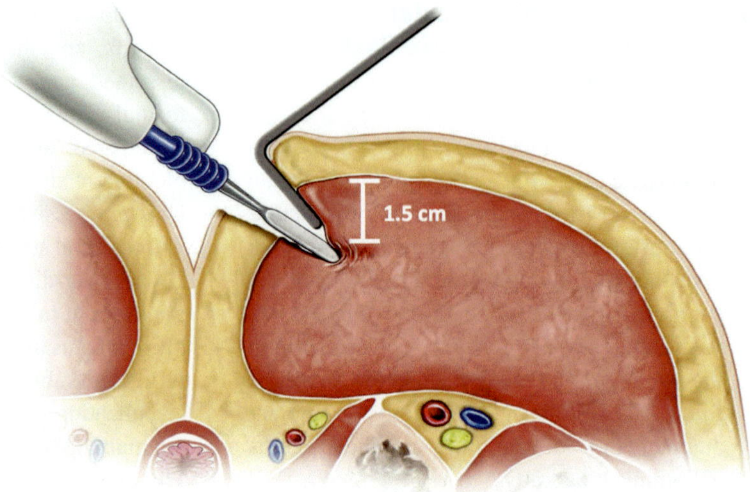

Fig. 31.17 While the assistant retracts the subcutaneous tissues, the surgeon marks vertical 2-cm incisions in the medial edge of the sub-fascial pocket. Once in the sub-fascial pocket, the assistant retracts as the surgeon gently maneuvers the folded implant into place

- The implant is then secured in its ideal position by placing a 3–0 Vicryl suture (Johnson & Johnson, New Brunswick, NJ) between the anterior surface of the implant and the overlying fascia of the implant pocket.
- The fascial incision is closed using a running 3–0 Vicryl suture.
- The preceding steps are then repeated for each subsequent abdominal implant to be placed.
- Reapproximate deep subcutaneous layer with a 3–0 Vicryl suture.
- Reapproximate skin with a running 4–0 Monocryl subcuticular suture.
- BodyBanking with lipocell transfer may then be performed (see section below) at the recipient sites overlying the implanted muscles that were marked preoperatively (Fig. 31.18).

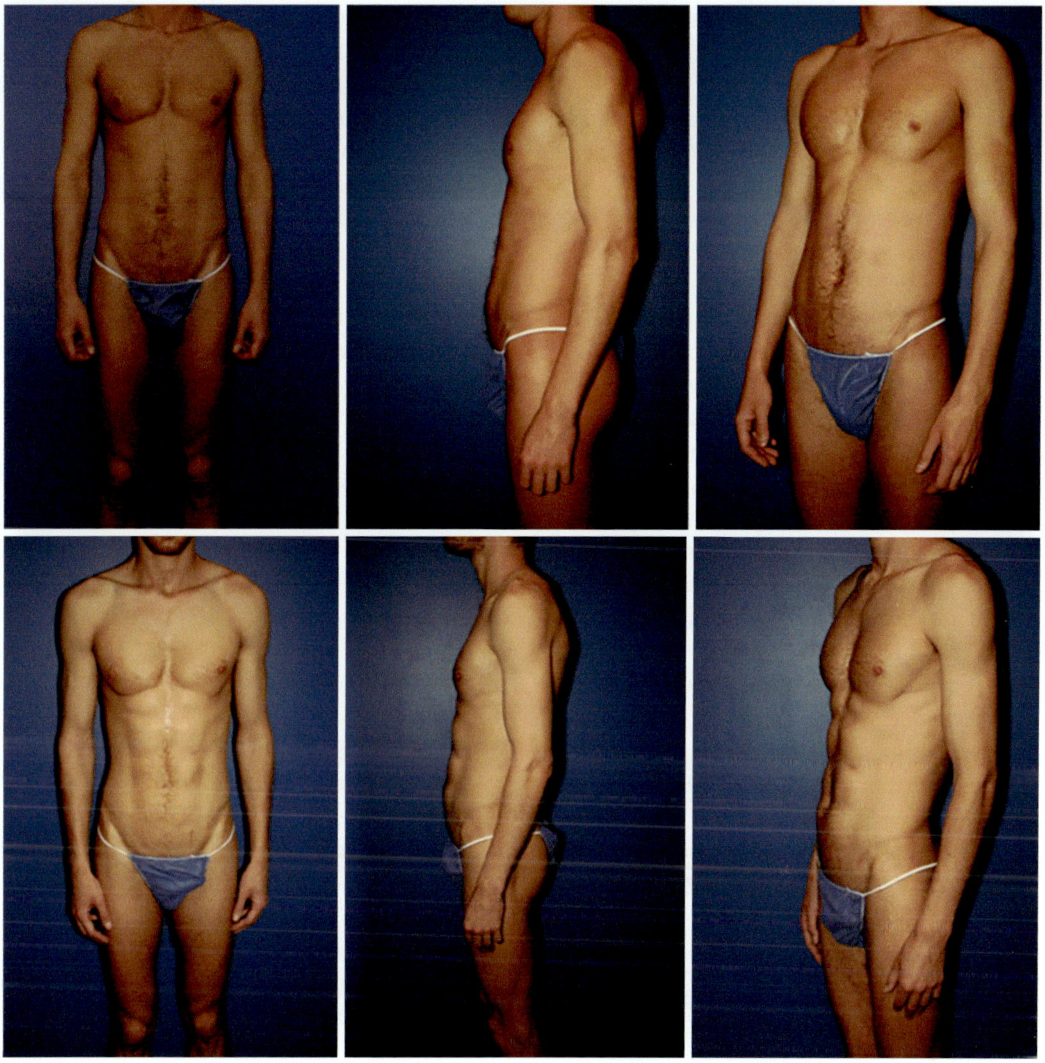

Fig. 31.18 A 27-year-old, 6 feet 3 inches, 159-pound, ectomorphic male model who presented with a request for more projection and definition to his abdominal musculature. He was very firm about his desire to have an eight-pack. Four sub-fascial implants were inserted via the "upper four" incision hidden in the midline shadows. The "lower four" were introduced by the deep hidden umbilical incision

31.8 Gluteal Augmentation with Implants

- Two 5–7 cm para-median incisions are placed in the intergluteal cleft, with the patient in a prone position (Fig. 31.19).
- Carry out subcutaneous dissection staying superficial to the fascia of the gluteus maximus muscle.
- The fascia of the gluteus maximus muscle is then incised at 2 cm from the midline.
- Intramuscular dissection using the cautery is then continued to an intermediate depth within the gluteus maximus that leaves 1.5 cm of muscle coverage superficial to the pocket.
- The thickness should be continuously checked by the surgeon using their thumb (Fig. 31.20).
- Dissection is continued in a lateral, superior, and inferior direction to create the implant pocket (Fig. 31.21).
- Direct visualization of dissection in this intramuscular plane is critical in order to avoid approximation to the sciatic nerve, which should always remain covered by muscle deep to the dissection plane.
- A more athletic contour is achieved by medial and lateral carving of the implant, allowing the implant to take the more vertical convexity characteristic of male buttocks aesthetics.
- The implant pocket is irrigated with betadine, triple-antibiotic, and bupivacaine.
- The surgeon's gloves are changed, and "no touch" introduction of the implant (AART, Carson City, NV) may be custom carved as needed and is placed into the intramuscular pocket using an Ioban™ drape and an optional Keller funnel™.
- Although the senior author (D.S.) no longer uses drains, a Jackson Pratt drain may be placed in each implant pocket and brought out laterally in the infra-gluteal fold through a separate stab incision.
- Closure of the implant pocket should be tension-free. The muscle fascial edges should approximate with ease, and a "watertight" closure is performed using 8–12 simple interrupted 0 or 2–0 Vicryl sutures (Johnson & Johnson, New Brunswick, NJ) (Fig. 31.22).
- Reapproximate the superficial fascial layer with a 2–0 Vicryl suture.
- Reapproximate the deep dermis with a 3–0 Vicryl suture.
- Reapproximate skin with a running 3–0 Monocryl subcuticular suture.
- BodyBanking with lipocell transfer is then performed (see section below) at the recipient sites overlying the implanted muscles that were marked preoperatively (Fig. 31.23).

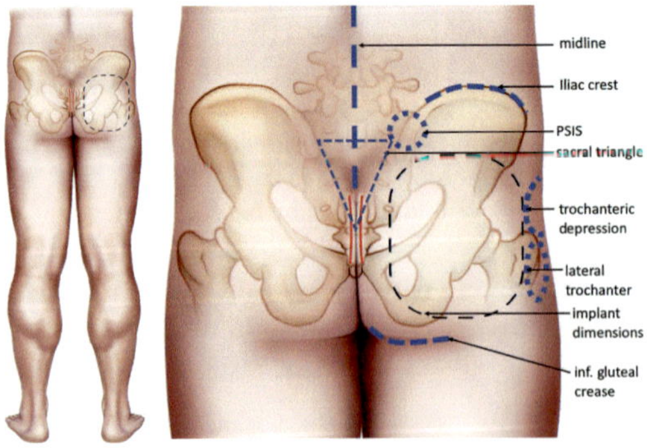

Fig. 31.19 Preoperative markings with the patient standing. The following landmarks are delineated: midline along the lumbar spinous processes, the sacral triangle, posterior superior iliac spine (PSIS), iliac crests, infragluteal creases, and lateral trochanters. The planned incision is marked at the natural gluteal crease (approx. 5 cm). Alternating between a flexed and in repose posture, the gluteal muscle groups and the proposed implant pocket dimensions are marked

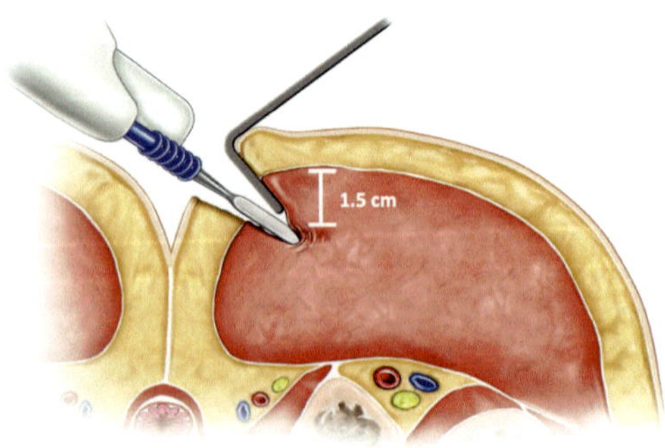

Fig. 31.20 Intramuscular dissection at an intermediate depth, leaving 1.5 cm of muscle coverage superficial to the implant pocket created

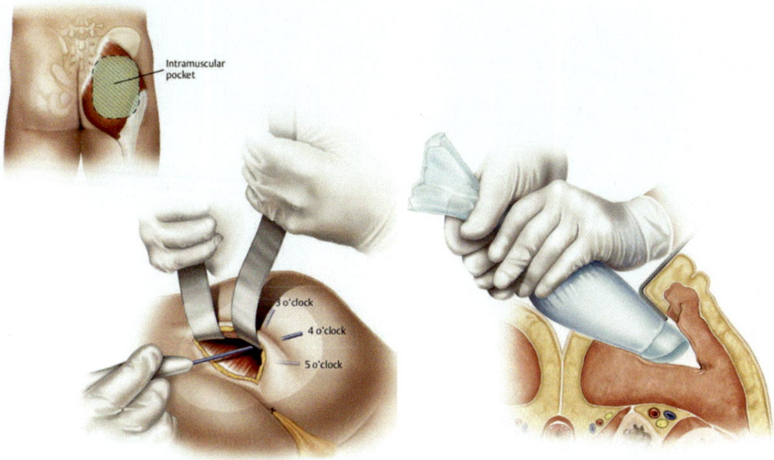

Fig. 31.21 The assistant holds the sweetheart retractor as the surgeon dictates "7 to 11 o'clock position." The surgeon self-retracts lower tissue with a malleable ribbon retractor and fully dissects the pocket with a headlight and Bovie under direct visualization. Placement of the gluteal implant. Using a "no-touch technique," the surgeon may use a funnel to aid in the placement of the implant

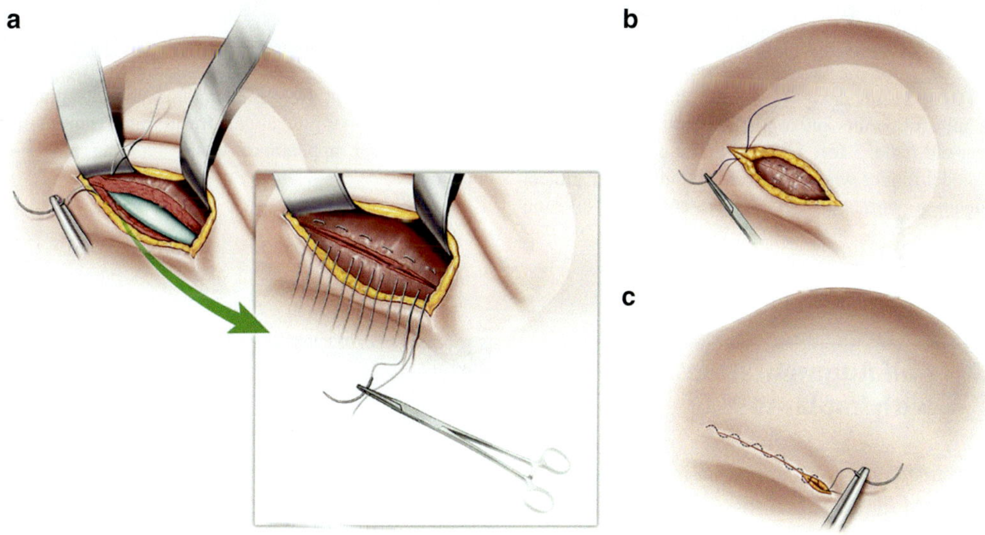

Fig. 31.22 "Watertight" closure of the muscle fascia (**a**), the superficial fascia (**b**), and dermis (**c**).

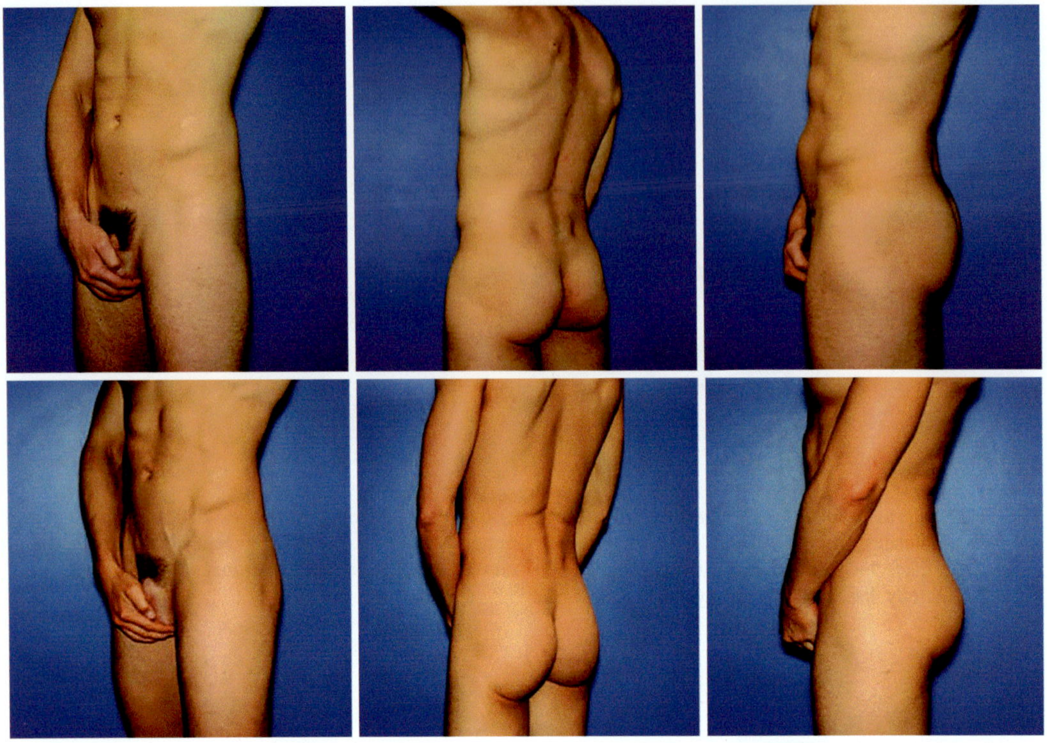

Fig. 31.23 Preoperative (top row) and postoperative 21-month follow-up photography (bottom row) of a 29-year-old male, 5 feet 11 inches, 165-pound, ectomorphic model/runner who underwent intramuscular gluteal implantation with a 276-cc custom-contoured silicone MuscleGel implant. BodyBanking fat was added cranially to define the upper gluteal pole, resulting in a more elongated muscular appearance while avoiding a step-off appearance

31.9 Calf Augmentation with Implants

- A transverse 4 cm incision is placed in the crease of the popliteal fossa with the patient in a prone position (Fig. 31.24).
- Carry out subcutaneous dissection using scissors and electrocautery heading in a caudal direction until the fascia of the gastrocnemius is reached.
- Identify the glistening muscle fascia by sweeping the areolar fascial tissue with a peanut.
- The small saphenous vein courses at the midline and runs superficially in the superficial fascial system; injury during dissection is avoided by retracting this structure either medially or laterally. The medial and lateral

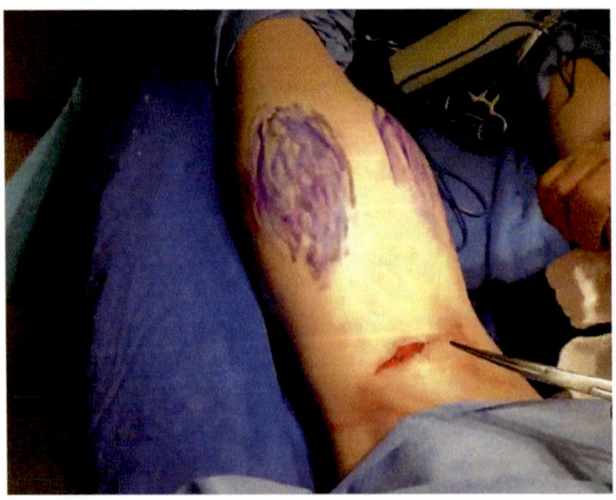

Fig. 31.24 Access incision for calf implant augmentation placed at popliteal fossa crease. The same incision is used for either medial or lateral calf augmentation

sural cutaneous nerves can also be encountered in this plane and typically follow the course of the small saphenous vein.

- Place a 3-cm incision in the fascia of the medial or lateral gastrocnemius muscles, depending on whether medial or lateral augmentation is desired.
- The sub-fascial plane is dissected using a tonsil clamp, followed by judicious pocket expansion with urethral sounds (Fig. 31.25), until a spatulated dissector can be inserted.

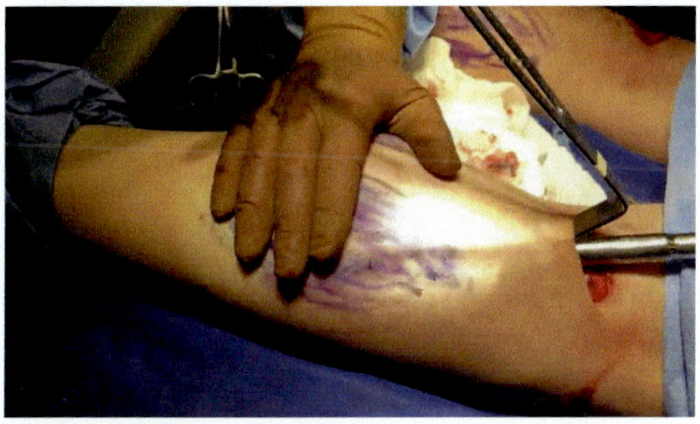

Fig. 31.25 Dissection of the sub-fascial implant pocket with urethral sound

- Be mindful not to over-dissect the implant pocket, as this can lead to implant malposition or migration.
- Observe for hemostasis and ensure the implant pocket is bloodless.
- The implant pocket is irrigated with betadine, triple-antibiotic, and bupivacaine.
- Change gloves for a "no touch" technique.
- Implant (AART, Carson City, NV) (Fig. 31.26) may be custom-carved as needed and is placed folded like a "taco" to avoid fracture of the implant.
- Manually range the ankle in order to ensure adequate dynamic implant position within the muscle complex.
- Close the muscle fascia with 3–0 Vicryl sutures (Johnson & Johnson, New Brunswick, NJ) on the muscle fascia.
- Reapproximate deep subcutaneous layer with a 3–0 Vicryl suture.
- Reapproximate skin with a running 3–0 Monocryl subcuticular suture (Fig. 31.27).

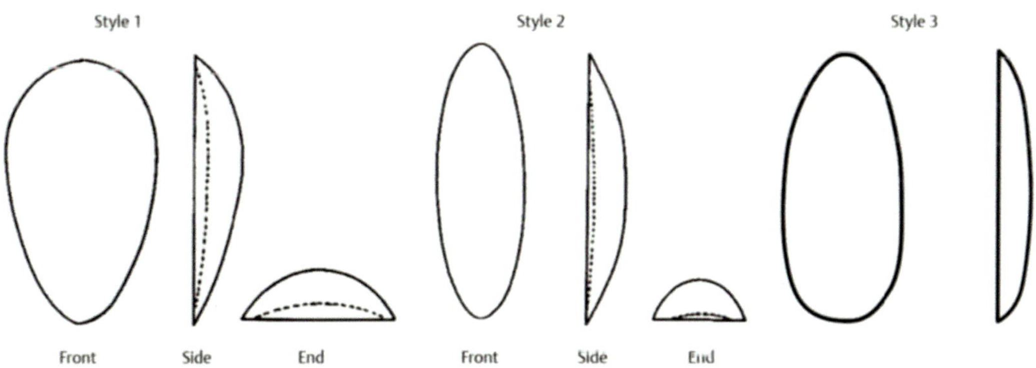

Fig. 31.26 Three commonly used styles of silicone calf implants. Aesthetic and Reconstructive Technologies, Inc., Reno, NV

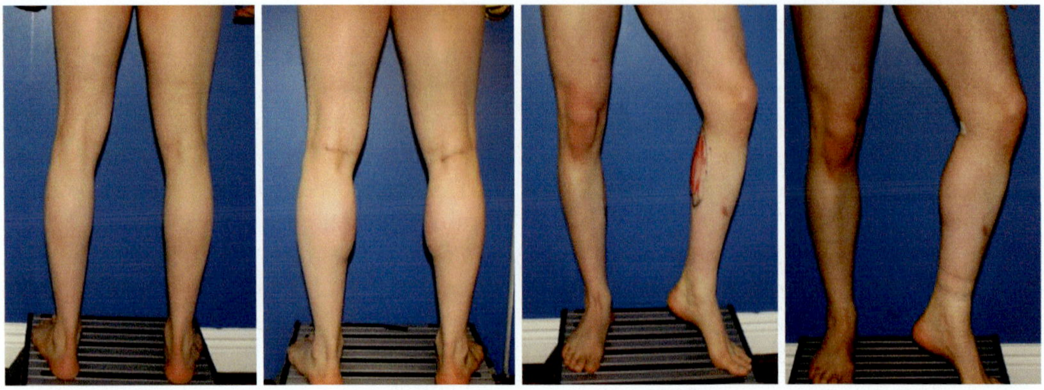

Fig. 31.27 A 32-year-old, 5 feet 9 inches, 155-pound, ectomorphic male with hypoplastic calves underwent augmentation of medial calf with placement of sub-fascial silicone implant

31.10 Bodybanking with Lipocell Transfer

- The fatty areas in the abdomen, the flanks, and the lateral chest in males typically yield enough lipocell aspirates to supplement the muscular augmentation that was performed with implants in the way of BodyBanking (Fig. 31.28).
- The lipocell aspirate is collected with the Microaire Power-assist Liposuction device (3590 Grand Forks Boulevard, Charlottesville, Virginia) and is strained or dry-rolled and placed into aliquot syringes for transfer (Fig. 31.29).
- The recipient areas must be selected and marked preoperatively.
- Lipocell transfer is performed using blunt tip cannulas in a subdermal plane; transfer to intramuscular planes should be avoided.
- A graded augmentation with lipocell transfer is recommended by constantly re-assessing the volume by palpation and inspection of the augmented area and using small, serial aliquots.
- In the chest, the clavicular head of the pectoralis muscle (parallel to the clavicle), as well as its medial aspect (parallel to the sternum) is augmented—forms a 90-degree angle at the level of the sternal notch.
- In the abdomen, the upper three (supra-umbilical) interval areas between the tendinous inscriptions of the rectus muscles are

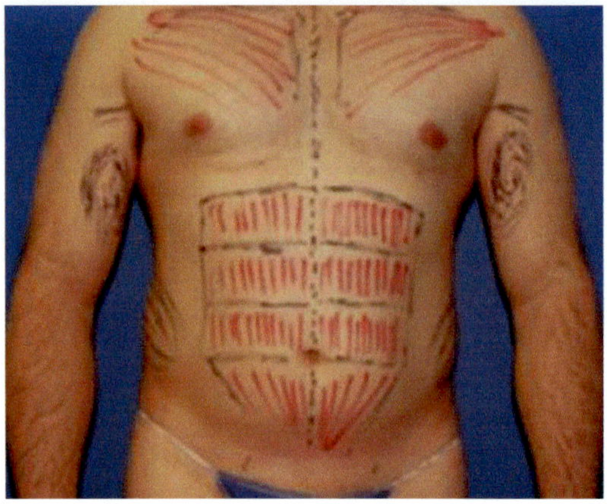

Fig. 31.28 BodyBanking preoperative markings for recipient sites of lipo-cell transfer

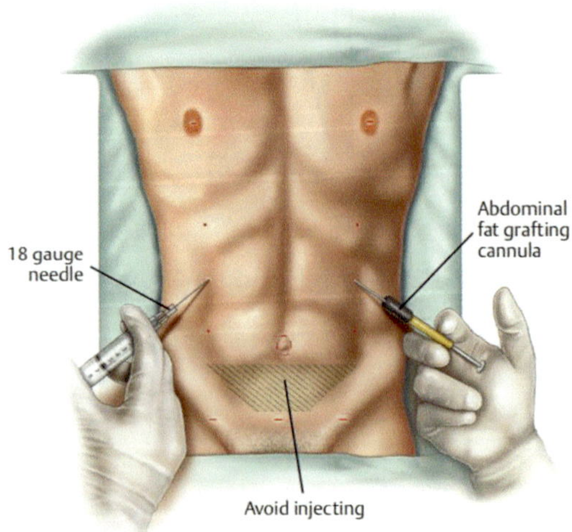

Fig. 31.29 The surgeon makes a nick incision with an 18-gauge needle and then uses a 2-mm abdominal fat grafting cannula in the subcutaneous, supra-fascial plane

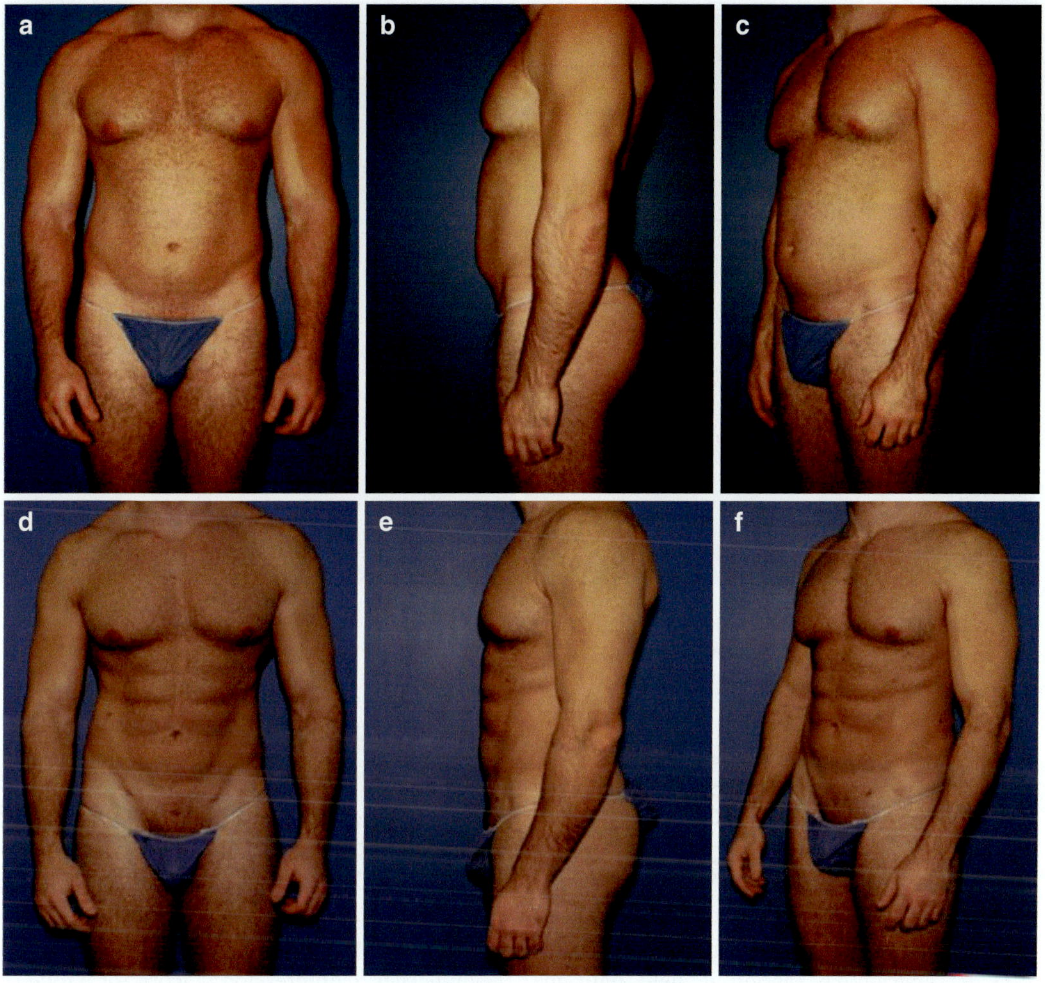

Fig. 31.30 A 32-year-old, 5 feet 11 inch, 220-pound, endo-mesomorphic amateur bodybuilder. Given the thickness of the subcutaneous fat of his anterior abdominal wall, he was not a good candidate for silicone "six-pack" MuscleGel implants. He underwent BodyBanking for "six-pack" projection and definition using lipo-cell transfer harvested from bilateral flanks and anterior abdomen

augmented sparingly in the subdermal plane (Fig. 31.30). The senior author typically does not perform lipo-cell transfer to the lower (infra-umbilical) abdomen, as this may result in bulging (Fig. 31.31).

- In gluteal augmentation, lipocell transfer is done superficial to the gluteal muscle fascia. The surgeon must be mindful of the safety zone triangle in order to avoid fat emboli into gluteal veins or injury to neurovascular structures. The apex of each triangle is the PSIS, with the lateral point located at the greater trochanter, and the medial point at the ischial tuberosity.

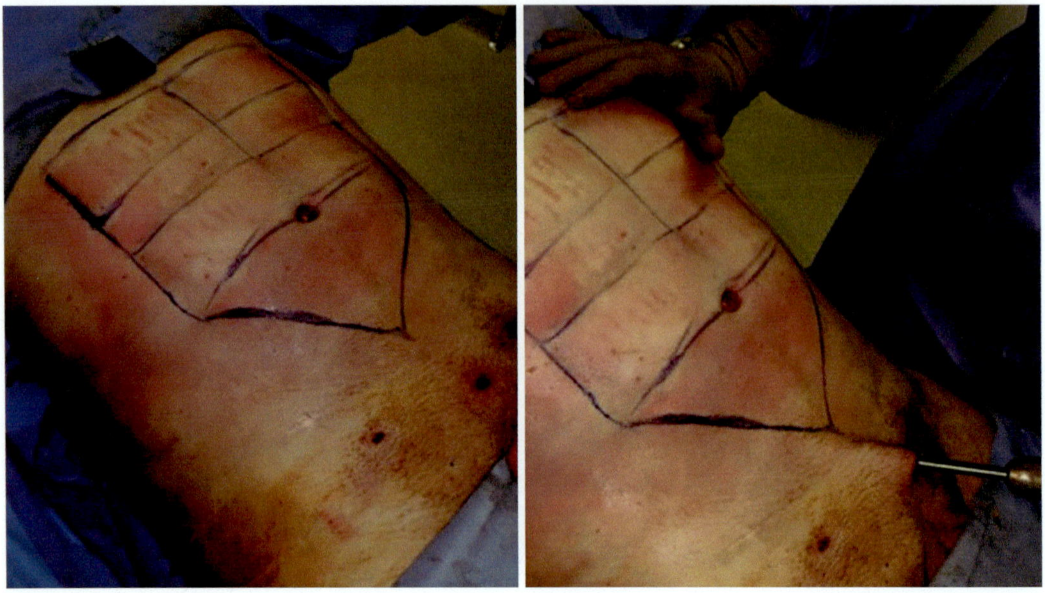

Fig. 31.31 The senior author's technique demonstrated in a 28-year-old patient through minimal scar access by using two, supra-pubic, 1 cm incisions below the belt line and one incision in the umbilical fold. All abdominal "six-pack" inscriptions can be accessed through these minimal access incisions

31.11 Postoperative Care

Patients are discharged home the same day of surgery once postoperative anesthesia care unit discharge criteria are met. Prior to their departure, an educational session is held with the patient and their designated care person in which drain care, dressing care, positioning, and activity restrictions are reviewed in detail. It is imperative to avoid positioning, manipulation, or activities that can displace the implant or hinder healing of the implant pocket (e.g., massages, sitting, and weightlifting). For pectoral, biceps, triceps, and forearm implants, activity instructions include: no pushing or pulling and no lifting anything heavier than 5–10 pounds for the first week, no overhead work, and no working out using the torso or upper extremities for 1 month. For pectoral implants, activity instructions include: no sitting for 2 weeks, squatting facing the commode in the restroom for 2 weeks, gym exercise is allowed at 2 weeks without using gluteus muscles, and mild exercise that uses gluteus muscles can begin at 4 months postoperatively.

For chest, gluteal, and abdominal "six-pack" augmentation, a compression garment with foam is worn for 3 weeks. It is important that the patient is compliant with compression and adjusts the foam pads in order to prevent creasing and asymmetries. Compression is worn for a total of 3 weeks. For forearm, biceps, triceps, and calf augmentation, ACE elastic bandages are worn for 2 weeks; patients are educated on how to change the bandages on a daily basis.

Antibiotic prophylaxis is continued postoperatively while drains are in place. Patients are allowed to shower, avoiding any immersion of incisions or drains in water. BodyBanking Penrose drains may be removed at 10 days. Although the senior author (D.S.) no longer uses drains for any implant pockets, if bulb drains are elected to be used in the implant pockets, they are removed when output reaches less than 30 ml/drain/day (varies with patient body habitus).

A Skype™ or Facetime® follow-up is done on postoperative day one to confirm correct dressing and drain care as well as re-enforcing positioning and activity instructions. The patient's first in-person follow-up visit is between postoperative day five to seven. Subsequent visits occur every one to two weeks during the first 6 weeks and every 3 months thereafter.

31.12 Complications

With refinement of technique, understanding of anatomy, and adherence to surgical principles, complications can be kept to minimum. Nevertheless, when complications arise, patients must be seen as frequently as needed in the office until resolution of the issue.

Wound dehiscence is prevented by appropriate implant size selection, tension-free closure, and adhering to postoperative activity restrictions. If small areas of dehiscence that do not go beyond the superficial fascia occur, these can be managed with local wound care. If the extent of the dehiscence is significant or if it involves the superficial fascial closure, washout and re-approximation of tissues is indicated, as long as the implant has not been exposed. When implant exposure occurs, salvage can be attempted with washout and implant exchange if exposure is minimal, coverage is feasible, and there is no evidence of implant pocket infection. Infection is a rare but troublesome complication. Localized, superficial cellulitis may be treated with a trial of antibiotics; however, any concern for deeper infection or implant pocket involvement warrants return to the operating room and, at a minimum, washout and possible implant removal. In cases of explanation, reinsertion (usually in 3 months) is delayed until there is no evidence of infection and a full antibiotic course has been completed. Although with adequate drain management, seromas are uncommon, if they are symptomatic and persistent, aspiration is warranted, and if it is believed the seroma has significantly encapsulated, it must be surgically evacuated. Implant malposition can be significantly decreased with appropriate pocket dissection and choice of implant. Although not a complication, temporary loss of sensation along the incision and overlying the implant pocket may occur, and patients must be counseled preoperatively. Specific to gluteal implant augmentation, temporary sciatic neurapraxia has been reported, generally subsides, and can be managed in the interim with Gabapentin and/or Ibuprofen.

When performing biceps, triceps, forearm, or calf augmentation, the patient must be monitored for compartment syndrome postoperatively. Pulses of the extremity (i.e., radial pulse, dorsalis pedis pulse) must be palpated before and after surgery, and the distal limb (i.e., hand, foot) must be assessed for adequate perfusion by monitoring capillary refill and temperature. Paresthesias or pain out of proportion to exam are the earliest signs of compartment syndrome. If the surgeon has high suspicion of compartment syndrome, the implant should be removed to prevent vascular and neurologic compromise of the extremity. This complication can be prevented with adequate implant selection by adjusting the implant size to the laxity of the skin and soft tissues, and by staging the procedure when more than one implant is desired, as reviewed in the previous section.

31.13 Conclusion

The senior author has found that success in male plastic surgery, and more specifically in this case of muscular enhancement, is achieved by adhering to thorough preoperative planning, understanding of patient expectations, comprehension of anatomy, systematic operative technique, and understanding of the unique aesthetics of males reviewed in this chapter. This yields effective, safe, and reproducible outcomes that keep patients happy and the surgeon busy.

32 Gluteal Implants

Rubem Lang Stümpfle
and Pedro Salomão Piccinini

32.1 Introduction

Gluteal augmentation is increasingly popular, with over 335,000 fat transfers to the buttocks and 36,859 buttock implant operations performed in 2017, according to statistics from the International Society of Aesthetic Plastic Surgery (ISAPS) [1]. This represents a 17% increase compared to 2016. Brazil leads in annual number of gluteal implants, with 8525 cases, followed by Mexico (3868), Colombia (3640), and the United States (1700), with other countries demonstrating much lower numbers. The same data show that only 6% of responding American plastic surgeons perform buttock implants, whereas 57% of Colombian plastic surgeons perform this operation, as do 42% of Mexican and 34% of Brazilian respondents. The low rate in the United States may be related to lack of exposure during residency training, concerns about reported high complication rates, or perceived disadvantages in using silicone elastomer gel implants which are currently available in the United States, as opposed to silicone gel implants, as well as the ease of gluteal fat grafting.

R. L. Stümpfle (✉)
Private practice, Clínica Nova Imagem, Santana, Porto Alegre, RS, Brazil

P. S. Piccinini
Division of Plastic Surgery, Montefiore Einstein, New York, NY, USA

With the widespread media emphasis on the buttocks, patients throughout the world have sought a shapelier gluteal region. The historical emphasis given to the buttocks in Brazil is related to the beach culture and ethnic miscegenation which have molded aesthetic values. Perhaps uniquely, alongside the well-known thong bikinis which are common in Brazil and other Latin American countries, it is common for men in Brazil to wear small swimming trunks (similar to "Speedos," derived from the sportswear brand), which emphasize the gluteal aesthetic unit. Many of our male patients often express frustration due to significant muscle hypertrophy gains with weight-lifting in the torso and arms, but limited gains in buttock volume, which leads to an imbalanced, "top-heavy" appearance.

While the term "Brazilian butt lift" (BBL) has been popularized, the very large volumes of grafted fat seen in this procedure when performed in some countries are not necessarily in line with the classic (or current) ideal of gluteal beauty. Shape, rather than volume, is the defining feature of beautiful buttocks; this is important to take into account when evaluating patients preoperatively, as patient and surgeon expectations need to find a common middle ground. In both social media and articles on gluteal fat grafting written by authors outside of Brazil, very large volumes of fat are often grafted into the gluteal muscles and lateral hips. This is mostly an African-

K. Jeffords et al. (eds.), *Aesthetic Surgery for Men*, https://doi.org/10.1007/978-3-032-03840-1_32

American or Caribbean aesthetic ideal [2, 3], distinct from the ideal gluteal aesthetics commonly sought by patients in Brazil or Europe. Indeed, Toledo, who started performing gluteal fat grafting in 1985 and from whom the term BBL derived, reported grafted volumes of at most around 500 mL to each buttock [4], with the goal being improved contours rather than very large volumes.

The first published report describing gluteal implants was the use of an implant for correction of gluteal muscle atrophy by Bartels et al. in 1969; the authors used a round Cronin breast implant to correct the patient's unilateral gluteal asymmetry, through an infragluteal fold incision.

In 1973, Cocke and Ricketson reported on the use of breast implants for correction of the lateral gluteal depression; implants were placed subcutaneously [5]. Posteriorly, in 1977, González-Ulloa also used a subcutaneous plane for implant placement, and described different incisions for pocket dissection: supragluteal, on either side of the coccyx; infragluteal fold; and intergluteal crease.

The subcutaneous pocket is of historical interest only, due to the required release of retaining ligaments and adhesions (aponeurotic expansions from the gluteal aponeurosis to the dermis) [6], which leaves the skin loose. Implants become unstable, may migrate, and capsular contracture is a real issue. Additionally, implant visibility and palpability are troubling.

Robles et al., in 1984, described submuscular implant placement [7] between the gluteus maximus and medius muscles, with the advantages of preserving the aponeurotic fixation between the skin and muscle, as well as decreasing the incidence of capsular contracture. The available space in this plane, however, is small, limiting implant size. Another significant issue is possible impingement or damage to the sciatic nerve (emerging caudal to the lower border of the piriformis) during pocket dissection; implants should not be placed lower than this level. This is especially problematic for men, in whom maximal gluteal projection should be at a lower point than in women.

The gluteus maximus fascia is not uniformly thick, and, thus, the subfascial pocket as described by De la Peña in 2004 offers little implant coverage [8]. The use of cohesive silicone gel, polyurethane-coated implants when performing subfascial implants helps decrease the risk of implant malposition and capsular contracture; however, even very slight asymmetries may be visible, due to the lack of tissue cover [9]. While subfascial gluteal implants may draw parallels to subfascial breast augmentation, the gluteal fascia, in our opinion, offers less support than the pectoralis major fascia, for which reason we do not use the subfascial plane for gluteal implants.

The intramuscular dissection for implant placement was published by Vergara and Marcos in 1996, using an intergluteal incision. The gluteus maximus fibers are divided, leaving approximately 2–3 cm of gluteus maximus fibers superficial to the implant. The fibers left deep to the implant protect the sciatic nerve, so the risk of symptoms from compression or direct damage to the nerve is greatly decreased. Intramuscular placement also decreases implant palpability and visibility of its edges. This is our preferred technique for gluteal implant placement, as well as being the most popular among a survey of 19 members of the American Society of Plastic Surgeons, with 68.4% of respondents favoring the intramuscular pocket [10].

32.2 Male Gluteal Aesthetics

Singh [11] proposed that the ideal, attractive female has full buttocks 1.4 times the circumference of the waist, or a waist-hip ratio of 0.7, while men have a ratio of 0.85–1.0. Although these strict numbers are rarely useful in clinical practice, they may help guide the novice surgeon with regard to ideal gluteal aesthetics in men, as there is a paucity of data on the ideal male buttock and gluteal evaluation in men [12], despite multiple depictions in arts, photography, and social media.

While an hourglass figure is a desirable characteristic in women [13], a more squared-off figure is desirable in men, with a higher WHR (waist–hip ratio). Men have a narrower pelvis than women and most commonly desire a slight increase in projection, not overall width. Since many patients who undergo gluteal implants also undergo liposuction, it is important not to excessively contour the lower back in men to avoid a decrease in WHR, which might lead to a more feminine appearance. The sculpted "V," or gull-wing shape at the superior border of the buttocks, leads to a feminine appearance [14] and should be avoided through judicious liposuction. Patients with a lot of flank or hip fat laterally will require larger volumes of liposuction in order to highlight the increased gluteal projection, as using implants only in patients who are significantly overweight or obese may not achieve the desired results.

The lateral depression is defined by the lateral edge of gluteus maximus, quadratus femoris, and vastus lateralis and gluteus medius insertions into the greater trochanter. In females, it is almost always necessary to fill this area, either with implant positioning or fat grafting to achieve adequate gluteal contour. In males, the main desire in gluteal contouring is to emphasize muscularity; therefore, maintaining the trochanteric depression is a desirable characteristic, as this gives a more athletic, muscular appearance to the region.

It is important to place implants slightly more caudally than in women, as the ideal point of maximal gluteal projection is more caudal in males than in females. Buttock projection on anterior-posterior view should also be less than in women, for which reason we opt for lower or medium profile implants. Patients should be examined in different positions and explanation given that the implants may become more visible or palpable depending on positioning of the lower body such as during exercise.

Ideal patients are those with a normal body mass index (BMI) or slightly overweight (BMI up to 30 kg/m^2), without skin laxity or gluteal ptosis. Exclusion criteria include medical conditions precluding general anesthesia, active infection, and gluteal ptosis.

32.3 Surgical Technique

Preoperative markings are done initially with the patient in profile view, standing; patients are asked to contract the gluteal musculature. The projected superior and inferior limits of the gluteal implant are marked on the patient, avoiding placing the superior aspect too cranially, which is more characteristic of women. The trochanteric depression is noted, and patient preference dictates whether this will be fat grafted or not. Next the buttocks are examined from a posterior view, and the medial and lateral limits for the dissection are marked. The estimated pocket diameter should be 1.5 cm larger than the implant base diameter in order to not compress the implants excessively.

In men we use both anatomical, nanotextured, medium-profile silicone gel implants, either 235 mL or 305 mL, and round, smooth silicone gel implants, between 240 and 300 mL. Anatomical implants are very useful in men as they offer good projection without excessive lateral size. We have not had any problems with implant rotation or malposition. In selecting implant size in men, since the goal of the operation is to increase gluteal projection anteroposteriorly, rather than laterally, the patient's hip width must be taken into account. Implants with wide bases should be avoided, as this may lead to more visible or palpable implant edges, especially when walking or performing other types of lower-body exercises.

We use general anesthesia in all cases. A 4–5 cm midline intergluteal incision is made with a 15 blade and carried down to the presacral area. Skin hooks are placed and the incision is continued down with electrocautery, angled at 45 degrees until the gluteus maximus aponeurosis is seen (Fig. 32.1). Infiltration of the gluteus maximus muscle with a solution of epinephrine, normal saline (1:200,000), and ropivacaine helps to hydrodissect the muscle fibers, making splitting of the muscle easier and less bloody. The fascia is incised and a subfascial dissection extends for

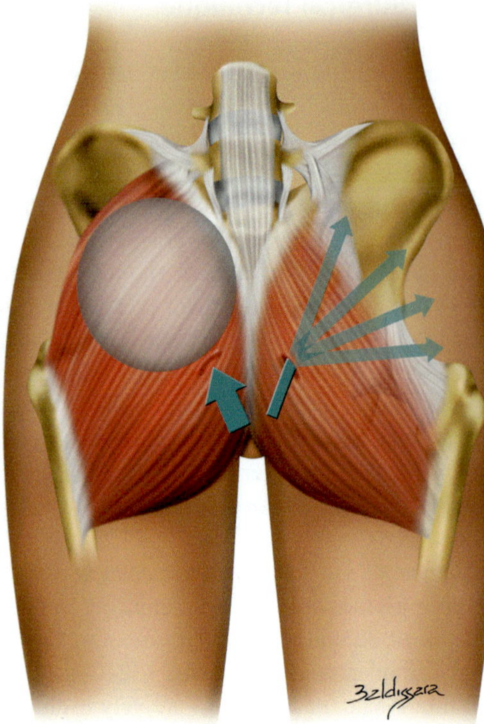

Fig. 32.1 Black line shows approximate line of initial muscle splitting. Blue lines show sweeping blunt intramuscular gluteus maximus dissection with malleable dissectors. Yellow arrow shows approximate access approach angle for implant placement. We stand on the contralateral side to dissect the pocket and introduce the implants

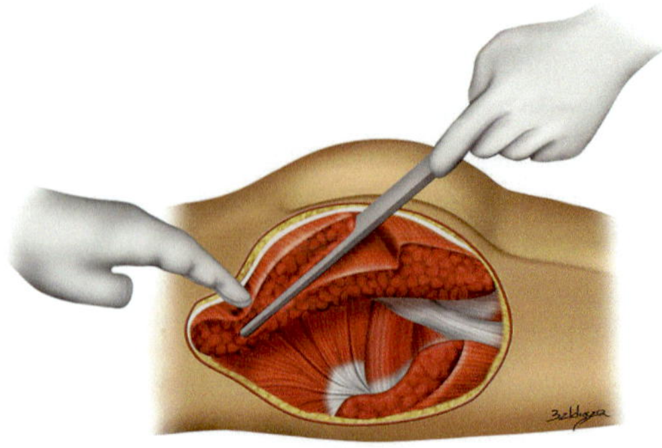

Fig. 32.2 The blunt spatula dissector has divided the gluteus maximus muscle, and limits of the pocket dissection are preserved by the surgeon's nondominant hand. A 2–3 cm thickness of gluteus maximus muscle is kept superficial to the implant to ensure adequate coverage. Dissection continues bluntly circumferentially until the pocket is complete. Care is taken to follow the curvature of the gluteus laterally, as inadvertent straight-line dissection can lead to popping through the muscle laterally, with subsequent subcutaneous implant placement and visibility. At this point of the operation, the lighted retractor is not very helpful

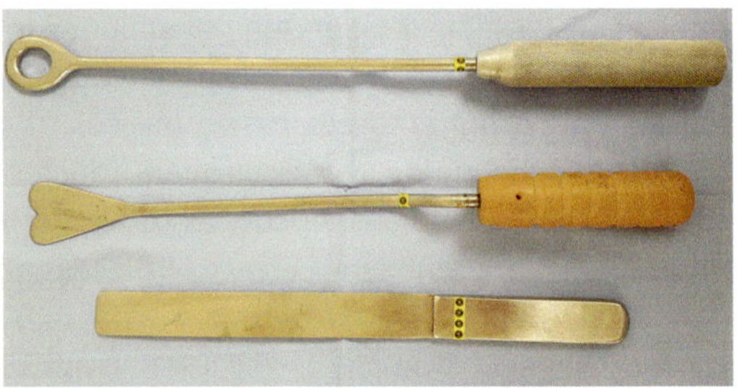

Fig. 32.3 Instruments used for blunt dissection

4 cm cranio-caudally and 4–5 cm laterally, angled toward the greater trochanter. Dissection is facilitated by use of a long lighted retractor. Bipolar cautery is used to simultaneously divide and cauterize the gluteus maximus muscle fibers, in a sweeping motion, leaving a thickness of 2–3 cm of gluteus maximus superficial to the implant pocket. Bipolar cautery assists in the initial intramuscular dissection, which is next performed bluntly (Fig. 32.2) with the use of malleable spatulas of differing widths and lengths (Fig. 32.3). The lack of an anatomical landmark to define the correct plane of dissection can make pocket creation difficult; the XYZ method described by Gonzalez [15] is a practical approach which may help surgeons who are starting gluteal implant surgery, as this potentially allows for more even intramuscular dissection. We have found it is helpful to never completely remove the lighted retractor or the dissection spatulas once the plane has been developed, to avoid creating a second, false pocket with the blunt dissectors; this has been described by Andrade et al. [16]. Care is taken to follow the natural gluteal curvature, especially supero-laterally, to avoid dissecting into the subcutaneous plane, which can easily happen if dissection is done in a straight line direction. Inadvertent pocket dissection too far cranially may lead to superior implant migration; as stated previously, the pocket should not be overdissected, and an approximately 1 cm greater overall pocket diameter than the implant base should be created. Infero-medially there are tight

adhesions of the gluteus muscle which should not be taken down or dissected; when checking the implant pocket with a fingertip, this area can be noted to be very adherent. Given the gluteus maximus muscle mass and strength, we cannot overemphasize the importance of precise pocket dissection, as attempting to close off an excessively large pocket with sutures tends to fail.

Prior to introducing the implant, a 2–0 Nylon suture is tied to reapproximate the divided edges of the gluteus maximus muscle. Next, the pocket and implants are washed with gentamicin + cefazolin solution in 200 cc of normal saline, the skin is cleansed with aqueous chlorhexidine, and gloves are changed. The implant is introduced, and the previously placed suture is used to close the gluteus maximus over the implant in a running fashion; contrary to what may be expected, closure can be performed without tension when adequate (not excessively large) size implants are used.

Progressive tension sutures (3–0 Vicryl) tied to the gluteal aponeurosis are used to slightly advance the dissected subcutaneous and superficial fascia to the midline, decreasing tension and dead space, and facilitating midline incision closure. In general, 3–4 sutures are used on either side. Non-absorbable, horizontal mattress sutures with 3–0 nylon, taking a bite of dermis and superficial fascia along with subcutaneous and the presacral tissue (including periosteum), help to maintain definition of the gluteal cleft and ensure a deep, well-hidden incision scar (Fig. 32.4).

Skin glue (Dermabond. Ethicon, NJ, USA) is placed over the midline incision; this gives mechanical support to the skin and acts as a barrier against superficial surgical site infection, factors which may contribute to a lower rate of wound dehiscence. Drains are used only in cases of hybrid gluteal augmentation. Figures 32.5, 32.6 and 32.7 show pre- and postoperative results in different patients.

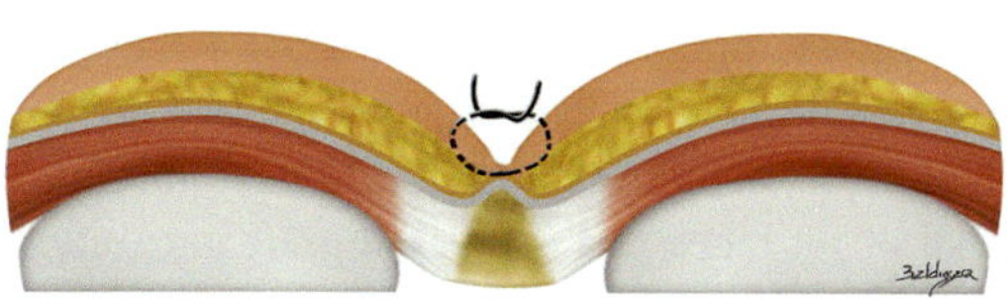

Fig. 32.4 Representation of midline wound closure. In order to decrease dead space in the area of subcutaneous undermining prior to division of the muscle, progressive tension sutures are used. Great attention to dermal closure is required, and bites should be taken of the presacral periosteum in order to deepen the intergluteal cleft

32.3.1 Hybrid Gluteal Augmentation

Fat grafting is not the topic of this chapter and is addressed in the appropriate section of the book; however, gluteal implants have two distinct advantages in comparison to gluteal fat grafting for buttock augmentation: greater predictability, since fat reabsorption rates from 24% to 50% are reported [17, 18], and the avoidance of the risk of fatal or nonfatal fat embolism (1:1449 over the prior 12 months) [19]. Staying subcutaneous (or, more precisely, suprafascial) during gluteal fat grafting is not a new concept and has been performed by surgeons all over the world for many years, but only now have attempts to systematically describe a reproducible and safe technique been performed by Del Vecchio et al. ("safe subcutaneous buttock augmentation") [20]. A very significant issue that is not described in the large Aesthetic Surgery Education and Research Foundation (ASERF) report is the correlation between fat graft volume and risk of pulmonary emboli. If the purported mechanism of fat embolism is damage to gluteal veins, which have a negative pressure relative to surrounding tissues and therefore "suck in" fat, it is reasonable to suppose that, as increasing volumes of fat are grafted to areas around these veins, the tissue pressure will increase, leading to an increased pressure gradient between the surrounding tissues and the gluteal veins, with resultant greater volumes of fat pulled into the venous system. As stated previously in this chapter, despite the "Brazilian Butt Lift" name, a majority of surgeons in Brazil do not perform fat grafting with large volumes (e.g., >500 mL), as the goal is always shape, rather than a set minimum volume (as requested by some patients); avoidance of creating excessively large buttocks, especially in men, is fundamental. Additionally, it is uncommon in Brazil to use pumps to reinject fat; this,

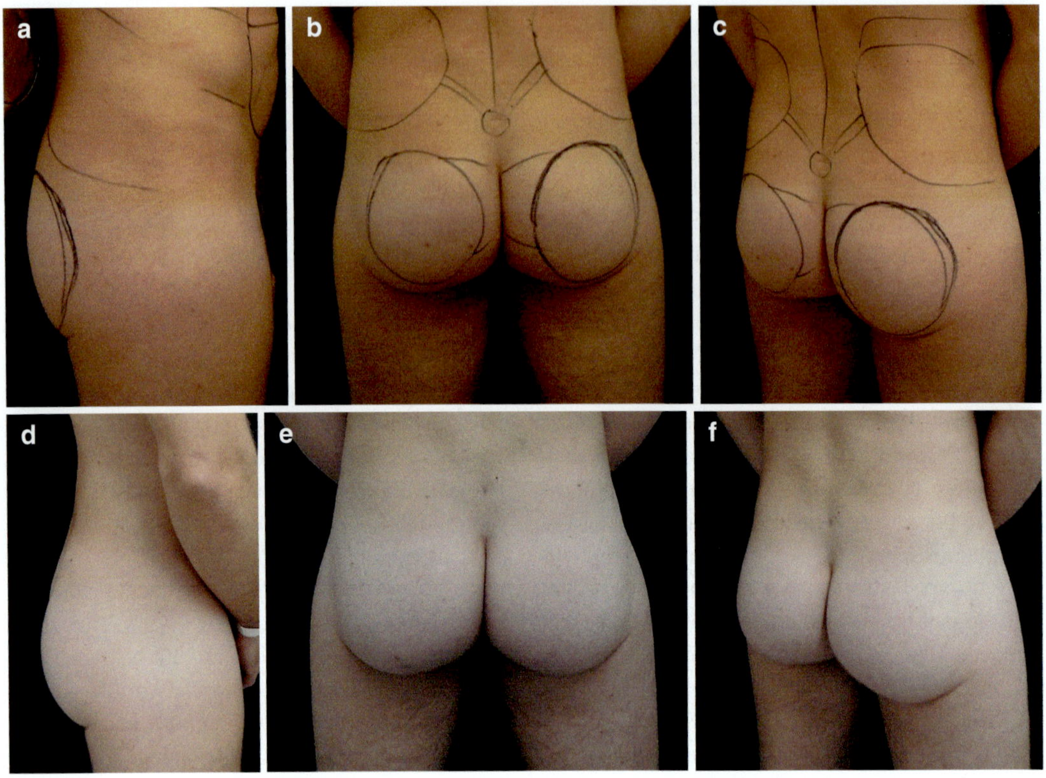

Fig. 32.5 (**a–c**) Preoperative (left) and (**d–f**) 12-month postoperative (right) views of a 37-year-old man who underwent intramuscular gluteal augmentation with 240 mL round, smooth, silicone gel implants. Increased gluteal projection is seen, and the importance of keeping the point of maximal gluteal projection in men is noted. Patient also underwent liposuction of the flanks

combined with the avoidance of excessive volumes, may be a contributing factor to fat grafting safety.

Hybrid gluteal augmentation [21] is commonly performed in our patients, especially in order to fill trochanteric depressions and, in association with subcision, to treat regions of cellulite depressions (the latter is almost never a problem in men). Additionally, the ischiatic region is often atrophic in patients with gluteal atrophy; when gluteal implants alone are used, this area can appear as a step-off or contour irregularity, especially in patients following weight loss. Fat grafting improves the contour and may decrease implant visibility. We perform liposuction in 85% of our male gluteal implant patients, of which 40% undergo adjunctive fat grafting. We have recently begun to use a closed system for fat aspiration and purification (Puregraft® and Motiva®, Establishment Labs, Costa Rica); possible benefits include decreased exposure of aspirated fat to the open environment, with lower risk of contamination, and increased fat retention rates [22].

Power-assisted liposuction (PAL) and fat grafting are performed after implant placement. The bottom layer of fat is discarded, and the remaining fat is injected at the subcutaneous level, using a 2 mm single-hole cannula and a 20 mL syringe parallel to the gluteal musculature. Multiple slow passes are made in a fanning technique, avoiding bolus injections to minimize risk of fat lakes and decreased graft integration. Care must be taken to follow the natural curvature of the buttocks, especially laterally, to avoid inadvertent penetration of the muscle or implant and potential risk of fat embolism. The average volume of fat used in hybrid cases is 120 mL per buttock.

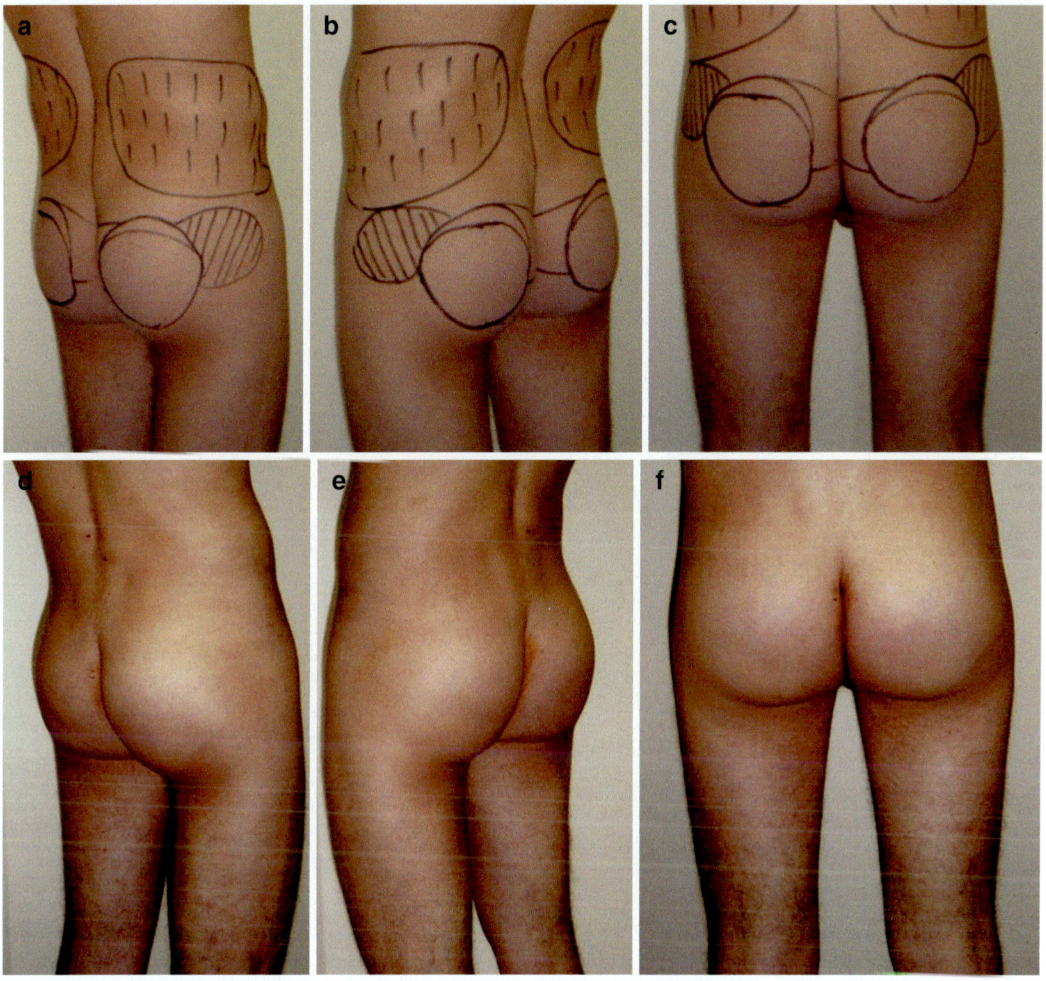

Fig. 32.6 (**a**, **b**) Preoperative (left) and (**c**, **d**) 6-month postoperative (right) views of a 29-year-old man with very little gluteal projection who underwent augmentation with 270 mL round, smooth, silicone gel implants, as well as liposuction of the flanks. (**e**, **f**) The hashed areas were grafted with 60 cc of fat to each side, to help ensure a smoother transition of the implants

32.3.2 Postoperative Care

Dressings are taken down 48 h postoperatively and then changed daily. We use either compressive shorts in case of isolated gluteal implants or a full postoperative compression garment in case of associated liposuction; these are used for 2 months. We do not use specific postoperative cushions. Patients are advised to avoid sitting for the first 4 days; after this period, we recommend chairs that have arms, allowing the patient to not force the gluteal muscles. We keep patients on sulfamethoxazole-trimethoprim or cefadroxil for 7 days postoperatively. Physical exercise can be started at 4 weeks, including squats with light weights, and running or elliptical exercise bikes after 6 weeks. We use enoxaparin 40 mg daily for 7 days in all patients unless there is a specific contraindication.

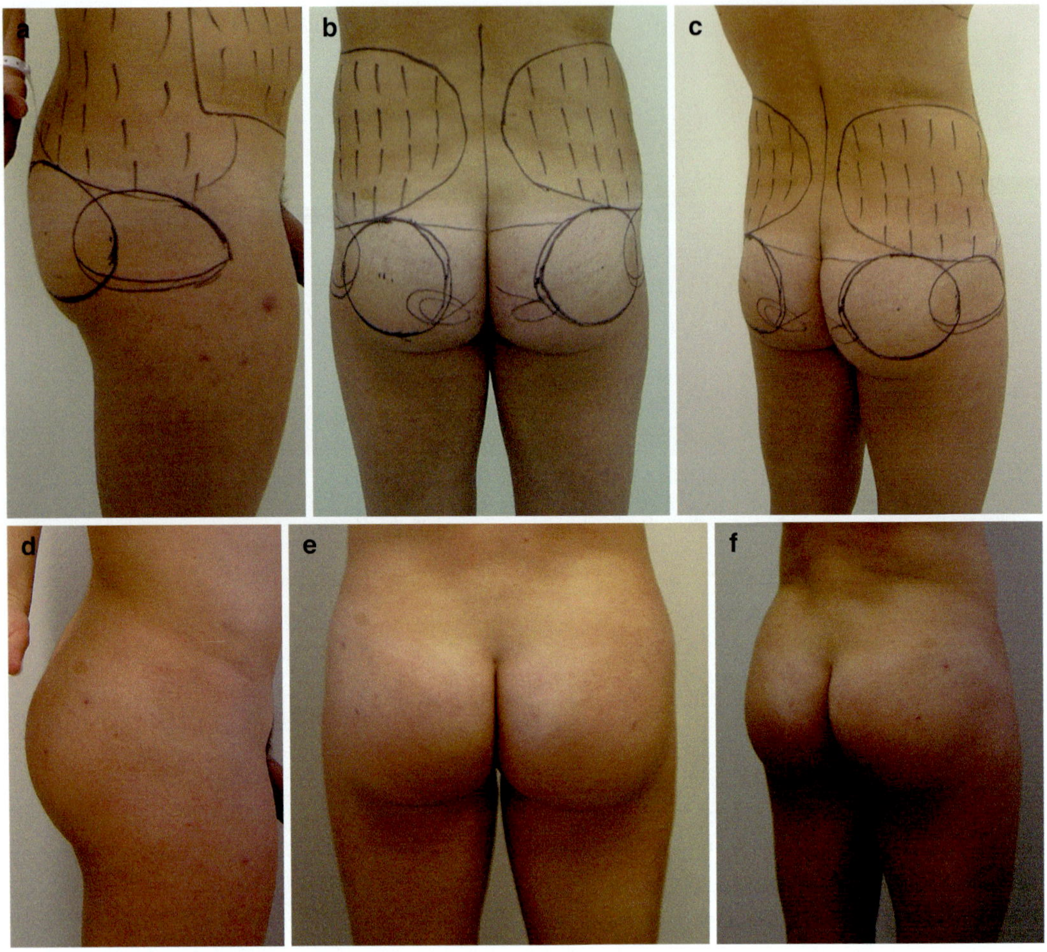

Fig. 32.7 (**a**–**c**) Preoperative (left) and (**d**–**f**) 18-month (right) postoperative views of a 34-year-old man who underwent gluteal augmentation with 235 mL, anatomic, nanotextured silicone gel implants, as well as liposuction of the flanks. Lateral trochanteric areas were grafted with 100 cc of fat to each side as the patient did not desire a trochanteric depression

32.3.3 Complications

Symptomatic seromas, which we define as those either palpable or visible by the patient or surgeon, are not uncommon, generally occurring between 7 and 14 days postoperatively. These are treated in the office with serial aspiration using a 1.8 mm multi-hole cannula, with gentle manual displacement of the implant. We do not routinely perform postoperative ultrasound to check for fluid collections, so smaller clinically insignificant seromas may be more common. We have not experienced any cases of capsular contracture, clinically significant hematoma requiring aspiration or surgical drainage, or need for implant revision or upsizing.

Wound dehiscence has occurred in <2% of our patients and is treated conservatively; unless there is evidence of surgical site infection, we do not use antibiotics prophylactically in case of dehiscence. The ensuing scar is generally of good quality and well hidden in the intergluteal crease, without a need for surgical revision.

32.4 Discussion

The increased emphasis by the media and consequently patients on the gluteal region is reflected in the large growth in gluteal augmentation operations, including fat grafting, gluteal implants, and poly-L-lactic acid injections.

Implants, with or without associated fat grafting, are our preferred approach, as the operation is safe, results are consistent, and the volume selected is maintained, contrary to fat grafting, in which rates and factors influencing retention are still incompletely understood and may be erratic, often leading to patient dissatisfaction due to undercorrection.

The intramuscular pocket, with limited subcutaneous undermining, has been shown to cause no change in postoperative buttock sensation (tactile, thermal, pain or pressure) [23]; however, because this study was performed in patients who underwent cohesive silicone gel implants, the results may not be applicable to solid elastomer implants, which are the most widely used type of implants in the United States and are firmer than silicone gel implants used elsewhere. Apart from the erogenous function of the buttocks, which has an important role in a patient's sexual life [24], impaired gluteal sensation could potentially lead to an increased risk of burns or pressure ulcers.

A common question, and potentially a limiting factor in more widespread patient desire for gluteal augmentation, is "will the implants feel like my own body at some point?" Aboudib et al. found that patients took between 7 and 90 days until they did not realize they had a gluteal implant, with an average time of 42 days [25]. This information is important during preoperative counseling.

A specific group of male patients who desire gluteal augmentation is those with human immunodeficiency virus (HIV), the overwhelming majority of whom are now on highly active antiretroviral therapy (HAART), which has some well-known untoward metabolic effects. Lipodystrophy caused by HAART results in fat redistribution, with loss of fat in the face, buttocks, legs, and arms. This has been shown to lead to low self-esteem and decreased compliance with HAART. Gluteal lipoatrophy is a bothersome aspect of HAART-related lipoatrophy, and can be successfully treated with gluteal implants, since many of these patients lack sufficient fat for autologous fat grafting (and questions remain as to the durability of results due to the ongoing metabolic changes related to grafted fat in patients with HAART-related lipoatrophy). These patients must be cleared preoperatively by their infectious disease physician; we use the same criteria as Andrade et al. [26]: use of HAART >12 months, CD4 count >200/mm^3, and an undetectable viral load. We have not had an increased complication rate in this group of patients and have experienced good satisfaction from the majority of the men whom we have operated.

High complication rates described in the literature [27, 28], including hematoma, infection, seroma, and dehiscence (up to 80% in overweight patients or those in which implants >350 mL are used), have been reduced by meticulous pocket dissection, use of bipolar cautery and rigorous hemostasis, and the use of adhesion sutures, to decrease dead space.

The CosmetAssure database [29], which covers 24 cosmetic surgery operations, showed an overall higher rate of hematoma in men compared to women (1.3% vs. 0.6%), between 2008 and 2013, in line with higher hematoma rates shown in the literature, but we have not noticed a gender difference in our experience. In this study, men represented 6.5% of patients, and buttock augmentation in men represented only 0.6% of body contouring procedures (32 patients). Whether these cases represented autologous fat grafting or buttock implants was not stated in this review; there was one complication in male patients. We have not seen differences in infections, seromas, hematomas, dehiscence, or need for surgical revision in our male patients as compared to our female patients.

With regard to incision placement, we prefer the midline intergluteal crease; in women, parasacral incisions such as proposed by González-Ulloa [30] and Mendieta [31] may become visible when wearing thong bikinis which are favored in Brazil. The wound dehiscence rate in the senior author's practice has been <1% using this approach. We have found no reason to modify this incision type in men, especially considering that implant sizes in our male patients are generally smaller than in women, varying from 200 to 280 cc. While authors such as Serra et al. advocate removal of a midline strip of skin and/or dermis in the intergluteal cleft [32], we believe that removing tissue in this area which is already under highest tension would increase the likelihood of dehiscence or hypertrophic scarring, for which reason we do not remove any skin. We agree with Senderoff [33] in that it is likely not an intrinsically lower vascular supply to the sacral midline which leads to dehiscence, but rather problems with adequate wound closure or excessively large implants.

As seen in Fig. 32.3, the use of progressive tension sutures [34] to decrease tension on the undermined subcutaneous pocket and advance the soft tissue to the sacral midline, as well as a layered closure including a horizontal, anchoring mattress suture with 3–0 Nylon incorporating both the superficial fascia at the incision edges, the deep dermis and, fundamentally, the sacral periosteum, has been our method of choice for closure and has led to <2% rates of dehiscence.

The question of whether there is a difference in complication rates between the solid elastomer implants available in the United States and cohesive gel implants which are used in countries with large numbers of gluteal implant patients, such as Brazil, Mexico, and Colombia, has not been adequately addressed. A review of gluteal augmentation using gluteal implants or autologous fat grafting by Sinno et al. [35] showed a complication rate of 21.9% for implants versus 9.9% for fat grafting. Most of the complications accounting for this higher number in the implant group were relatively minor, including wound dehiscence and seroma. Interestingly, the rate of sciatic pain tended to be higher in the fat grafting group. We consider that implants have two inherent and evident advantages over fat grafting: predictability and no risk of fat embolism [36]. With adequate training and anatomical knowledge, as well as bringing patient expectations in line with safe surgical practice, we have not encountered some of the problems described in the literature such as implant palpability and patient dissatisfaction [37]; in fact, we find gluteal implant surgery to be one of the operations which we least frequently need to revise, at <1%. Judicious and targeted use of fat grafting in hybrid cases may help improve outcomes of gluteal implants while increasing safety compared to large-volume fat grafting.

As with breast implants, there is some degree of gluteal muscle atrophy related to the pressure exerted by the implants; however, with intramuscular gluteal augmentation, this is almost negligible, at 4.3% and 2.6% atrophy by volume, on the right and left buttock, respectively [38]. Interestingly, in this study, all oval base implants, which were initially placed in a vertical position, turned obliquely in the direction of the gluteus maximus fibers at 3 months.

As noted by Serra et al. [32], a modified intramuscular technique with a smaller area of subcutaneous undermining, use of adhesion sutures, and least interruption of the midline soft tissue all contribute to a decreased risk of wound healing complications, including dehiscence. The authors noted a decreased complication rate in two groups of patients which were compared, from 35% to 5%. This complication rate is in line with or lower than autologous fat grafting for buttock augmentation.

Further studies are needed to compare aesthetic and patient satisfaction outcomes of gluteal implants versus fat grafting; additionally, ideal male gluteal aesthetics have still not been completely defined. With the growing number of male aesthetic operations, we should turn more attention to this large potential patient group.

32.5 Conclusion

The buttocks are a huge source of media attention, and demand for gluteal augmentation is likely to grow for the foreseeable future. Accordingly, it is worthwhile for plastic surgeons to learn and dominate both implant and fat-based gluteal augmentation to attend to the full spectrum of patients desiring posterior body contouring. The use of silicone gel gluteal implants in an intramuscular pocket is safe and effective, without the risk of fat emboli associated with gluteal fat grafting. Targeted, precise gluteal fat grafting to smooth contour irregularities is an excellent adjunct. Patient satisfaction is high when the difference between male and female gluteal aesthetic goals is respected and expectations are realistic.

References

1. International Society of Aesthetic Plastic Surgery 2017 Statistics. 2017. https://www.isaps.org/wp-content/uploads/2019/03/ISAPS_2017_International_Study_Cosmetic_Procedures_NEW.pdf). Accessed 28 Mar 2019.
2. Roberts TL, Weinfeld AB, Bruner TW, Nguyen K. "Universal" and ethnic ideals of beautiful buttocks are best obtained by autologous micro fat grafting and liposuction. Clin Plast Surg. 2006;33:371–94.
3. Lee EI, Roberts TL, Bruner TW. Ethnic considerations in buttock aesthetics. Semin Plast Surg. 2009;23:232–44.
4. Toledo LS. Gluteal augmentation with fat grafting: the Brazilian Buttock technique: 30 years' experience. Clin Plast Surg. 2015;42:253–61.
5. Abel de la Peña J, Rubio OV, Cano JP, Cedillo MC, Garcés MT. History of gluteal augmentation. Clin Plastic Surg. 2006;33:307–19.
6. Ghavami A, Villanueva NL, Amirlak B. Gluteal ligamentous anatomy and its implication in safe buttock augmentation. Plast Reconstr Surg. 2018;14:363–71.
7. Robles J, Tagliapietra J, Grandi M. Gluteoplastia de aumento: implante submuscular. Cir Plast Iberolatinoamericana. 1984;10:365–9.
8. De la Peña JA. Subfascial technique for gluteal augmentation. Aesthetic Surg J. 2004;24:265–73.
9. Aiache AE. Gluteal recontouring with combination treatments: implants, liposuction, and fat transfer Clin Plastic Surg. 2006;33:395–403.
10. Mofid MM, Gonzalez R, de la Peña JA, Mendieta CG, Senderoff DM, Jorjani S. Buttock augmentation with silicone implants: a multicenter survey review of 2226 patients. Plast Reconstr Surg. 2013;131:897–901.
11. Singh D. Adaptive significance of female physical attractiveness: role of waist-to-hip ratio. J Pers Soc Psychol. 1993;65:293–307.
12. Mendieta CG, Sood A. Classification system for gluteal evaluation revisited. Clin Plastic Surg. 2018;45:159–77.
13. Singh D. Universal allure of the hourglass figure: an evolutionary theory of female physical attractiveness. Clin Plastic Surg. 2006;33:359–70.
14. Cuenca-Guerra R, Lugo-Beltran I. Beautiful buttocks: characteristics and surgical techniques. Clin Plastic Surg. 2006;33:321–32.
15. Gonzalez R. Augmentation gluteoplasty: the XYZ method. Aesth Plast Surg. 2004;28:417–25.
16. Andrade GA, Coltro PS, Andó A, et al. Gluteal augmentation with silicone implants: a new proposal for intramuscular dissection. Aesth Plast Surg. 2017;41:872–7.
17. Wolf GA, Gallego S, Patrón AS, et al. Magnetic resonance imaging assessment of gluteal fat grafts. Aesth Plast Surg. 2006;30:460–8.
18. Carpaneda CA, Ribeiro MT. Study of the histologic alterations and viability of the adipose graft in humans. Aesth Plast Surg. 1993;17(43):47.
19. Mofid MM, Teitelbaum S, Suissa D, Ramirez-Montañana A, Astarita DC, Mendieta C, Singer R. Report on mortality from gluteal fat grafting: recommendations from the ASERF Task Force. Aesthet Surg J. 2017;37:796–806.
20. Del Vecchio DA, Villanueva NL, Mohan R, Johnson B, Wan D, Venkataram A, et al. Clinical implications of gluteal fat graft migration: a dynamic anatomical study. Plast Reconstr Surg. 2018;142:1180–92.
21. Lee JW, Kang MG, Park SS. Secondary gluteal augmentation: surgical technique and outcomes. Plast Reconstr Surg. 2018;141:1371–82.
22. Gerth DJ, King B, Rabach L, Glasgold RA, Glasgold MJ. Long-term volumetric retention of autologous fat grafting processed with closed-membrane filtration. Aesthet Surg J. 2014;34(7):985–94.
23. Serra-Guimarães F, Venturini De Barros MA, Aboudib JH, et al. Does intramuscular gluteal augmentation using implants affect sensitivity in the buttocks? J Plast Reconstr Aesthet Surg. 2017;70:801–5.
24. Senderoff DM. Aesthetic surgery of the buttocks using implants: practice-based recommendations. Aesthet Surg J. 2016;36:559–76.
25. Aboudib JH, Serra-Guimarães F, Sampaio FJB. Profile of patients undergoing gluteoplasty. Aesth Plast Surg. 2016;40:30–7.
26. Andrade GA, Coltro PS, Barros ME, Müller Neto BF, Lima RV, Farina JA Jr. Gluteal augmentation with intramuscular implants in patients with human immunodeficiency virus with lipoatrophy related to the use of antiretroviral therapy. Ann Plast Surg. 2017;79:426–9.
27. Bruner TW, Robert TL, Nguyen K. Complications of buttocks augmentation: diagnosis, management, and prevention. Clin Plastic Surg. 2006;33:449–66.
28. Oranges CM, Tremp M, di Summa P, et al. Gluteal augmentation techniques: a comprehensive literature review. Aesthetic Surg J. 2017;37:560–9.
29. Kaoutzanis C, Winocour J, Yeslev M, Gupta V, Asokan I, Roostaeian J, Grotting JC, Higdon K. Aesthetic surgical procedures in men: major complications and associated risk factors. Aesthet Surg J. 2018;38:429–41.
30. González-Ulloa M. Gluteoplasty: a ten-year report. Aesth Plast Surg. 1991;15:85–91.

31. Mendieta CG. Intramuscular gluteal augmentation technique. Clin Plastic Surg. 2006;33:423–34.
32. Serra F, Aboudib JH, Marques RG. Reducing wound complications in gluteal augmentation surgery. Plast Reconstr Surg. 2012;130:706–13.
33. Senderoff DM. Commentary on: gluteal augmentation techniques: a comprehensive literature review. Aesthet Surg J. 2017;37:570–2.
34. Baroudi R, Ferreira CA. Seroma: how to avoid it and how to treat it. Aesthet Surg J. 1998;18:439–41.
35. Sinno S, Chang JB, Brownstone ND, Saadeh PB, Wall S Jr. Determining the safety and efficacy of gluteal augmentation: a systematic review of outcomes and complications. Plast Reconstr Surg. 2016;137:1151–6.
36. Kalaaji A, Dreyer S, Vadseth L, Maric I, Jönsson V, Haukeboe TH. Gluteal augmentation with fat: retrospective safety study and literature review. Aesthetic Surg J. 2019;39:292–305.
37. Shah B. Complications in gluteal augmentation. Clin Plastic Surg. 2018;45:179–86.
38. Serra F, Aboudib JH, Marques RG. Intramuscular technique for gluteal augmentation: determination and quantification of muscle atrophy and position by computed tomographic scan. Plast Reconstr Surg. 2013;131:253–9.

Male Abdominoplasty

33

Alan Matarasso and Darren M. Smith

33.1 Introduction

The abdomen plays a major role in determining an individual's overall appearance. A fit midsection projects health and strength. Abdominoplasty has received a great deal of attention in the literature, especially in the context of post-partum body contouring in women, and our techniques have evolved substantially over time to offer better results with safer procedures. While male abdominoplasty has received less academic attention (which is proportionate as the procedure is performed much less frequently in men than in women), abdominoplasty remains a very powerful procedure in properly selected male patients. The basic principles of abdominoplasty are similar in men and women, as are the essential goals of the procedure. These are to achieve a firm, flat abdomen with the least prominent scars possible. There are, however, differences between male and female core composition that dictate distinctions between abdominal contouring procedures in men and women. We will begin by first highlighting these differences and follow with a discussion of techniques designed to maximize success in abdominoplasty.

A. Matarasso (✉)
Department of Plastic Surgery, Hofstra University/Northwell School of Medicine, Manhattan Ear, Eye and Throat Hospital, Lenox Hill Hospital, New York, NY, USA
e-mail: receptionist@drmatarasso.com

D. M. Smith
Private Practice, New York, NY, USA

33.2 Distinguishing Characteristics of Male Abdominoplasty

As in women, abdominoplasty in men is focused on addressing three treatable layers of soft tissue: skin, fat, and muscle. Abdominoplasty is most frequently performed in postpartum women who have undergone specific anatomical changes after pregnancy. The skin becomes more lax due to excess from expanding to accommodate a once enlarged uterus and often develops stretch marks in the process. The defining change of the muscle layer is the development of a rectus diastasis, another adaptation to allow for uterine expansion. Finally, after pregnancy and with increasing age, the amount of intra-abdominal fat generally increases. Pregnancy is also often associated with an accumulation of subcutaneous fat.

Males, of course, do not undergo pregnancy; however, the same three treatable soft tissue layers of the abdomen undergo changes over time and with weight fluctuation, and efforts to improve the male patient's abdominal contour again target the skin, fat, and muscle of the region. There are several differentiating characteristics of the male and female abdomen that

K. Jeffords et al. (eds.), *Aesthetic Surgery for Men*, https://doi.org/10.1007/978-3-032-03840-1_33

bear mentioning in this context. First, women tend to have thinner skin with a greater tendency towards laxity and striae, whereas men have thicker skin less susceptible to the development of stretch marks. Next, while women tend to develop a rectus diastasis that is most prominent inferiorly, men tend to develop a rectus diastasis that is widest superiorly. Finally, with regard to fat distribution, women tend to have less visceral fat until it accumulates after pregnancy and menopause, while men begin accumulating this deep fat in their mid-twenties. In women, subcutaneous fat is thicker with a less uniform distribution (it is primarily prominent peripherally and below the iliac crest. In men, the abdominal subcutaneous fat layer is thinner in general but with relative central accumulation. There is also more flank accumulation of subcutaneous fat in men. Taken together, these anatomical differences contribute to an average waist-to-hip ratio of 0.66 in women and 0.90 in men.

In reviewing a series of his male abdominal contouring patients, the senior author found that of 58 males, 84% underwent suction-assisted lipectomy alone, while only 16% "open" abdominoplasty (Fig. 33.1). Of men undergoing full abdominoplasty, it was further noted that rectus muscle plication was frequently not performed—in contrast, this is a mainstay of full abdominoplasty performed in women (with the exception of massive weight loss patients). Additionally, pregnancy in some cases causes abdominal con-

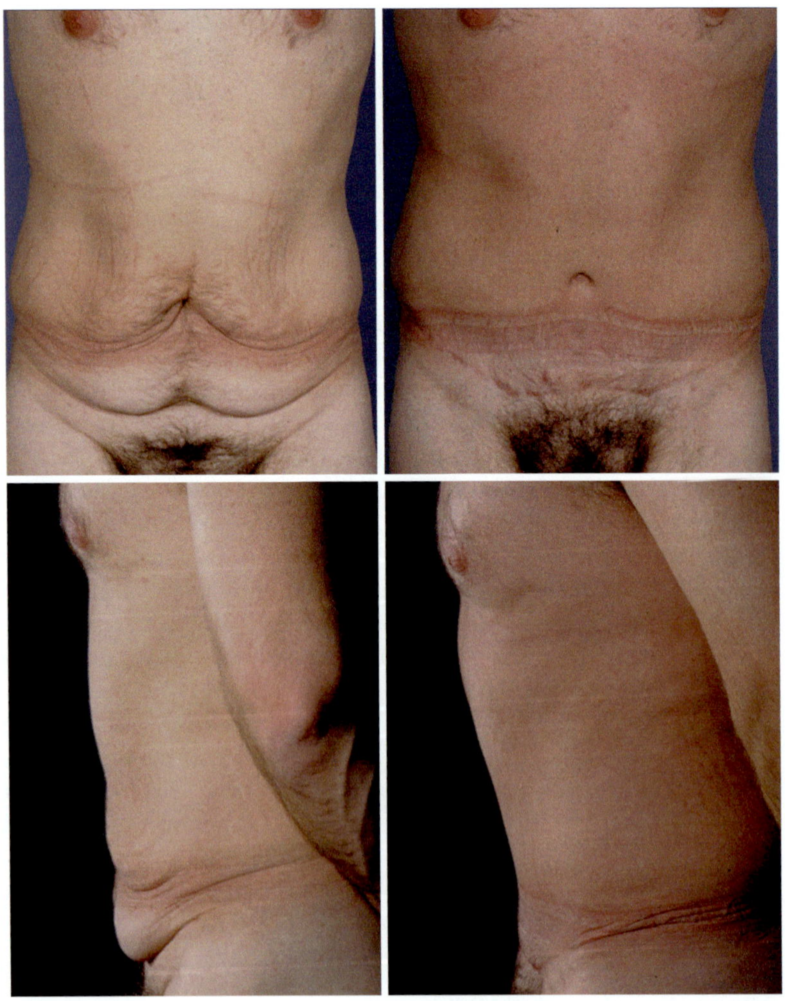

Fig. 33.1 A 29-year-old male before (left) and after (right) abdominoplasty

tour deformities limited to the infra-umbilical region, which can be effectively managed with a mini abdominoplasty. A localized lower-abdominal contour deformity such as this is unusual in males, and therefore so is the indication for a mini abdominoplasty. Analogously, pregnancy may result in isolated skin laxity in the supra-umbilical region, which some may choose to address with a reverse abdominoplasty. This is not a frequently indicated procedure in general, and its indications in male patients are limited even further.

Whereas in female abdominal contouring patients, it is not unusual to perform the entire procedure in a supine position, we find that male abdominal contouring procedures are frequently enhanced by adjunctive interventions to address the flanks (excisional flankplasty with or without liposuction) and liposuction of the lumbar roll (localized adiposity on the back from approximately L2 to L4). Therefore, when planning male abdominal contouring procedures, we often perform these portions of the operation in a lateral decubitus or prone position before returning to the supine position for the abdominoplasty.

33.3 Preoperative Considerations

33.3.1 Patient Selection

Abdominoplasty should be performed on healthy, low-risk individuals. Special vigilance is required when considering abdominoplasty in the massive weight loss population due to unique risk factors [1]. Aside from ensuring overall good health in abdominoplasty patients, additional attention should be paid to evaluating their risk for VTE (venous thromboembolism) given the relative prevalence of this potentially devastating complication in abdominoplasty [2]. As a point of reference, a survey of over 1100 plastic surgeons on venous thromboembolism in their practice found that VTE was most frequently reported in association with abdominoplasty and abdominoplasty combined with other procedures (there was no significant difference in VTE frequency between the these two groups) [3]. Therefore, a comprehensive history must be taken in abdominoplasty patients that allows for a data-based, patient-specific risk reduction strategy to be employed [4]. One important historical feature that may be reported by a woman and would alert one to a propensity for VTE is the occurrence of unexplained miscarriages. This data point will, of course, not be available in men, further underscoring the necessity of vigilance and directed history taking. Patients deemed to be at high risk for VTE will be referred for a hematologic workup. Patients can also be screened by blood tests for prothrombogenic genetic risk factors.

To complement any physical or pharmacological VTE chemoprophylaxis that may be indicated by the date-driven, patient-specific approach mentioned above, our female patients our advised to discontinue the use of female hormones in the preoperative period. While much less common in men, estrogen therapy may be employed for some conditions [5]. It should similarly be discontinued in men prior to undergoing abdominoplasty, as should testosterone. Nicotine is also discontinued in the preoperative period.

Aside from a personal or family history of VTE, additional red flags in the medical history include pulmonary conditions, cardiac insufficiency, peripheral vascular disease, hypertension, obesity, bleeding disorders, smoking, exposure to secondhand smoke, and diseases affecting the microcirculation (diabetes, lupus, chronic fatigue syndrome). Any such issues must be identified and resolved in conjunction with an appropriate specialist prior to performing an abdominoplasty.

33.3.2 Preoperative Evaluation

After the patient has been determined to be a medically sound candidate for abdominoplasty, a thorough physical exam is the next step in setting up a successful abdominal contouring procedure. The exam should be considered in terms of the three treatable layers of the abdomen discussed above. The degree of skin laxity should be assessed, and the location of any stretch marks should be identified. Stretch marks superior to the umbilicus will likely not be amenable to removal with abdominoplasty, and this should be reviewed with the patient to avoid disappointment in the postoperative period. The relative proportion of visceral abdominal fat to subcutaneous fat should be assessed, and the distribution of superficial fat should be evaluated to design an approach to incorporate suction-assisted lipectomy into the procedure. The anatomy of the abdominal wall should be examined, and the presence of rectus diastasis or true hernias (e.g., ventral, umbilical, or inguinal) should be noted. If a true hernia is identified, a plan to manage this should be devised (a general surgeon can be consulted to address hernias in conjunction with abdominal contouring procedures, and the use of a Ventralex patch may be indicated [6]). Any scars present on the abdominal wall should also be identified and assessed with regard to their potential impact on the blood supply of the abdominoplasty flap. Any low transverse scars (more common in women in the form of Cesarean section scars) should be assessed for incorporation into the abdominoplasty incision if they cannot be excised.

Identification and discussion of non-treatable causes of abdominal contour deformity is also an integral portion of the preoperative evaluation so as to properly manage expectations and maximize postoperative patient satisfaction. Specifically, skeletal issues such as lumbar lordosis or scoliosis may contribute to the persistent appearance of an abdominal bulge or an asymmetric result, respectively. Hip asymmetry may also cause persistent postoperative asymmetry and should be identified and brought to the patient's attention.

After evaluation of the abdomen is completed, assessment of surrounding areas should be performed. Specifically, the flanks in men frequently contain deposits of stubborn adipose tissue relatively recalcitrant to diet and exercise. Suction-assisted lipectomy of this region is therefore frequently performed in concert with an abdominoplasty. Moreover, men frequently develop a dorsal lumbar roll of adipose accumulation from approximately L2 to L4, and treatment of this adiposity with suction-assisted lipectomy at the time of abdominoplasty can significantly improve the overall result by contributing to a global improvement in core contour. Additionally, depending on the relative excess of skin with respect to adipose tissue in the flanks, the abdominoplasty incision may be carried further laterally to constitute a true flankplasty (a 270-degree lift). Inclusion of flank liposuction or flankplasty will necessitate prone or lateral decubitus positioning, while suction-assisted lipectomy of a lumbar roll will mandate prone positioning. These requirements should be assessed ahead of time, included in the operative plan, and clearly communicated to the operating room team.

33.4 Preoperative Preparation

33.4.1 Preoperative Decision-Making

We use the abdominolipoplasty system of classification and treatment as a framework for evaluating, counseling, and treating patients (Fig. 33.2) [7]. By way of review, a Type I procedure includes liposuction alone and is appropriate for those with minimal skin laxity, excess adiposity, and minimal rectus diastasis. In short, this is the abdominal contouring procedure of choice for most men (recall from above that only 16% of male abdominal contouring patients undergo "open" surgery). The Type II procedure consists of a mini abdominoplasty and is indicated in individuals with minor skin laxity, excess adiposity, and a lower rectus diastasis. Consistent with the anatomical considerations discussed earlier, this procedure is rarely performed in men. A Type III procedure consists of a modified abdominoplasty designed to address moderate skin laxity, excess adiposity, and a lower (with or without an upper) rectus diastasis. This has also been referred to as a lower abdominoplasty, where essentially, instead of removing half of the abdominal skin as in a full abdominoplasty, one quarter of the abdominal skin is removed, and the umbilicus is left intact. This can be an option for patients who have less skin excess and prefer to avoid umbilical scarring. Finally, a Type IV (full standard abdominoplasty) is indicated in the presence of

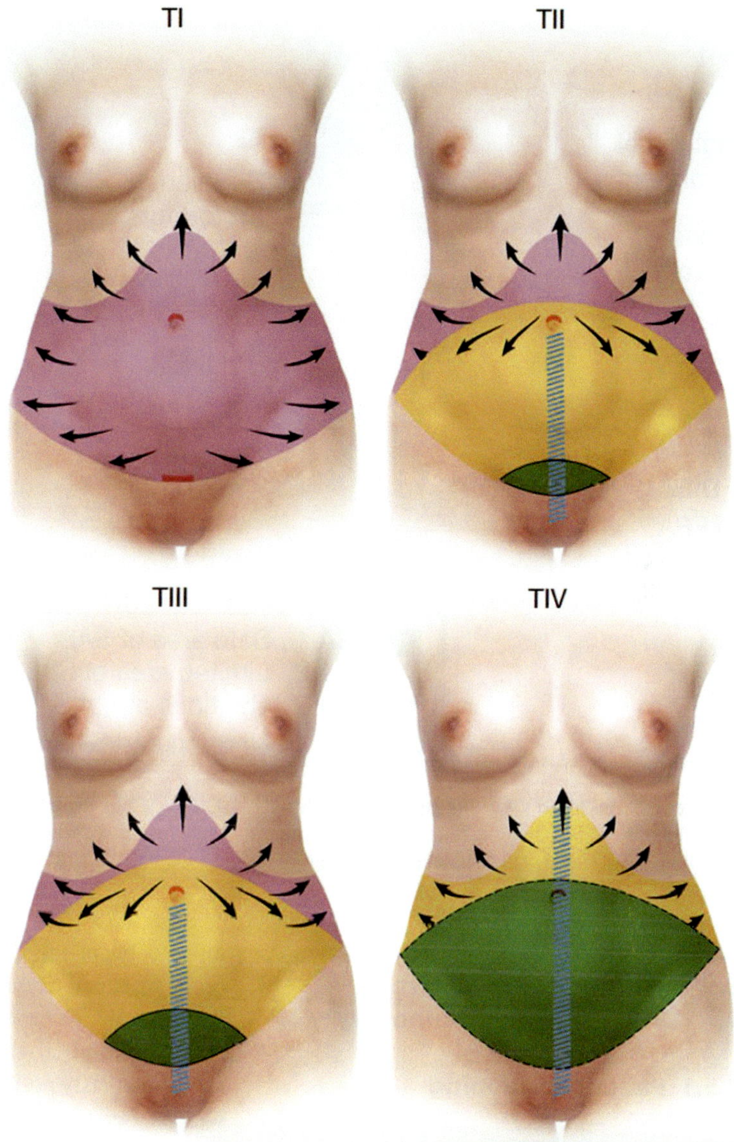

Fig. 33.2 The abdominolipoplasty system of classification and treatment. This classification schema includes (clockwise from top left): Type 1, liposuction alone; Type 2, mini abdominoplasty; Type 3, modified abdominoplasty (with Types 1 and 2 being limited abdominoplasties); and Type 4, a full standard abdominoplasty, which may or may not include liposuction. SAL suction-assisted lipectomy. Pink: liposuction. Yellow: undermining. Green: excision. Cross-hatching: fascial plication

severe skin laxity, excess adiposity, and complete rectus diastasis. When considering open procedures, this is the most common procedure performed in males, although males rarely require rectus plication. When performing any of these procedures, it is critical to keep the abdominal blood supply in mind (Fig. 33.3).

33.4.2 Preoperative Optimization

Once medically cleared to undergo an abdominoplasty, several steps are taken to further reduce the risk of perioperative complications. Abdominoplasty patients should be well-hydrated, and compression stockings and sequential compression devices are placed prior to the induction of anesthesia. Any history of surgical site infection (especially involving MRSA) is identified and appropriately accounted for. Nostril mupiricin ointment (GlaxoSmithKline, Research Triangle Park, NC) is routinely used in the perioperative period, as are oral and intravenous antibiotics and antimicrobial body scrubs. We prefer alcohol-based prep solutions at the time of surgery.

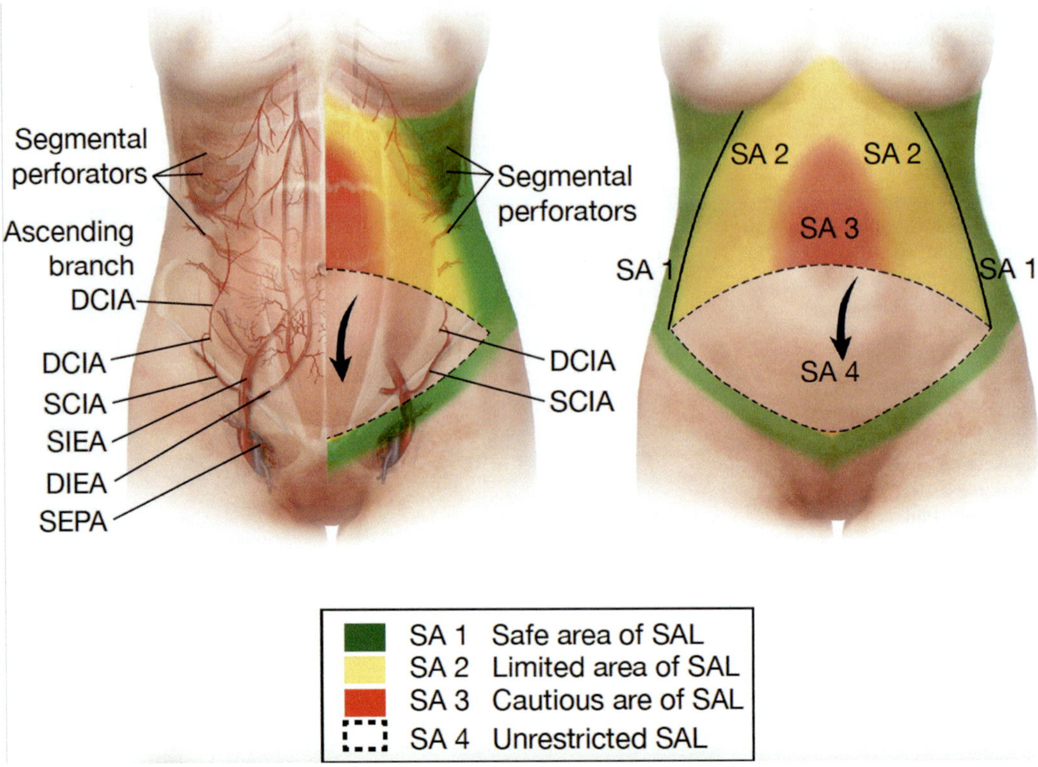

Fig. 33.3 (**a**) The blood supply of the abdomen before (left) and after (right) abdominoplasty. (**b**) A depiction of the suction areas (SA 1–4) of the abdomen, which are determined by these patterns of blood supply. SA 4 is not suctioned; it is excised

33.5 Techniques to Maximize Success in Abdominoplasty

33.5.1 Patient Positioning

Excellent results in abdominoplasty are especially dependent on the adequacy of patient positioning. As closure after appropriate skin excision requires that the operating room table can reach a full "beach chair" position, this is tested prior to the outset of the procedure. The symmetry of the skin excision is also reconfirmed with 0 silk sutures after liposuction is performed (see Operative Technique below). Similarly, symmetrical patient positioning is critical in achieving a symmetrical result. As such, the arm board angle and position along the side of the table are confirmed to be symmetrical prior to beginning the procedure. While in male patients, it is very common to begin the case with the patient in the prone or lateral decubitus position to address the flanks or lumbar roll. When the patient is ultimately placed in the supine position for the abdominoplasty portion of the procedure, a gauze wrap is used to secure the arms to the arm boards. Finally, the scrotum should be checked for pressure and position.

33.5.2 Approach

We perform this procedure under systemic anesthesia (most frequently spontaneous ventilation, general anesthesia, or spinal/epidural anesthesia in selected cases) administered by a board-certified anesthesiologist, in a certified ambulatory surgery facility. We regularly use a Foley catheter for fluid monitoring and bladder decompression. In cases involving multiple procedures, the abdominoplasty is generally performed last.

The patient wears his preferred undergarment at the outset of the markings to ensure the proposed incision is covered by the undergarment. The abdominal excision is gauged by assessing the ease with which the lower abdominal skin (from umbilicus to hairline) can be excised after grasping the pannus with both hands in an attempt to touch the thumbs with the fingers. In this manner, an abdominal excision is marked that is comprised of an ellipse of tissue between the umbilicus and the mons pubis. The lower incision is designed (with the pannus held slightly upward) to traverse the natural lower skin crease, slightly below its normal position to account for superior scar migration. Points just lateral to the bilateral lateral extents of the lower skin crease are noted with the patient in the sitting position at the outset of the marking process and delineate the lateral extents of this incision. The upper incision is designed to pass just over the umbilicus, so the excision encompasses the old umbilical site. This upper mark is brought further superior only if there is clearly sufficient skin excess to allow for closure. Laterally, this upper incision meets the lower incision to form an ellipse. It may be useful to trace the lower incision with a flexible ruler and subsequently flip this ruler along its horizontal axis to assess the path of the upper incision. Next, vertical lines can be marked through the planned abdominal excision, which can be later used to line up the skin edges for closure. Finally, the umbilical incision is drawn in a circumferential fashion, and its four quadrants are marked for reference.

33.5.3 Operative Technique

We begin by infiltrating the abdomen with approximately 1 liter of superwet anesthesia (1 L Ringer's lactate, 1 mL 1:1000 epinephrine, 20 mL 1% lidocaine). All sites of planned liposuction accessible from the supine position are infiltrated with tumescent solution at this point as well. Next, the patient is turned to address any portions of the procedure necessitating lateral or prone positioning (such as flankplasty or suction-assisted lipectomy of a lumbar roll). These sites are infiltrated, the tumescent is allowed to act for 10–15 minutes, and then suctioned as indicated. We then return the patient to the supine position. Liposuction of sites accessible from the supine position is then performed. Next, the abdominoplasty incisions are checked for symmetry by anchoring 0-silk sutures in the midline at the xiphoid and the mons below the lower incision. These sutures are crisscrossed and grasped with a clamp in such a fashion that the incisions' symmetry can be confirmed by moving the clamp to either side of the midline at various points on the upper and lower skin incision lines. The lower silk suture and the midline of the mons are used as reference points towards the end of the procedure when determining the midline position for exteriorization of the umbilicus.

We begin the procedure by circumscribing the umbilicus and thereby freeing it from the planned abdominoplasty excision. The pannus excision begins by sharply incising the upper limb of the ellipse to the level of the rectus fascia. The cut is beveled inward at a 45-degree angle. Sharp dissection and electrocautery are then used to undermine the upper abdominoplasty flap in a narrow tunnel. This is depicted as the zone of complete undermining in Fig. 33.4. The zone of selective undermining (indicated in orange in Fig. 33.4) surrounds this tunnel and is undermined as necessary to decrease skin bunching after muscle closure. By following this pattern of dissection, we are maintaining the intercostal blood supply (Fig. 33.3) and likely also preserving the deep superior epigastric blood supply (Fig. 33.3). This pattern of dissection also preserves a broad intact subcostal perforator blood supply in the zone of discontinuous undermining (green area in Fig. 33.4) that has been suctioned. This sequence allows for the entire flap and adjacent areas to be suctioned during a full abdominoplasty. This sequence represents a standard template and can be adjusted to meet individual patient needs. Liposuction can be omitted when it is not necessary.

At this point, the operating room table is flexed, and the upper skin flap is pulled over the

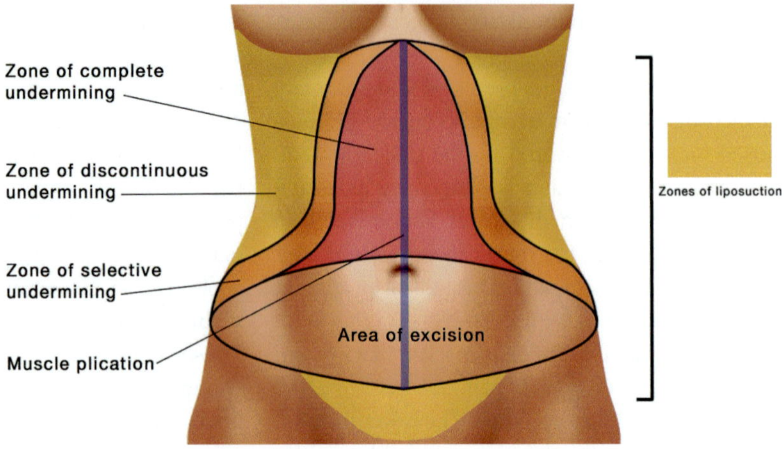

Fig. 33.4 The types of undermining in abdominoplasty may be divided into zones. Complete undermining is performed only as much as is required to allow for rectus muscle plication. Note how these zones correspond to the abdominal blood supply detailed in Fig. 33.3

pannus to verify that it reaches the lower skin incision as marked. If the flap does not reach the proposed lower incision (an extremely rare scenario), the flap can be stretched, further undermined as appropriate, Scarpa's fascia scored, or the lower incision can be raised. Once the final position of the lower incision is confirmed, it is made to the level of the fascia. We then grasp the pannus with Allis clamps and excise it en bloc, from right to left. We do not attempt to leave a thin layer of fibro-fatty tissue on the fascia with this excision, although some choose to do so in an effort to reduce seroma formation. Next, an ocular conformer is sutured to the umbilicus so as to facilitate later identification; this is removed when the umbilicus is later exteriorized. Hemostasis is actively achieved by the surgeon and assistants at each step of the procedure. This is the point of the operation at which we would turn our attention to plicating the rectus diastasis in women [8]; however, this maneuver is infrequently indicated in males. The cavity is irrigated, and final inspection and hemostasis are performed. Exparel is then widely injected in the surgical field [9].

The table is then returned to the beach chair position to facilitate wound closure. We begin the closure with a 2–0 Vicryl suture placed in the midline. Closed suction drains are placed within 5–8 cm from the lateral extent of each side of the incision and secured with 3–0 nylon sutures. We staple from lateral to medial to align the wound edges and minimize dog-ear formation. Next, a 2–0 PDO bidirectional barbed suture (Quill SRS, Angiotech, Vancouver, Canada) is used to close the deep layers from Scarpa's fascia to the dermis on either side of the midline. After closing most of the wound, we mark the site of the planned exteriorization of the umbilicus. The ocular conformer is palpated below the flap, and the new position of the umbilicus is marked on the skin in the midline, slightly cephalad to its natural position. We next run a second layer of 3–0 monoderm Quill in the subcuticular layer.

Before exteriorizing the umbilicus, we first verify the patient's midline using the silk marking sutures and our preoperative drawings. After confirming the new site of the umbilicus, the exteriorization is marked as a 2.5-cm inverted V in the midline. We defat the upper and (more so) the lower skin edges of the umbilical opening to provide a refined umbilical contour. The umbilicus is then exteriorized, and the ocular conformer removed. Deep absorbable sutures are used to sew the umbilicus to the skin flap, and the umbilical skin is closed with 3–0 nylon sutures. We no longer secure the umbilicus to the fascia. The umbilicus is packed with a strip of xeroform gauze. The abdominoplasty incision is covered with antibiotic ointment and covered with a Telfa dressing. The patient is transferred to a bed or stretcher pre-flexed to maintain the patient's positioning used for closure. We do not place the patient in an abdominal binder until the early postoperative period. Another male abdominoplasty patient is shown in Fig. 33.5.

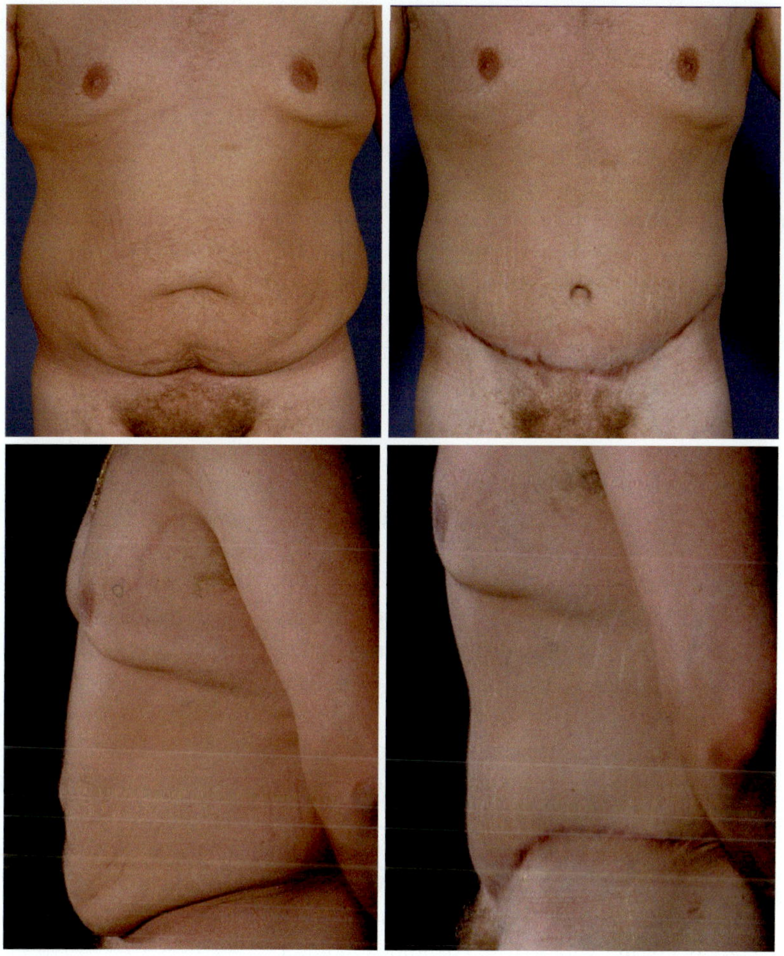

Fig. 33.5 A 22-year-old male before (left) and after (right) abdominoplasty

33.6 Other Considerations

33.6.1 Postoperative Care

Vigilance and adherence to protocol are essential in the immediate postoperative period. Patients should ambulate on the day of surgery, bent over as if they were using a walker. When in bed, they should flex and extend the knees and ankles and move the legs. Over the next few days to a week, their posture should gradually normalize. An experienced registered nurse should spend the first 24–48 hours after surgery with the patient to allow for close observation. Vital signs, pain control, intake and output, hygiene, and pulmonary care are closely monitored. Bowel function is followed carefully, and an over-the-counter regimen is used to avoid constipation.

In the days and weeks following the procedure, the incisions and abdominoplasty flap are frequently inspected for evidence of wound healing difficulties, and any necessary treatments are initiated as indicated. Drainage is followed closely, and the drains are removed (usually one at a time) as permitted by the volume and character of the drainage. As untreated seromas can result in a variety of sequelae, including infection and late contour irregularities due to pseudobursa formation, immediate drainage is advised should one arise. Patients are educated regarding the signs of possible thromboembolic events (e.g., shortness of breath, anxiety, leg or chest pain, palpitations, unilateral lower extremity swelling), and any concern is carefully evaluated. We also encourage a postoperative venous Doppler study. It is critical to adequately and appropriately treat postoperative pain not only to enhance patient comfort but also to avoid potentially severe complications such as paralytic ileus and hematoma formation [10]. A bowel movement is an important milestone that we monitor and treat constipation if necessary, because increased pressure and straining can result in an untoward series of events, such as hematoma formation.

33.6.2 A Brief Overview of Complications and Their Management

Abdominoplasty carries a relatively high complication rate (4.7%), necessitating meticulous attention to detail in all phases of the procedure, from patient selection through the operating room and into the postoperative period [10]. The most common complication after abdominoplasty is seroma [10]. The risk of seroma is reduced by using closed suction drains, quilting sutures, or a combination of the two, surgical sealants, and perhaps technical factors such as avoiding cutting with Bovie. Fastidious monitoring in the postoperative period is also critical. Pulmonary embolism, occurring in 0.19% of abdominoplasties, is the most dangerous complication of this procedure. The importance of the anti VTE measures discussed earlier cannot be overemphasized [10]. Wound healing problems and tissue ischemia (including damage to or even loss of the umbilicus) are minimized by paying close attention to the method and extent of undermining, an understanding of the abdominoplasty flap's blood supply, and prudent decision-making in reconciling the tension on wound closure with the extent of liposuction performed. All incisions are inspected on the night of surgery and the following morning for any signs of ischemia. Should any issues be identified, any reversible causes such as fluid collection, infections, or wound tension (that can be relieved by suture removal) are addressed. Progressing ischemia is treated with topical therapies including dimethyl sulfoxide (DMSO) or nitroglycerine ointment. Any frank necrosis that develops is managed with standard wound care principles, including allowing the tissues to demarcate before any debridement is performed [11].

33.7 Conclusion

Abdominoplasty is a comprehensive procedure that addresses skin laxity, abdominal adiposity, and laxity of the abdominal wall, yielding great patient satisfaction. While more frequently performed in women, appropriately selected male patients can benefit a great deal from this procedure as well. The basic principles are similar between male and female abdominoplasty. The recognition of anatomical differences between men and women dictates the variations in technique we have discussed here. Taken together, these principles should provide a path for success in male abdominal contouring characterized by excellent outcomes and a minimized complication profile.

References

1. Michaels J, Coon D, Rubin JP. Complications in postbariatric body contouring: strategies for assessment and prevention. Plast Reconstr Surg. 2011;127:1352–7.
2. Matarasso A, Smith DM. Combined breast surgery and abdominoplasty: strategies for success. Plast Reconstr Surg. 2015;135:849e–60e.
3. Spring MA, Gutowski KA. Venous thromboembolism in plastic surgery patients: survey results of plastic surgeons. Aesthet Surg J. 2006;26:522–9.
4. Friedman T, et al. Hereditary coagulopathies: practical diagnosis and management for the plastic surgeon. Plast Reconstr Surg. 2010;125:1544–52.
5. Kulkarni J, Gavrilidis E, Worsley R, Van Rheenen T, Hayes E. The role of estrogen in the treatment of men with schizophrenia. Int J Endocrinol Metab. 2013;11:129–36.
6. Neinstein RM, Matarasso A, Abramson DL. Concomitant abdominoplasty and umbilical

hernia repair using the Ventralex hernia patch. Plast Reconstr Surg. 2015;135:1021–5.
7. Matarasso A. Abdominolipoplasty: a system of classification and treatment for combined abdominoplasty and suction-assisted lipectomy. Aesth Plast Surg. 1991;15:111–21.
8. Matarasso A, Smith DM. Strategies for aesthetic reshaping of the postpartum patient. Plast Reconstr Surg. 2015;136:245–57.
9. Constantine FC, Matarasso A. Putting it all together: recommendations for improving pain management in body contouring. Plast Reconstr Surg. 2014;134:113S–9S.
10. Matarasso A, Matarasso DM, Matarasso EJ. Abdominoplasty: classic principles and technique. Clin Plast Surg. 2014;41:655–72.
11. Matarasso A. Traditional abdominoplasty. Clin Plast Surg. 2010;37:415–37.

Penis Enlargement with Fat Transfer

34

Tim Neavin and Keith Jeffords

The majority of men believe that the average length of an erect penis is greater than 6 inches (15.24 cm) [1]. Yet, many studies prove this estimate to be a stretch, with average measured sizes in the erect state as small as 13.61 cm to 14.15 cm [2, 3]. In part due to these hyperinflated dimensions, many men wish to increase the size of their penis, whether it be length or girth or both. Yet, most men who desire surgery for a larger penis actually have a normal-sized penis [3] and often are unaware that they are endowed at least with an average size until counseling with their surgeon.

Men's satisfaction over their size and their own estimated ability to perform sexually is impacted by not only the true size of their penis but also their *perceived* size of their penis. That is, even if men possess a penis that is larger than average, they often feel inadequate because they believe they are too small to satisfy their partner, a condition termed penile dysmorphia (PD) or small penis anxiety (SPA) [4]. Perhaps not surprisingly, men who are satisfied with their penile length generally overestimate their size, whereas men who are dissatisfied consistently underestimate [5]. Despite reassurance to patients who exhibit signs of PD or SPA that their penis is of at least normal size, often there is minimal help alleviating these concerns even in the face of hard facts [6]. As such, patients who express signs or symptoms of PD or SPA may not be particularly ideal candidates for penis enlargement surgery since their dissatisfaction resides more inside their head than within their physical attributes. So, who are the ideal candidates for penile fat transfer?

34.1 Ideal Candidates for Penile Fat Transfer

The patients who are best suited for fat transfer to the penis are adult persons who wish to improve the girth of their penis and are willing to accept both the limitations of what can be achieved with fat transfer and the potential complications and postoperative sequela and have realistic expectations as to what can and cannot be achieved with this procedure. Patients should otherwise be healthy and not suffer from any overt signs of PD or SPA. While those who have never had sexual intercourse are not necessarily ruled out as potential candidates, it is the author's strong recommendation that such patients are not ideal candidates, since the authors believe that patients should first experience sex with what they were ascribed by genetics before entering into a

T. Neavin (✉)
Private Practice, Plastic/Reconstructive Surgery, Beverly Hills, CA, USA

K. Jeffords
Private Practice, Paramount Plastic Surgery, Smyrna, GA, USA

K. Jeffords et al. (eds.), *Aesthetic Surgery for Men*, https://doi.org/10.1007/978-3-032-03840-1_34

surgery where very real complications exist. This is especially the case if the patient reports they have avoided sex because they are uncomfortable with their size.

Importantly, patients who wish to see improved lengths after surgery should also be cautioned to proceed with fat transfer since any gains in length are small at best.

Circumcision is not a prerequisite for penile fat transfer, but in the author's experience circumcised penises tend to have more predictable outcomes with respect to symmetry of fat retention and appear to less commonly form undesirable nodule formation or exhibit prolonged swelling, but more on this below.

Erectile dysfunction (ED) is a relative contraindication to penile fat transfer because postoperative massaging protocols are often best employed with erections. Any history of preexisting ED should be documented in the chart.

Patients in poor health, immunocompromised, with significant peripheral arterial disease, or who have diabetes are not good candidates for fat transfer given the fear of Fournier gangrene.

34.2 Permanent Penile Enlargement Options

While this chapter's focus is penile fat transfer, it is helpful for the surgeon to know what other options exist for the patient so the patient can make an informed decision before surgery, understanding what other procedures exist in this arena, as well as their respective risks and benefits.

34.2.1 Suspensory Ligament Release

Surgical division of the suspensory ligament is the most commonly accepted surgical technique to permanently increase penis length [7]. The suspensory ligaments are best considered a system comprising the fundiform ligament of the penis, the suspensory ligament of the penis, and the arcuate pubic ligament [8, 9].

Various penis-lengthening procedures with ligament release have been described [10–12]. However, the most commonly used technique utilizes a transverse incision of the fundiform ligament and partial division of the suspensory ligament from the pubic symphysis, resulting in a displacement of the root of the penis forward from the pubic body [13]. The procedure achieves an appearance of a longer penis, but it may come at a cost of destabilization, losing its upward orientation, and even complicating vaginal penetration [14]. Generally, the gains in length (or perceived length) is modest, averaging 1.2 to 1.6 cm with ligament division [15]. However, perhaps its greatest limitation is its relatively low (30–65%) satisfaction rate, although many of these studies were performed prior to the more common use of buffers to reduce postoperative shortening [15].

The addition of buffers interposed between the divided tissues has to some effect reduced the unfavorable outcome of postoperative penile shortening. Described buffers include, silicone, a vascularized flap from the lipomatous tissue of the spermatic cord or a small testicular prosthesis, or V-Y advancement with subsequent silicone sheath insertion [7, 14, 16, 17].

34.2.2 Suprapubic Lipectomy

Suprapubic lipectomy describes the removal of fat and skin above the penis to improve penis show. This procedure is often best suited for patients with a hidden penis or patients with redundant mons tissue related to either obesity or massive weight loss.

The skin excision is performed with a trapezoid incision, with the inferior portion of the incision marked 2 cm above the penis to allow closure of the base of the penis to the pubic symphysis periosteum, and the superior portion should not interfere with the waistline sulcus [18]. This technique increases the exposed penile length, hence improving the perceived length of the penis. Suprapubic lipectomy can be combined with suspensory ligament release [19].

34.2.3 Suprapubic Liposuction: Liposuction of the Mons

Liposuction of the area above the penis can improve penile aesthetics by increasing the visibility of the penis, making a buried penis look more prominent. Often, the spermatic cord contributes to much of this protrusion inferolaterally, so men must be counseled on the limitations of liposuction. Likewise, the surgeon must be cognizant of the anatomy to avoid injury to it. Compression in this area is difficult, and the additional liposuction will amplify swelling of the penis. Nonetheless, suprapubic liposuction in conjunction with fat transfer is often combined and can provide superior results than if performed alone.

34.2.4 Silicone Penile Implants

Inflatable or malleable penis implants are most commonly indicated for patients with erectile dysfunction refractory to oral medications or injections or Peyronie's disease and have a very high satisfaction rate for these indications [20, 21]. Less frequently, they are placed exclusively to improve penis size. Up to 12% of patients with penile implants require a revisional surgery due to erosion, mechanical failure, floppy glans, and infection, among other known complications [22]. Fibrosis, penile shortening from infection or extrusion, and erectile dysfunction have also been reported [23].

34.3 Pertinent Penile Anatomy

The penis is fully developed by the end of puberty. In adulthood and advancing age, the size of the penis can decrease in both flaccid and fully erect states, albeit this loss is generally minimal. Vascular disease can negatively impact this trend.

The penis has three parts: root (radix), body (shaft), and glans.

The anatomy of the penis is best thought of as a series of cylinders: 2 corpus cavernosa on the dorsal aspect and the corpus spongiosum centrally wherein the urethra resides. The corpus cavernosum houses the erectile tissue and plays the largest role in erections. All three columns are enveloped by fascial layers containing lymphatics, vessels, and nerves.

The skin functions as both a protective layer and a source for pleasure, harboring nerve endings with the most concentration in the region of the glans and frenulum. In circumcised men, it is important to note that the most sensitive location on the circumcised penis is the circumcision scar on the ventral surface—and that circumcision therefore ablates some of the most sensitive parts of the penis [24]. Thus, adults wishing to undergo circumcision should be counseled that sensation may be altered.

On the dorsal surface exist the superficial dorsal vein of the penis and the deep dorsal vein of the penis, which reside in the space beneath Dartos fascia and the deeper Buck's fascia. This space is pertinent to this procedure, as this is the space where fat is to be injected. The superficial dorsal vein of the penis drains the prepuce and skin, lying outside the deep fascia (Buck's fascia) within the subcutaneous tissue as it trails backward, opening into the superficial external pudendal vein, a tributary of the great saphenous vein.

Beneath Buck's fascia runs the deep dorsal vein, communicating with the glans penis and corpora cavernosum. As it courses backward in the middle line between the dorsal arteries, it passes between the two parts of the suspensory ligament by the root of the penis. It then continues through an aperture between the arcuate pubic ligament and the transverse ligament of the pelvis, eventually dividing into two branches entering into the vesical and prostatic plexuses. Below the pubic symphysis, the deep vein of the penis also communicates with the internal pudendal vein (Fig. 34.1).

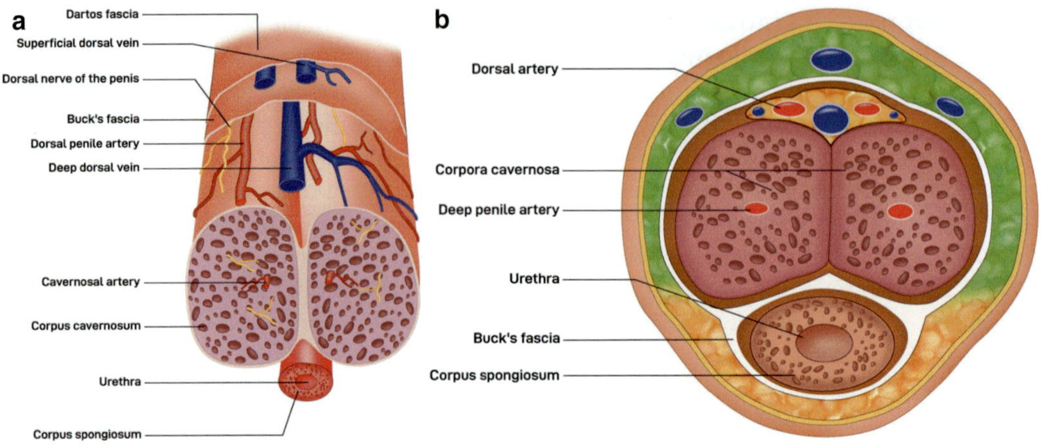

Fig. 34.1 Penis anatomy

34.4 Operative Approach: The Author's Technique

Patients are counseled on the risks of infection, nodule formation, asymmetry, unpredictable retention of fat, skin loss, prolonged edema, and the possibility for a need of series of triamcinolone acetonide and/or 5-flourouracil injections to reduce nodules and/or the possibility of surgical revisions to improve size and/or symmetry. Importantly, *if any one of these undesirable outcomes would be too much for the patient to handle, they are not a good candidate*. In fact, it is wise to ask the patient point-blank if they could tolerate any of these potential complications before proceeding with surgery.

Importantly, out-of-town patients should stay in town for at least one week—and be willing to visit the surgeon as necessary to optimize the outcome even if that means multiple trips within the following six months after surgery.

Patients are photographed in three views: front, and left and right three-quarter. Areas for fat harvest are marked and most often include the abdomen, flanks, mons pubis, or inner thigh.

If the patient is overweight, the mons pubis may be considered the superior harvest site (with additional machine-assisted liposuction) to improve penis show. After marking is complete, topical anesthesia (benzocaine 20%, lidocaine 10%, tetracaine 4%) is applied to the penis and wrapped in cling film, such as Saran Wrap ®.

The procedure is generally performed under local anesthesia. 10 mg Diazepam, one Percocet ® 5/325, and 1 gram of Keflex ® are taken by the patient 45 minutes prior to surgery. The patient is prepped and draped above the waist while the anesthetic sits in place, caking on the penis during the first part of the procedure: fat harvest.

If no machine-assisted liposuction is performed, then approximately no more than a total of 500 cc of tumescent is used, comprising one ampule of epinephrine 1/1000 (1 mg/ml) and 40 cc 1% lidocaine HCl (10 mg/ml). The abdomen, flank, lower back, or inner thighs are generally good harvest sites.

Fat is harvested with 10 cc syringes on gentle negative pressure using fat harvesting cannulas with harvest holes no greater than 1.5 mm. It should be noted that even if machine-assisted liposuction is performed, it is still preferable to collect the fat for transfer using negative pressure and a harvesting cannula with openings no greater than 1.5 mm.

The collected harvest is emptied onto an abdomen pad (Covidien ™ Abdominal Pad 5″ × 9″) and strained via absorption of fluid onto the pad as the fat is pushed along the pad with a spoon (Fig. 34.2).

Alternatively, the fat can be allowed to separate by gravity before straining onto the pad. The authors do not centrifuge. The rinsed and filtered fat is then placed in a small basin, where 3 cc of Gentamycin (80 mg per 2 ml) solution is added

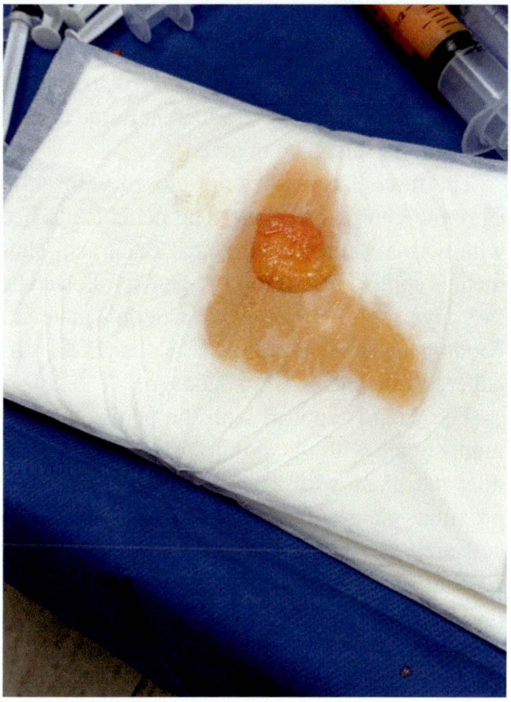

Fig. 34.2 Pad and fat

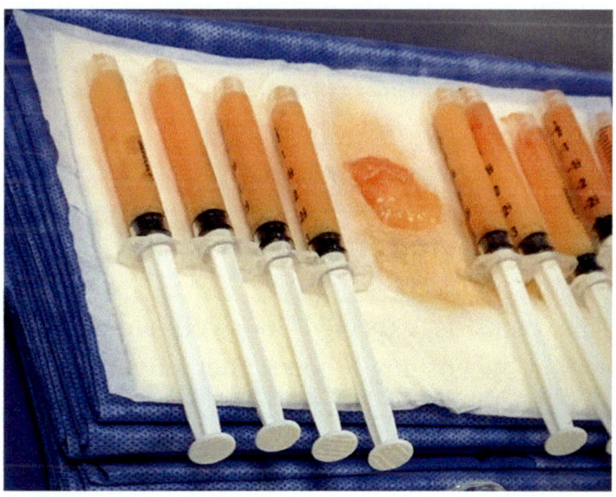

Fig. 34.3 Fat in syringes

and mixed. The fat is then transferred to 3 cc syringes for injection (Fig. 34.3).

As the fat harvest access incisions are being closed, 10 cc of 1% lidocaine HCl (10 mg/ml is injected with a 1.5″ 27 g needle above the root of the penis deep to Buck's fascia, fanning from 10 o'clock to 2 o'clock. No epinephrine is used in this block (Fig. 34.4).

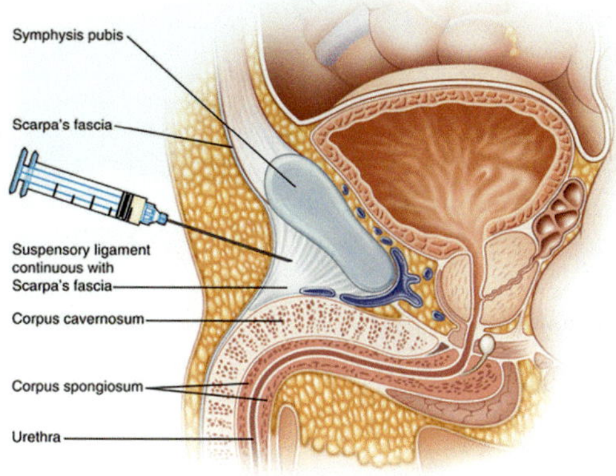

Fig. 34.4 Cartoon of injection

The penis is then prepped and draped, wiping away the anesthetic cream.

Three sites are marked just proximal to the glans dorsally and injected with 1–2 cc of 1% lidocaine HCl (10 mg/ml). Using an 18 g needle, three punctures are made into the skin to access the subcutaneous plane for fat injection. Of note, epinephrine is avoided in all injections into the penis or at its root.

From the puncture size, fat is injected retrograde from the root of the penis to the glans from 4 o'clock to 8 o'clock, sparing the region of the urethra with a 16 or 18 gauge single-port cannula above and below Dartos fascia and Buck's fascia within the plane of areolar tissue—essentially just beneath the skin in a smooth, gliding plane (Fig. 34.5).

To assist in injection, the technician grabs the glans of the penis with a gauze and pulls it straight, stretching the penis from the body. Importantly, the length of the cannula must be long enough to reach the root of the penis with the penis on stretch (Fig. 34.6).

It is important for the surgeon to tent the skin with the cannula and see the tip to ensure the cannula is just beneath the skin to avoid any vein injury or intra- venous injection.

On average, 25 cc to 80 cc is injected in total with a 16 or 18 gauge, 10 cm Coleman cannula, depending on initial penis size. Generally, the amount of fat injected is divided equally into three zones from root to puncture size. The larger

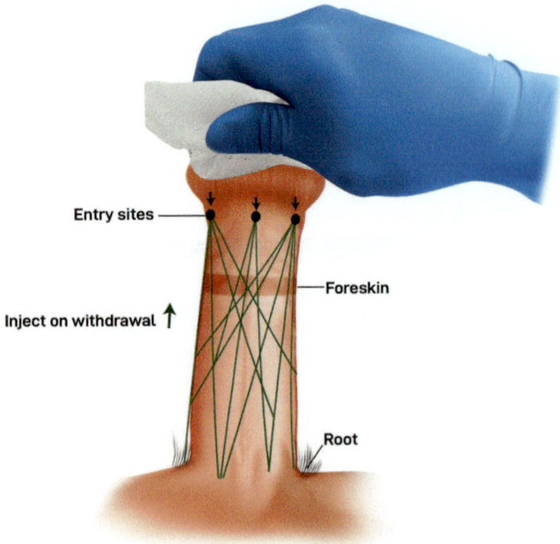

Fig. 34.5 Illustration of injection paths

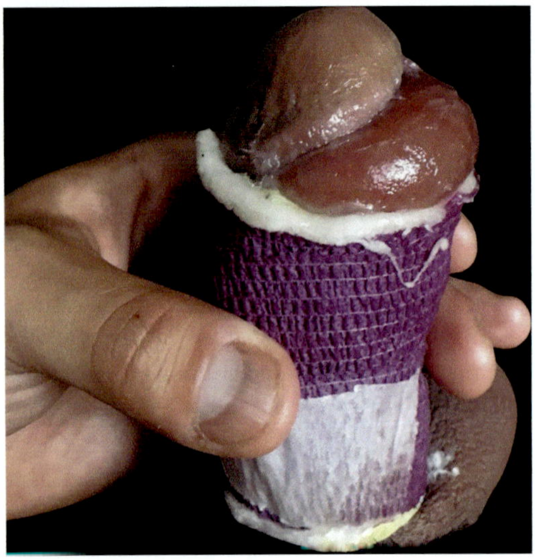

Fig. 34.6 Swelling can be alarming within the first 24–36 hours after surgery. Note that the elastic wrap in this photo does not have the radial cuts now recommended by the author to accommodate the ventral edema. Any tape applied to secure the elastic wrap should be placed at the base and not exceed more than 25% of the circumference of the wrap

the penis, the more fat can be accommodated. The technician grabs the glans of the penis with a 4 × 4 gauze and pulls the penis up 45 degrees toward the patient's feet to expose the 3 entry sites. With the penis taught, the injections proceed with "caissons of fat" being delivered from the root to just beneath the glans. Through these entry sites, fat is also injected in a cross-hatching fashion. Fat is injected from 4 o'clock to 8 o'clock, sparing the more adherent tissue around the urethra (illustrated in green).

The three access sites are closed with a 5-0 Chromic Gut (Ethicon ®). The penis is cleaned with normal saline, then topical Bacitracin ointment is applied over the entire penis, followed by 2–3 layers of 2" Webrill ® Cotton Undercast Padding and one layer of 1" Coban® ® self-adherent stretchable wrap bandage.

The wrap is applied with the penis on maximum stretch with the aid of the technician grabbing the glans with a gauze, from root to just proximal glans. At its leading edge, six 5 mm cuts are made into the stretchable wrap bandage circumferentially to afford extra room for swelling. Importantly, the stretchable wrap should not be applied tight. It should be under very little tension—just enough to keep the cotton padding in place. A Q-tip ® is placed under the wrap from the root to assess proper fit. It should pass easily between the wrap and the skin. Importantly, *the cotton gauze should extend slightly beyond the elastic wrap to avoid injury to the skin of the penis when swelling ensues.*

34.5 Postoperative Care

The penis is expected to swell significantly within the ensuing 8 hours after surgery. While the idea of the wrap is to stabilize fat migration, it is not without its own set of risks. For one, they often fall off in patients with micropenis or hidden penis the evening after surgery. In patients who are not circumcised, swelling can be more intense and must be monitored more closely. If the dressing falls off, do NOT allow the patient to rewrap their own penis. That only invites problems. Instead, rewrap it yourself within twelve hours if possible. If the patient had a prior fat transfer, then the matrix from the prior transfer is generally sufficient to prevent fat migration, and these patients are often not wrapped.

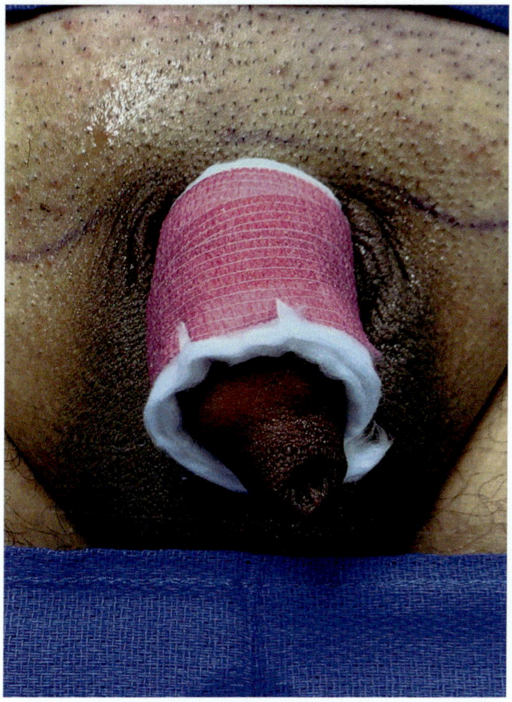

Fig. 34.7 Note the radial cuts into the leading edge of the elastic wrap to accommodate swelling

The author instructs the patient the evening after surgery to send a photo to their phone or email to evaluate the swollen tissue since on more than one occasion superficial skin loss resulted from tissue injury against the bandage. Thus, if any signs of significant mushrooming out of tissue outside are evident the evening after surgery—or the ensuing few days—the patient is instructed to remove the dressing and visit the office within 24 hours for a re-wrap (Fig. 34.7).

Ideally, the penis should remain wrapped between 3 and 7 days. However, it is preferable for the surgeon to receive daily images when first performing this surgery. The edema can be alarming to both you and the patient, and it befits the surgeon to know what to expect.

Patients are seen the following day for a wrap check. If the wrap appears too tight or loose, the penis is rewrapped. Uncircumcised penises will complicate the picture since swelling can become much more intense than in the circumcised. Experience will help determine acceptable from unacceptable wrap pressure. In many cases, such as in patients with micropenis or a heavy mons pubis or in some uncircumcised men, wrapping may just not be feasible.

The patient is seen again at 5–7 days to remove the wrap and assess the penis. Somewhere between the second and the fourth week post-op, the patient is evaluated for lumpiness or asymmetric firmness. In about 20 percent of patients, one or more areas of fat will clump up and become more firm and prominent. In such instances, patients are instructed to massage any irregularities for 3 minutes 3 times a day either flaccid (or, more preferably, erect) with lubrication. In most cases, massaging alone will flatten and soften any irregularities. If nodules persist 6 weeks after surgery, then patients are instructed to purchase a tissue massage gun. The author's preferred device is Sharper Image Power Percussion Deep Tissue Massager ®.

At two months post-op, any visible firm nodules are injected with 0.1 to 0.2 Kenalog®-10 (triamcinolone acetonide injectable suspension) with a ½" 30-gauge needle +/− 5 Fluorouracil. Secondary and tertiary injections are performed at the following three and six weeks, respectively. Concentration, if necessary, can be increased to Kenalog® 20 if injections fail to reduce the irregularity after three injections. It is rare that a series of injections and massaging fails to significantly flatten any nodule. The author has never had to surgically remove any nodules to obtain patient satisfaction.

Patients are instructed to refrain from oral sex for three weeks and penetrative sex for six weeks. They are prescribed broad spectrum oral antibiotics for a total of seven days.

On average, approximately 20 to 25 percent of fat should survive. Secondary fat transfer sessions for additional global volume enhancement of the penis or revisions for symmetry can be performed after 3 months and often yield better fat survival rates (Figs. 34.8, 34.9, and 34.10).

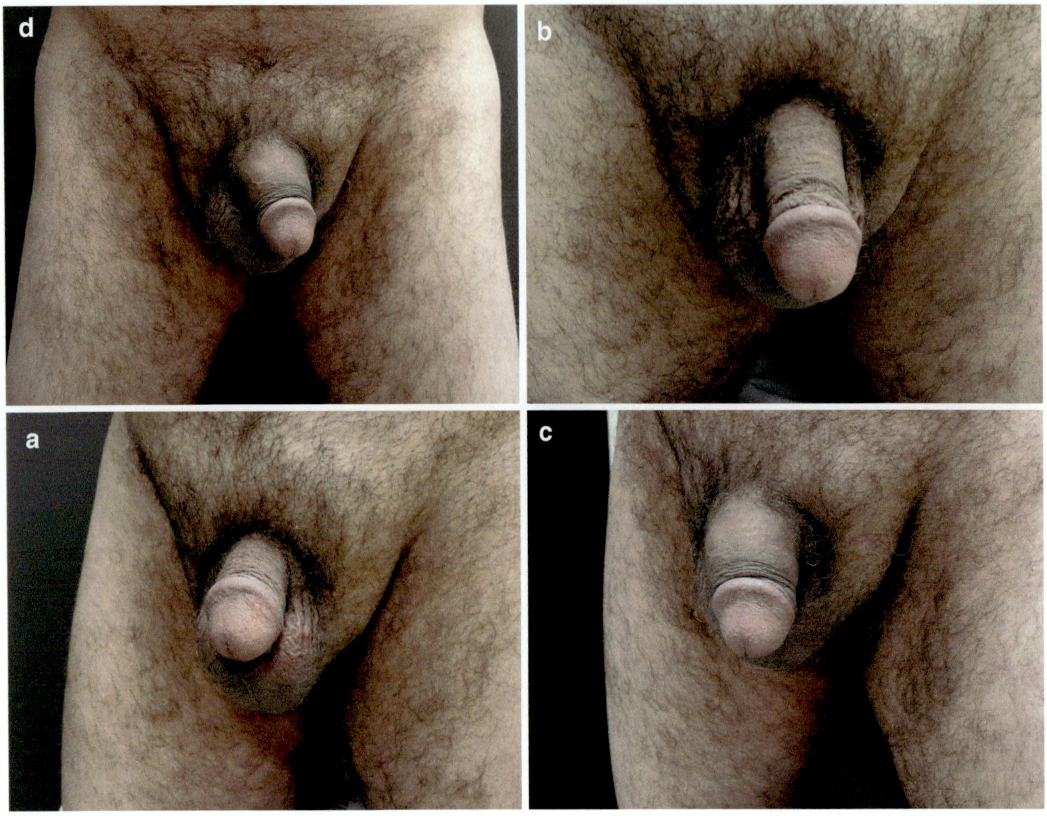

Fig. 34.8 Before (left view, **a**; front view, **b**) and after (left view, **c**; front view, **d**) 44 cc fat transfer to the penis

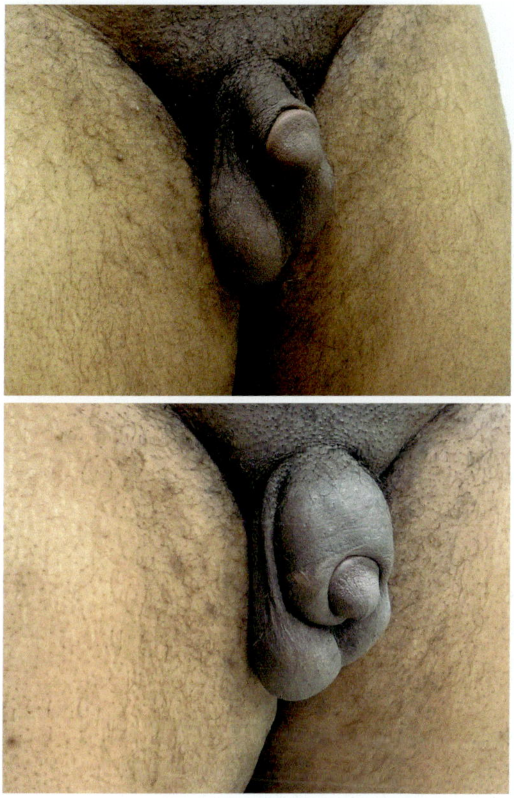

Fig. 34.9 Before (right view, **a**; front view, **b**) and after (right view, **c**; front view, **d**) two fat transfer sessions to the penis with 44 and 60 cc of fat

1. Before and after 55 cc five months after fat transfer. This photo represents a standard, expected result after a primary transfer.
2. Before and after 2 high-volume fat transfers, 60 cc and 85 cc. Retention is generally better on subsequent procedures, and more volume can be placed due to larger surface area for fat.
3. Before and after 3 high-volume fat transfers, with the third transfer approaching 100 cc. While this case is unusual in that the patient had a penile implant removed, this case is presented to illustrate the enormous size that can be achieved with this procedure with multiple transfers.

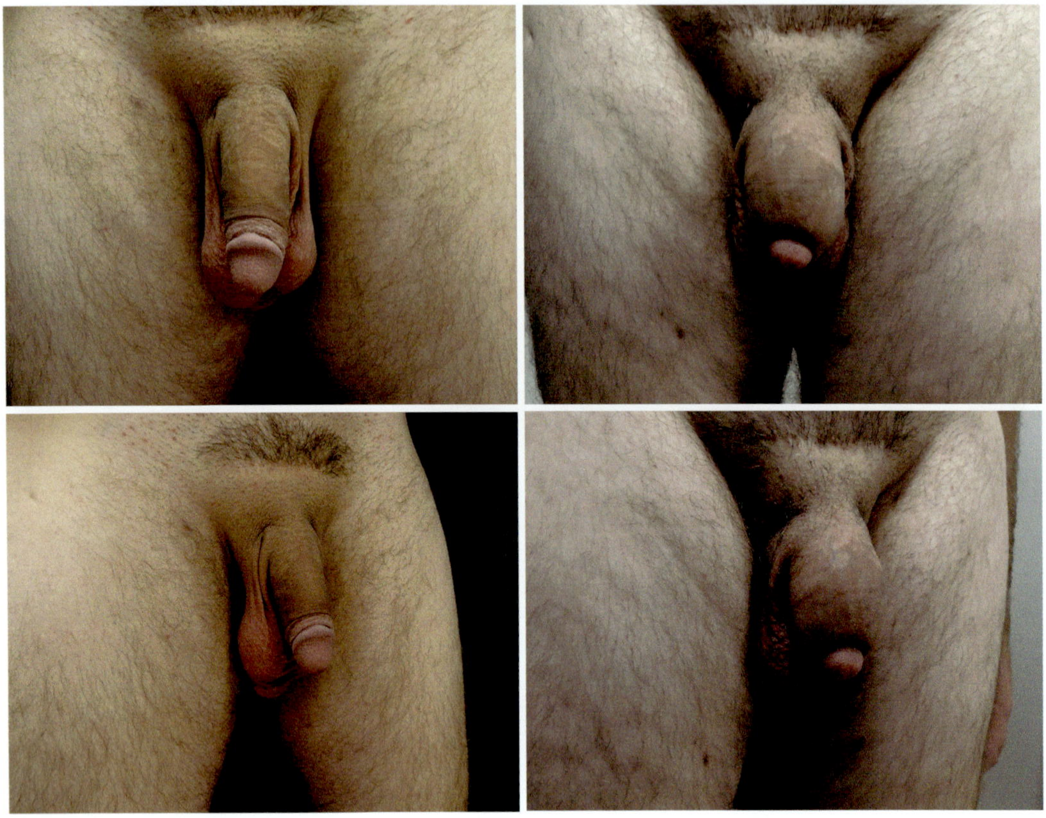

Fig. 34.10 Before (left view, **a**; front view, **b**) and after (left view, **c**; front view, **d**) three fat transfer sessions to the penis with volumes ranging from 80 to 90 cc per session

34.6 Complications

34.6.1 Skin Injury

Skin injury from edema versus compression wrap generally occurs within the first 48 hours after surgery and can be mitigated (or even avoided totally) with a photo evaluation within the first eight hours after surgery and again within 24 hours. If there is any concern about edema formation relating to the wrap, it is best to just have the patient remove the wrap and re-evaluate within 24 hours. Multiple cuts into the Coban ® wrap at its most distal end help accommodate edema, which is particularly more intense in uncircumcised patients.

34.6.2 Asymmetry and Nodule Formation

In the author's experience, approximately 20% of patients will develop a noticeable asymmetry or nodule. Most of the time, massaging protocols, and if necessary, a series of steroid injections (see prior section) will reduce or eliminate any lump or nodule. Larger, firm nodules may represent oil cysts and often respond to a combination of steroid injections and aggressive massaging. In rare instances, the author has attempted aspirations on the cysts to help break up the mass. While a small incision can be made to excise any nodule or cyst, the author has never had to resort to this method.

Injections, if necessary, are generally begun after 4 weeks post-op.

Asymmetry is often addressed with a secondary fat transfer, but not before three months from the prior surgery. Most often, patients will want more fat globally—not just in the deficient area—which is fine to offer and often makes the revision more palatable for the patient. Secondary procedures are discounted for the patient. Secondary procedures can camouflage smaller, stubborn nodules.

34.6.3 Penis Infection

Given the high vascularity of the penis, infections are rare. Patients who develop increased pain after one week of surgery should be suspected of infection. Photos or in-person evaluations are necessary. Antibiotic coverage can be expanded to include gram-negative bacteria, and a low threshold should exist to initiate therapy.

34.7 Other Considerations

This is not a penile lengthening procedure. If patients want a longer penis, they should be advised that this is the wrong procedure.

The skin at the root of the penis is tighter than the skin in the center of the shaft. Augmentation at the root is more difficult because of these tissue dynamics—fat will tend to migrate along the path of least resistance. Patients should be counseled that the root of the penis—and just beneath the glans—may not enlarge as much as the shaft.

The glans cannot easily be augmented with fat, and it is not advisable to inject fat into the glans.

Fat should never be injected with anything but large, blunt cannulas. The cannula should be passed slowly in the subcutaneous plane, not in quick back-and-forth motions as is commonly done for facial fat transfer. Fat should be injected only on withdrawal.

One should always see the tip of the cannula at all times when injecting.

Measuring the width or circumference of the penis is difficult and unreliable due to a host of factors. Thus, photos are the best comparison tool.

More isn't always better. In smaller than average penises, it is advisable to not exceed 60 cc of fat given the propensity for asymmetry and nodule formation with greater transfer volume:penis size ratios.

The final results are generally evident by 3 months.

The steepest learning curve will likely be wrapping and managing nodules.

References

1. King B. Average-size erect penis: fiction, fact, and the need for Counseling. J Sex Marital Ther. 2021;47(1):80–9.
2. Herbenick D. Erect penile length and circumference dimensions of 1,661 sexually active men in the United States. J Sex Med. 2014;11(1):93–101.
3. Mondaini N, Ponchietti R, Gontero P, et al. Penile length is normal in most men seeking penile lengthening procedures. Int J Impot Res. 2002;14:283–6. https://doi.org/10.1038/sj.ijir.3900887.
4. American Psychiatric Association. Diagnostic and statistical manual of mental disorders. 5th ed. Arlington: American Psychiatric Publishing; 2013.
5. Veale D, Miles S, Read J, et al. Sexual functioning and behavior of men with body dysmorphic disorder concerning penis size compared with men anxious about penis size and with controls: a cohort study. Sex Med. 2015;3:147–55.
6. Veale D, Miles S, Read J, et al. Penile dysmorphic disorder: development of screening scale. Arch Sex Behav. 2015;44:2311–21.
7. Li CY, Kayes O, Kell PD, et al. Penile suspensory ligament division for penile augmentation: indications and results. Eur Urol. 2006;49:729–33.
8. Spyropoulos E, Christoforidis C, Borousas D, et al. Augmentation phalloplasty surgery for penile dysmorphophobia in young adults: considerations regarding patient selection, outcome evaluation and techniques applied. Eur Urol. 2005;48:121–8.
9. Li CY, Agrawal V, Minhas S, Ralph DJ. The penile suspensory ligament: abnormalities and repair. BJU Int. 2007;99:117–20.

10. Yongsheng S, Qingping Y, Yiyang J, et al. Clinical experience of penile elongation: a comparison of four different operative approaches. Zhonghua Zheng Xing Wai Ke Za Zhi. 2015;31:411–3.
11. Egydio PH, Kuehhas FE. Penile lengthening and widening without grafting according to a modified 'sliding' technique. BJU Int. 2015;116:965–72.
12. Mertziotis N, Kozyrakis D, Bogris E. Is V-Y plasty necessary for penile lengthening? Girth enhancement and increased length solely through circumcision: description of a novel technique. Asian J Androl. 2013;15:819–23.
13. Vardi Y, Har-Shai Y, Gil T, Gruenwald I. A critical analysis of penile enhancement procedures for patients with normal penile size: surgical techniques, success, and complications. Eur Urol. 2008;54:1042–50.
14. Protogerou V, Anagnostopolou S, Venierates D, et al. Penis ligaments: their use in "increasing" the size of the penis in penile augmentation procedures. Anatomical description in human cadavers and clinical results of a phalloplasty series. Ann Ital Chir. 2010;81:199–204.
15. Metro M. Division of the penile suspensory ligament often leads to less than satisfactory results in augmentation phalloplasty. Eur Urol. 2006;49(3):729–33.
16. Alter GJ, Jordan GH. Penile elongation and girth enhancement. AUA Update Ser. 2007;26:229–37.
17. Srinivas BV, Vasan SS, Mohammed S. Penile lengthening procedure with V-Y advancement flap and an interposing silicone sheath: a novel methodology. Indian J Urol. 2012;28:340–2. https://doi.org/10.4103/0970-1591.102722.
18. Figler BD, Chery L, Friedrich JB, et al. Limited panniculectomy for adult buried penis repair. Plast Reconstr Surg. 2015;136:1090–2.
19. Pestana IA, Greenfield JM, Walsh M, et al. Management of "buried" penis in adulthood: an overview. Plast Reconstr Surg. 2009;124:1186–95.
20. Rodriguez KM, Pastuszak AW. A history of penile implants. Transl Androl Urol. 2017;6(S5):S851–7. https://doi.org/10.21037/tau.2017.04.02. PMC 5715175. PMID 29238664.
21. Krzastek SC, Smith R. An update on the best approaches to prevent complications in penile prosthesis recipients. Ther Adv Urol. 2019;11:1756287218818076.
22. Jorissen C, De Bruyna H, Baten E, Van Renterghem K. Clinical outcome: patient and partner after penile implant surgery. Curr Urol. 2019;13:94–100.
23. Furr J, Hebert K, Wisenbaugh E, Gelman J. Complications of genital enlargement surgery. J Sex Med. 2018;15(12):1811–7.
24. Sorrells ML, Snyder JL, Reiss MD, Eden C, Milos MF, Wilcox N, Van Howe RS. BJU Int. 2007;99(4):864–9.

35 Male Body Contouring After Massive Weight Loss

Amy S. Colwell and Avery C. Capone

35.1 Introduction

Body contouring following massive weight loss is associated with high rates of patient satisfaction [1, 2] and improved long-term weight control after bariatric surgery [3, 4]. A comparatively greater risk of complications following these operations has inspired comprehensive and evidence-based approaches to surgical technique and perioperative care.

Massive weight loss (MWL) is defined throughout surgical literature as an absolute weight loss in excess of 50 pounds, or an excess body mass index loss of 30% or more. The vast majority of patients with MWL undergoing body contouring procedures have achieved weight loss through bariatric surgery [5]. There has been a tremendous increase in the utilization of weight loss surgery throughout the United States. Census data and estimates provided by the American Society for Metabolic and Bariatric Surgery suggest that 5.1 weight loss surgeries were performed for every 10,000 individuals in 2011. 6.7 procedures were performed for every 10,000 individuals in 2016, representing a 32% increase in bariatric surgery procedures during this five year interval [6, 7]. The prevalence of adult obesity during this same interval increased by only 4.7% based on the National Health and Nutrition Examination Surveys [8, 9]. Given this considerable rise in weight loss surgery utilization, it is not surprising that the number of lower body lift and upper arm lift procedures performed in the United States saw the greatest interval increase between 2000 and 2018 than any other cosmetic or reconstructive procedure, 4295% and 5030% respectively, compared to 845% increase in botulinum toxin procedures during the same interval [10].

Men appear to pursue weight loss surgery less frequently than women, and, furthermore, they appear less likely than women to pursue body contouring following bariatric surgery. A review of New York State Department of Health data from 2004 to 2010 found 20.3% of 37,802 bariatric surgeries were performed on men. Within this cohort, 6.3% of female patients underwent body contouring surgery following bariatric surgery compared to 2.9% of male patients [11]. Similarly, a review of the National Health System of France between 2007 and 2013 found that 10.6% of 150,808 women undergoing bariatric surgery later underwent body contouring surgery whereas only 5.5% of 30,736 men did the same [12]. Despite their smaller constituency, male body contouring patients present unique challenges following massive weight loss. Male

A. S. Colwell (✉)
Division of Plastic Surgery, Massachusetts General Hospital, Harvard Medical School, Boston, MA, USA
e-mail: acolwell@mgh.harvard.edu

A. C. Capone
Private Practice, Pittsburgh, PA, USA

K. Jeffords et al. (eds.), *Aesthetic Surgery for Men*, https://doi.org/10.1007/978-3-032-03840-1_35

gender has been identified as a risk for perioperative morbidity [13–15]. In addition, some techniques met with success in female patients must be reconsidered in men given fundamental differences in aesthetic goals and anatomy [16]. As such, the approach to male body contouring following MWL warrants comprehensive consideration and planning. This review outlines our approach to the male body contouring patient with emphasis on the torso and underscores those strategies which we have found successful in their care.

35.2 Patient Selection and Assessment

In addition to a complete surgical history, a weight history is imperative in the assessment of male body contouring patients. Peak and trough weights as well as recent weight changes and trends are documented. Body mass index (BMI) is identified throughout the literature as an independent predictor of postoperative morbidity in these patients [14, 17–19]. BMI in excess of 35 is typically considered a contraindication to body contouring surgery, although functional panniculectomy may be considered in select patients with class II or III obesity [20]. Those patients with class I obesity (BMI between 30 and 35) are considered higher risk, although not necessarily ineligible for body contouring, depending on other risk factors, physical exam, and surgical goals. Weight stability for less than 3 months or bariatric surgery within 12 months is absolute contraindication to body contouring. Ideally, the male body contouring patient has achieved a stable, goal weight with BMI less than 30 for at least 6 months, and he is at least 12 to 18 months out from his weight loss surgery.

A comprehensive medical history is also obtained. The American Society of Anesthesiologists' physical status classification is considered a predictor of morbidity following body contouring surgery [21]. Rohrich and colleagues considered ASA class greater than two to be a contraindication to circumferential body lifting in their published series of 151 patients [22]. Nutritional history is also imperative as protein and micronutrient deficiencies are known to be prevalent following MWL [23]. Noncompliance with post-bariatric surgery nutritional supplementation regimens is considered a contraindication to body contouring surgery. While we do not routinely perform nutritional testing in our clinic, those weight loss surgery patients under consideration for body contouring are evaluated by their multidisciplinary bariatric service. Nutritional bloodwork is collected at these visits, and nutritional deficiencies are addressed. Iron deficiency is especially common in this cohort, and correction of microcytic anemia is required prior to body contouring.

Tobacco or nicotine use within 4 weeks of surgery is considered an absolute contradiction to body contouring surgery. A retrospective, single-center review of 470 ambulatory plastic surgeries found the complication rate of patients using non-smoked nicotine sources to be comparable to that of smoked nicotine [24]. As such, we advise our patients to discontinue all nicotine sources perioperatively, including electronic cigarettes and patches.

Venous thromboembolism (VTE) is of important concern during preoperative assessment. A personal history of blood clots, blood disorders, leg swelling, congestive heart failure, lung disease, inflammatory bowel disease, lupus, varicose veins, or hormone use is obtained. Immobility related to skin redundancy is not uncommon in this group and is also explored. Any family history of blood clot, rheumatologic disease, lupus, or miscarriage is also noted. We utilize the Caprini score during preoperative risk stratification [25]. While all of our patients will receive intermittent pneumatic compression and chemical prophylaxis while hospitalized, the role of preoperative and extended postoperative chemoprophylaxis remains undefined. The Michigan Bariatric Surgery Collaborative found superior thromboprophylaxis with low molecular weight heparin (LMWH) compared to unfractionated heparin (UH) in bariatric surgery patients without differences in bleeding complications [26], whereas Rohrich et al. found an increase in bleeding complications when LMWH was used preoperatively [21]. Altieri et al. reviewed 11,860 bariatric patients and observed more transfusions with preoperative chemoprophylaxis than with post-operative prophylaxis alone without significant difference in VTE [27]. In the absence of firm guidelines, we will consider preoperative and/or postoperative subcutaneous UH or LMWH in MWL patients presenting for body contouring depending upon Caprini score and combined procedures [28, 29].

35.2.1 Preoperative Assessment

Patients are examined in the supine and standing positions. Preexisting scars are noted and assessed for hernia. Inguinal and umbilical hernias are also noted. Rectus diastasis and stretching of the rectus muscle are sometimes found in the male MWL patient. Valsalva maneuver in the standing position and straight leg raise in the supine position can aid in this hernia and diastasis assessment.

The degree of skin redundancy, ptosis, and lipodystrophy is noted throughout the torso, pelvis, extremities, face, and neck. Rashes, skin ulceration, and intertrigo are documented when present. While an overhanging and redundant panniculus is routine, a supraumbilical panniculus is typically not seen. However, suprapubic skin excess in addition to the abdominal pannus is common.

Pelvic examination should include assessment of the suprapubic skin and penis. Burying of the penis should be noted and assessed. Penile skin irritation, balanitis, and phimosis are documented when present as is the presence of penoscrotal webbing. Extremity examination should make note or preexisting edema, varicose veins, leg swelling, and asymmetries in the limbs.

35.2.2 Operative Staging

It is important that the patient prioritize his anatomic areas of concern, as it is rare for ptosis and lipodystrophy to arise in anatomic isolation following MWL. In general, our male MWL patients tend to prioritize their abdomen and chest over arms, buttocks, thighs, face, and back.

Staging body contouring procedures after massive weight loss must be tailored to the individual patient. Coon et al. reviewed 661 cases (comprised of 1070 body contouring procedures) and found no increased rate of complications on a per-procedure basis when comparing single procedure cases to combined cases [30]. In our experience of 770 abdominoplasties, there was no increased risk of overall complications in combined abdominal surgeries, with the exception of truncal contouring and medial thigh lift [31]. Other single-center reviews have identified increased length of stay and transfusion requirements with combined procedures [13], while operative time has been identified as an independent predictor for morbidity in another review [21].

While combined procedures in body contouring may not increase the per-procedure incidence of complications, experts agree that duration of surgery should be limited. It is our practice to limit the duration of surgery to 6–7 hours in most patients. We might further limit our procedural scope in the setting of increased preoperative risk, high BMI, increased age, or in patients wherein large amounts of tissue excision are anticipated [32].

When combining procedures it is common to perform circumferential lower body contouring separate from upper body contouring. It has been suggested that a lower body lift should be performed separate from medial thigh lifts secondary to competing vectors; however, any combination of procedures may be performed effectively in experienced hands. It is rarely necessary for medical or surgical reasons to stage a lower body lift into two surgeries; however, this can be performed for patient or surgeon preference or financial reasons. If upper back lift and lower body lift are to be combined, we typically proceed first with the more severe deformity, then recheck the marks for the secondary procedure as the amount of redundancy may change. If gynecomastia is combined with abdominoplasty, the chest surgery is done first. Face and neck lift is typically performed as an isolated procedure or with other facial rejuvenation surgery.

35.2.3 Surgical Options for the Lower Torso

35.2.3.1 Panniculectomy

A panniculectomy alone addresses the infraumbilical skin excess. Although technically a panniculectomy does not involve the umbilicus, umbilical transposition may be considered to allow increased skin removal and to allow more separation from the umbilical position to the transverse scar. A panniculectomy is often considered a medically necessary procedure to help avoid rashes and infections and therefore may be covered by insurance.

35.2.3.2 Abdominoplasty

An abdominoplasty includes removal of excess infraumbilical and supraumbilical skin with umbilical transposition, rectus diastasis and abdominal wall correction, and flank liposuction. A suprapubic lift is often considered part of the abdominoplasty to remove the excess suprapubic skin. This procedure is recommended for patients who want an improved cosmetic appearance to their abdomen in addition to the functional improvement seen with a panniculectomy. An abdominoplasty does not address the redundant flank and buttock skin.

35.2.3.3 Lower Body Lift

The gold standard in truncal contouring after massive weight loss is the lower body lift, which removes circumferential torso excess. A lower body lift combines an abdominoplasty with a buttock lift and lateral thigh lift, leaving a low circumferential scar. This procedure is recommended over abdominoplasty for patients who also have loose skin of their flanks, lateral thighs, and buttocks. In contrast to female MWL patients, a fleur-de-lis or corset approach is rarely needed.

35.2.3.4 Suprapubic Lift

The excess suprapubic skin, equivalent to the female mons region, is typically addressed with an abdominoplasty or lower body lift procedure by marking the inferior incision 5–6 cm above the base of the penis to remove this skin. If this was not performed in the primary abdominal contouring procedure, a secondary procedure may be planned to remove the redundant skin. Liposuction may be used sparingly to remove excess fatty tissue in this region; however, direct fatty tissue excision is avoided inferior to the spermatic cord to avoid arterial or nerve injuries.

35.3 Surgical Technique: Lower Body Lift

35.3.1 Preparation and Marking

The patient is marked in the standing position. Posterior marking begins with a vertical midline reference line along the spinous processes. The lower incision line of the lower body lift is marked at the superior border of the commissure of the gluteal cleft. This line is extended transversely sloping inferior along the gluteal margin toward the flanks. Using a pinch test, the superior incision line is marked on one side and then a symmetric superior mark is placed on the opposite side. Typically, the least amount of tissue is resected centrally to minimize tension on this area and to avoid gluteal crease elevation. Vertical hash marks at fixed intervals can assist with symmetry. Flank lipodystrophy to be targeted with liposuction is marked with concentric ovals and circles at this time. The posterior incision may be designed more superiorly to optimize flank lipectomy. However, superior design may leave a scar that is visible above underwear and bathing suits. These conflicting options should be discussed with the patient.

Anterior markings begin with a vertical midline reference mark extending from the sternum to the symphysis pubis. The anterior, low transverse incision mark is made 5–6 cm superior to the penopubic junction on stretch at the midline. It is important to keep this mark low to address the redundant skin superior to the penis. This mark is extended in a gradual line toward the lower flanks and posterior marks with minimal superior curvature. A straight line will help avoid waist accentuation and feminization. Any areas of lipodystrophy to be targeted with liposuction are marked with concentric ovals and circles.

The superior line of the anterior dermatolipectomy is then estimated based on a pinch test and connected to the superior mark of the posterior marking. However, this line of resection will be checked after undermining the anterior flap. Vertical lines are placed at the mid-axillary line. This lateral vertical line will denote the limit of the posterior lower body lift prior to position change from prone to supine.

35.3.2 Surgical Procedure

Pneumatic compression devices are applied in the preoperative holding area and maintained throughout the hospitalization. Preoperative acetaminophen and gabapentin are administered as part of an enhanced recovery after surgery (ERAS) pain program, and 5000 units of heparin are given for DVT prevention. The patient is placed prone and then supine to maximize abdominal skin resection. A foam face pad and two longitudinal gel chest rolls support the body. Care is taken to ensure the superior aspect of the chest roll does not rest within the axillae to avoid nerve compression. A pillow is placed under the calves for modest knee flexion, and gel pads support the anterior knees. Arms are positioned on padded arm-boards in the "super-man" position with shoulder abduction and flexion of the elbows at 90 degrees. The bed is placed in 10 degrees of reverse Trendelenburg to minimize intraocular pressure. An upper body and lower body forced air warming blanket are applied. When turned supine, an underbody warming blanket is placed. The skin is prepped with chlorhexidine, and intravenous antibiotics are administered.

Tumescent fluid is instilled into the lower back and flank above the excisional marks and into the lateral thighs if needed. Traditional or ultrasonic liposuction is performed. All surgical marks are rechecked and infiltrated with local anesthetic. The inferior incision is made with a 10-blade scalpel and extended through Scarpa's fascia using electrocautery. The superior mark may be checked by splitting the excision vertically to ensure closure if desired. The superior mark is then incised and the tissue removed at the level below Scarpa's fascia. For excessively flat buttocks, the central fatty tissue of the excision may be retained for autoaugmentation. The incisions are closed in layers using 2–0 PDS Scarpa sutures followed by 3–0 monocryl deep dermal and running sutures. Two #15 drains are placed laterally and sewn in using 2–0 nylon sutures. Incisions are sealed with surgical glue, steri-strips, and Tegaderm.

The patient is transferred to a second operating room table in the supine position with a pillow beneath the knees and arms on padded arm-boards. He is reprepped and draped. The umbilicus is then incised in a circular fashion, and the stalk is dissected widely down to abdominal wall fascia. The low transverse incision is placed, and dissection is beveled superiorly to the anterior abdominal wall fascia. Initial superficial dissection avoids the spermatic cord. The adipocutaneous abdominoplasty flap is elevated with cautery, leaving a thin subscarpal fat layer adherent to the abdominal wall fascia to help prevent seroma formation and minimize nerve injury. Supraumbilically, dissection is carried toward the xiphoid in the midline. The rectus diastasis and rectus muscle widening is corrected with fascial 0-Ethibond figure of eight sutures conservatively to avoid waist accentuation. The patient is flexed in the midline, and the superior mark is checked with revision as necessary. In the setting of a buried penis, penopubic tacking of Scarpa's layer to the anterior abdominal wall fascia is performed. The umbilicus is brought out through an inverted U-shaped incision and inset. The excess skin is resected and the incision closed in three layers using 2–0 PDS and 3–0 monocryl. Two #15 drains are placed and brought out through the incision laterally, approximately 4 cm from the posterior drains. Incisions are dressed with surgical glue, steri-strips, and Tegaderm.

35.4 Postoperative Care

Patients are placed in a three-paneled supportive abdominal binder upon transfer to their hospital bed in beach chair position. In the case of simultaneous brachioplasty or gynecomastia procedures, compressive sleeve garments or a supportive vest is placed, respectively. Patients are typically observed in our extended recovery unit overnight, but outpatient procedures may be performed in cases of abdominoplasty alone and in select lower body lifts. Chemoprophylaxis with unfractionated heparin continues twice daily throughout the hospitalization. Patients are discharged to home on postoperative day 1 with abdominal binder, a ledger to record drain outputs, and prescriptions for gabapentin, oxycodone, and cefadroxil for the duration of surgical drains. Patients are encouraged to ambulate daily at home and are permitted to shower after 48 hours.

Patients are evaluated in clinic at 1 week and at 2 weeks postoperatively for wound healing and drain removal. Drains are removed when output is less than 30 mL over 24 hours. Patient typically returns to work 2 weeks postoperatively, and exercise is limited for at least 6 weeks following surgery. If surgical staging was planned, 3–6 months of uneventful healing is recommended prior to the second procedure.

35.5 Outcomes

Surgical outcomes are excellent (Figs. 35.1 and 35.2). However, revisions are sometimes required. The most common areas for revision include the suprapubic region and the flanks. In the suprapubic region, designing the incision to fall just beneath the abdominal pannus without

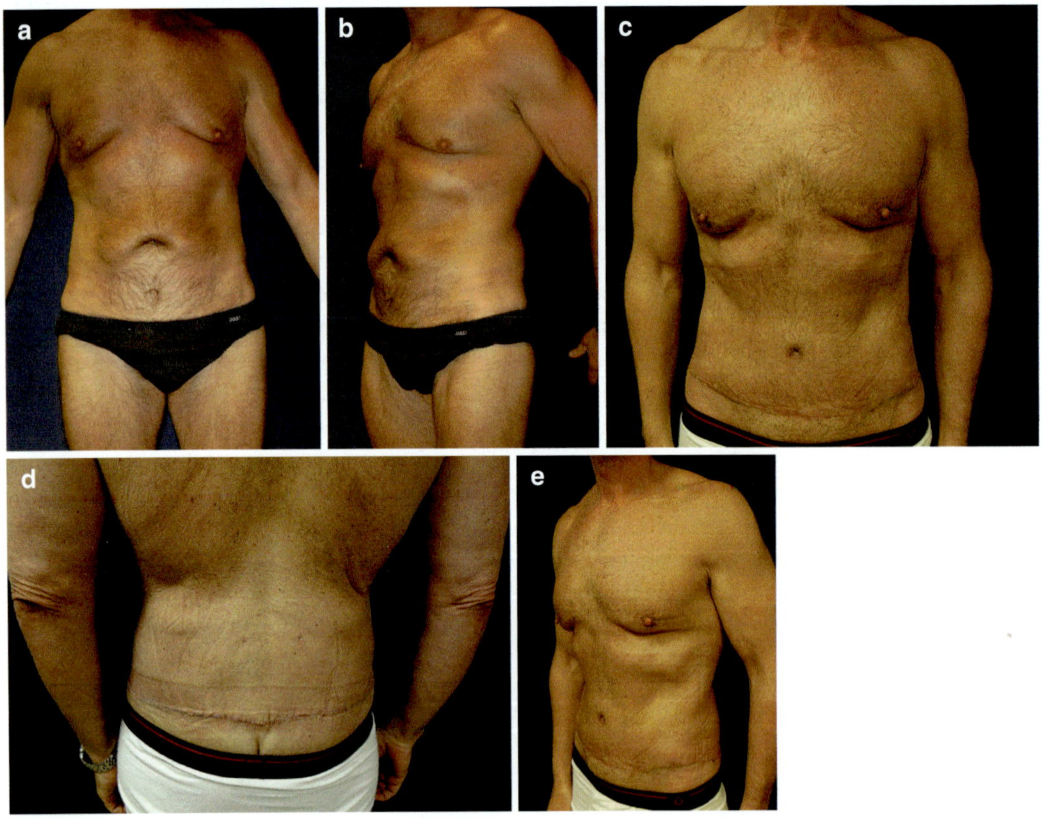

Fig. 35.1 (**a**, **b**) This 45-year-old man had a history of an 80-pound weight loss. Although he was otherwise healthy, he was bothered by the excess skin at the level of the umbilicus and buttocks. His exam was remarkable for skin laxity and a small amount of fatty tissue. (**c**–**e**) He underwent a lower body lift procedure with a low straight transverse scar

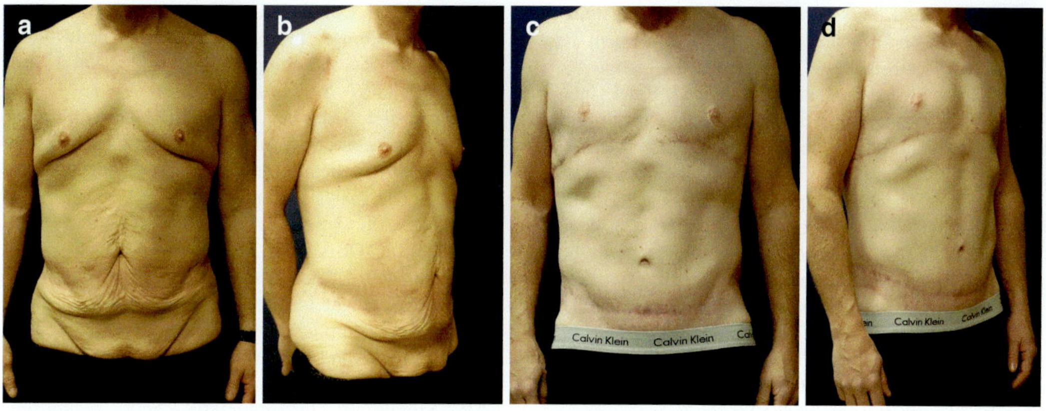

Fig. 35.2 (**a**, **b**) This 46-year-old male had massive weight loss. He complained of excess skin circumferentially. In addition, he had excess suprapubic skin. (**c**, **d**) He underwent a lower body lift with a low transverse scar and gynecomastia correction

recognizing and addressing suprapubic skin will inevitably lead to a secondary deformity. Placing the incision low will allow simultaneous correction of abdominal and suprapubic deformities. For the flanks, desire for a low transverse straight incision may not allow complete correction of the flank deformity. If persistent skin and/or fatty tissue remains, secondary ultrasonic liposuction may allow additional fatty tissue removal, and consideration is given for skin removal with shifting of the posterior incision slightly superior. Design of the original posterior incision more superior can remove more of this tissue and improve contour; however, the scar may be visible above underwear and bathing suits. Scar placement should be specifically discussed with the patient preoperatively, and shared decision-making can help determine the best placement for each individual patient. Although an oblique flankplasty completely removes the skin and fatty tissue in the region, the patient is left with a permanent scar traversing the middle back which many patients find objectionable.

35.6 Complications

Seroma is the most common complication and is treated with compression and serial aspiration. Although infection is uncommon, it is most often treatable with an oral course of antibiotics. Other complications include bleeding, wound breakdown, and hypertrophic scar. Hypoesthesia is expected following surgery and typically takes months to normalize.

35.7 Conclusions

Weight loss surgery is utilized by a growing number of Americans, and body contouring after massive weight loss is one of the fastest-growing realms within plastic surgery. Although men appear less likely than women to pursue weight loss surgery and subsequent body contouring, they present special challenges to the surgeon. The operative plan and staging must be considered in the context of each individual patient. Circumferential ptosis and skin redundancy are best addressed with lower body lifting procedures.

References

1. Klassen AF, Cano SJ, Scott A, Johnson J, Pusic AL. Satisfaction and quality-of-life issues in body contouring surgery patients: a qualitative study. Obes Surg. 2012;22:1527–34.
2. Gilmartin J, Bath-Hextall F, Maclean J, Stanton W, Soldin M. Quality of life among adults following

bariatric and body contouring surgery: a systematic review. JBI Database System Rev Implement Rep. 2016;14:240–70.
3. Balague N, Combescure C, Huber O, Pittet-Cuenod B, Modarressi A. Plastic surgery improves long-term weight control after bariatric surgery. Plast Reconstr Surg. 2013;132:826–33.
4. Wiser I, Heller L, Spector C, Fliss E, Friedman T. Body contouring procedures in three or more anatomical areas are associated with long-term body mass index decrease in massive weight loss patients: a retrospective cohort study. J Plast Reconstr Aesthet Surg. 2017;70:1181–5.
5. Gusenoff JA, Coon D, Rubin JP. Implications of weight loss method in body contouring outcomes. Plast Reconstr Surg. 2009;123:373–6.
6. English WJ, DeMaria EJ, Brethauer SA, Mattar SG, Rosenthal RJ, Morton JM. American society for metabolic and bariatric surgery estimation of metabolic and bariatric procedures performed in the United States in 2016. Surg Obes Relat Dis. 2018;14:259–63.
7. U.S. and World Population Clock. 2019, at https://www.census.gov/popclock/.
8. Ogden CL, Carroll MD, Kit BK, Flegal KM. Prevalence of obesity among adults: United States, 2011-2012. NCHS Data Brief. 2013:1–8.
9. Hales CM, Carroll MD, Fryar CD, Ogden CL. Prevalence of obesity among adults and youth: United States, 2015-2016. NCHS Data Brief. 2017:1–8.
10. Surgeons ASoP. 2018 National Plastic Surgery Statistics. 2018.
11. Altieri MS, Yang J, Park J, et al. Utilization of body contouring procedures following weight Loss surgery: a study of 37,806 patients. Obes Surg. 2017;27:2981–7.
12. Lazzati A, Katsahian S, Maladry D, Gerard E, Gaucher S. Plastic surgery in bariatric patients: a nationwide study of 17,000 patients on the national administrative database. Surg Obes Relat Dis. 2018;14:646–51.
13. Shermak MA, Chang D, Magnuson TH, Schweitzer MA. An outcomes analysis of patients undergoing body contouring surgery after massive weight loss. Plast Reconstr Surg. 2006;118:1026–31.
14. Momeni A, Heier M, Bannasch H, Stark GB. Complications in abdominoplasty: a risk factor analysis. J Plast Reconstr Aesthet Surg. 2009;62:1250–4.
15. Vieira BL, Dorfman R, Turin S, Gutowski KA. Rates and predictors of readmission following body contouring procedures: an analysis of 5100 patients from the National Surgical Quality Improvement Program Database. Aesthet Surg J. 2017;37:917–26.
16. Hurwitz D. Enhancing masculine features after massive weight loss. Aesth Plast Surg. 2016;40:245–55.
17. Nemerofsky RB, Oliak DA, Capella JF. Body lift: an account of 200 consecutive cases in the massive weight loss patient. Plast Reconstr Surg. 2006;117:414–30.
18. Arthurs ZM, Cuadrado D, Sohn V, et al. Post-bariatric panniculectomy: pre-panniculectomy body mass index impacts the complication profile. Am J Surg. 2007;193:567–70; discussion 70.
19. de Kerviler S, Husler R, Banic A, Constantinescu MA. Body contouring surgery following bariatric surgery and dietetically induced massive weight reduction: a risk analysis. Obes Surg. 2009;19:553–9.
20. Colwell AS. Current concepts in post-bariatric body contouring. Obes Surg. 2010;20:1178–82.
21. Greco JA 3rd, Castaldo ET, Nanney LB, et al. The effect of weight loss surgery and body mass index on wound complications after abdominal contouring operations. Ann Plast Surg. 2008;61:235–42.
22. Rohrich RJ, Gosman AA, Conrad MH, Coleman J. Simplifying circumferential body contouring: the central body lift evolution. Plast Reconstr Surg. 2006;118:525–35; discussion 36–8.
23. Agha-Mohammadi S, Hurwitz DJ. Nutritional deficiency of post-bariatric surgery body contouring patients: what every plastic surgeon should know. Plast Reconstr Surg. 2008;122:604–13.
24. Michaels BM, Craft P, Michaels JA, Csank GA. Is nicotine replacement a safe alternative to smoking in plastic surgery patients? Plast Reconstr Surg Glob Open. 2018;6:e2017.
25. Pannucci CJ, Bailey SH, Dreszer G, et al. Validation of the Caprini risk assessment model in plastic and reconstructive surgery patients. J Am Coll Surg. 2011;212:105–12.
26. Birkmeyer NJ, Finks JF, Carlin AM, et al. Comparative effectiveness of unfractionated and low-molecular-weight heparin for prevention of venous thromboembolism following bariatric surgery. Arch Surg (Chicago, Ill : 1960). 2012;147:994–8.
27. Altieri MS, Yang J, Hajagos J, et al. Evaluation of VTE prophylaxis and the impact of alternate regimens on post-operative bleeding and thrombotic complications following bariatric procedures. Surg Endosc. 2018;32:4805–12.
28. Colwell AS, Borud LJ. Optimization of patient safety in postbariatric body contouring: a current review. Aesthet Surg J. 2008;28:437–42.
29. Reish RG, Damjanovic B, Colwell AS. Deep venous thrombosis prophylaxis in body contouring: 105 consecutive patients. Ann Plast Surg. 2012;69:412–4.
30. Coon D, Michaels JT, Gusenoff JA, Purnell C, Friedman T, Rubin JP. Multiple procedures and staging in the massive weight loss population. Plast Reconstr Surg. 2010;125:691–8.
31. Seth AK, Lin AM, Austen WG Jr, Gilman RH, Gallico GG 3rd, Colwell AS. Impact of patient subtype and surgical variables on abdominoplasty outcomes: a 12-year Massachusetts General Hospital experience. Plast Reconstr Surg. 2017;140:899–908.
32. Pajula S, Jyranki J, Tukiainen E, Koljonen V. Complications after lower body contouring surgery due to massive weight loss unaffected by weight loss method. J Plast Reconstr Aesthet Surg. 2019;72:649–55.

Part V

Hair

What Causes Male Pattern Hair Loss?

36

Ernest K. Manders

36.1 From Antiquity

Baldness is no stranger to those in the medical profession. It is all around us. Doctors still stand and recite the Hippocratic Oath at graduation from medical school, recalling Hippocrates who himself was bald. And there is another association: many of our learned teachers, friends, and colleagues show a hair pattern like that is featured on the bust of Hippocrates, a swath of hair bearing scalp stretching over the ears and the occiput with a bald vertex. Today this hair pattern is referred to as "Hippocratic baldness." It is said that Hippocrates himself did not like it! Whether this is true or not, it is a common appearance among mature men, and a familiar feature of our grandfathers, judges, institutional presidents, and statesmen. Far from being a liability, it may indeed be a positive asset in the right setting and at the right age. We do not know how it happened that we acquired baldness as a secondary sex characteristic but can speculate that there may have been a survival advantage from this appearance. Perhaps it was a signal of age, leadership, experience, and fitness for parenthood and family leadership.

E. K. Manders (✉)
Department of Plastic Surgery, University of Pittsburgh, Pittsburgh, PA, USA
e-mail: mandersek@upmc.edu

36.2 The Natural History of Hair Loss: Androgenetic Alopecia

In normal healthy men, hair loss is a normal part of life. With puberty the forehead and temple hairlines recede. Seeing a man of 30 years of age with a low forehead hairline and no temple recession is distinctly unusual and looks abnormal. Generally one may anticipate that a man will lose about 10% of his hair per decade past puberty. The amount parallels the number of the decade. Thus, an average man of 70 years of age might be expected to have only about 30% of the hair that he had in his 20s. Of course, this is a rule of thumb, and some men are blessed with full heads of hair until their passing. The rule, though, is to anticipate gradual, relentless hair loss as a man ages, unless the natural history of hair loss is interrupted by medical intervention.

Baldness is a non-scarring miniaturization of the hair follicle. Normal hair growth includes about 90% of the scalp hair follicles at any one time, and a hair shaft normally lengthens about ½ inch per month. About 10% of the hair follicles are in a dormant phase. Periodically hair follicles shift phase in the life cycle of the structure. The growth phase is the anagen phase and lasts 2–6 years on average. Eventually the follicle enters the catagen phase for 1–2 weeks, followed by the telogen phase of 5–6 weeks duration when the papule of the hair follicle separates from the hair bulb and the base of the hair shaft forming a

K. Jeffords et al. (eds.), *Aesthetic Surgery for Men*, https://doi.org/10.1007/978-3-032-03840-1_36

club hair. In time the shaft will be lost. Normally we shed about 100 so-called club hairs a day. As we age, the hairs grown out with follicle regeneration are more vellus in character, and the ratio of terminal hair shafts to vellus hairs falls. Eventually diminutive hair shafts occupy the hair shaft canal in the skin but do not emerge.

The number of stem cells in scalp skin is undiminished in the balding scalp, but fewer stem cells are observed moving toward hair follicle progenitor cells. Thus, fewer follicles with the potential for long-term anagen phase hair shafts are present in the scalp with androgenetic alopecia.

A number of hair loss classification schemes are available on the internet and in textbooks. The Hamilton-Norwood classification is most familiar. Also available but not so often used by surgeons are the 3-point Ludwig scale and the 5-point Sinclair scale [1].

36.3 A Multifactorial Problem

Genetics do play a role, and at least 12 genetic loci have been implicated in the process of male pattern baldness [2, 3]. It has been observed that the mother's father's hair pattern will often predict that of her son. This is because androgen receptors are related to the X chromosome conferred by the mother. However, autosomes are also important as a number of factors have been implicated in the complex process of male pattern hair loss. The androgen receptors of balding men are different and more numerous than those of men with no hair loss.

Ethnic groups do vary profoundly in their hair-bearing scalp's natural history. Men of Peru and Ecuador of Incan ancestry have famously dense black hair until the day they die. Contrast this with the expected gradual hair loss and graying of those of European descent. Environmental factors do not seem to play any role; our hair destiny is in our genes.

36.4 Testosterone and Its Metabolism

Testosterone is linked to hair loss. The hormone circulates and is metabolized to dihydrotestosterone (DHT) by the enzyme 5-α-reductase in the region of the hair bulb. This DHT metabolite is the active principle that causes atrophy of the hair bulb and eventual loss of its shaft. In this activity it is five times more potent than testosterone itself. Only 5% of circulating testosterone becomes DHT, which is active in the scalp. A group of dermatologists in Miami mapped the distribution of 5-α-reductase in the scalps of men and women. They accomplished this with small cylindrical biopsies of the skin as one obtains with a Baker punch. The scalps of fresh cadavers were biopsied in closely spaced rows from forehead to the nape of the neck. Women were found to have a fairly uniform distribution of the enzyme, but men had distinctly higher levels in the anterior hairline area, the temple areas, and at the vertex, with lower levels in the areas above the ears and over the occiput. The 5-α-reductase distribution predicted and coincided with the normal pattern of male pattern baldness and provides a potential target for drug therapy.

36.5 The Diagnosis of Male Pattern Hair Loss

The diagnosis of normal male pattern hair loss is usually an easy one to make with few alternatives in the differential diagnosis (Table 36.1). That said, a few questions to insure the correct diagnosis are in order before treatment decisions are made. Questions regarding the history of the hair loss should include when it started and how it has progressed. Has there been any intercurrent illness? Did the hair loss follow and illness? Are there any dermatologic diagnoses that the patient bears? What is the family history of hair loss, if it is known?

Table 36.1 Differential diagnosis of baldness

Disease entity or cause	Description
Trichotillomania	Focused loss and history of pulling hair
Tight hair styles, excessive tension of hair shafts	History and observation
Following major illness and surgery; Telogen effluvium	History; hair pull test positive
Side effect of medications	Anticoagulants, Vitamin A supplements, and retinoids
Malnutrition	By history and observation
Lupus	History, physical exam, blood work
Thyroid dysfunction	History and TSH
Alopecia areata	History of others in family; hair loss elsewhere; nail changes
Frontal fibrosing alopecia	Frontotemporal with band-like scarring and loss of eyebrows; biopsy helpful
Hypotrichosis simplex	Diffuse loss of body and scalp hair from childhood with normal nails, skin, teeth
Cytotoxic chemotherapy	History

36.6 Approaches to Non-operative Non-medical Therapy

Many patients are not candidates for medical and surgical therapies. They may simply not want to use medicines or have surgery. Financial resources may be a concern. Some want a "quick fix." How important can this be to a man? Imagine having Hippocratic baldness for years and then showing up at work with a hairpiece that suggests you have never had significant hair loss! Despite what must be quite an awkward moment—possibly for several days—men do this! It is a testament to the importance of this appearance in some men's lives. Those of us who have seen this can recall few such dramatic aesthetic changes in any patients we have seen.

Hair pieces, additions, toupees, wigs, and weaves are the choice of many men. The results in the hands of a skilled hairpiece professional are little short of amazing. It is important for the plastic surgeon who wishes to treat patients with male pattern baldness to have hair professionals with whom he or she regularly works. The patient meets the hair professional, talks about styling and hair color, a sample of hair is obtained for matching color and texture, and then the appropriate hairpiece is ordered from a place of manufacture. On its arrival its color should accurately match that of the patient. It is then placed on the patient and styled with scissors to fit the patient's head with the hairstyle that produces the appearance desired. Hairpieces are made with human hair or synthetic fibers. Human hair is superior in look and feel, and it lasts longer. It may be washed, permed, and styled like native human hair. The patient interested in an addition should be encouraged to seek a human hair replacement if possible.

Attaching the hairpiece to the head is a challenge that can be met in several ways. Some full wigs fit like a swim cap, and no adhesive means of fixation are needed. Some patients have actually had metal rings inserted through the anterior and vertex scalp to which a clip on the underside of the hairpiece attaches. This is now quite uncommon.

A very common method is using adhesive to attach a hairpiece with a polymer underside to the scalp. This is usually accomplished with double-sided sticky tape. The process is lengthy, taking up to 4 hours, but once in place the hairpiece will stay in place for a week. This duration of fixation is of course dependent on temperature, humidity, and perspiration. Vigorous activity can dislodge it, and this is a frequent worry of men choosing this option.

The process of reattaching the hairpiece requires a demanding ritual of first removing the hairpiece in place without damaging it. Then the scalp is cleaned—perhaps with a shampoo in the shower. When dry, the skin is covered with a good adhesive. The silicone adhesive Uro-Bond® is frequently applied to the skin, and a silicone double-sided sticky tape is meticulously cut and laid down on the bald scalp with mirror vision control. After this the hairpiece itself is very carefully positioned and lowered into place on its adhesive bed. Needless to say, it needs to be right the first time! It takes some practice, but the patients doing this get very good at it. It does take about 4 hours of care a week. Periodically the patient will return to the hair professional who has helped with the hairpiece to get a haircut of the remaining growing hair so that hair sits well with the hairpiece.

Cost is a significant factor. Hairpieces can cost from several hundred dollars to easily $1500 or more each. Note that the patient will ideally have two identical hairpieces. This allows one to be sent out for cleaning every 6 months at a cost of more than one hundred dollars. Depending on wearing conditions, especially heat and humidity and activity, hairpieces have a finite lifetime. They must be replaced at least every few years.

Another type of hairpiece is that which is fixed to the head with a weave into adjacent hair. This requires a skilled technician and must be repeated every 6 weeks or so because the hair to which the hairpiece is attached is growing with the result that the addition is loosened in its fixation to the head. A session to have the weave adjusted may cost $200–300 and is a recurring charge.

36.7 Medical Therapy

Medical therapy has only two pharmacologic treatment possibilities with a third treatment consisting of light therapy showing perhaps some benefit (Table 36.2). Minoxidil (Rogaine®) has been around the longest and was discovered quite by accident when the drug was being tested as an antihypertensive agent, for which it is still prescribed. Hair growth was noted in the clinical trial, and the focus of usefulness was shifted to treating male pattern hair loss. Minoxidil requires once or twice daily application of an oil-based solution that is applied directly to the scalp. The directions are to apply 1 ml of 2% or 5% solution q12h, usually morning and evening, every day. The application per day is not to exceed 2 ml. The treatment should persist for at least 4 months to assess the response, if any. Hair loss is prevented or retarded with the greatest effect noted at the vertex scalp. Perhaps 60% of patients with vertex loss see significant hair regrowth. Once begun, the minoxidil must be used regularly for as long as hair loss is to be avoided. Once the drug is stopped, hair loss will occur to approximate that which would have occurred in the absence of the foregoing minoxidil therapy. A wide variety of circulatory system and other side effects have been reported, but the drug seems generally well tolerated.

Table 36.2 Medical interventions to treat androgenetic hair loss

Medication	Dose/application	Beware
Minoxidil	Apply 1 ml of 2% or 5% solution to the affected areas of the scalp q12h (don't exceed 2 ml/24 hours)	Variety of side effects reported
Finasteride	1 mg po qd	Variety of sexual side effects
Dutasteride	0.5 mg qd	Variety of side effects including sexual and other

Finasteride (Propecia®) was developed to inhibit 5-α-reductase in the prostate, thereby counteracting the effect of testosterone in causing benign prostatic hypertrophy (BPH) and urinary obstruction. The knowledge of the action of the 5-α-reductase enzyme at the level of the hair follicle prompted trials to determine if it could inhibit 5-α-reductase in the scalp and thereby prevent hair loss. Indeed used customarily at 1 mg po per day, a dose that is one-fifth that used to treat BPH, a salutary effect has been demonstrated. Perhaps 30% of patients will have a salutary effect. Finasteride at 1 mg per day is said to reduce the activity of 5-α-reductase by 70%. As for minoxidil, as long as the effect is desired, the patient is committed to taking the medicine. Undesirable sexual side effects have been reported. There is no quick effect, and the trial of the drug must persist for 6–12 months. If there is no response, then the drug dutasteride (Avodart®) may be prescribed at a dose of 0.5 mg qd for off-label use. There may be a response to this 5-α-reductase inhibitor [4].

Lately interest in energy transfer and methods to treat the skin and hair with light has shown that near infrared low-level light will excite metabolic pathways, including NFκB activation. This apparently encourages hair growth, leading to increased shaft diameter, which is relatively more important than absolute number of hairs. This modality is reported to stop hair loss by 90%. A red light laser cap used as little as 6 minutes per day has been reported to reduce hair loss by 90% and to increase growth up to 60%. Several products are on the market now with little hard evidence from supervised trials (DiBernardo, 2019, personal communication).

36.8 Surgical Therapy

Surgical therapy has enjoyed a revolution in concept and success in recent decades. Since donor dominance was described by Dr. Norman Orentreich in the 1950s, which led to the strategy of hair transplantation from an area destined to not lose hair to one of recent or impending hair loss, hair transplantation has been a common treatment for male pattern baldness. As an alternative, flap surgeries with and without tissue expansion have been utilized, at times with outstanding aesthetic results. Today single follicular unit hair transplantation with single unit harvest over the donor area has so changed both the donor site and the recipient site that flap surgeries will likely only be of historical interest henceforth. Subsequent chapters will discuss these modern methods of hair transplantation.

36.9 A Word About Hair Loss in Women

Women do also suffer hair loss. In younger women, especially, endocrine conditions with greater than usual testosterone production should be ruled out. Polycystic ovary syndrome is one fairly common example leading to male pattern hair loss in a young woman. Adrenal and thyroid dysfunctions are other possibilities that cause hair loss. Few young women are affected, but estimates are that 29–42% of women age 70 or older suffer significant hair loss. In older patients the pattern is generally not that seen in males but a more diffuse, wide vertex thinning.

Minoxidil and finasteride can be used for women, too. Finasteride should not be used in reproductively active women. (Men on finasteride should not donate blood.) In women otherwise normal in endocrine terms, who will not conceive (on birth control or post-menopausal), finasteride can be tried starting with the conventional dose 1 mg po qd. If there is no response, this can be increased to 5 mg po qd.

Women have an option for wigs and additions that men generally do not. One option that is very effective for thinning hair is the hair net addition prosthesis. In this device, hair is bonded to a net with interstices of perhaps 5–7 mm. The net is placed upon the crown of the patient's head, and then a stylist patiently combs the patient's native hair through the interstices to join the matched hair of the addition. The patient can wear this for weeks with no attention given to the device and may shampoo, swim, and exercise as if wearing no addition at all. The results are stunning, and the freedom and independence this device gives the patient are simply wonderful. Plastic surgeons will occasionally see women with hair loss, and knowledge of this alternative will help many patients.

References

1. Blume-Peytavi U, Blumeye A, Tosti A, et al. S1 guideline for diagnostic evaluation in androgenetic alopecia in men, women and adolescents. Br J Dermatol. 2011;164(1):5–15.
2. Nyholt DR, Gillespie NA, Heath AC, et al. Genetic basis of male pattern baldness. J Invest Dermatol. 2003;121(6):1561–4.
3. Heilmann-Heimbach S, Hochfeld LM, Paus R, et al. Hunting the genes in male-pattern alopecia: how important are they, how close are we and what will they tell us? Exp Dermatol. 2016;25(4):251–7.
4. Blume-Peytavi U, Kanti V. Androgenetic alopecia. In: Kang S, Amagai M, Bruckner AL, Enk AH, Margolis DJ, Mcmichael AJ, Orrigner JS, editors. Fitzpatrick's dermatology. 9th ed. New York: McGraw-Hill Education; 2019.

37 Follicular Unit Transplantation (FUT): Hair Restoration

Alfonso Barrera

Hair is and has always been a very important component of facial aesthetics in both males and females. Considering the significance placed on hair, it is easy to understand why hair loss often causes severe emotional distress and why many people seek hair restoration.

There are two main schools of thought today as to techniques for hair restoration:

- Follicular Unit Transplantation (FUT) involves harvesting an ellipse of donor hair from the occipital and or temporal donor site areas, closing primarily and carefully under magnification and background lighting accurately dissecting the ellipse into 1–2 mm slices and subsequently into individual hair follicular unit grafts, which are then transplanted one by one into the recipient site.
- Follicular Unit Extraction (FUE) involves individual follicular units harvested directly from the donor site in a random fashion by using round, very small, sharp punch (0.85–1 mm in diameter) blades. Without the need to harvest a horizontal donor hair ellipse of scalp, no linear incisions.

My personal preference over the past two and a half decades has been doing primarily Follicular Unit Transplantation (FUT). I will describe here details about patient selection, preoperative care, technique, after care, and long-term follow-up. Although, I do feel that FUE is a great option for patients who plan on keeping their donor area hair very short.

About 25 years ago, I incorporated hair transplantation into my practice, initially treating primarily cases of Male Pattern Baldness, but soon thereafter, I started finding other applications as in enhancing aesthetics in the reconstruction of the face and scalp, such as in scarring alopecia after facial rejuvenation surgery (the loss of the temporal hairline and sideburn), alopecia due to trauma, burns, radiation therapy, and even congenital defects (such as in cutis aplasia, or on the male patient, bilateral cleft lip) enhancing significantly their final aesthetic outcome.

My interest in hair transplantation began when I became aware of the work of Carlos O. Uebel from Brazil [1]; he was the first one to do follicular unit grafting (1–2 hair follicular unit grafts) in large numbers, 1000 or more per session, and his technique allowed finally for natural-looking results. He harvested a horizontal ellipse of scalp out of which he dissected the follicular units. This is what we know today as FUT.

I met Dr. Carlos O. Uebel personally in a live demonstration course he gave in San Diego, CA, organized by Dr. Carson Lewis at his private clinic. I believe in 1994, Dr. Uebel did a great job

A. Barrera (✉)
Department of Plastic Surgery, Baylor College of Medicine, Houston, TX, USA
e-mail: abarrera@lookinggood.com

K. Jeffords et al. (eds.), *Aesthetic Surgery for Men*, https://doi.org/10.1007/978-3-032-03840-1_37

demonstrating his technique. Very soon after that I went to visit him in Brazil to learn more about his technique, and I also had him do the procedure on me. Then I came back home (to Houston) and started little by little doing hair transplantation in my private clinic. A few years later it became the most frequent procedure in my practice.

37.1 Brief Historic Review on Hair Transplantation

Initially Norman Orentreich [2] from New York in 1959 introduced his technique of hair transplantation, the so-called "Punch Grafts" (Hair plugs); soon it became the standard in hair transplantation. The problem then was that the grafts were too large, often creating an artificial, pluggy, clumpy appearance. The grafts at that time were extracted from the donor areas by using round 4–5 mm in diameter punches containing multiple follicular hair units. However, we learned a lot from him, particularly the "Donor Dominance" concept, which is key to successful hair transplantation today. It basically states that each individual hair follicle has its own unique genetic features. When transplanted to another site, these unique genetic properties are preserved regardless of the recipient transplantation site, enabling the hair to grow in the recipient area with the characteristics and longevity of the hair from the donor site. What we then needed was a technique that would allow for these grafts to provide a natural, aesthetically pleasing result. Thanks to Rolph E. Nordstrom [3] from Helsinki, Finland, who described in 1981 the use of very small grafts (individual follicular units) to the frontal hairline to camouflage the PLUG LOOK. It was a very laborious job to do this, so at this time only the front hairline was being treated. Subsequently, as mentioned above Carlos O. Uebel described his technique FUT, by transplanting much larger number of individual hair follicles (over 1000) over the entire area of baldness. Finally natural and aesthetically pleasing results were possible.

37.2 Patient Selection

To date, we have no method to create new hair follicles. All current techniques for hair restoration involve only a redistribution of the patient's own existing active hair follicles. Therefore, to be a candidate for hair transplantation, we need to have a good supply and demand ratio. Ideally we want a donor area (occipital and temporal areas) with a high density of healthy growing hair so we have enough hair follicles to distribute over the affected area of baldness. Unfortunately male pattern baldness is a progressive condition. The rate of hair loss may slow down after the age of 40, but it never stops completely. Therefore, the preoperative plan must ensure natural results, both short- and long-term. Good communication with patients is essential to establish realistic expectations. Also, there is only so much density we can accomplish on the grafted area in one session, so it is important that the patient understands that, and it is not uncommon to do more than one session, especially as time goes along and we age.

Most experts today agree that the average healthy full head of hair has a density of about 200 hairs/cm^2 (range 130 to 280). We have learned that about 50% of this number is what we needed to give an appearance of aesthetically pleasing density; that is, about 100 hairs/cm^2 (in the range 65–140 hairs/cm^2) looks reasonably good. To accomplish this it will take at least two procedures. I recommend to wait a year between procedures (a minimum of 10 months). This must be explained to our patients as it helps to give them realistic expectations.

Finally in view that my preferred technique is FUT, I harvest a horizontal ellipse from the donor area and do a very careful aesthetic closure, almost always this results in a minimally detectable scar, even when looking for it. However, if the patient plans to shave the donor area or wear the hair very short, I then alert them that the donor scar may be slightly detectable, especially after multiple procedures. Fortunately most of my patients wear hair at least three-fourths of an inch or an inch long on the donor areas (me included), and this is not a problem. If they do plan on wearing very short hair, then they should definitely undergo the FUE technique.

As with any other elective procedure, make sure the patient is in good health and not on any blood thinners.

37.3 Preoperative Marking

It is important to be conservative in the design of the frontal hairline. We all age, and we should plan on a mature hairline; some degree of fronto-temporal recession is key (Fig. 37.1a).

As to the donor ellipse, I generally make it 1 cm in width and often 20 cm in length, sometimes longer up to 28–30 cm depending on the number of grafts planned. This way it closes with minimal to no tension without the need to undermine, resulting in a minimally detectable scar even when looking for it (Fig. 37.1b, c, d).

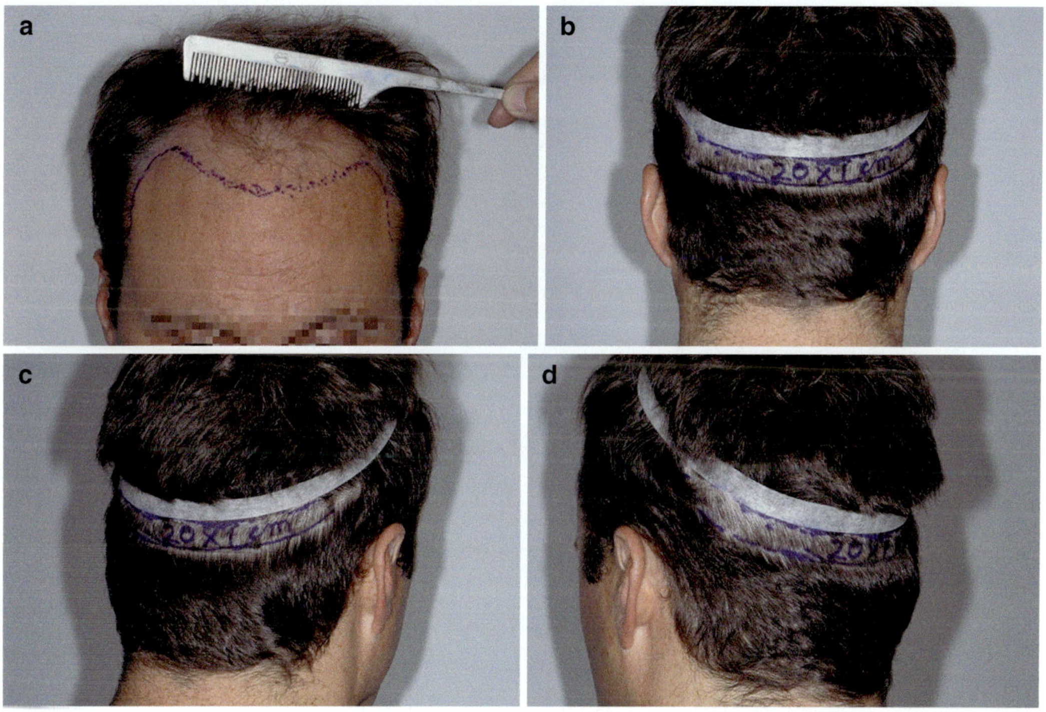

Fig. 37.1 (**a**) Preoperative markings. Here is an outline of the design of the proposed hairline. It is important to be provide a mature hairline with some degree of fronto-temporal recession. This may vary depending on the supply and demand factor. (If the degree of baldness is mild and there is plenty of donor hair a more aggressive design may be done.) (**b–d**) Outline of the donor site elliptical incision. The length will vary depending on the number of grafts planned. As far as the width I usually make it 1 cm, and sometimes up to 1.5 cm if the donor site scalp is lax and mobile. I want to be able to close with minimal to no tension at all and without even the need to undermine the edges

37.4 Technique

I will now describe my preferred technique (FUT) [4–8].

With the patient in the supine position and under I.V. sedation with midazolam (Versed) and Sublimaze (Fentanyl), we comfortably localize the operative areas by doing occipital and supra-orbital nerve blocks with 0.5% Bupivacaine (Marcaine) with epinephrine 1:200,000 (Fig. 37.2a, b).

Once the area is locally well anesthetized, we use tumescence infiltration into and along the donor ellipse; this provides hemostasis, and we feel it assists in the graft dissection.

My tumescence solution consists of: 120 cc of Normal Saline with 20 cc of 2% plain Xilocaine plus 1 cc of Epinephrine 1:1000 plus 40 of

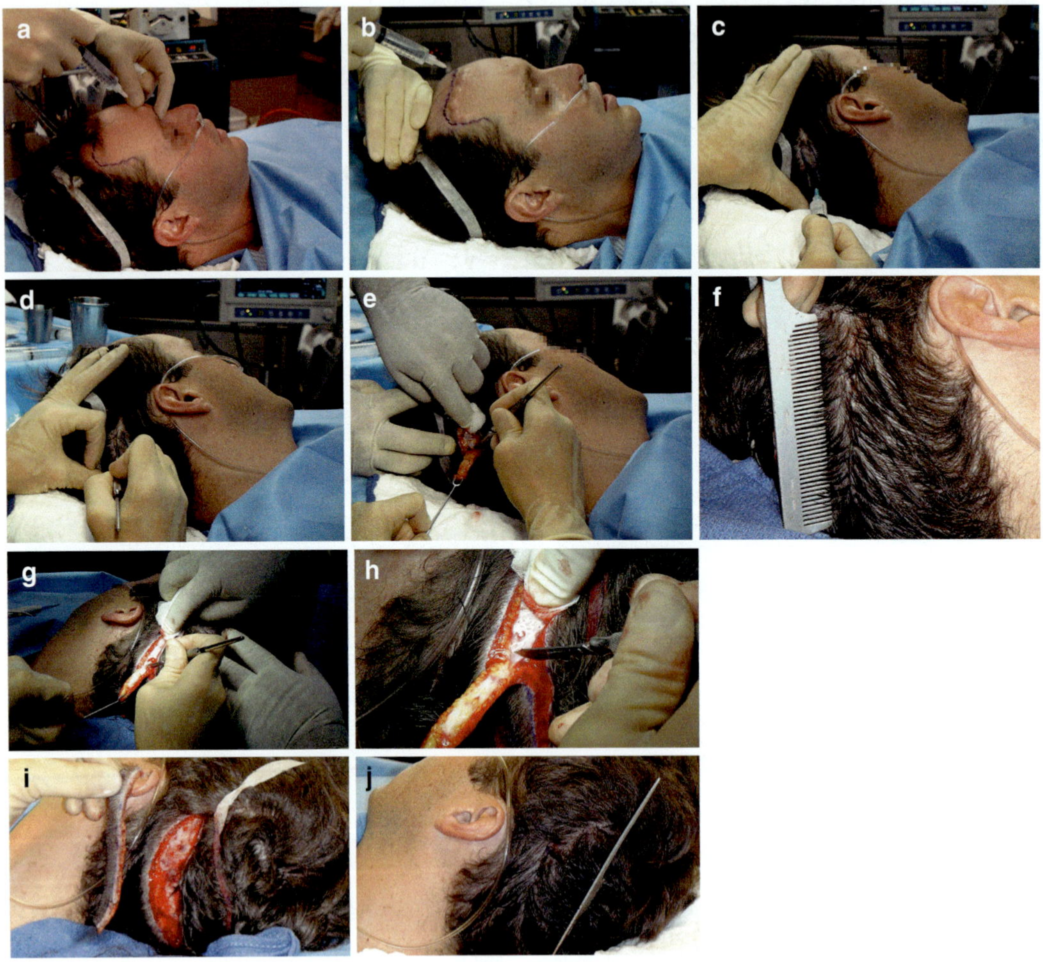

Fig. 37.2 (**a**) With the patient very comfortable under I.V. Sedation (Versed and Fentanyl) here doing Supraorbital and Supratrochlear nerve blocks with 0.5% Marcaine with epinephrine 1:200.000 (2–3 cc). (**b**) Plus 12 cc of the same just in front of the proposed hairline, reinforcing the block. (**c**) Then I inject the caudal margin of the donor ellipse 15–20 cc of the same local (0.5% Marcaine with epinephrine 1:200.000). (**d**) With the patient in supine position and his or her head is turned to the left. We inject intradermically and small amount subcutaneously about 20 cc of tumescence solution, I harvest the right half of the donor ellipse first. Very carefully under 3.5 loupe magnification incising parallel to the hair follicles. (**e**) Harvesting at a depth barely deep to the hair roots and superficial to the underlying fascia, sensory nerves and vessels. (**f**) Donor site closure, without the need to undermine, I use a continuous running 3"0" Prolene suture. (**g–j**) Then we harvest the left half in the same fashion closing with continuous 3"0" Prolene suture

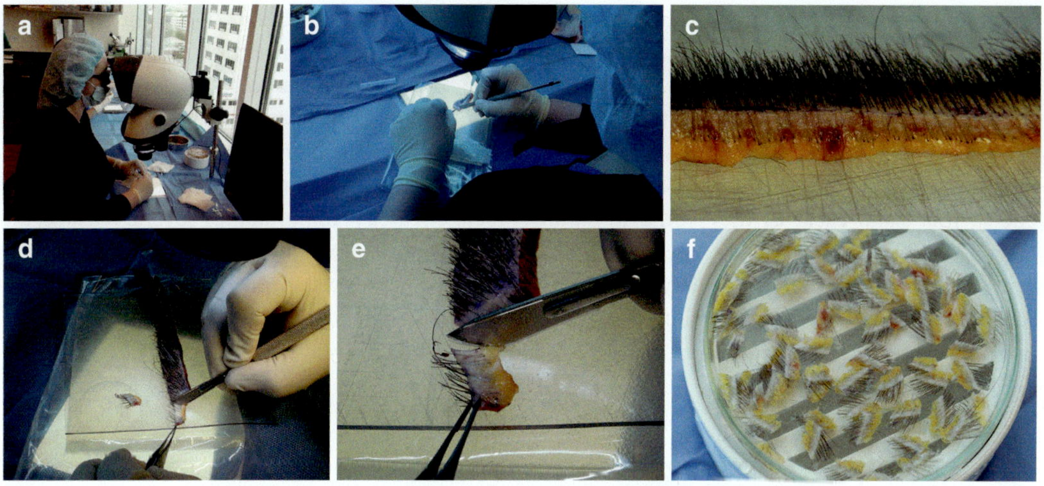

Fig. 37.3 (**a, b**) My surgical team using MANTIS Microscopes under 10 × magnification and background lighting. (**c**) A close-up of the donor ellipse, notice the accurate margin incision. (**d, e**) Carefully dissecting the ellipse into 1–2 mm thick slices with # 10 blades incising parallel to the hair follicles and maintaining them intact from top to bottom. (**f**) Slices are then placed in Petri dishes in chilled normal saline

Triamcinolone (Kenalog). The same solution is used to infiltrate both the donor and the recipient area (Fig. 37.2c). By adding Kenalog we have found significantly less postoperative pain and significantly less postoperative edema.

A horizontal ellipse of scalp is harvested from the occipital area, often extending to the temporal areas, frequently from above the ear on one side to above the ear on the other side. I look for the area of highest density, staying away from the cephalic potential progression of the hair loss margin, as well as the caudal margin of the donor area. I harvest the right side first (Fig. 37.2b) and close (Fig. 37.2c). The patient's head is then turned to the right and the left half of the ellipse is harvested (Fig. 37.2d, e, f) and then sutured (Fig. 37.2g–j).

The ellipse dimensions will vary depending on the number of grafts planned and the density of the donor site. When planning on 2000 or more grafts in my practice, generally the ellipse will measure 20–25 cm by 1 cm. You want to always avoid tension at the closure, allowing for optimal healing (Fig. 37.2d). After injecting tumescence solution, I use a # 10 Scalpel blade to harvest the donor ellipse by using under 3.5× loupe magnification and very carefully incise precisely parallel to the hair shafts (Fig. 37.3a, b).

As far as depth, the plane of dissection is just deep to the hair follicles and superficial enough to avoid injury to significant vessels and sensory nerves, often leaving a little subcutaneous fatty tissue over the galea or fascia.

We make sure to always do the closure without undue tension and without the need to undermine the incision edges. We use 3"0" Prolene simple running sutures. There is no need for buried sutures (Fig. 37.2f).

We usually harvest the right half and close, while my assistants start dissecting follicular unit grafts from it, we proceed to harvest the left half and close in the same fashion.

My assistants under microscope at 10× magnification (Mantis Microscope) process the donor ellipse into 1.5 mm thick slices and dissect it into follicular unit grafts (Fig. 37.3a–e) as the surgeon continues the donor site harvesting and closure.

The harvested scalp and all grafts are kept chilled in normal saline (4 °C) until transplanted (Fig. 37.3f).

Careful dissection of the thin slices into 1–2 hair follicular unit micrografts and 3–4 hair follicular unit minigrafts continues and is done with background lighting and using # 10 scalpel blades and magnification. This is the most tedious part of the procedure and one of the most important steps; the grafts obviously need to be handled gently and atraumatically. The darker and thicker the individual hair shafts, the easier it is to dissect the grafts. The ideal grafts have intact hair shafts all the way from the subcutaneous fatty tissue to the scalp surface and contain from one to four hairs each, as they come in nature (Fig. 37.4a, b, c).

Several hundred grafts will have been dissected at this point. They are lined up in rows on a wet green or blue surgical towel and are now ready for insertion (Fig. 37.4d). The process of graft dissection and insertion continues until all the grafts are transplanted.

It is imperative to keep the grafts wet; desiccation damages the hair bulbs (Fig. 37.4e).

Infiltration of tumescent solution into the recipient area is important for several reasons, the most important of which are to promote hemostasis and to produce temporary edema of the scalp, which facilitates graft insertion (Fig. 37.5a).

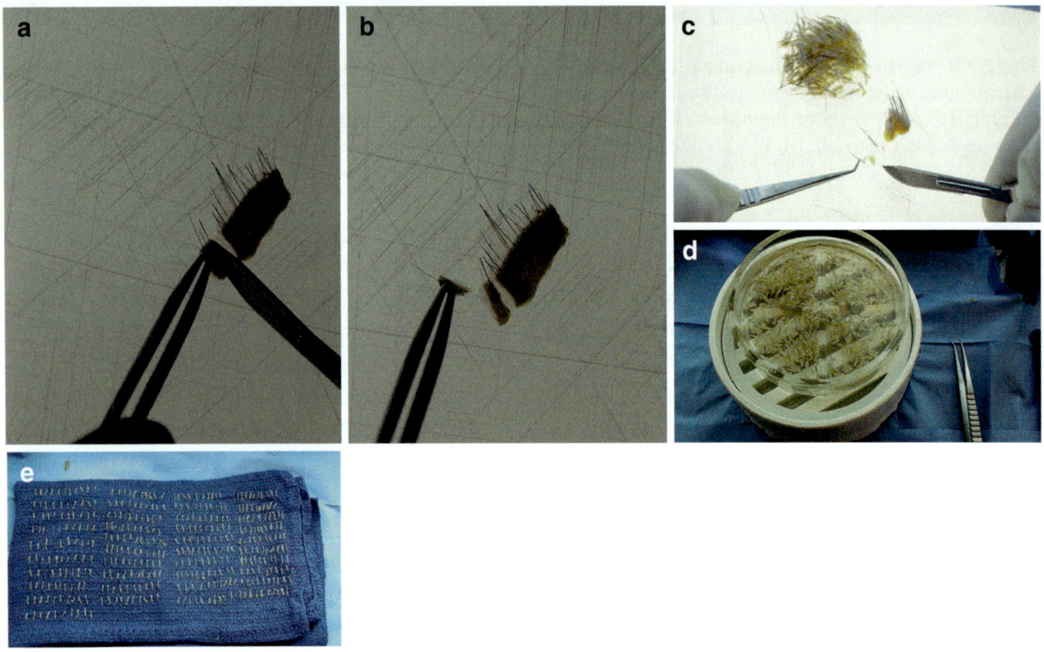

Fig. 37.4 (**a**) Subsequently we dissect the slices into individual hair follicular units under the Manthis Microscopes (10×) or 3.5 × magnifying loupes. (**b**) The surgeon inserts the 15-degree Sharpoint blade creating a recipient site for each graft, then (**c**). The assistant inserts the graft using jeweler's forceps, so on and so forth until all grafts are inserted. (**d**) Then the grafts are lined up on groups of 10 by 10 (100) on a wet surgical towel ready for insertion. (**e**) We keep them chilled in normal saline

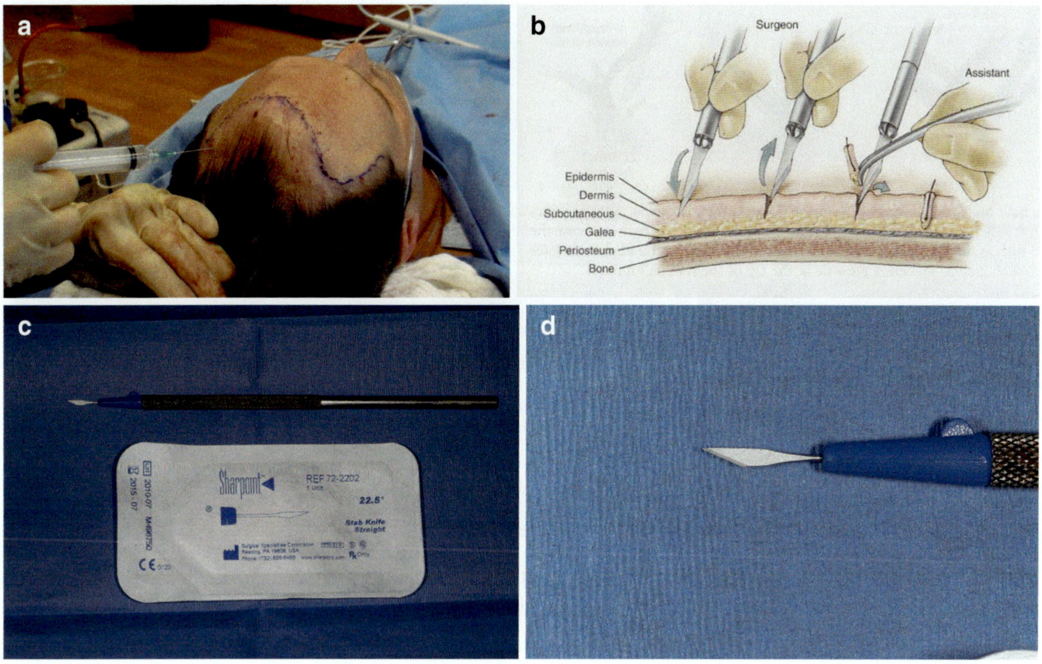

Fig. 37.5 (**a**) Infiltration of tumescent solution into the recipient area is important for several reasons, the most important of which are to promote hemostasis and to produce temporary edema of the scalp, which facilitates graft insertion. (**b**) Illustration of the Stick and Place technique, in which the surgeon makes the recipient site incision, and the assistant immediately inserts the graft (from Barrera [7]; and Barrera and Uebel [8]). (**c, d**) My preferred surgical blade is the 22.5 Sharpoint blade

37.5 Stick and Place Technique

As to the graft insertion into the recipient site, my preference is the Stick and Place technique. A small incision is made in the direction in which I want the hair to grow and immediately the graft is inserted (Fig. 37.5b).

In a given case we generally use a total of about 150 ml of tumescence solution throughout the procedure including both the donor and recipient site.

My preferred surgical blade is the 22.5 Sharpoint blade (Fig. 37.5c, d).

On the front 10–15 mm of the hairline we should only use 1–2 hair follicular unit grafts (micrografts). Posterior to that and in the crown area, we can use a mixture of follicular units with 1–2 or 3–4 hairs (minigrafts).

I carefully create each recipient site inclining the blade in the direction I want the hair to grow (Fig. 37.6a, b); as the blade is in the scalp, it is inclined a little, creating an opening for the graft to be inserted, and my assistant inserts the graft with jewelers forceps as I come out with the blade (Fig. 37.6 c, d, e). This is the *stick and place technique*.

It is very important to have a good surgical team to have these cases go smoothly and obtain great results. I have two RNs and one surgical assistant on my team, with me personally inserting every single graft on all my patients.

I harvest the donor strip with one assistant, then I usually see some follow-ups for an hour or so, while my assistants dissect grafts; then once they have 500 grafts ready and lined up, we start transplanting them. I am there for every single graft insertion, and I select where the grafts go and incline the blade in the direction I want it to grow. I create the recipient incision and one of my assistants inserts the graft. You continue this

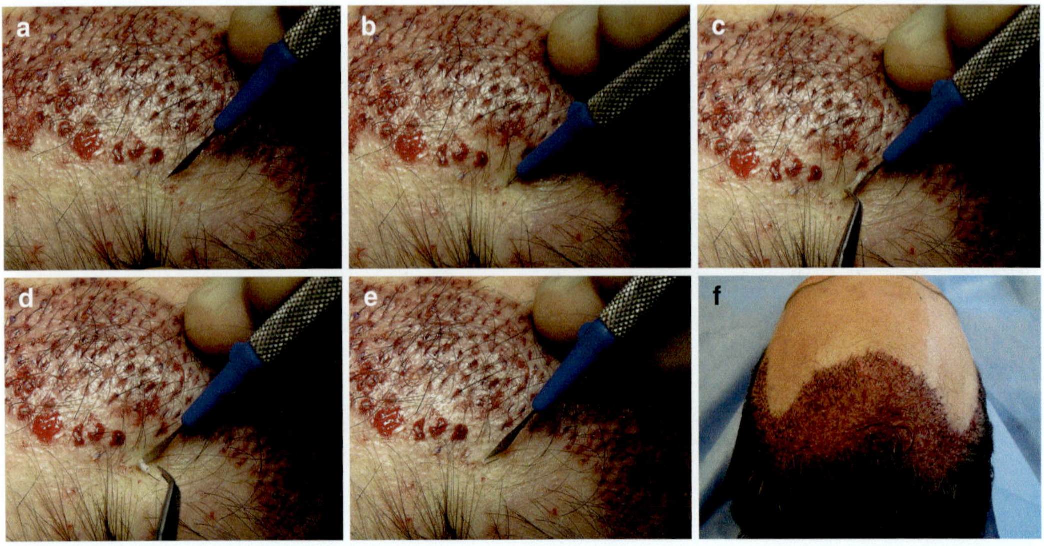

Fig. 37.6 (**a–e**) Here is a demonstration of the Stick and Place technique using 22.5 Sharpoint blade and jeweler forceps. (**f**) Appearance at the end of the procedure, about 25 grafts per square cm

process until all the grafts are in. It usually takes us 4–6 hours depending on the number of grafts being performed, we typically do 1500 to 2800 per session, depending on the size of the area being grafted and the amount of donor hair available. You can't be in a rush; we enjoy (my assistants and I) this procedure. Often we, including the patient depending on the length of the procedure, will take a short lunch break and then continue with the procedure. Patients are ready to leave our surgical suite as soon as we finish.

37.6 Postoperative Care

For dressing we use Adaptic impregnated with Polysporin or Bactroban Ointment, Kurlex, and a 3 inch Ace bandage for the first 48 hours, after which we allow the patient to gently shampoo daily. The sutures are removed after 10–12 days (Fig. 37.7).

The aftercare is simple and safe, and the main thing is to instruct the patient on being gentle with his or her scalp for the first 2 weeks; after that, nothing special is needed, just time. A lot of the transplanted hair will go into telogen (rest phase) and will shed in the first 2–3 weeks; clearly it is important to make sure the patient understands that. Then at about 12–14 weeks it shifts into anagen (growth phase) and the hair begins to grow; by 3–4 months it becomes evident that hair begins to grow, and after 6 months generally we see a very nice improvement as far as hair growth, length, and thickness. The final result usually occurs at about a year postoperatively; subsequently if the patient desires greater hair density, an additional session can be done.

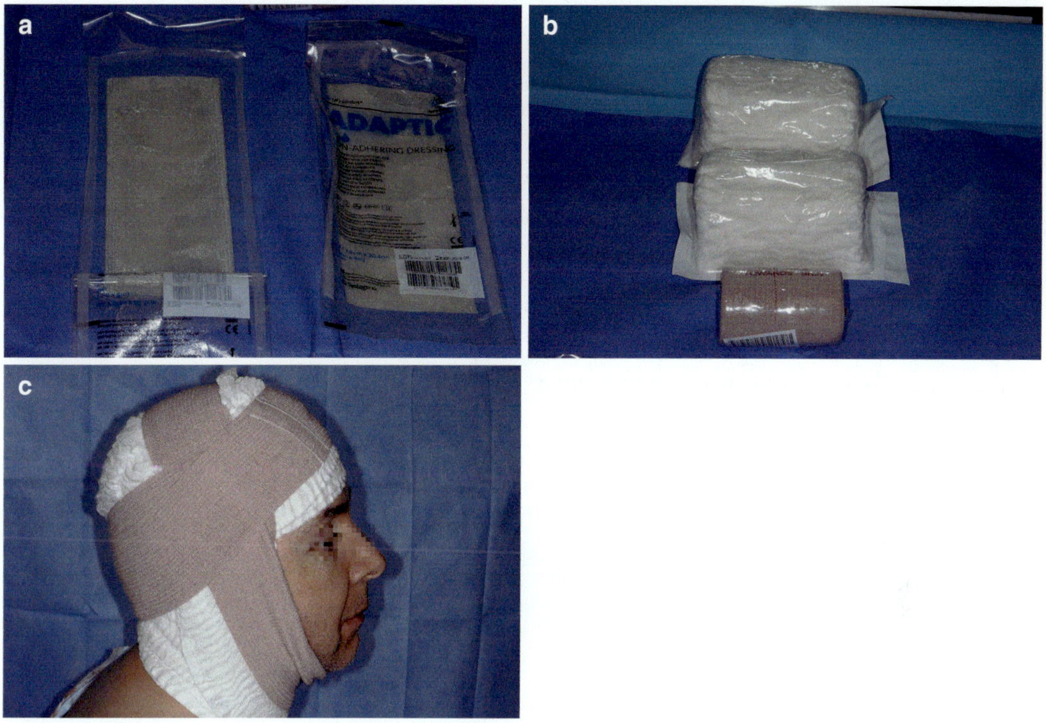

Fig. 37.7 (**a–c**) We use Adaptic, with bactroban or polysporin ointment, 2–3 kurlex bandages, and an ace bandage for 48 hours, after which the patient self-removes the bandage at home and starts gently shampooing

37.7 Advantages of This Technique (FUT)

The length of the donor ellipse will vary depending on the number of grafts needed for each patient. This donor site, by the way, is completely concealed immediately (same day) covered by hair. I like the fact that by accurately observing the direction of the hair follicles in the donor area under 3.5× power magnification, I can harvest the donor ellipse by making my incisions quite parallel to the hair shafts; this way having minimal damage or wastage of hair follicles at the edges of the ellipse. The closure is then done without the need for undermining. The actual follicular unit grafts are the subsequently dissected under the Mantis Microscope (10× magnification) and 3.5 loupe magnification, again with minimal collateral damage and or wastage of neighboring hair follicles.

37.8 Disadvantages of FUT

If the patient wears his hair very short, particularly on the donor areas, to not have any risks of a detectable linear scar, a well-performed FUE technique would certainly be a better option.

37.9 Examples

Figure 37.8 shows a 61-year-old patient with MPB V who underwent a single session of hair transplantation using a total of 2600 follicular unit grafts.

Figure 37.9 shows 29-year-old male patient with MPB V, who had two sessions of hair transplantation a year apart with a total of 4000 follicular unit grafts.

A 58-year-old man with MPB VI underwent two sessions of hair transplantation a year apart for a total of 5300 follicular unit grafts (Fig. 37.10).

Figure 37.11 shows the results of hair transplantation to the crown area on a 54-year-old man.

Figure 37.12 shows the view of the donor ellipse (Fig. 37.12a) and immediately after harvesting and closure (Fig. 37.12b) and a second example (Fig. 37.12c,d). Notice how the donor area can be well camouflaged immediately.

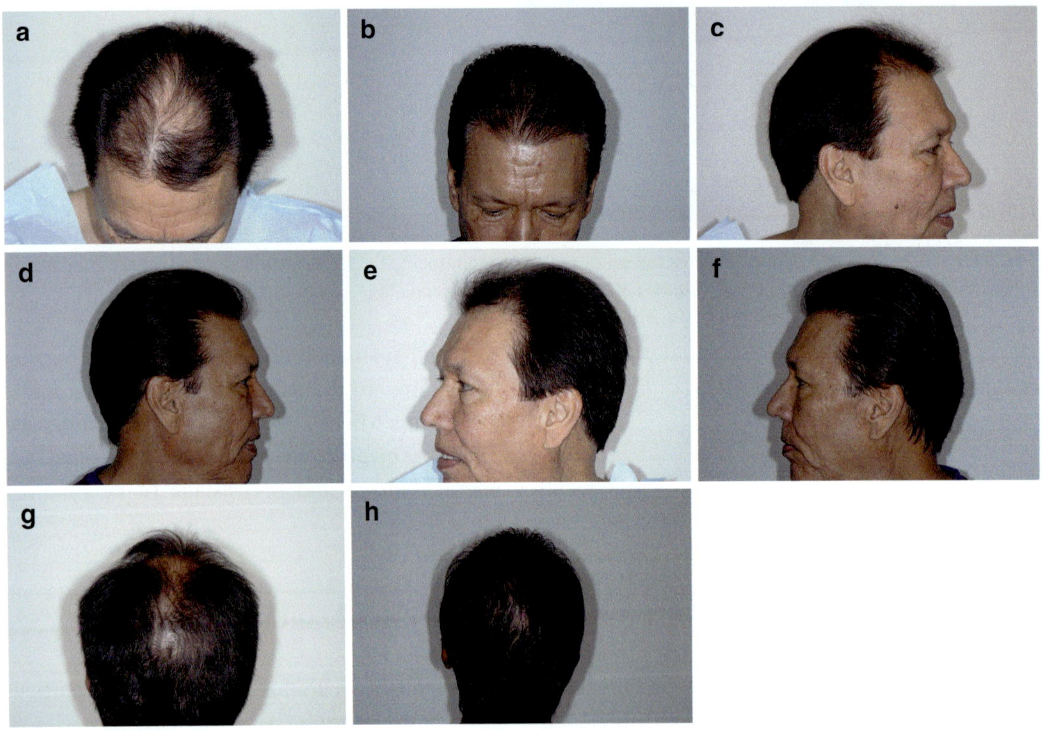

Fig. 37.8 Sixty-one-year-old man MPBV before and a year after a single session of 2600 grafts. (**a**) Preoperative appearance looking down; (**b**) results 1 year postoperatively; (**c**) right side preoperatively; (**d**) right side postoperatively; (**e**) left side preoperatively; (**f**) left side postoperatively; (**g**) crown view preoperatively; (**h**) crown view postoperatively

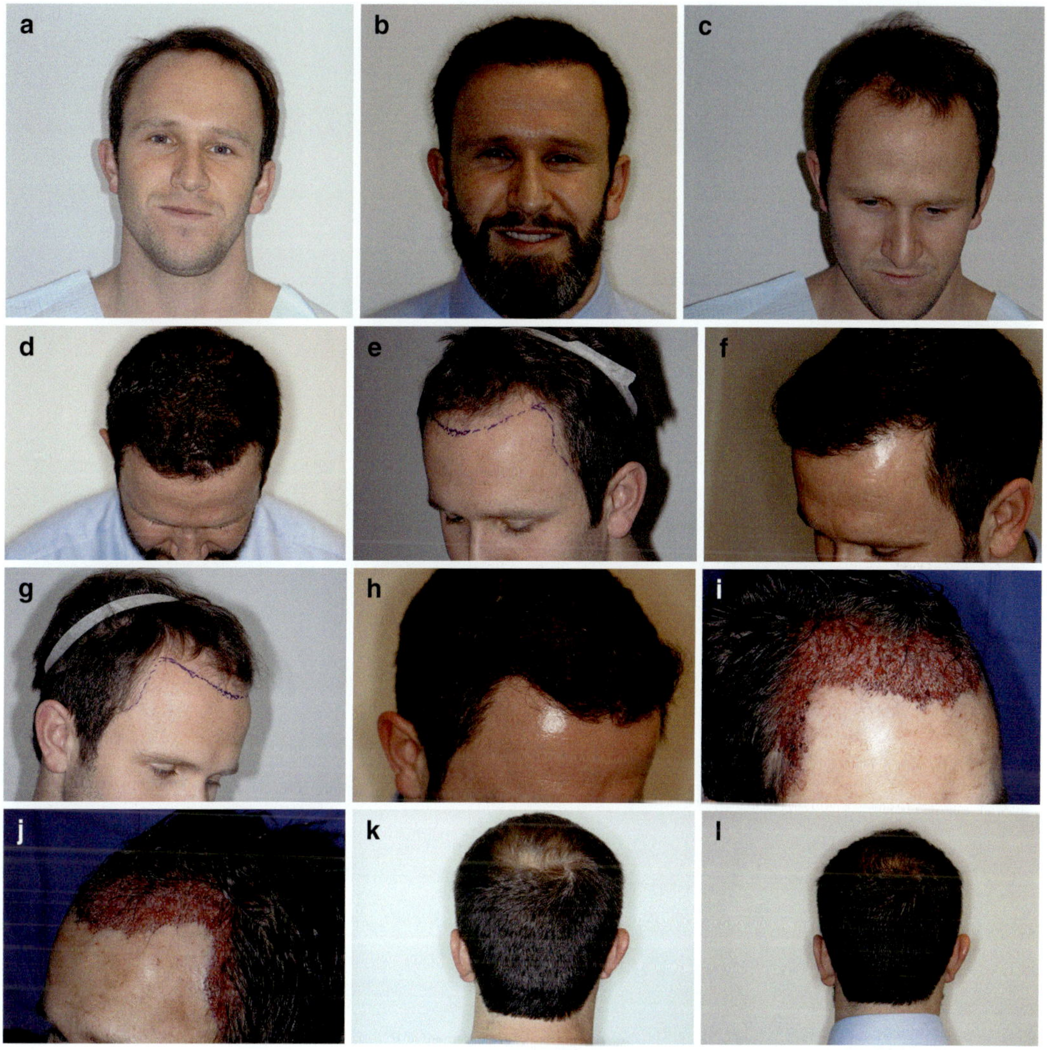

Fig. 37.9 Twenty-nine-year-old young man MPB V. Before and a year after his two sessions of hair transplantation, approximately 4000 grafts. (**a**) Preoperative front view; (**b**) front view 1 year after the second session; (**c**) preoperative view looking down; (**d**) Postoperative view looking down; (**e**) left side looking down preoperatively; (**f**) left side looking down postoperatively; (**g**) Preoperative looking down; (**h**) postoperative looking down; (**i**) Left side view of the grafted area immediately postoperatively; (**j**) right side view of the grafted area immediately postoperatively; (**k**) view of the crown area preoperatively; (**l**) view of the crown area immediately postoperatively

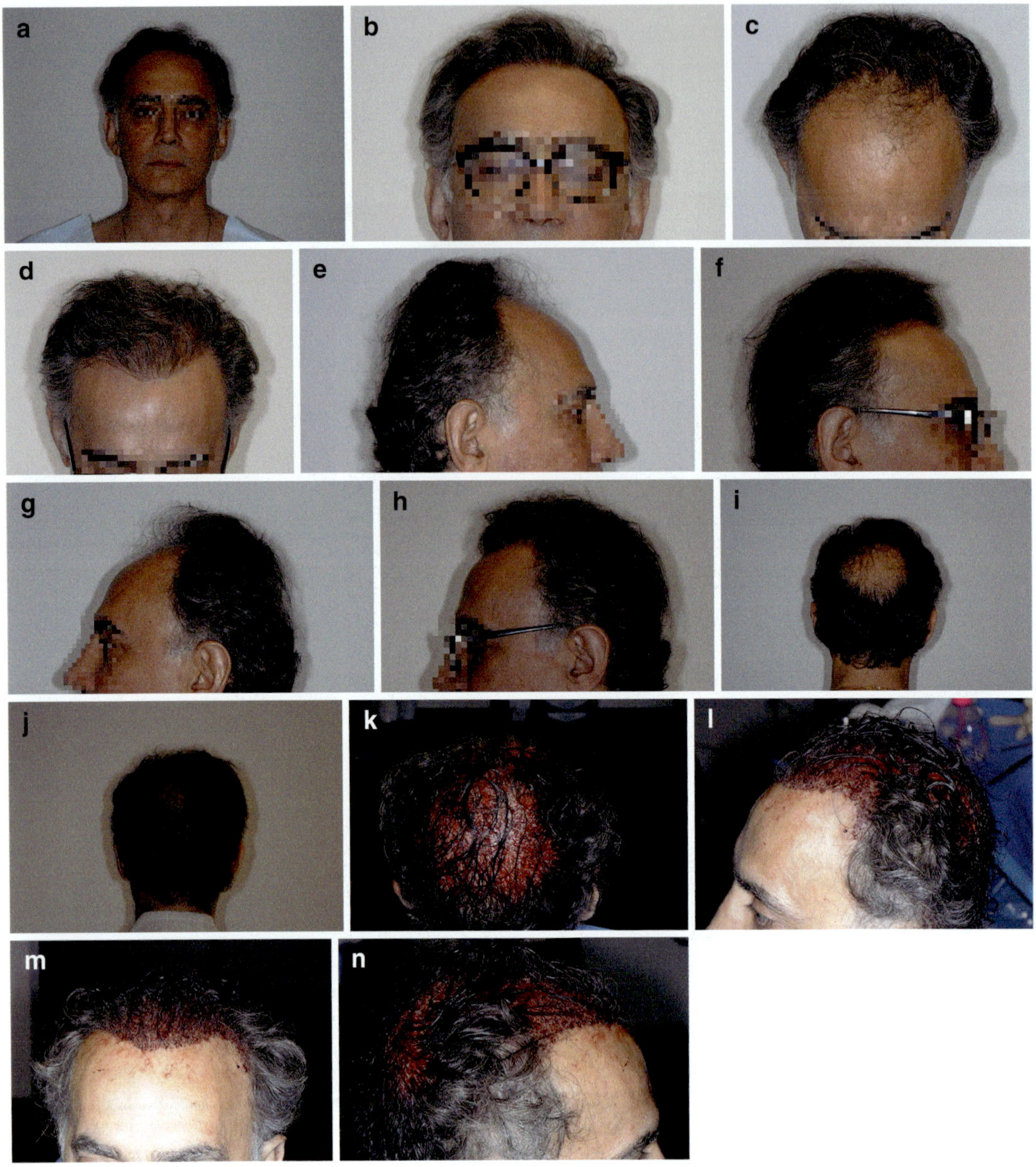

Fig. 37.10 Fifty-eight-year-old man MPB VI before and 1 year after two sessions of hair transplantation, a total of 5300 grafts. (**a**) Here you can see his front view preoperative appearance, (**b**) the result a year after the second session. (**c**) preoperative, looking down. (**d**) postoperative. (**e**) right side preoperatively, (**f**) postoperatively. (**g**) preoperative, left side. (**h**) postoperatively. (**i**) crown area preoperatively (**j**) crown area postoperatively. (**k**) View of the crown area immediately postoperatively. (**l**) shows left side immediate postoperative view. (**m**) front view immediately postoperatively. (**n**) finally right side immediately postoperative appearance

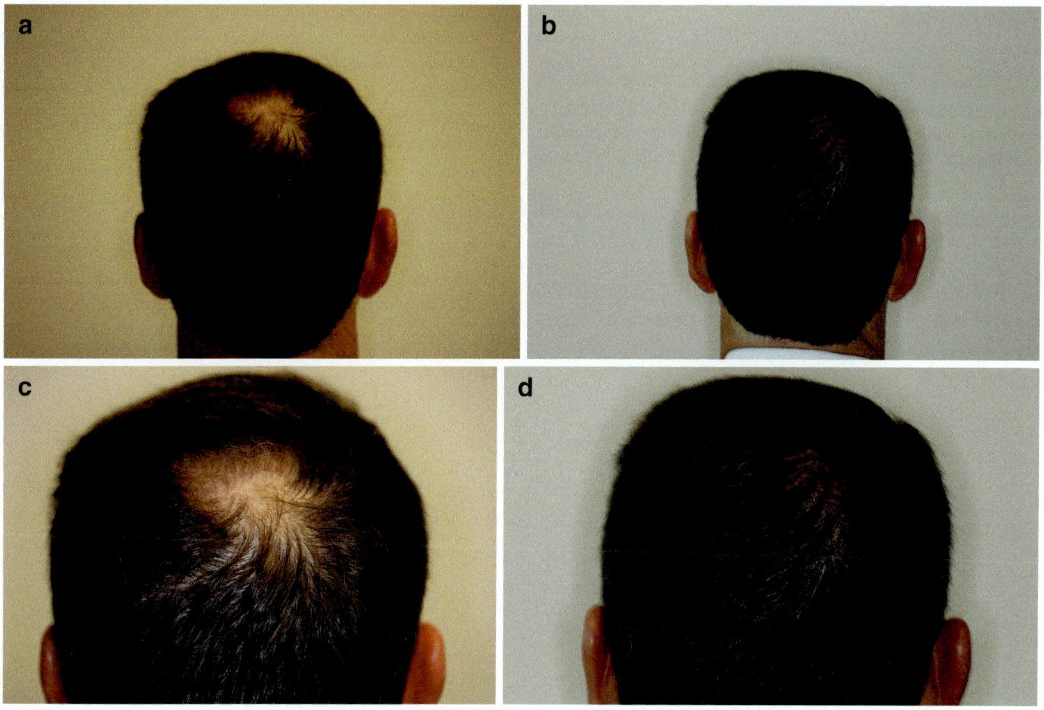

Fig. 37.11 (**a**) Crown pattern alopecia, before. (**b**) A year after 1200 grafts in a single session. (**c**) Before, close-up view. (**d**) After close-up view

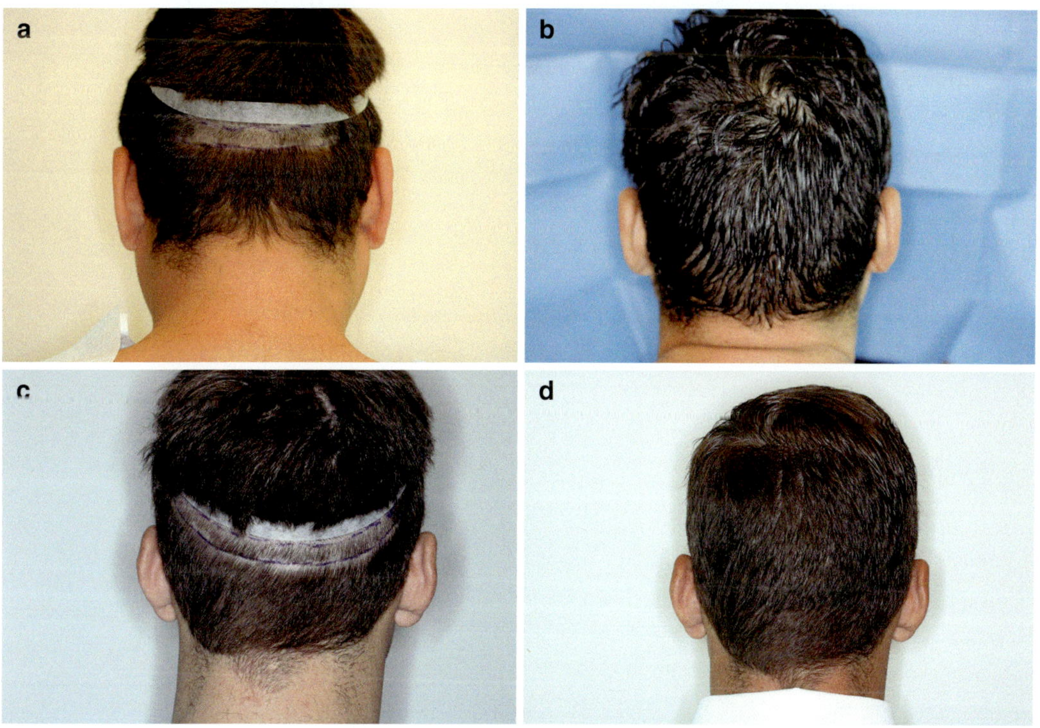

Fig. 37.12 (**a**) Donor site markings, just prior to starting the procedure. (**b**) Typical appearance at the end of the procedure (same day). (**c**) Example of the donor site markings. (**d**) Typical appearance 2 weeks postoperatively

References

1. Uebel CO. Micrografts and minigrafts: a new approach to baldness surgery. Ann Plast Surg. 1991;27:476.
2. Orentreich N. Autografts in alopecias and other selected dermatological conditions. Ann N Y Acad Sci. 1959;83:463.
3. Nordstrom REA. Micrigrafts for improvement of the frontal hairline after hair transplantation. Aesth Plast Surg. 1981;5:97.
4. Barrera A. Micrograft and minigraft megasession hair transplantation: review of 100 consecutive cases. Aesthet Surg J. 1997;17(3):165.
5. Barrera A. Micrograft and minigraft megasession hair transplantation results after a single session. Plast Reconstr Surg. 1997;100(6):1524.
6. Barrera A. Refinements in hair transplantation: micro and minigraft megasession. Perspect Plast Surg. 1998;11(1):53.
7. Barrera A. Hair transplantation - the art of micrografting and minigrafting. 1st ed. St. Louis: Quality Medical Publishing Inc; 2012.
8. Barrera A, Uebel C. Hair transplantation - the art of follicular unit micrografting and minigrafting. 2nd ed. St. Louis: Quality Medical Publishing Inc; 2014.

Robotic FUE Hair Transplantation

38

Zakery Austin Koban and Brian Vassar Heil

38.1 Introduction

The integration of medical expertise with robotic technology has been transforming healthcare for nearly two decades. Applications range from the Xenex® Robot for ultraviolet disinfection of healthcare facilities, to Aethon's Tug® Robot for automated transport of supplies and medications, to Intuitive's Da Vinci® Surgical System for minimally invasive surgery. In parallel, the exponential growth of artificial intelligence (AI) has advanced clinical decision-making, enhancing both technical precision and higher-order processes such as diagnosis and treatment selection [1]. The last half century of advancement in hair restoration has been primarily in pursuit of limiting invasiveness, enhancing harvest precision, improving graft survival, reducing graft size to more accurately model nature, and refining recipient site creation, all to achieve the ultimate goal of undetectable and natural aesthetic outcomes. According to the ISHRS, there has been an undeniable shift in procedure share from Follicular Unit Transfer (FUT) to Follicular Unit Extraction (FUE) over recent years. "In 2006, follicular unit transplantation accounted for 91% of procedures, while follicular unit extraction represented only 7%. By 2016, this trend had reversed, with FUE comprising 55% and FUT 45% of cases [2]. The 2025 ISHRS Practice Census reports that while FUE now accounts for the majority of procedures worldwide (85% in men, 68% in women), robotic-assisted FUE represents only 1.3% of cases, underscoring both its underutilization and the significant opportunity for growth given its potential advantages over manual and motorized techniques [3]. The inherent human error and surgeon fatigue associated with manual FUE introduced limitations in efficiency and consistency, setting the stage for a paradigm shift in hair restoration surgery—first through automated FUE devices (e.g., NeoGraft™, SmartGraft™, Auragraft™), and more recently through robotic FUE [4]. The authors anticipate that procedure share will continue to shift away from manual and automated FUE toward robotic-assisted FUE, as improvements in efficiency, precision, and reproducibility become more widely recognized and economic barriers lessen. The application of robotics, high-definition 3D vision, and AI into one platform has already resulted in an efficient, accurate, and reproducible process capable of achieving the goals above. The ARTAS® Hair Restoration system represents one of the most significant advances in hair restoration history, revolutionizing the world of aesthetic plastic surgery through its seamless integration of robotic precision with surgical artistry [5] (Fig. 38.1).

Z. A. Koban (✉) · B. V. Heil
Premier Plastic Surgery, PC, Wexford, PA, USA

K. Jeffords et al. (eds.), *Aesthetic Surgery for Men*, https://doi.org/10.1007/978-3-032-03840-1_38

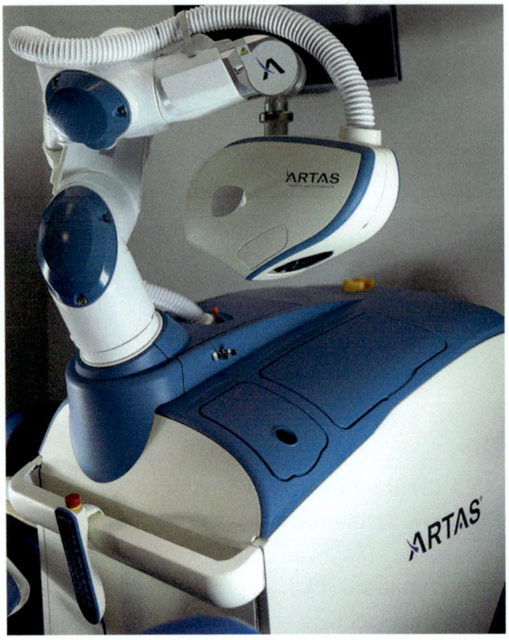

Fig. 38.1 The ARTAS® 9X robotic FUE system

38.2 The Robotic FUE Revolution

The initial conception of applying robotic technology and AI to hair restoration is credited to Dr. Philip Gildenberg, who extrapolated design concepts from the CyberKnife® system that he used for external radiation as a neurosurgeon in Houston, Texas. *Restoration Robotics* was founded in 2002, and a prototype FUE robot was developed. In 2006, human testing trials began under internal review board control, and FDA clearance was achieved in 2011 for the first and only robotic FUE system now known as ARTAS® [6]. In addition, several major system upgrades were developed and integrated into the ARTAS® system over the following decade [7].

The first significant development in robotic graft extraction is the two-step automation process known as the SAFE (Surgically Advanced Follicular Extraction) technique. SAFE uses a sharp needle to breach the superficial scalp surface, immediately followed by a blunt punch dissection of the targeted follicular unit [8]. The first robotic system performed this via computer control and physician assistance using a three-dimensional optical system to locate, select, and harvest follicular units from the donor scalp [9–11]. Robotic recipient site creation was then developed in 2013, adding uniformity to the depth and distribution of the grafting and the ability to avoid injury to existing follicles [12]. In 2016, the AI advanced again with the ability to select follicular units (FU's) based on the number of grouped follicles, maximizing the total number of hairs grafted while simultaneously reducing the required graft quantity [13]. In addition, the scalp stabilization system (Skin Tensioner or ST) has evolved to optimize the consistency of the scalp surface tension and visual tracking of the target follicular units.

The evolution of robotic FUE has further escalated since 2017. Harvesting accuracy and efficiency have dramatically increased, and the avoidance of potential over-harvesting has improved. Greater sophistication and customized digital design of site-making plans through AI developments are the hallmarks of the ARTAS® 9X system. This includes harvesting capability in the range of 1200–1800 grafts/hour with faster FU alignment, improved robotic arm range, advances in lighting, and a high-definition multi-camera stereoscopic vision system with 44 μm resolution. The ARTAS® 9X can also perform FUE with 1.0 mm, 0.9 mm, or 0.8 mm punch systems to minimize harvest site trauma and produce pinpoint scars [14, 15]. The most recent advancement is robotic graft placement, now possible with the ARTAS® iX System (Fig. 38.2). Graft placement is accomplished simultaneously with site creation through a cannulated needle. The grafts are pre-loaded into a 25-graft cartridge that is auto-advanced with each site creation. This has made complete robotic FUE hair transplantation a reality that will undoubtedly be perfected in future system iterations (Fig. 38.3).

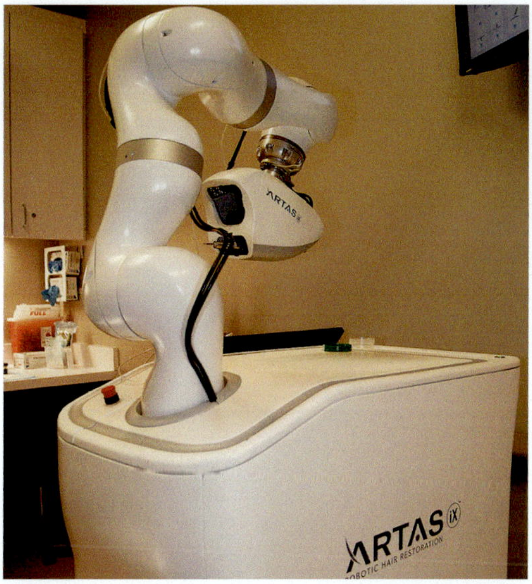

Fig. 38.2 The ARTAS® iX Robotic FUE system

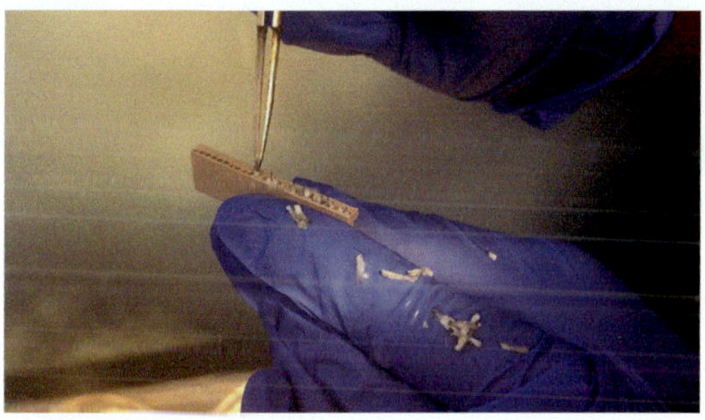

Fig. 38.3 Robotic graft implantation is now possible with using the ARTAS® iX system. Graft insertion is accomplished simultaneously with site creation through a cannulated needle. The grafts are pre-loaded into a 25-graft cartridge that is auto-advanced with each site creation

38.3 Patient Selection

The broad candidacy for FUE in the general hair loss population directly translates into similar eligibility for robotic FUE hair restoration. Some have tried to relegate FUE procedures to just addressing those patients who wish to wear their hair short or to others who have sustained multiple FUT strip scars to the occipital donor site and present as poor candidates for further FUT. In our practice view, all patients who may benefit from a hair transplant are considered valid candidates until proven otherwise. Some of the contraindications for robotic FUE include excessive skin laxity or dermatofibrosis, use of anticoagulant medications or supplements, history of bleeding diathesis or autoimmune disorders, very tightly coiled hair (e.g., Type VI-VIII hair pattern per L'Oréal classification), heavily pigmented scalp color serving as the optical backdrop to dark donor hair (e.g., Fitzpatrick skin type V–VI with dark hair shafts), patient inability to maintain the required positions for harvest or graft placement, and absolute contraindications to hair restoration surgery such as scarring alopecia [16–18].

38.4 The Robotic FUE Procedure: Harvesting

The transplant procedure begins with the preparation of the donor region by trimming the occipital hair to 1.0–1.2 mm in length with a no-guard clipper (Fig. 38.4). Patients with medium-to-long hair often choose to prepare for the process by having a "transitional" haircut with short sides and back a few weeks or months in advance of their upcoming treatment date. This is done to obscure the impact of their sudden change of hairstyles upon post-procedural return to work and social encounters (Fig. 38.5). When the patient has blonde, red, gray, or white hair, the clipped hair must be dyed brown to achieve the required color contrast against their scalp to

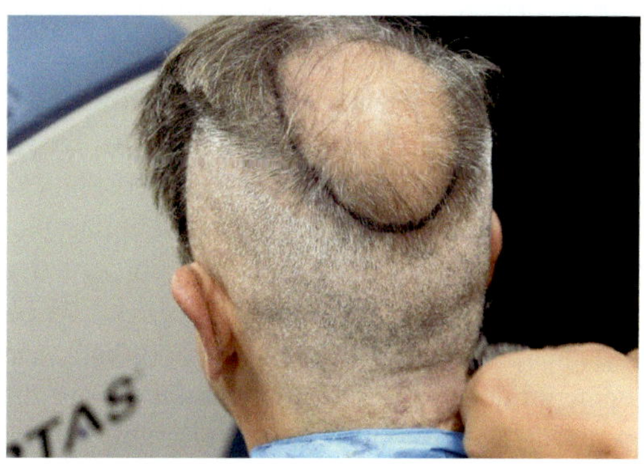

Fig. 38.4 Preparation for robotic FUE harvesting requires clipping of the donor scalp to 1.0–1.2 mm length, allowing the artificial intelligence to accurately assess follicular density and hair exit angle

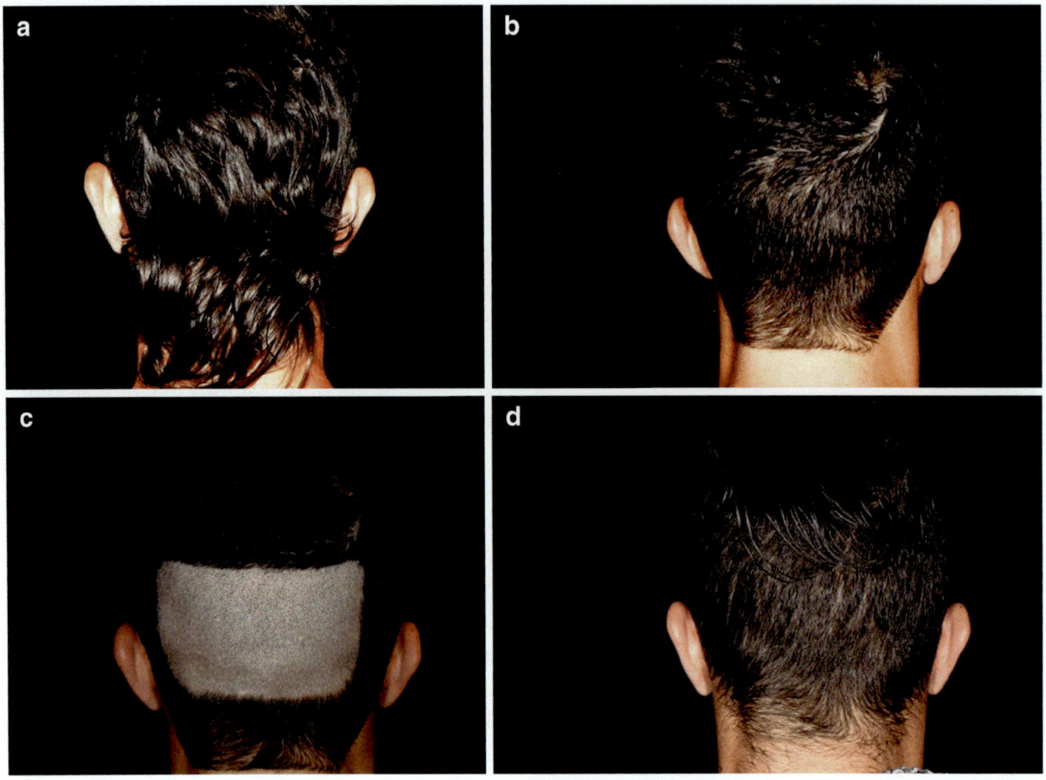

Fig. 38.5 Transitional hair styles can help patients prepare for surgery, obscuring the impact of a suddenly short hair style on procedure day. Clipping of the sides and back with a number one or two-guarded clipper is ideal. (**a**) Preoperative view of donor site at consultation, (**b**) transitional hair styling, (**c**) immediate preoperative clipping, (**d**) postoperative view of donor site

enable proper follicle identification by the robotic camera system throughout the harvesting phase. The patient is given an oral anxiolytic and narcotic dose at the start of the process after written informed consent has been obtained. These medications are in effect by the time the donor site is anesthetized with local anesthetic (dilute lidocaine with epinephrine and sodium bicarbonate) infiltration and appropriate localized nerve blocks with bupivacaine. The administration of anesthesia is followed by infiltration of a conservative amount of tumescent solution (Fig. 38.6). Adequate time is allowed for full anesthetic and epinephrine effects. The patient then uses the restroom and is positioned comfortably in the robotic treatment bed in the prone position for the start of the harvest.

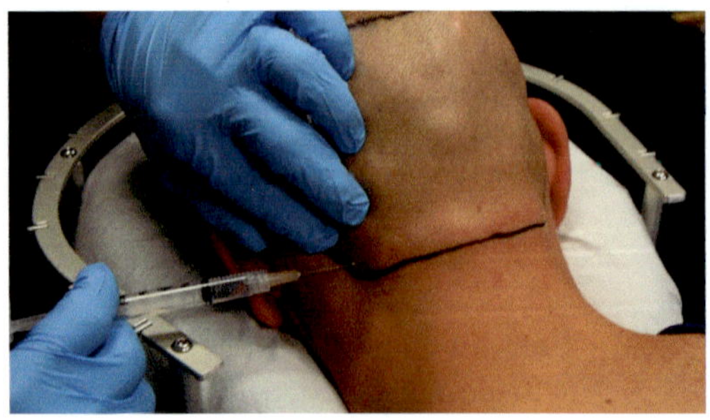

Fig. 38.6 Administration of local anesthesia is performed following written informed consent, dosing of oral anxiolytic and narcotic medications, and proper preparation of the donor scalp

The patient's headrest is oriented directly in front of the robotic arm, with the adjustable procedure bed about one foot away from the system cart. The bed position is adjustable for comfort and minimization of movement. The robotic harvesting system requires stabilization of the patient's head and the scalp skin to achieve precise interaction with the follicle unit and accurate insertion of the harvesting mechanism. This is accomplished with a 12 cm^2 Skin Tensioner (ST) inserted into the target area, inducing a stretch force on the skin via its perimeter of pins (Fig. 38.7). The ST, and thereby the targeted grid of follicular units, is then stabilized with flexible elastic bands anchored to a frame around the patient's head in a face-down position on an open-center prone pillow. Proper ST placement must be verified for minimal superior movement, skin blanching and firmness, and pin engagement with the scalp. Tumescent is then injected within the corners of the grid to maintain consistent graft quality. No more than 2.0 mL of tumescent per grid is recommended.

The *Acquire Tensioner* icon is activated on the user interface (UI) or remote control (ARTAS® Hair Pendant) to start the automatic tensioner reading. This activates the robotic system to locate the ST automatically, move the needle mechanism to a position over the patient, and acquire the ST by analyzing and mapping its peripheral fiducials (Fig. 38.8). The artificial intelligence automatically performs follicular unit density and hair length calculations. Harvesting, or automation, is initiated by selecting an FU and pressing *Begin* on the UI. The robotic system performs graft extraction using a two- or four-prong sharp inner needle. The needle functions to breach the skin surface with a shallow 1.5–2 mm deep incision, facilitating the entry of a dull, rotating punch (5000 revolutions/min) to dissect the follicle free from the surrounding tissue gently. Light suction aids in the elevation of the liberated follicular unit (Fig. 38.9). The needle and punch are available in 18-, 19-, and 20-gauge options to address the varying FU characteristics among patients. The robotic approach angle (off-set angle), hair exit angle, punch/core depth, punch spacing, and applied scalp force are monitored continuously throughout the extraction phase via the user interface. Intergrid density variations are monitored automatically by the AI and can be adjusted accordingly with the surgeon's input. The surgeon monitors and controls all aspects of the harvesting procedure through the touch-screen user interface and hand-held remote control. The UI uses the three-dimensional camera system and harvesting mechanism to control and adjust the space between harvests, needle angle and depth, and harvest area. The AI allows the surgeon to employ advanced algorithms to choose optimal FUs, randomizing the pattern of harvest sites while choosing higher follicle-count units to achieve higher hair-count restorations with the least number of FUs required (Fig. 38.10). Any punch depth, core depth, and off-set angle parameter adjustments are made in response to visual cues from the UI and microscopic graft assess-

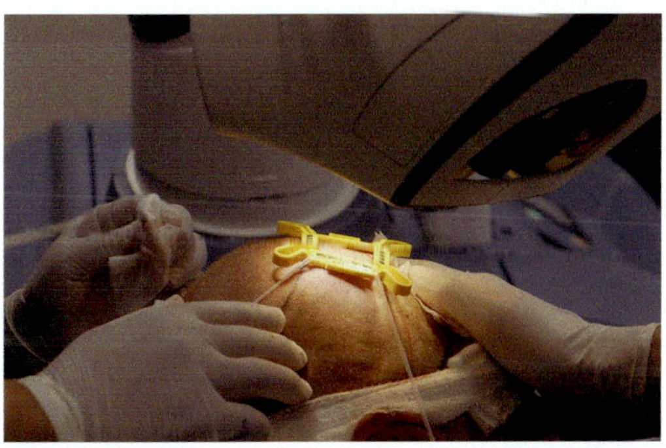

Fig. 38.7 The robotic harvesting system requires stabilization of the patient's head and the scalp skin to achieve precise interaction with the follicle unit and accurate insertion of the harvesting mechanism. Proper ST placement must be verified for minimal superior movement, skin blanching and firmness, and pin engagement with the scalp. Tumescent is then injected within the corners of the grid to maintain consistent graft quality

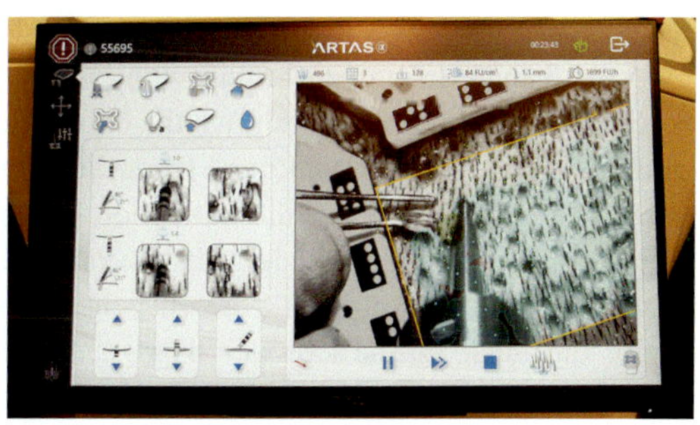

Fig. 38.8 The robotic user interface provides magnified and standard views of the robotic stereoscopic visual field. Note the peripheral fiducials along the ST grid margin used for ST alignment

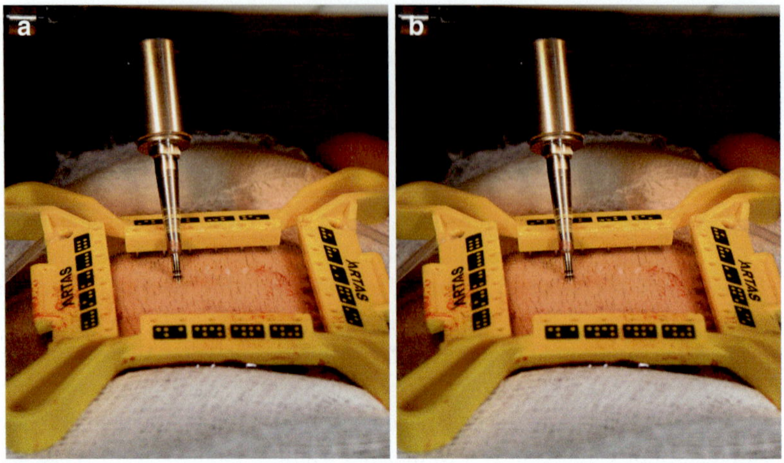

Fig. 38.9 Robotic extraction using the ARTAS® 9x system. Follicular units are analyzed and extracted by first analyzing the position of the fiducials located on the Skin Tensioner perimeter

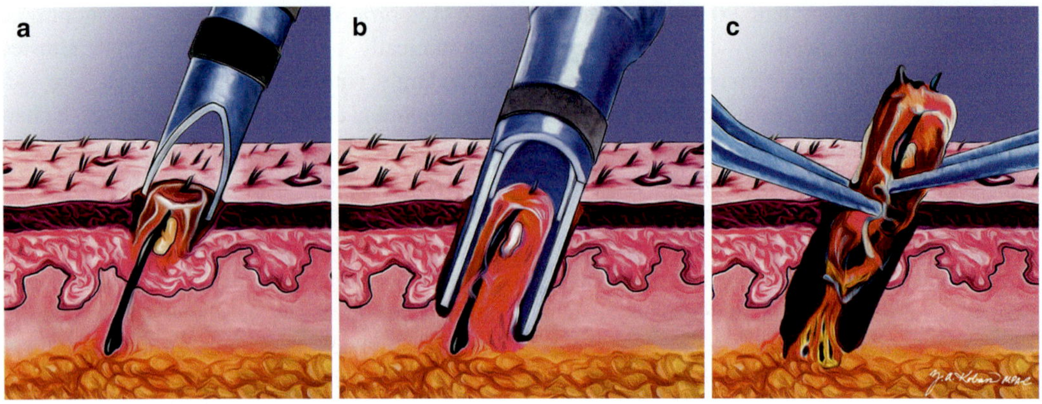

Fig. 38.10 The SAFE Technique. (**a**) A sharp two- or four-pronged needle is first deployed to score the superficial scalp surface, (**b**) immediately followed by blunt rotating punch dissection of the targeted follicular unit. (**c**) Light suction aids in FU elevation, and the graft is removed using the recommended two-hand extraction technique

ment, which can be performed simultaneously during the harvesting phase by another technician.

A two-hand extraction technique with *Forester* forceps is recommended to remove the extracted grafts from the grid region. Loupe magnification should be used throughout the extraction phase (Fig. 38.11). After the first few dissections are performed, automation should be suspended to verify the inner needle's proper depth and the coring depth of the dissection punch. Microscopic graft inspection and counting under 10× magnification is recommended. Quality grafts are identifiable by the presence of well-centered hairs with cylindrical epidermal and dermal cell casings,

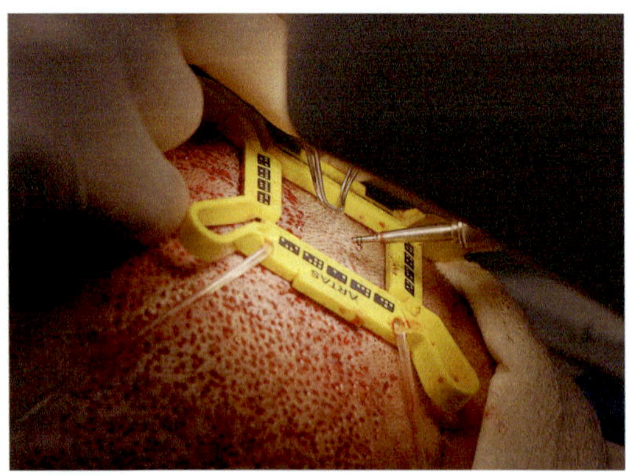

Fig. 38.11 Robotic FUE harvesting and simultaneous graft extraction using the recommended two-hand technique with *Forester* forceps

intact bulbs with protective root sheaths, and adipocytes in the deep segment of the grafts. Follicular units can be separated and categorized based on shaft groupings (F1–F4) to accelerate the speed of later graft placement. Any transected, incomplete, or damaged grafts (J-shaped or bent follicles, crushed or spun follicles) must be discarded and excluded from the total graft count (Fig. 38.12). The grafts are maintained in chilled saline or preservative agent throughout this process until placement. Once graft quality, core depth, and punch depth are assessed, automation can resume.

Upon completing the first grid, the robotic arm and needle mechanism will assume the "Safe Position" oriented over the system cart. The ST is then removed and prepared for placement in the following grid location. The grid zone is moved from position to position with proper overlap allowing for the even harvest of the required quantity of FUs. Appropriate grid overlap is necessary to prevent gaps in the donor area, and grid borders can be further adjusted via the UI. The harvest density along the donor site's grid perimeter may be reduced to taper the decrement in remaining hair density and avoid a detectable margin. Depending on donor density, the average quantity of harvest from each grid can range from 60 to 120 FUs. Extraction from the superior occipital scalp should be avoided due to the possible presence of androgen-sensitive hairs in the lower fringes of the vertex. Vellus hairs in the nape of the neck should also be avoided (Figs. 38.13, 38.14 and 38.15).

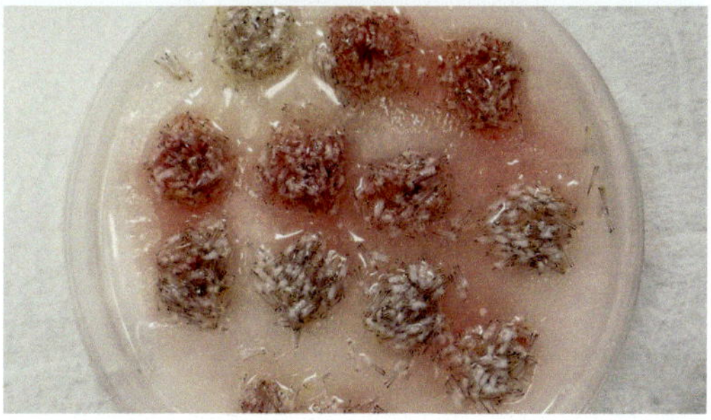

Fig. 38.12 Quality grafts are identifiable by the presence of well-centered hairs with cylindrical epidermal and dermal cell casings, intact bulbs with protective root sheaths, and adipocytes in the deep segment of the grafts

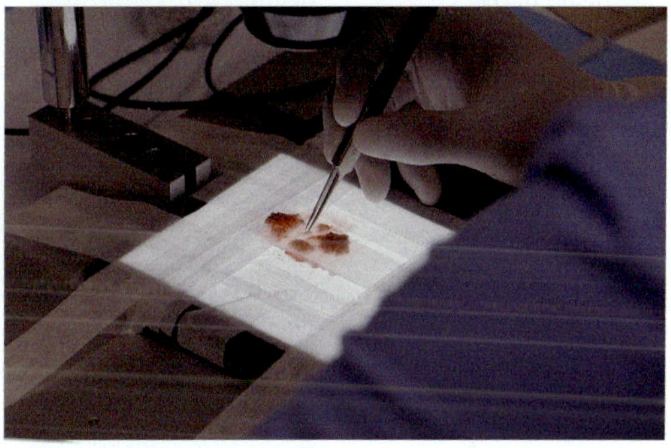

Fig. 38.13 Microscopic graft assessment under 10× magnification is recommended and should proceed simultaneously with the robotic harvesting phase. Follicular units can be separated and categorized based on shaft groupings (F1–F4) to accelerate the speed of later graft placement

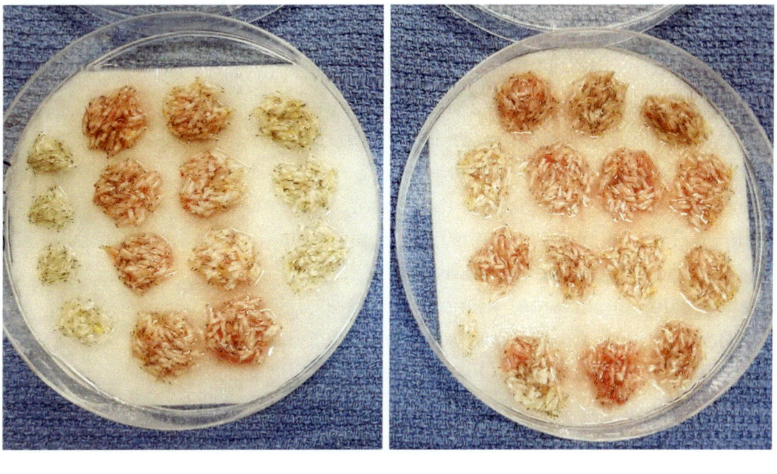

Fig. 38.14 An image of 2908 FUs fully prepared for the insertion phase. The grafts are maintained in chilled saline or preservative agent throughout this process until placement

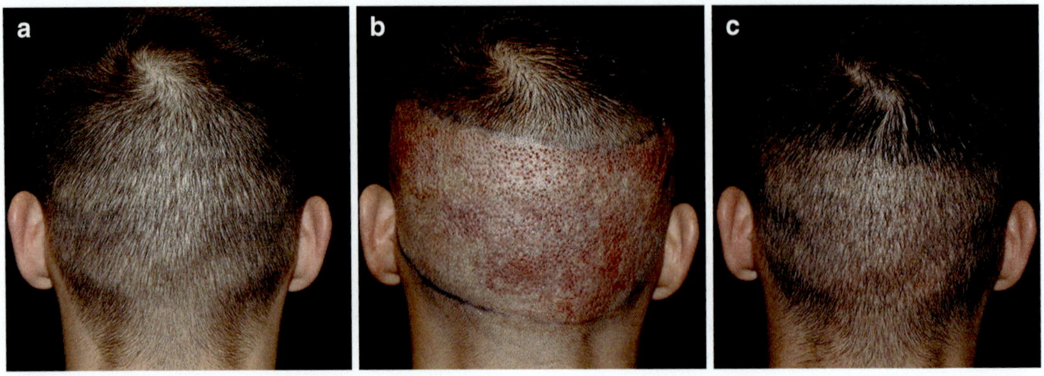

Fig. 38.15 Extraction from the superior occipital scalp should be avoided due to the possible presence of androgen-sensitive hairs in the lower fringes of the vertex. Vellus hairs in the nape of the neck should also be avoided. Recovery of the donor scalp is rapid: (**a**) image of the donor zone preoperatively, (**b**) image of the donor zone immediately post-operative, (**c**) image if the donor zone at 1 week post-operative

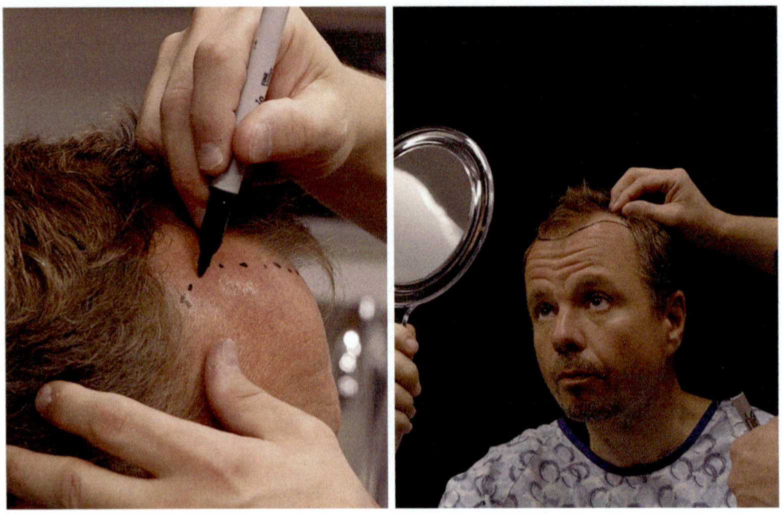

Fig. 38.16 The graft placement plan is decided upon during the preoperative consultation and designed on the patient's head together with the patient's input at the start of the case before the donor site is clipped

38.5 The Robotic FUE Procedure: Site Creation and Graft Placement

The graft placement plan is decided upon during the preoperative consultation and designed on the patient's head together with the patient's input at the start of the case before the donor site is clipped (Fig. 38.16). This consultation and planning process can be facilitated using the ARTAS® Hair Studio® application, which provides a digital simulation of various scenarios and outcome models [19] (Fig. 38.17). On treatment day, the

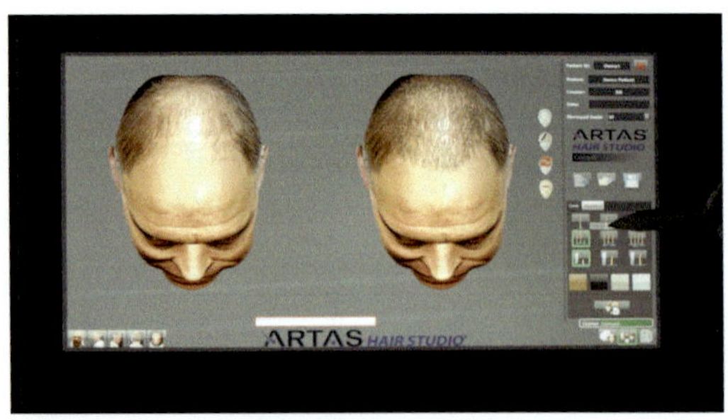

Fig. 38.17 ARTAS® Hair Studio® application provides a digital simulation of various scenarios and outcome models

hair transplant plan can be realized by either manual or robotic site creation. The manual method involves creating graft recipient sites with 18-, 19-, or 20-gauge needles or 1.0–1.3 mm Minde blades. The sites are made only to the depth necessary to insert the graft bulbs back to the level from which they are harvested. This reduces the overall amount of trauma in the treatment zone. The sites are also angled to match the naturally occurring angles of the original recipient site hair to achieve cohesive hair restoration.

Following the harvest and processing of the grafts, the administration of local anesthetic into the recipient region is performed. At this stage, whole blood is drawn from the patient via standard phlebotomy, and autologous platelet-rich plasma (A-PRP) is then prepared and injected into the dermis of the recipient scalp, where site creation is planned. Specific details regarding transplant supplementation with A-PRP will be addressed later. The surgeon then has the option of robotic site creation, which requires a digital photograph of the plan drawn on the patient's scalp and clipping the hair in the recipient region. The clipped recipient region is required by the ARTAS® visual system in order to identify the precise location of each graft site while avoiding injury to existing follicles in the same area (Fig. 38.18).

The manual creation of sites is always done with the best effort to avoid injury to these bulbs; however, the 3D vision system and AI can better assess and calculate the ideal distribution of sites. The prime limitation of robotic site-making is the reluctance of many patients to clip their entire head of hair. For this reason, most patients may have reservations about proceeding with site creation robotically. Thus, in the author's experience, most cases are executed with manual site creation, but this may vary from practice to practice. Furthermore, some surgeons choose to decrease the time between the completion of harvesting and initiating graft insertion by pre-making recipient sites. Pre-made sites can be prepared after the hair design is completed immediately before the harvesting phase or on the day before treatment altogether [20] (Fig. 38.19). Just

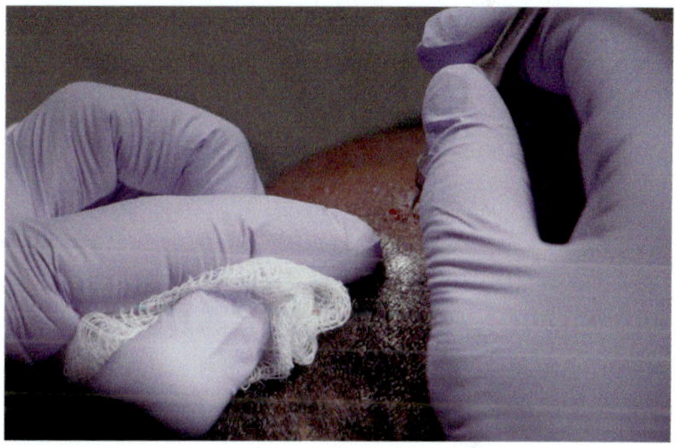

Fig. 38.19 Manual site creation. Recipient sites may be prepared at different stages: after robotic FUE harvesting, immediately before harvesting once the hairline design is completed, or on the day before the procedure

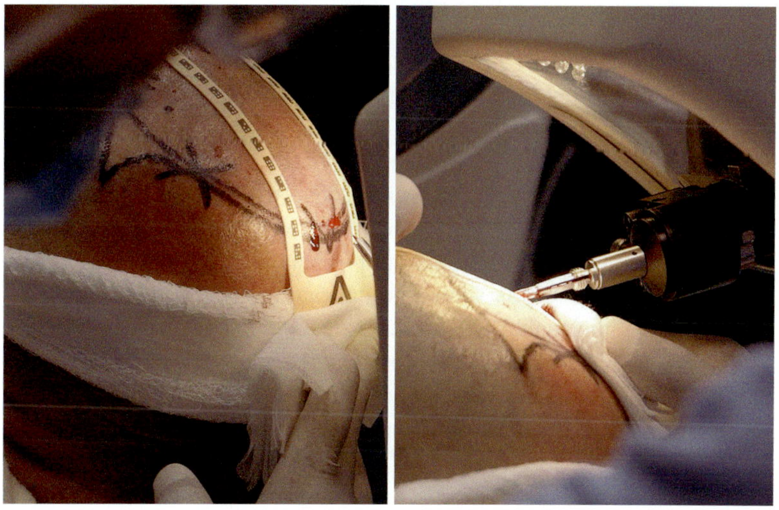

Fig. 38.18 Robotic site creation requires a digital photograph of the plan drawn on the patient's scalp and clipping the hair in the recipient region. The clipped recipient region is required by the ARTAS® visual system in order to identify the precise location of each graft site while avoiding injury to existing follicles in the same area

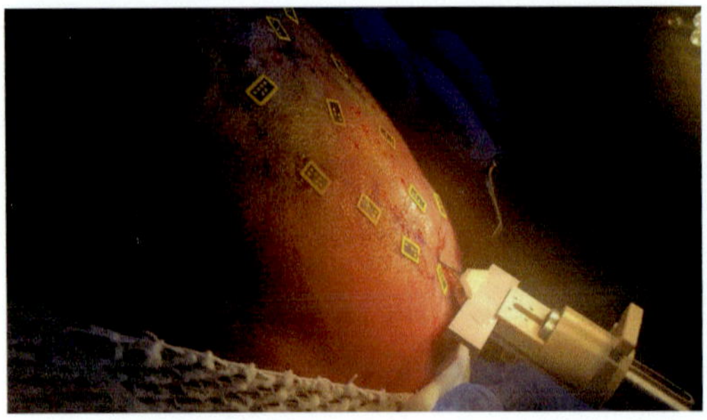

Fig. 38.20 Robotic graft insertion using the ARTAS® iX robotic system

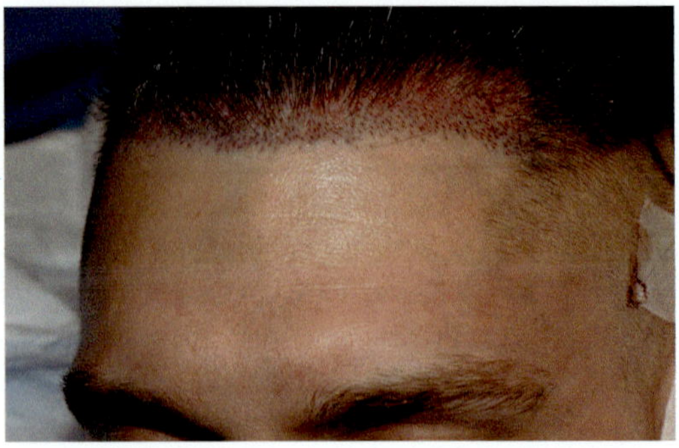

Fig. 38.21 Sites created along the frontal hairline and temporal regions prior to graft insertion

as the graft sites can be created manually or robotically, the insertion or placement of the FUs can be accomplished in the same manner. The current ARTAS® iX model can robotically insert grafts from a pre-loaded cartridge simultaneously with site creation using a cannulated needle system (Fig. 38.20).

Manual site creation and placement should follow the pre-marked recipient site layout exactly. The treatment zones are prepared to receive grafts by making micro-slits in the skin with 18- to 19-gauge needle tips on a *Lightning* handle. Site depth must be set to the depth of the native follicles extracted from the donor regions. Region-specific slit angle and orientations must be set to match the natural hair angulations. Care must be taken to avoid any injury to the preexisting hair in the recipient zones, thus reducing the likelihood of shock trauma. All sites should be made with the application of appropriate skin tension (Fig. 38.21). The posterior and lateral margins of the treatment zones should be feathered into adjacent regions of the scalp that were not planned for restoration at this stage. Any frontal hairline sites should be created with tight density but in irregular alignment to effectively model a natural hairline. Jeweler-type microforceps are recommended for manual graft implantation (Fig. 38.22). Grafts should be delicately but efficiently implanted into each recipient site bulb first, avoiding over-insertion and forceful manipulation that might injure the grafts and thus decrease viability. This process is repeated until implantation of the entire recipient area is complete.

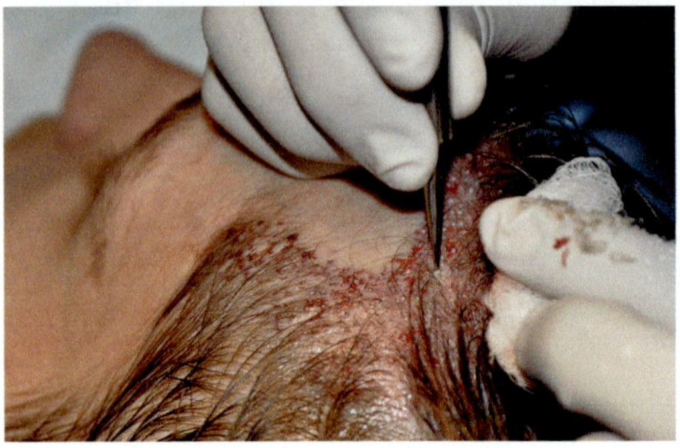

Fig. 38.22 Manual placement of grafts into pre-made insertion sites using Jeweler-type microforceps

Upon completion of graft placement, the recipient and donor zones are cleansed with saline solution. A light, non-adhesive pressure dressing with topical antibiotic ointment (Bacitracin®) is applied and secured with a Coban® wrap to the donor site. The recipient zones are left uncovered (Fig. 38.23). The dressing is removed after 36 hours, and Bacitracin® ointment is applied twice daily for three additional days and then discontinued. The grafted region is misted with saline while the dressing is in place. After dressing removal, the scalp is cleansed with cups of baby shampoo solution and water, avoiding pressure sprays. The patient may return to regular scalp cleansing on day ten and total physical activity, including strenuous exercise, on day 14 post-transplant (Fig. 38.24).

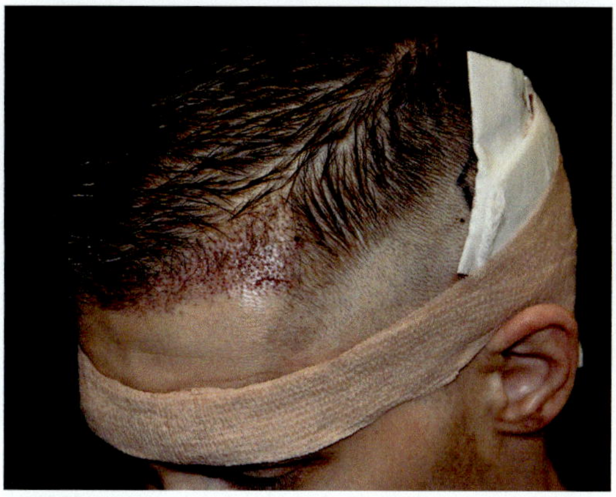

Fig. 38.23 A light, non-adhesive pressure dressing with topical antibiotic ointment (Bacitracin®) is applied and secured with a Coban® wrap to the donor site. The recipient zones are left uncovered, and the dressing is removed after 36 hours

38.6 Autologous Platelet-Rich Plasma (A-PRP): A Stand-Alone Therapy and Supplement to Robotic FUE

Autologous platelet-rich plasma (A-PRP) is a cellular biotherapy of heightened interest in treating androgenetic alopecia (AGA). The treatment is an autologous preparation of blood plasma with concentrated platelets [21]. It is performed by obtaining a sample of whole blood (typically 15–30 mL) via standard phlebotomy using a blood collection system intended for use with PRP (e.g., ProGen PRP™ Eclipse System by Crown Aesthetics or Healeon HD PRP™). Erythrocytes are eliminated, and the plasma is

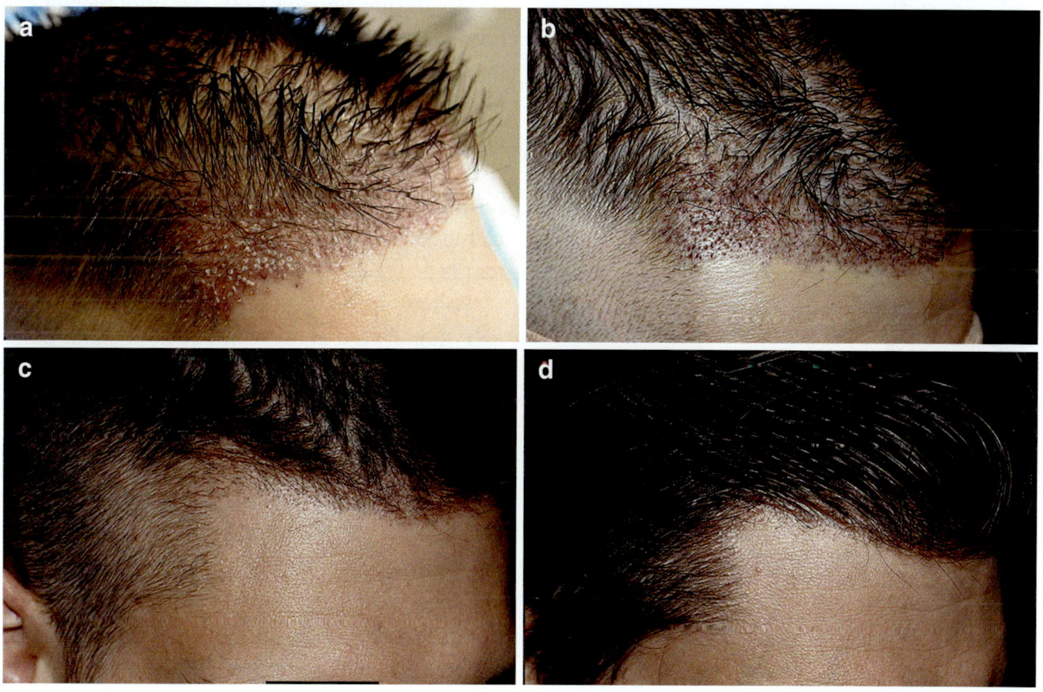

Fig. 38.24 Recipient site recovery: (**a**) post-op day 0, (**b**) post-op day 2, (**c**) 2 weeks post-op, (**d**), post-op 1 year

concentrated 4–6 times above baseline through centrifugation. Newer collection systems include prepared anticoagulants and utilize gel medium separators. Higher quality systems boast around 90% platelet retention (Fig. 38.25). Centrifugation protocols vary based on the collection system, the quantity of whole blood collected, and the intended platelet concentration.

The platelet-rich plasma is then injected into regions of the balding scalp at a dose of 0.1 mL/cm^2 at a target depth of 2-5 mm based upon scalp thickness and follicular depth. Mechanical controlled injections (i.e., Ultim® Mesogun, AAMS, Montrodat, France) allow for precision dosing and better scalp coverage [22] (Fig. 38.26). Platelets are inherently rich in proteins and growth factors that act upon numerous targets, including the stem cells within the pilosebaceous unit. The platelets can be chemically activated (autologous-activated or AA-PRP) or activated naturally upon scalp collagen exposure (A-PRP). Platelet activation results in the alpha-granule release of growth factors which interact with their respective tissue receptors, resulting in angiogenesis and initiation of the healing and growth of organic structures [23]. Three primary growth factors involved in the treatment of AGA are platelet-derived growth factor (PDGF), transforming growth factor (TGF-β), and vascular endothelial growth factor (VEGF). These growth factors activate stem cells within the hair structure, potentially stimulating vellus to terminal hair transformation. PRP is also believed to prolong the anagen phase and increase follicular cell survival by inhibiting cellular apoptosis that occurs during telogen [24]. An improvement in hair quality and density is typically reported following a series of treatments. Patients with earlier hair loss have better results than those with a more advanced Hamilton-Norwood pattern [24]. In addition, those with vellus hair have better results than those with few but normal hairs, indicating that PRP may act on the hair shaft diameter [24].

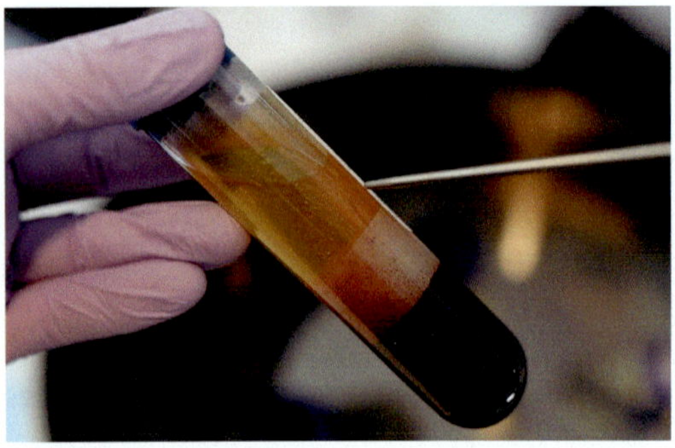

Fig. 38.25 Whole blood collection system for use with autologous platelet-rich plasma. Newer collection systems include prepared anticoagulants and utilize gel medium separators. Higher quality systems boast around 90% platelet retention

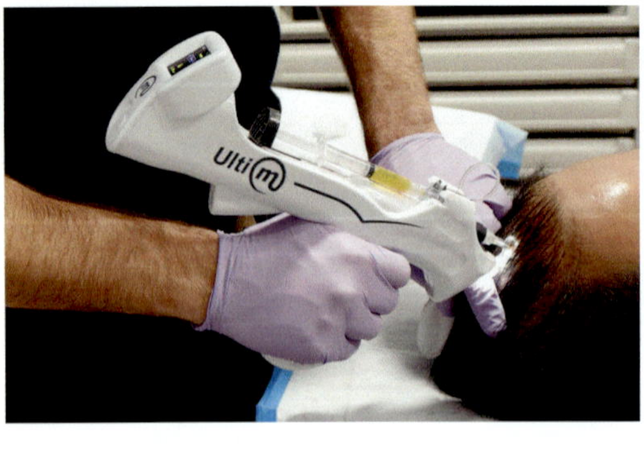

Fig. 38.26 Mechanical controlled injections (i.e., Ultim® Mesogun, AAMS, Montrodat, France) of A-PRP allow for precision dosing and better scalp coverage

Follow-up studies on the long-term effects of PRP therapy are underway. For now, stand-alone PRP therapy is performed in our practice as an initial series of three treatments at 1-month intervals. Results are typically assessed 90 days following the initial treatment series via photographic comparison and software-based trichoscan analysis (e.g., HairMetrix®, Canfield Scientific) (Fig. 38.27). If results are clinically significant, or androgenetic alopecia appears to be stabilized, patients are encouraged to continue booster treatments every 6–12 months to maintain a continued response (Figs. 38.28 and 38.29). Aside from use as a stand-alone therapy, studies have demonstrated a decisive role for PRP during the transplantation procedure by improving FU survivability and post-transplant capillary density. Split-head FUT studies in 2006 observed a 15.1% increase in hair density and growth when follicular units were pre-treated with AA-PRP prior to implantation [23]. PRP is not currently

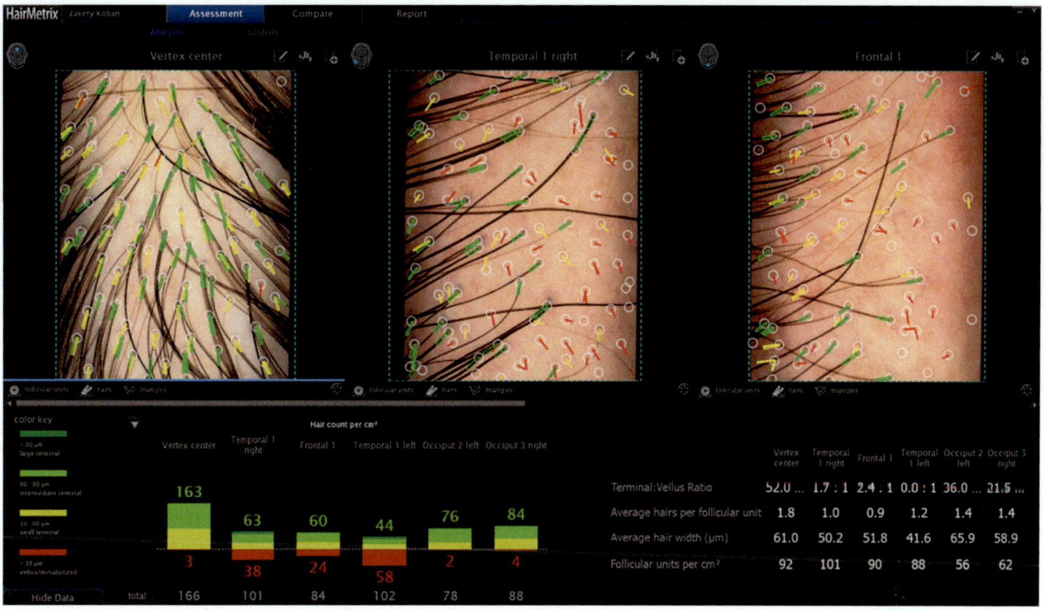

Fig. 38.27 Software-based trichoscan analysis (e.g., HairMetrix®, Canfield Scientific) allows for superior assessment of treatment efficacy

Fig. 38.28 Before and after image of A-PRP injection series in the frontal hairline, temples, forelock, and anterior vertex regions. Performed as a stand alone therapy

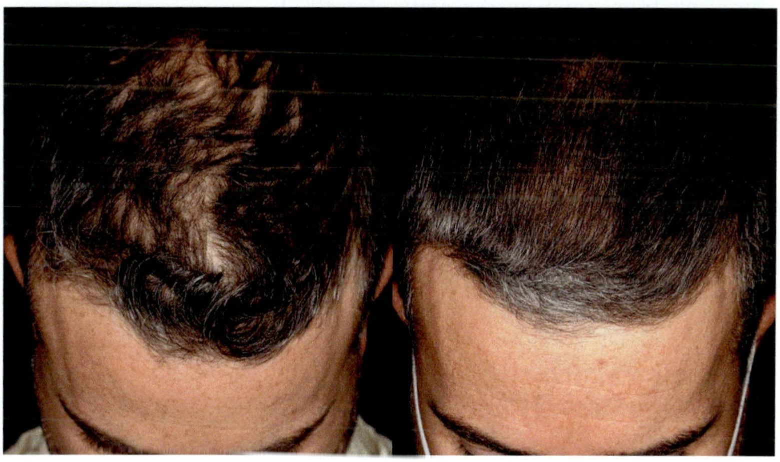

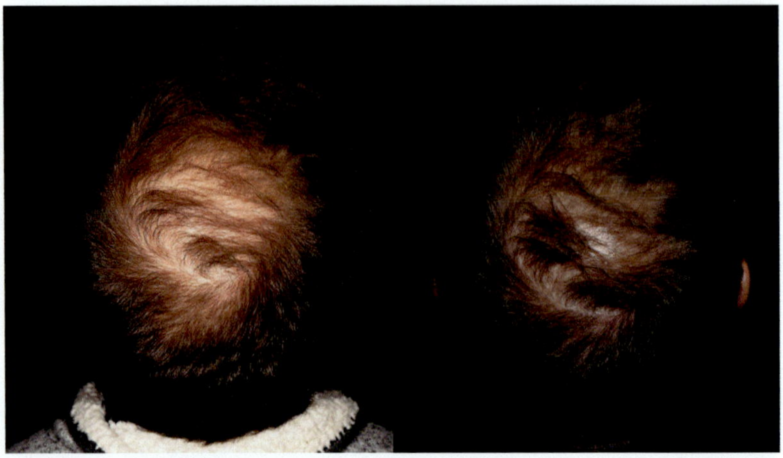

Fig. 38.29 Before and after image of A-PRP injection series in the vertex, performed as a stand alone therapy

approved by the FDA for the treatment of androgenic alopecia or its use in transplantation surgery. However, given numerous studies with clinically significant outcomes, we recommended including PRP as part of the robotic transplantation procedure. PRP can be collected, prepared, and injected into the recipient scalp before site creation to avoid the fibrin glue-like effect that can result from imbibing the grafts directly. It should be noted that platelet count for the treatment of AGA has not yet been optimized; however, a platelet concentration of more than one million platelets per microliter is generally accepted as the therapeutically effective concentration of PRP [10].

38.7 Clinical Results

It is the author's experience that patients typically report a high degree of satisfaction and comfort following robotic FUE. The enhanced harvesting precision, minimal manipulation of FU grafts, and reduced procedure time of robotic FUE contribute to improved graft viability and better clinical outcomes relative to other harvesting methods. Routine follow-up assessments and standard photographic documentation reveal definite improvements in hair quality and scalp coverage (Fig. 38.30). Correction of frontotemporal hairline recession can restore facial framing, resulting in a more youthful appearance. The total number of robotic FUE sessions required depends on the patient's Hamilton-Norwood (HN) pattern and his individual goals and expectations regarding the outcome. There is a proportional relationship between HN classification and the required number of grafts. The same is true for the total number of grafting sessions. Robotic FUE sessions may range in graft quantity from 700 to 4000 grafts (Figs. 38.31 and 38.32). Many patients elect to proceed with high-volume cases (2500 grafts or more in a single sitting) in order to limit the interruption of work and familial and social activities. Cases over 3000 FUs may or may not require additional tools to obtain grafts from the posterior parietal scalp zones. The hair exit angle in these regions can be exceedingly acute and potentially challenging to extract robotically. Automated FUE technology (e.g., NeoGraft®) is an excellent supplementary resource for harvesting from these zones. Robotic FUE *can* be used for secondary grafting procedures as well. Automated follicular unit density calculations by the AI and physician control over harvest spacing parameters significantly reduce the risk of over-extraction. However, patients with severe or significant scarring in the mid-occipital zones from repeated FUT or outdated punch grafting methods may better benefit from automated FUE technology alone. This is due to ease of use in the posterior parietal scalp to avoid further harvesting from the mid-occipital region.

Multiple grafting sessions may be required for patients with an advanced HN pattern to accomplish the desired degree of scalp restoration. The

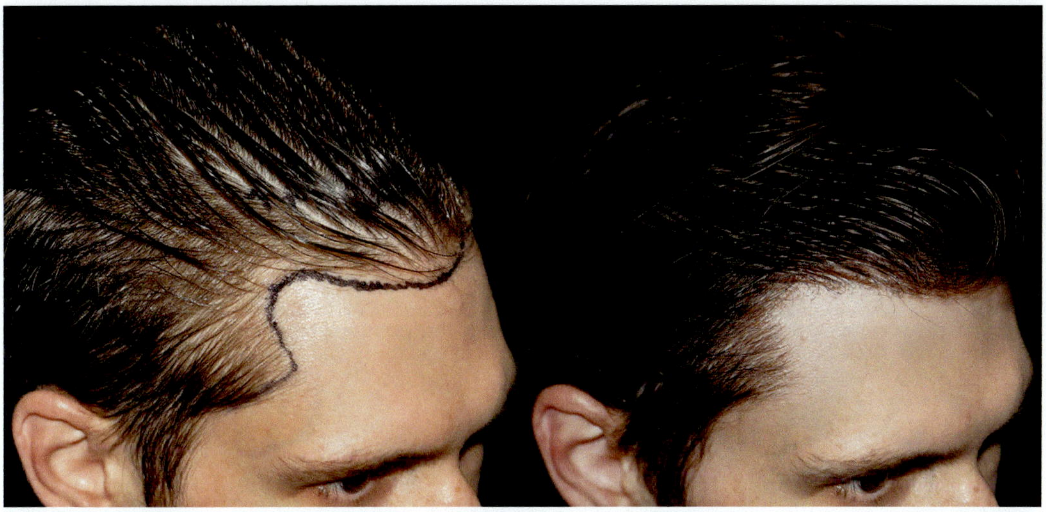

Fig. 38.30 Correction of front temporal hairline recession with robotic FUE can restore facial framing, resulting in a more youthful appearance; 1323 grafts

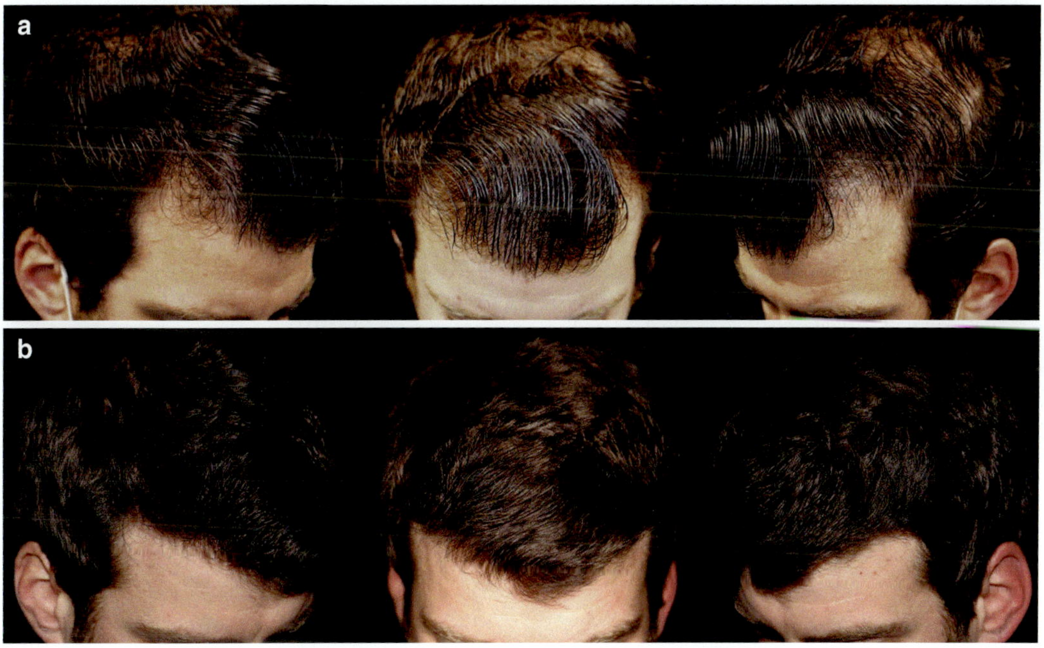

Fig. 38.31 Before and 1-year after image of single-session robotic FUE result with 1758 grafts

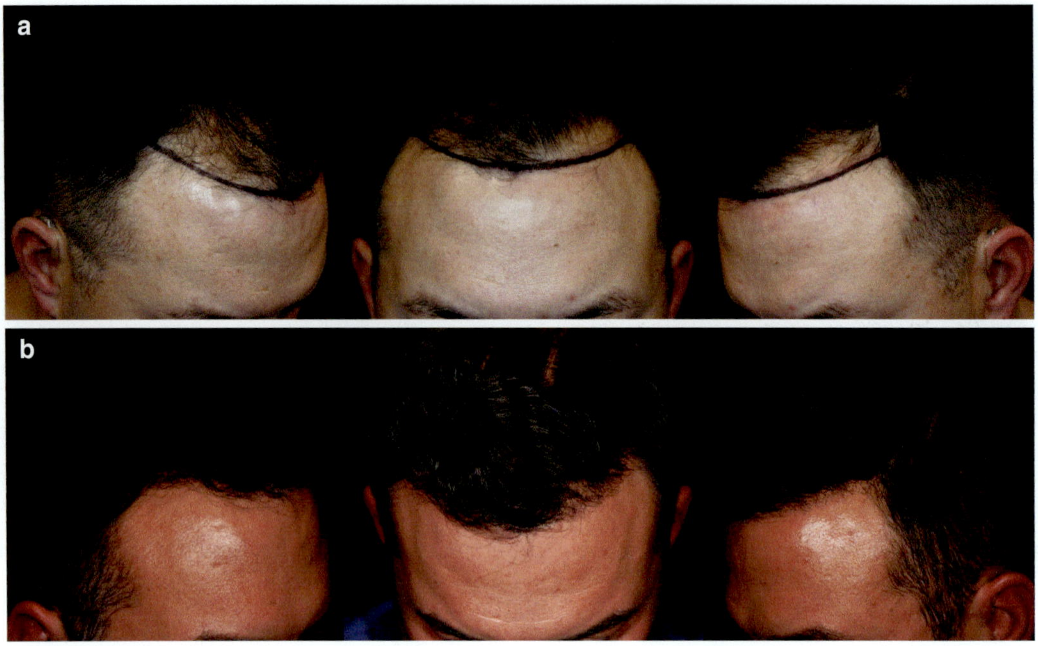

Fig. 38.32 Before and 1-year after image of single-session robotic FUE result with 2804 grafts

SAFE harvesting technique employed by robotic FUE is highly preservative of the donor zone, making repeat transplantation possible. Patients can potentially accumulate upwards of 10,000 grafts over multiples in the presence of adequate donor scalp size and follicular density (Figs. 38.33a, b, 38.34 and 38.35a, b).

Patients typically report procedural ease, limited social and physical downtime, minimal post-operative discomfort or sensory disturbances, and rapid recovery. Anagen-to-catagen phase conversion of grafted FUs occurs within the first 2 weeks following implantation, marked by an inflammatory process in which mild scalp erythema and shaft shedding are reported. The proceeding telogen phase persists for the next 3–4 months, followed by a latency period. Finally, emergence into a new anagen phase results in visible growth of the grafted hair [23]. Notable improvement is present 6 months post-transplant, and final results can be assessed at 12–15 months (Fig. 38.36). Procedural supplementation with PRP has been shown to reduce FU loss due to apoptosis during the telogen phase of graft recovery [23]. Post-transplant low-level light therapy (e.g., NeoLTS) may help accelerate donor and recipient site recovery by stimulating adenosine triphosphate production within follicular cells and by increasing tissue oxygenation [25] (Fig. 38.37).

a

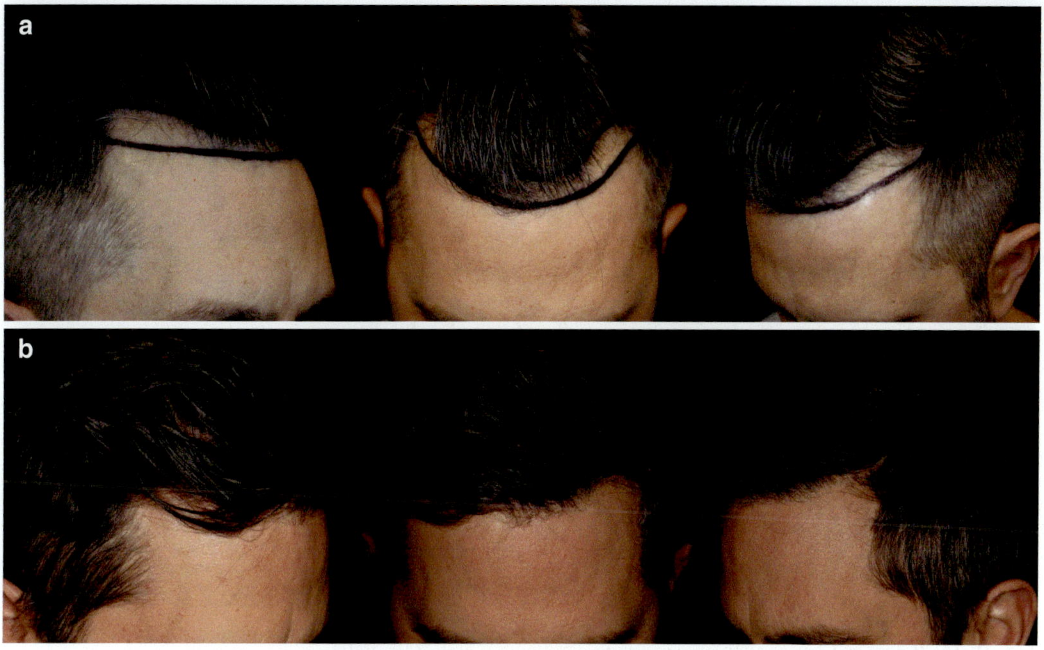

b

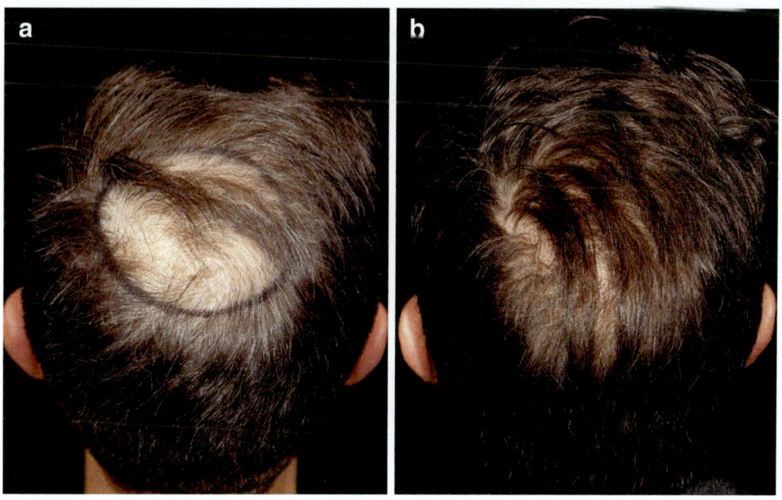

Fig. 38.33 (**a**) Before and 1-year after image of single-session robotic FUE result with 3010 grafts, anterior views. (**b**) Posterior view

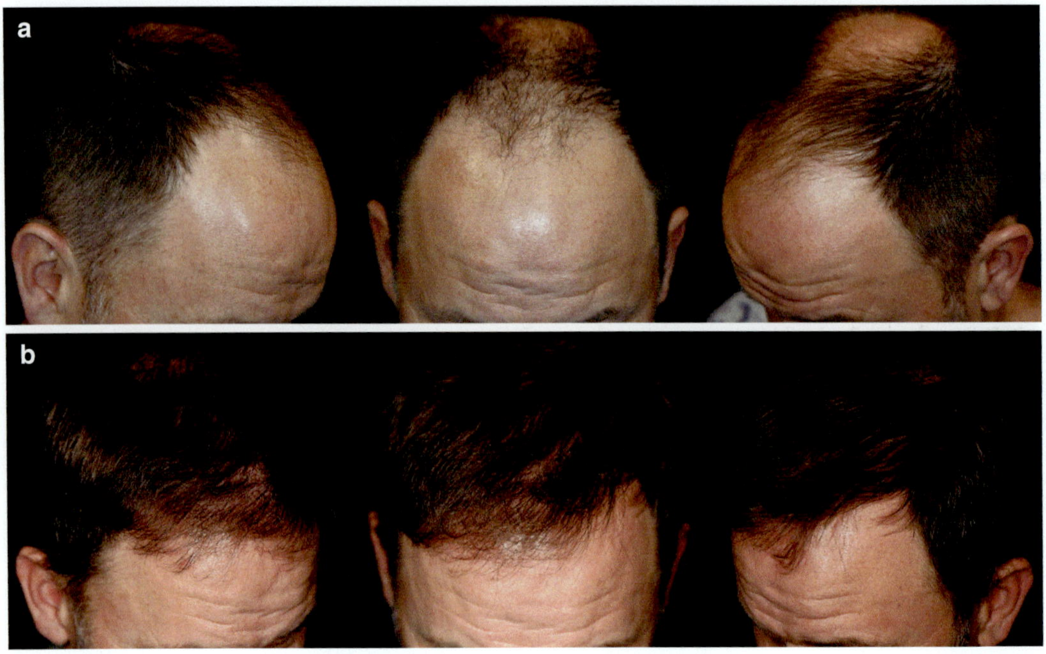

Fig. 38.34 Before and 1-year after single-session robotic FUE with 4005 grafts

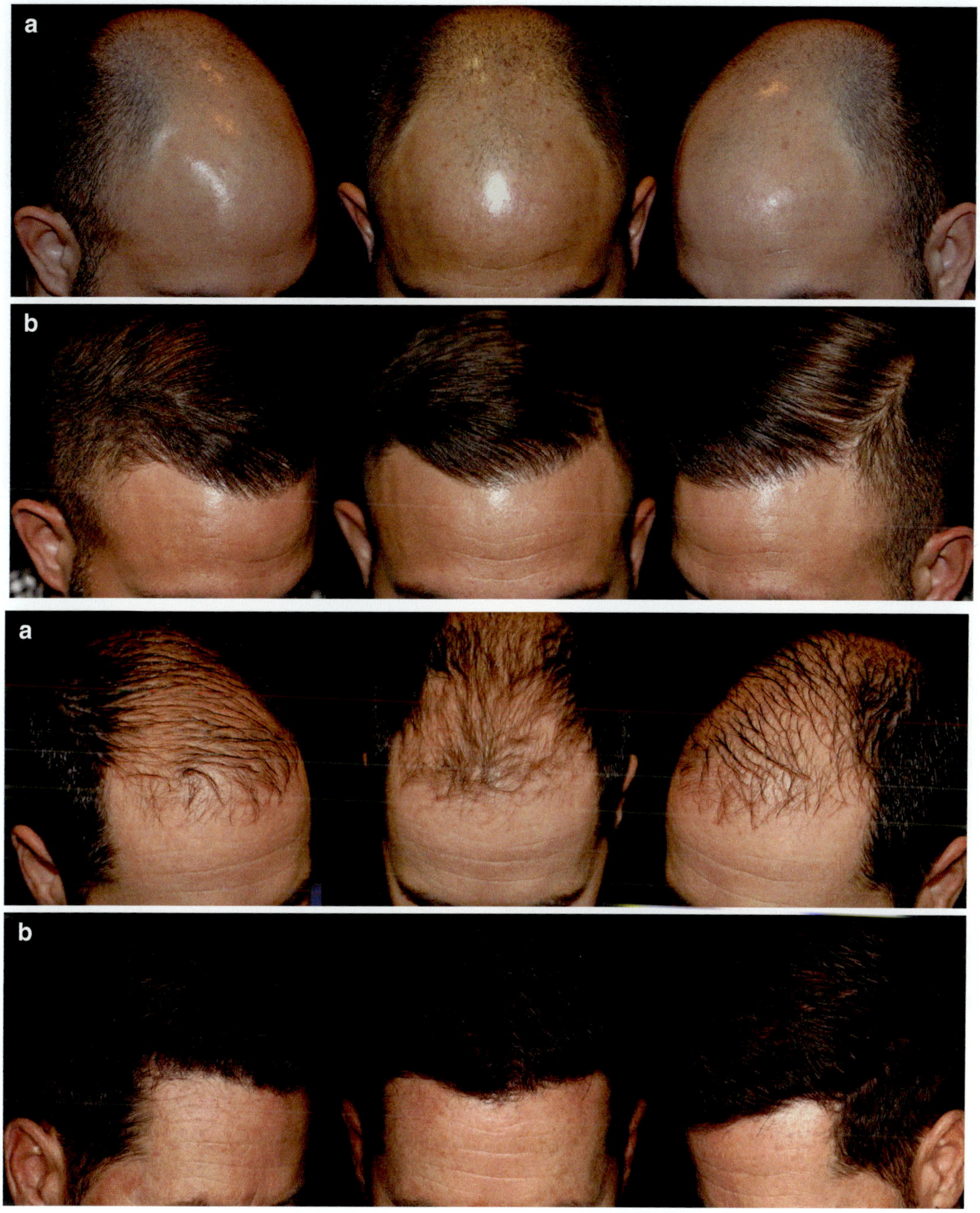

Fig. 38.35 (**a**) Before and after image of multi-session grafting, total 7489 grafts over three automated FUE sessions. Multiple grafting sessions may be required for patients with an advanced HN pattern to accomplish the desired degree of scalp restoration. Additionally, hybrid cases utilizing both robotic and automated FUE technologies may be required based on donor scalp size and natural follicular density. (**b**) Before and after image of multi-session grafting case, total 10,218 grafts over 5 sessions. Automated follicular unit density calculations by the AI and physician control over harvest spacing parameters significantly reduce the risk of over-extraction. However, patients with severe or significant scarring in the mid-occipital zones from repeated FUT or outdated punch grafting methods may better benefit from automated FUE technology alone. This is due to ease of use in the posterior parietal scalp to avoid further harvesting from the mid-occipital region

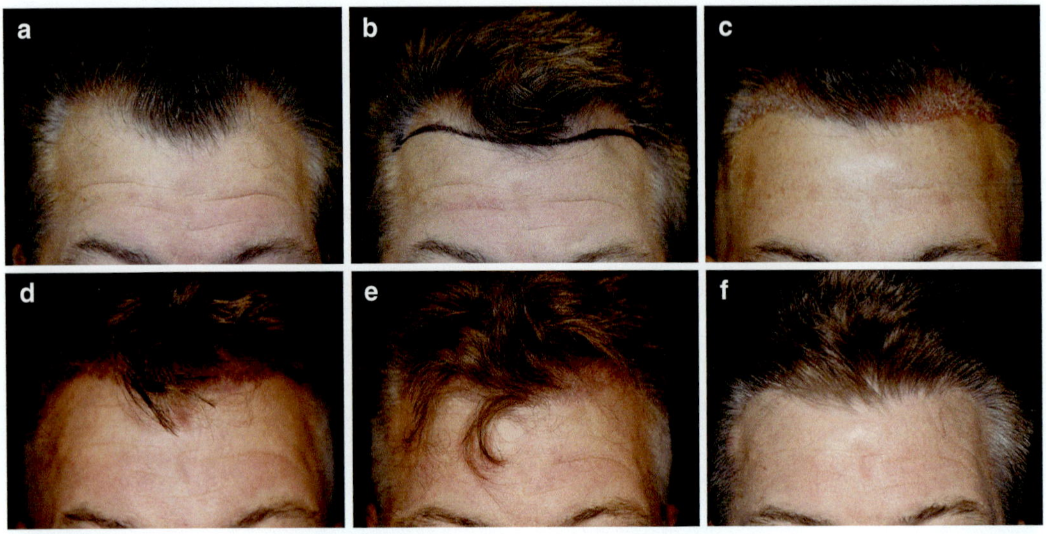

Fig. 38.36 Example of robotic FUE recipient area growth over the first year: (**a**) pre-op, (**b**) immediate pre-op, (**c**) immediate post-op, (**d**) post-op Day 4, (**e**) post-op Day 14, (**f**) post-op 1 year, 4 months

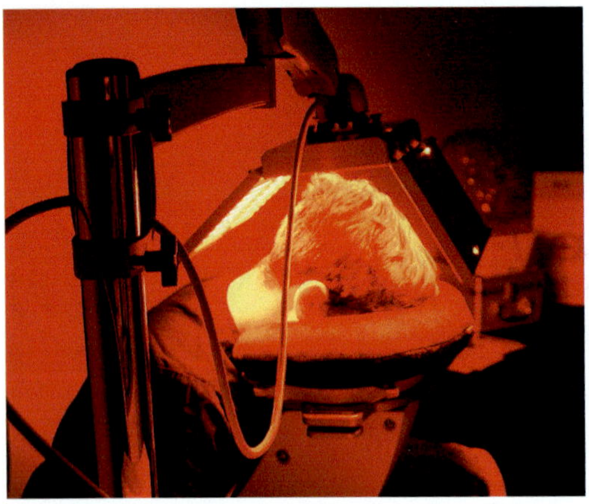

Fig. 38.37 Low-level light therapy

38.8 Risks and Potential Complications

Robotic FUE is indicated for the treatment of androgenetic alopecia (AGA) only. Patients suffering from other forms of hair loss, such as telogen effluvium, alopecia areata, and lichen planopilaris (scarring alopecia), are not suitable candidates for transplantation and should be referred to the appropriate resource for medicinal management. Patients with atypical presentation of hair loss may benefit from laboratory evaluation and scalp biopsy to confirm diagnosis of AGA before investing financially in aesthetic surgery. The authors recommend collecting at least two 4 mm punch biopsies, one from the region of concern and another from the potential donor scalp as the control (androgen-insensitive hairs). Global scalp photos and any unique historical factors should be included with the biopsy specimens to assist pathology in diagnosis.

Small donor site size, donor site skin laxity, poor donor hair quality, and preexisting donor site scarring may present additional challenges in robotic FUE harvesting. Proper preoperative counseling and patient expectation management can help these patients prepare for the possibility of harvesting challenges, limited graft quantity, inability to meet aesthetic goals, and the potential need for staging further surgery to prevent over-harvesting of the donor scalp or exposure of pre-existing donor scarring.

Patients who present with early HN pattern AGA should be counseled on the possibility of further hair loss progression and the potential need for further grafting in the future. Additionally, hair preservation options such as prescription finasteride, topical or oral minoxidil, low-level light therapy, autologous platelet-rich plasma therapy, and nutritional supplementation systems should be discussed as options to potentially slow the progression of AGA and partially reverse balding in regions of early miniaturization. Because of the androgen-insensitive nature of the donor hairs, they can generally be regarded as permanent in the treatment of AGA. Therefore, it is critical in surgical planning to consider the patient's potential for further hair loss, with planned feathering of FUs into adjacent regions of the scalp that are predicted to regress over time.

Complications following robotic FUE are rare and similar to other forms of FUE. Although minimally invasive, mild post-operative bleeding and scalp swelling is possible following robotic FUE. Transient post-operative scalp tenderness, paresthesia, pruritis, erythema, and dandruff are the most commonly reported adverse events and typically resolve spontaneously within 10–14 days. Mild post-transplant folliculitis (i.e., intermittent ingrown hairs) is more common in acne-prone patients, and more significant cases are typically managed with oral doxycycline, topical antibiotics (e.g., erythromycin), steroids when indicated (e.g., topical clobetasol), and ketoconazole or ciclopirox shampoos. Significant skin infection following robotic FUE is extremely rare and has never been encountered by the authors. Patients with psoriasis and seborrheic dermatitis history may require closer clinical observation post-operatively and treatment with topical steroids when indicated. Donor site alopecia areata (AA) following FUE has been observed. Smaller regions of AA are treatable using triamcinolone acetonide (Kenalog-10) diluted with lidocaine 1% with epinephrine 1:100,000, in a 1:1 ratio. The mixture can be injected intradermally in the affected region at a dose of 0.1 mL/cm^2 and repeated every 4–6 weeks as needed. Minimal therapeutic dosing and careful titration should be considered to avoid scalp atrophy. Most cases can be resolved in as little as 2–3 months without further complication. Larger or refractory areas may require systemic pulse-dosed corticosteroids, and dermatology referral is recommended for consideration of advanced therapies such as JAK inhibitors or biologics (Fig. 38.38).

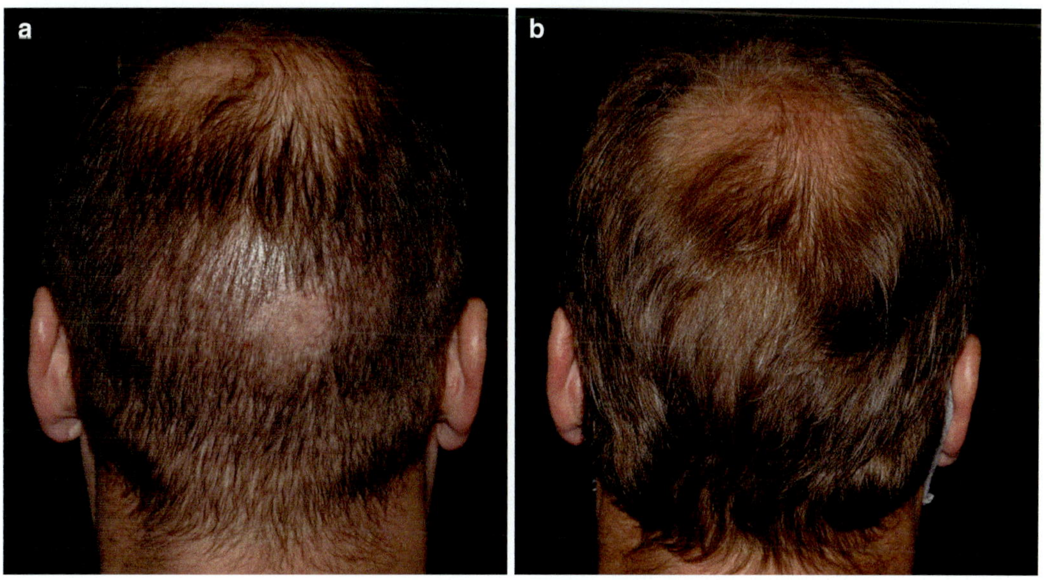

Fig. 38.38 Correction of post-transplant donor site alopecia using injectable triamcinolone acetonide (Kenalog-10) diluted with Lidocaine 1% with epinephrine, 1:100,000. (**a**) Before and (**b**) after injection treatments

38.9 Conclusions

Robotic FUE provides a superior alternative for plastic surgeons relative to outdated hair transplantation methods. The integration of robotic technology, high-definition visual systems, and artificial intelligence into a single platform has resulted in an efficient, accurate, and reproducible process capable of reducing procedural invasiveness, enhancing harvest precision, improving graft survival, minimizing graft size, refining recipient site creation, and protecting native follicles of the recipient regions. Robotic FUE can be supplemented with the injection of autologous platelet-rich plasma to improve scalp capillary density and reduce cellular apoptosis during the post-transplant telogen phase, thereby improving graft survival. With the ARTAS® iX system, plastic surgeons now have the option of complete robotic transplantation due to the capability of site creation with simultaneous graft insertion. Manual site creation and graft placement remains a viable option for patients who may be reluctant to clip the entire scalp. Complications following robotic FUE are rare, treatable, and similar to other forms of FUE. With little discomfort, minimal downtime, and natural results, robotic FUE offers an attractive option for male patients seeking a superior experience and clinical outcome. Undoubtedly, continued advancements in robotic technology and growth in artificial intelligence will produce unprecedented surgical sophistication in future robotic FUE models.

References

1. Calderone L. The Most Important Robots in Medicine, Robotics Tomorrow, 20 June 2017.
2. I. Relevant Research. ISHRS practice census results. Geneva: International Society of Hair Restoration Surgery; 2017.
3. International Society of Hair Restoration Surgery (ISHRS). 2025 ISHRS Practice Census Results. Chicago, IL: ISHRS; 2025. Available from: https://ishrs.org/2025-practice-census/.
4. Frentzen J. ARTAS hair studio and ARTAS robotic system signal a paradigm shift in hair restoration, The Aesthetic Guide, No. March/April, pp 1–2, March/April 2014.
5. Bishara M. The ARTAS robotic system is transforming the hair restoration industry- physicians are leading the way. San Jose: Restoration Robotics; 2013.
6. Harris J. Robot-assisted FUE may be the future of hair transplantation. Natl Hair J. 2011:1–6.
7. Harris J. Automated FUE. In: Hair transplant 360: follicular unit extraction (FUE). Jaypee Brother Medical Publishers; 2016. p. 309–27.
8. Harris J. New methodology and instrumentation for follicular unit extraction: lower follicle transection rates and expanded patient candidacy. Dermatol Surg. 2006;32(discussion 2):55–61.
9. Berman D. New computer assisted system may change the hair restoration field. Pract Detmatol. 2011;2011:32–5.
10. Avram M. Robotic follicular unit extraction in hair transplantation. Am Soc Dermatol Surg. 2014;40:1319–27.
11. Lewis W. Robotic surgery revolutionises the treatment of hair loss. Prime J. 2014:68–9.
12. Bernstein R, Wolfeld M. Robotic recipient site creation in hair transplantation. Hair Transplant Forum International; 2014. p. 95–7.
13. Bernstein R. Robotic follicular unit graft selection. Am Soc Dermatol Surg. 2016;42:710–4.
14. Ziering C. Does size matter in hair transplant cases. Aesthetic Insights; 2018. p. 5–7.
15. Bernstein R, Wolfeld M. Innovations in robotic hair restoration. Aesthetic Insights; 2018. p. 1–2.
16. Bishara M. Robotic hair restoration & male aesthetic market opportunities. Aesthetic Insights; 2018. p. 3–4.
17. Loussouarn G, El Rawadi C, Genain G. Diversity of hair growth profiles. Int J Dermatol. 2005;44 Suppl 1:6–9. https://doi.org/10.1111/j.1365-4632.2005.02800.x.
18. Fitzpatrick TB. The validity and practicality of sun-reactive skin types I through VI. Arch Dermatol. 1988;124(6):869–71. https://doi.org/10.1001/archderm.124.6.869.
19. Berman D. The ARTAS hair studio technology is a powerful tool integral to the patient consultation experience. Restoration Robotics; 2015.
20. Bernstein R, William RR. Pre-making recipient sites to increase graft survival in manual and robotic FUE procedures. Hair Transplant Forum International; 2012. p. 128–30.
21. Cervantes J, Jimenez J. Effectiveness of platelet-rich plasma for androgenetic alopecia: a review of the literature. Skin Appendage Disord. 2017; https://doi.org/10.1159/000477671.
22. Gentile P, Garcovich S, Scioli MG, Bielli A, Orlandi A, Cervelli V. Mechanical and controlled PRP injections in patients affected by androgenetic alopecia. J Vis Exp. 2018;131:e56406.
23. Uebel CO, Braga da Silva J, Cantarell D, Martins P. The role of platelet plasma growth factors in male pattern baldness surgery. Plast Reconstr Surg. 2006:1458–6.
24. Kachhawa D, Vats G, Sonare D, Rao P, Khuraiya S, Kataiya R. A Split head study of efficacy of placebo versus platelet-rich plasma injections in the treatment of Androgenic alopecia. J Cutan Aesthet Surg. 2017; https://doi.org/10.4103/JCAS.JCAS_50_16, Wolters Kluwer Medknow Publications
25. Pillai JK, Mysore V. Role of low-level light therapy (LLLT) in androgenic alopecia. J Cutan Aesthet Surg. 2021;14:385–91.

Automated Follicular Unit Extraction

39

Alan H. Chen, Brian V. Heil, and Matthew O'Brien

39.1 Introduction

Throughout history, hair has been associated with youth, beauty, and vitality. The account of Samson in the Hebrew bible, an individual who lost his physical strength after his hair was cut, supports the idea that hair has been an item of intense obsession in society for many years. Hairstyles can communicate an enormous amount of information. They portray religious practices, beliefs, and help construct identities. A particularly egregious example of the social implications of hair can be illustrated by the systemic humiliation and exploitation of Jewish people by Nazi Germany. In concentration camps, Jews were stripped of their hair to control, dehumanize, and identify prisoners. Hair can also be associated with success in life, and it is believed that an individual with a full head of hair is more electable for political roles in western society. Observations largely support this idea, as office positions are more commonly occupied by persons with full heads of hair [1].

Androgenetic alopecia (AGA) is an extremely common form of hair loss that may threaten identity and well-being. Approximately 50% of men over the age of 50 have some degree of thinning [2]. Characteristically, men lose hair in the temporal peaks followed by the crown. The extent of hair loss is popularly described by the Hamilton-Norwood staging system [3]. Patients who are afflicted by androgenetic alopecia can experience anxiety, depression, and reduced self-esteem [4, 5]. Unfortunately, males who have hair loss often suffer without emotional support, due to the observation that individuals without hair loss are quick to dismiss the negative impact of alopecia [6]. Importantly, for men afflicted by AGA, several measures exist for treatment. Medical therapies, including minoxidil and finasteride, are effective for many patients (Fig. 39.1) in hair preservation and slowing AGA [7, 8]; however, surgical therapies such as follicular unit transplantation (FUT) and manual and automated follicular unit extraction (FUE) are the best options for permanent hair restoration for AGA in most patients (Figs. 39.2 and 39.3).

A. H. Chen (✉)
Division of Plastic Surgery, University of Chicago Pritzker School of Medicine, Midwestern University Chicago College of Osteopathic Medicine, Chicago, IL, USA

Division of Plastic Surgery and Hand Surgery, Silver Cross Hospital, Chicago, IL, USA
e-mail: alanchenmd@uchicago.edu

B. V. Heil
Premier Plastic Surgery, Wexford, PA, USA

M. O'Brien
Division of Plastic Surgery, University of Chicago Pritzker School of Medicine, Midwestern University Chicago College of Osteopathic Medicine, Chicago, IL, USA

Division of General Surgery, SSM Health, Janesville, WI, USA

K. Jeffords et al. (eds.), *Aesthetic Surgery for Men*, https://doi.org/10.1007/978-3-032-03840-1_39

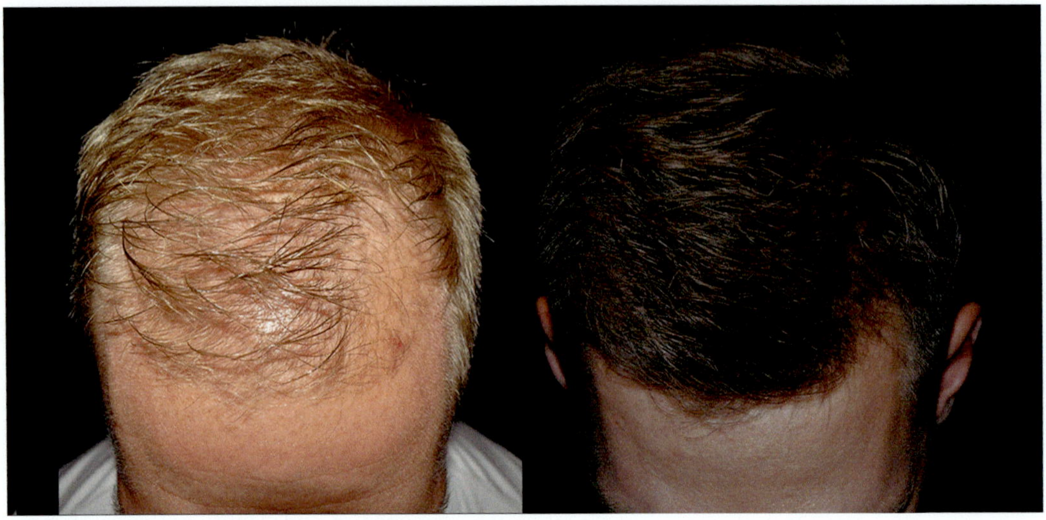

Fig. 39.1 Effective hair preservation in AGA using therapy with finasteride (1 mg po daily) and minoxidil (foam topical twice daily), start of treatment and after 5 years of treatment

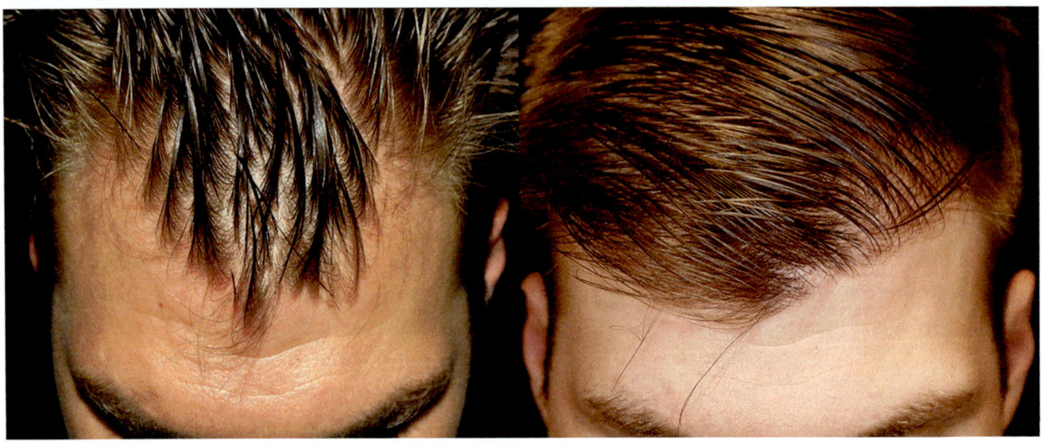

Fig. 39.2 Neograft automated FUE transplantation for AGA with 3623 grafts, before and 1 year post transplantation

In this chapter, the patient selection, technique, advantages, and outcomes are discussed for automated follicular unit extraction. Notably, for those experiencing hair loss, FUE remains an overwhelmingly successful option for cosmesis and offers the opportunity to regain self-esteem and individual identity. Data have demonstrated that men who have undergone hair transplantation are graded as younger, more attractive, and approachable [9].

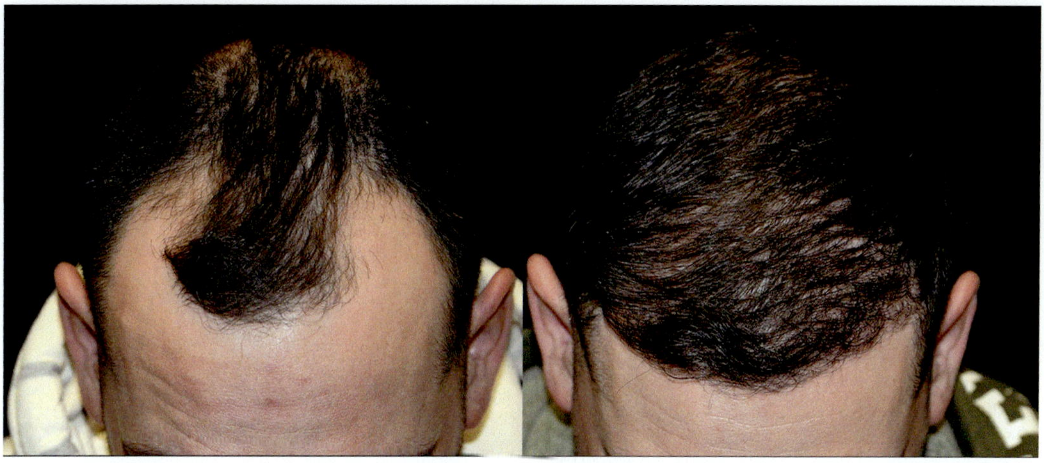

Fig. 39.3 Neograft automated FUE transplantation for advanced AGA, before and 1 year post 3000 grafts

39.2 Transplantation

Through analysis of the past two centuries of hair transplant research, one can gain significant insight into how FUE was developed. Hair transplant was initially documented in 1822 as a doctoral thesis written by J. Dieffenbach, who experimented with hair autografts on animal models [10]. Nearly a century later, a Japanese Dermatologist, Dr. Okuda, utilized grafts of 2-4 mm in size in an effort to fix cicatricial and pubic alopecia [11]. Shortly after, in 1943, another Japanese Dermatologist named Dr. Tamura updated Dr. Okuda's technique by utilizing smaller grafts. Dr. Tamura's grafts were typically 1–3 hairs in size. This technique is similar to the FUE procedure in use today, but due to WWII, his work was not fully recognized in Western Medicine until recently. The first Westerner to popularize hair transplant was Dr. Orentreich in the 1950s. He made popular the use of 4 mm punches [12]. He also coined the term, "donor dominance theory" which states that hair from the back of the head, when transplanted, will grow without hindrance in regions previously affected by androgenetic alopecia. The large 4 mm grafts remained in use throughout the 1960s and 1970s, but fell out of favor due to the unnatural, plug-like appearance, high transection rate, and poor graft survivability. In 1987, Dr. Bobby Limmer introduced the use of the microscope while preparing grafts for transplant [10]. Under magnification, a surgeon could better visualize the course of the follicle through the skin and avoid damage to the hair. With the aid of magnification to improve graft preparation, follicular unit transplantation became very popular. In 2002, Rassmen et al. developed FUE, in which individual grafts are removed from the donor area instead of a strip of tissue [13]. This is essentially a refinement of Dr. Okuda's technique, and remains extremely popular today.

39.3 Patient Selection

Patients who elect to undergo FUE should be in relatively good health, as is the case with any surgical procedure. All blood-thinning medications, including over-the-counter medications, such as aspirin and vitamin E, should be discontinued. If the patient is on prescription anticoagulants such as warfarin or clopidogrel, they should obtain clearance from the prescribing physician to discontinue the medication before proceeding. There is no universal protocol for perioperative antibiotics, though one office stated that they routinely utilize Omnicef 300 mg 1 h before the start of the procedure, as well as 6 h later [14]. It is also recommended that patients wash and shampoo their hair prior to the start of the procedure.

Table 39.1 Preoperative considerations for FUE

Surgeon factors
Proper surgeon experience and training
Physical stamina to endure many hours of tedious work
Capabilities and experience of transplant team
Incorporate patient desires into operative plan
Manage expectations, if necessary
Medical history and examination
Discontinue blood thinning medications such as vitamin E and ASA
Adequate donor density, preferably >40 FUs/cm^2
Patient selection factors
Preference for the option to wear a short hairstyle
Desire to avoid FUT permanent linear scarring
Willing to endure longer treatment case time
Preference for a less invasive procedure
Inadequate laxity of donor scalp for FUT strip harvest
Limited or exhausted occipital donor site grafts leaving only off-scalp sites (beard or body) as donor options

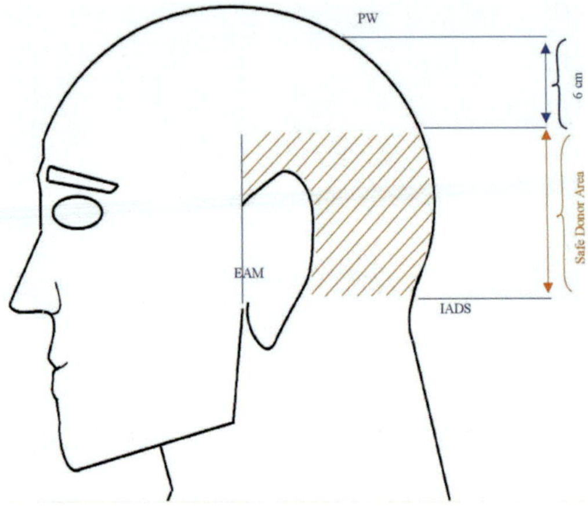

Fig. 39.4 The three boundaries of the safe donor area are adapted from Unger (1994) and Park (2014). A vertical line from the external acoustic meatus (EAM) signifies the anterior boundary, superior boundary is located 6 cm inferior to the parietal whorl (PW), and the inferior aspect of the donor site (IADS) is defined previously by Unger in 1994 as a lower limit density of 10 hairs/4 mm2 circle

Before discussing requirements for transplantation, it is important to define a few of the terms used in donor assessment. Follicular unit density refers to the number of follicular units located in a specific segment scalp. The number of hairs in each follicular unit may vary; 1, 2, or 3 hair FUs are common. Hair density refers to the amount of hair strands in the area of interest. If the term measured density is used, it refers to the average number of hairs per follicular unit.

Specific selection factors for follicular unit extraction are listed in Table 39.1. Patients must have an adequate donor site density and size for the procedure. Average donor hair density in American Caucasians is 200 hairs/cm^2 [15]. If density is <40FUs/cm^2, the patient is likely a poor candidate for the procedure. Patients presenting to address extensive alopecia can require upwards of 3000–4000 grafts, and a poor donor density and long case duration limit procedure success if manual FUE were to be used. For patients without adequate donor density, it may be beneficial to extract donor hair from another location on the body. However, this is less efficient and not commonly performed with manual FUE technique.

In some younger patients who have not finished losing hair, it can be difficult to estimate the progression of their alopecia. It is important to take grafts from a site on the occiput that will not be affected by AGA. In a study of Korean men who underwent transplantation, the authors attempted to define a specific donor area that was safe from progression of AGA. Their findings illustrated that the parietal whorl can be helpful in determining a safe donor site [16]. They suggested that a safe donor area involves three boundaries. Superiorly, the boundary was 6 cm inferior from the parietal whorl, anterior boundary was the external acoustic meatus, and the inferior boundary was less defined due to migration of the hair fringe with age. To define an inferior boundary, one can look to the safe donor site defined by Unger in 1994 [17], which delineates the inferior boundary as the location of a lower limit density of 10 hairs per 4 mm circle. These boundaries are summarized in Fig. 39.4.

For individuals who have incomplete but progressive alopecia, attention should be focused on restoration of the anterior hairline, temples, and forelock instead of the crown (Fig. 39.5). This is the suggested plan of action because continued hair loss threatens the long-term result of the transplant. If hairs were grafted tightly over the crown, most young patients would end up with a donut of alopecia surrounding an area of transplanted hairs. The crown is also significantly

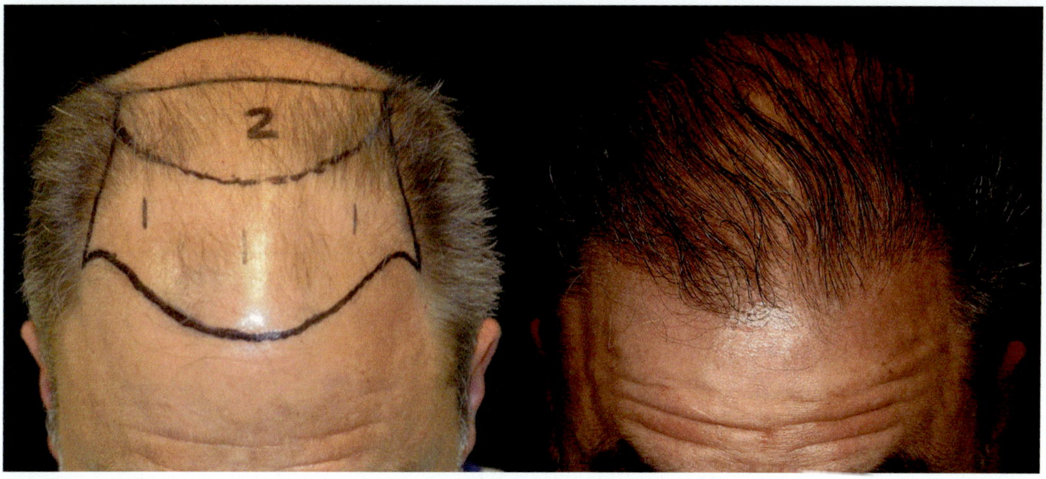

Fig. 39.5 Preoperative view with treatment plan focusing on frontal hairline, temples, and forelock, leaving crown treatment for later stage and view at 6 months post Neograft Automated FUE (4163 grafts)

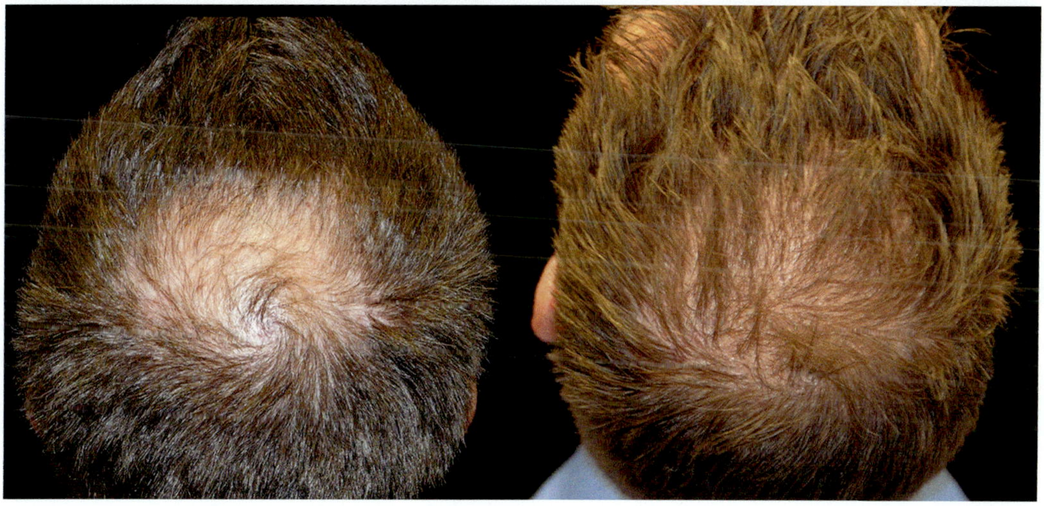

Fig. 39.6 Crown restoration with Neograft Automated FUE with 1529 grafts, before and 20 months post transplantation

more difficult to design with transplantation due to the complexity and orientation of hair in the whorl (Fig. 39.6). The anterior hairline is composed from fine hair oriented in a similar direction and plays a significant role in framing of the face. Leonardo DaVinci suggested that the hairline is the superior boundary in his "thumb rule" of human beauty. His rule postulates that the face is divided into equal thirds; the top extending from the anterior hairline to glabella, middle from glabella to tip of nose, and bottom from nose to the chin. It is referred to as the thumb rule because each section of the face should be equivalent in size; approximately the length of the thumb, extending from metacarpophalangeal (MP) joint to distal fingertip. These proportions are often used by artists to ensure proper human form, but the cosmetic surgeon should also be familiar with beauty standards to ensure an optimal cosmetic outcome. Studies have illustrated that the "thumb rule" is an objective method in the determination of proportions of the human face [18]. Alopecia threatens the balance of the face by enlarging the size of the superior third, from glabella to hairline. It should also be noted that a high forehead is a frequently recognized sign of aging [19]. Therefore, in individual situations without other significant deformities, it can be reasonably inferred that restoration of the anterior hairline has a larger impact on overall beauty as compared to the vertex.

Patients who choose manual FUE as their procedure for restoration should be willing to sit for multiple hours before the procedure is complete. If a large case is planned, patients should also be aware that it may take multiple sessions before optimal cosmesis is achieved. Due to the possibility of long procedures, physicians should provide an adequate atmosphere for patient relaxation. This can include movies, books, music, or an environment conducive to relaxation. The level of experience of the surgeon and transplant team plays a role in determining the length of the operation. Due to the learning curve associated with FUE, novice surgeons may be extremely slow at removal of FUE grafts, taking longer than 1 h to remove 100 grafts. Automation has reduced some of the learning curve, inefficiency, and graft waste of manual FUE, allowing a harvest rate of 500 or more grafts per hour with transection rates of 1–7% [20].

Although thin caliber of hair is not a contraindication to follicular unit extraction, expectations of patients who have thin hair should be managed during the consultation. Coarse hair types tend to have better visual scalp coverage following transplantation. Thin hair types may require additional grafts or transplant sessions to achieve the visual coverage desired.

Lastly, the patient who chooses FUE should be willing to cut their hair to a 1.2–1.4 mm length using a no-guard clipper. If a patient has excessively long hair and is opposed to shaving more broadly, the more focused donor area alone may be shaved, and the patient can wear the rest of their hair at length to cover the donor site post-operatively. Also two or three horizontal zones of donor hair can be shaved inferior to moderate length zones of hair left to conceal the harvest clipping, and the opposite zones can be harvested at a subsequent session to balance donor region density. Although unshaved FUE is possible, the majority of surgeons ask patients to shave the donor site so that the hair shaft can be visualized as it tracks through the skin for more accurate harvest technique.

39.4 Follicular Unit Extraction Technique

Local anesthesia is first administered over the entire donor area. Options for local anesthesia include Xylocaine 1% diluted with saline or 2% lidocaine with 1/100,000 epinephrine, among others. Following anesthesia, donor hair is extracted with micro-punches under 2.5–5× magnification. There are many tools available with a variety of sizes for extraction. In general, the smaller punches of 0.6–1.0 mm, which may include 1–4 hairs per graft, appear the most natural post-operatively. The size of the punch is largely determined from follicular unit density of the donor site [21]. Punches larger than necessary increase the risk of post-operative, "buckshot" appearing scars of the donor site. The patient may be placed prone or seated erect for the extraction phase of the operation, but the prone position provides the physician with the most stability and best angle of harvest approach.

Hand-held devices were the first instruments utilized for extraction in FUE. The original piece of equipment is the manual punch, which is a circular, hollow scalpel similar to the instrument used for a punch biopsy. The proper method for a right-handed individual involves a short punch into the lower dermis followed by a clockwise twisting motion to release the follicle. The amount of force required to release the follicle from the surrounding connective tissue will vary from patient to patient. There are multiple techniques advocated for in the literature, and two will be discussed here.

The first technique is known as the two-step procedure. First, a well-aligned, sharp punch is performed to release the follicle. This should be performed in one motion and must be well positioned to follow the hair shaft through the dermis.

If the punch is not well aligned, the result could be a transection injury. Forceps are then used to extract the hair follicle, being careful not to squeeze too firmly and damage the graft [13].

The second technique is known as the three-step technique, or the SAFE system [22]. The sharp punch is used to score the follicle, then the blunt instrument is used to carry out the dissection and release the follicle. The tightest segment to release before removal is the arrector pili [12]. It is believed that using a blunt instrument to carry the dissection through the dermis lowers the risk of transection. Lastly, jeweler's forceps are used to remove the follicle. Bernstein and Rassman [23] discovered that the three-step technique could increase hair yield from 74% to 93%. The downsides to the three-step technique are that the process is more time consuming, and it may result in an increased incidence of buried grafts. This is because the downward motion of the blunt instrument can jam follicular units into the dermis. Buried grafts are at risk of forming inflammatory cysts [22].

Since extraction is the most time-consuming step of the procedure, additional tools have been developed to automate the process. For physicians who are less experienced with FUE, this can significantly improve outcome and operative times [24]. There are several manufacturers that offer FDA-approved automated FUE devices, including NeoGraft, Smartgraft, and Auragraft. The term automated FUE applies to technology that combines several steps of the procedure to save time. For example, some technologies allow a motorized punch to be delivered from a hand-held device. The graft is then removed via a pneumatic tube, and they are stored in a chamber with saline to prevent desiccation. The pneumatic tube removal additionally eliminates the step of jeweler's forceps which reduces potential handling damage. The motorized hand-held devices boast an extraction rate of approximately 400 grafts per hour with a transection rate below 10% [24]. A study of 40 FUE cases comparing manual and powered FUE punches confirmed this assertion, finding a mean harvest time of 100 grafts per 8.9 ± 1.3 min with a transection rate of 5.5% [25]. With an increased speed of harvest, it is important for physicians to remember that graft extraction sites must be spaced out adequately to avoid noticeable thinning of the donor site. It is recommended to only remove 12–20% of grafts from available donor site during the first harvest to avoid detection of thinning by the human eye (Fig. 39.7). Postoperative discomfort is minimal and most commonly referred to by patients as

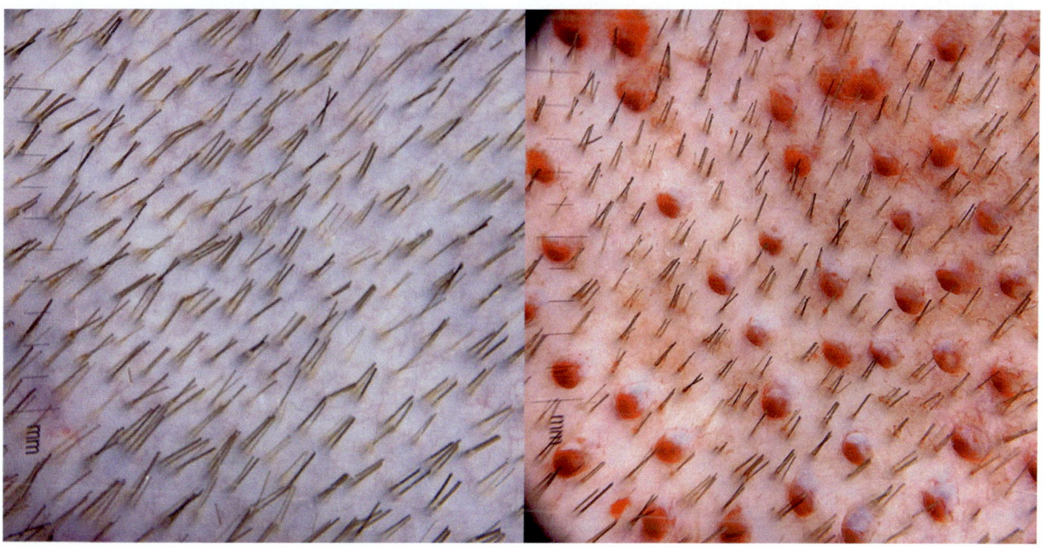

Fig. 39.7 Magnified view of donor follicles clipped to 1.2 mm ready for Automated FUE harvest and immediately after completion of harvest

"sensitive like a sunburn feeling" and requires little analgesia. The clipped donor site heals very quickly, and the remaining hair grows out to a socially acceptable length over 7–14 days, allowing the patient to return to social and professional settings in an acceptable time frame.

Robotic FUE is also a recent advancement in the field of FUE (The Artas), which has technology to identify follicular units with a 3-D imaging system and artificial intelligence software and then frees them from the donor scalp using a computer-controlled robotic tool with a dual sharp and dull coring tool. Since extraction does not require a handheld device, this removes significant physical strain from the surgeon and speeds operative times. A robotic FUE system often integrates imaging, touch-screen video control user interface display, a robotic arm, and artificial intelligence algorithms to produce a successful procedure. The robotic system is capable of more randomly spreading out follicular harvest and automatically adjusting to variances in donor density and scar tissue present, so that donor sites are less detectable when patients choose to wear their hair very short. The robotic system can also create recipient sites at 3000 sites per hour following a digital surgical plan designed by the surgeon and automatically avoid injury to existing follicles that it recognizes in the treatment zones. Graft insertion at the time of each site creation is also now possible with the most recent version of the robotic system.

After grafts are extracted, they are examined, counted, sorted into groups, and placed in cool unbuffered saline, Plasma-Lyte A, or lactated Ringer's solution (Fig. 39.8). This is done to prevent dehydration which is often the most important factor causing damage to grafts. It may be beneficial to group the grafts by color, texture, and caliber while they are stored, so the proper graft can be selected with ease during the implantation stage. It is estimated that grafts can be stored for 6–8 h in solution before there is a decrease in graft survival [25]. There have been numerous publications suggesting the use of additives to chilled saline or lactate Ringer's to improve graft survival. Antioxidants and various buffers can markedly reduce shedding of transplanted hair post-operatively [26]. A common solution used today is 1 mL of ATP added to 100 mL of hypothermosol, which may have some benefit in longer operations [24].

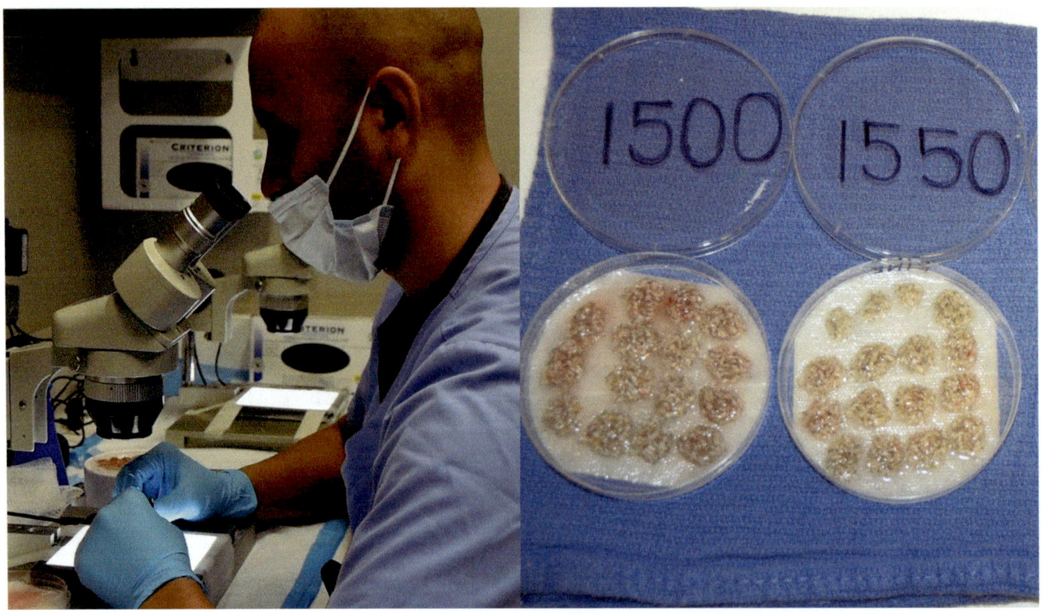

Fig. 39.8 Magnified graft inspection, sorting and counting, and close-up view of prepared grafts in saline ready for implantation

The recipient site can be prepared as the extraction stage is nearing an end. The first step in implantation is design of the anterior hairline, if this is being treated. While designing the anterior hairline, it is important to be familiar with the anatomic components. The hairline can be broadly divided into five segments. From medial to lateral, these are: frontal area (FA), frontotemporal recess (FTR), temporal peak area (TPA), infratemporal area (ITA), and the sideburn area (SA). The frontal area is often the most anterior portion of the hairline, and if it is deviated to the right or left, it should be brought midline. To make the face appear shorter, the FA can be brought to a lower point, and the FTR should be near as possible to the FA. To make the face appear longer, the FTR should be placed laterally away from the FA. According to a study performed on 200 Turkish individuals without alopecia, the face appears slimmer when the TPA is closer to the ITA; therefore, if the goal is to shrink the overall facial profile, the more lateral aspects of the hairline can also play a crucial role [27]. Cultural and ethnic background should also be taken into consideration when designing a hairline for patients, as preferences can differ by the country in which FUE is practiced.

Once the design has been marked, the recipient site can be infiltrated with lidocaine 2% with 1/100,000 epinephrine. This provides anesthesia as well as tumescence for the graft sites. As the anesthesia and edema dissipate, graft sites will shrink closer together for improved density. Goal density of the transplanted hairs is generally 25–40 FUs/cm^2 [25]. Some sites can be packed more densely with FUs if desired. Typically, sites for graft placement can be created with an 18- to 21-gauge needle or fine grafting blades. As a general rule, the size of the follicular unit determines which gauge needle will be employed for site creation. If a graft contains only one hair, then the recipient slit may be created by a 20- to 21-gauge needle, or a 0.7–0.9 mm microblade. If two to three grafts are contained in an FU, an 18-gauge needle or 1.0 mm mini-blade may be used. For frontal hairlines, slits should be made in a slightly irregular alignment, and single hair FUs should be placed most anteriorly. Once the initial hairline is created with single hairs, FUs containing more hairs should be placed behind to generate volume. The angle at which the hairs are placed into the scalp is extremely important for the final result, and if the patient still has hair within the

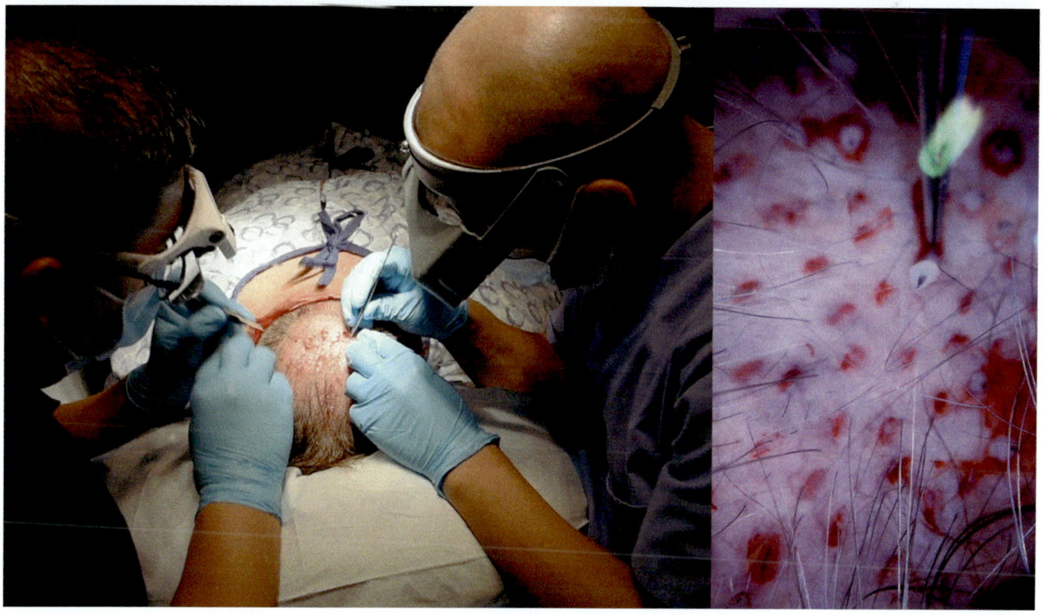

Fig. 39.9 Team of two technicians placing grafts and close-up of graft placement

recipient site, attention should be given to match the other hairs for a natural result.

For implantation, a single site may be made and then immediately filled with a follicular unit, the "stick and place method," or all sites can be made first followed by total implantation. The latter method is more efficient and allows multiple assistants to place grafts into the sites simultaneously. Traditionally, surgeons utilized jeweler's forceps to place the grafts. Substantial care is required to avoid manipulative damage to the grafts. The top of the FUs should sit slightly above the epidermis so that as the FU site heals and the anesthesia dissipates, the graft will sit flush with surrounding skin (Fig. 39.9). Teamwork significantly accelerates the process. Roles are assigned to assistants, reducing confusion on how the workflow proceeds (Fig. 39.10). Following implantation, the donor sites and grafted sites are thoroughly rinsed clean with saline spray and a light pressure dressing is applied to the donor site with topical antibiotic ointment, non-adherent gauze, padding gauze, and elastic wrap (Fig. 39.11). The dressing is removed in 36 h, and topical antibiotic is applied for 3 more days. Clipped hair in the donor region grows in over the next couple weeks adding to

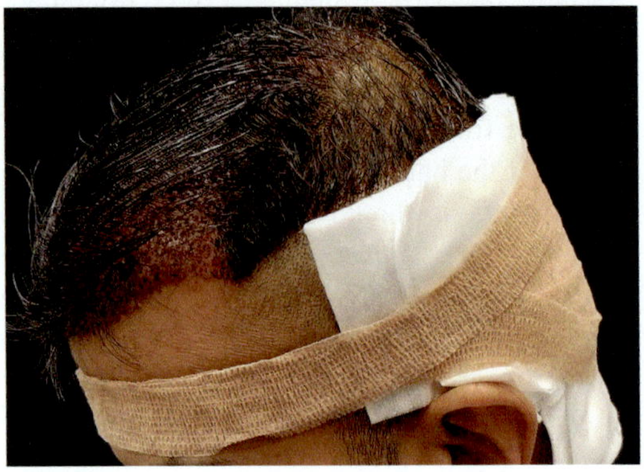

Fig. 39.11 Donor site dressing in place following automated FUE harvest and grafting

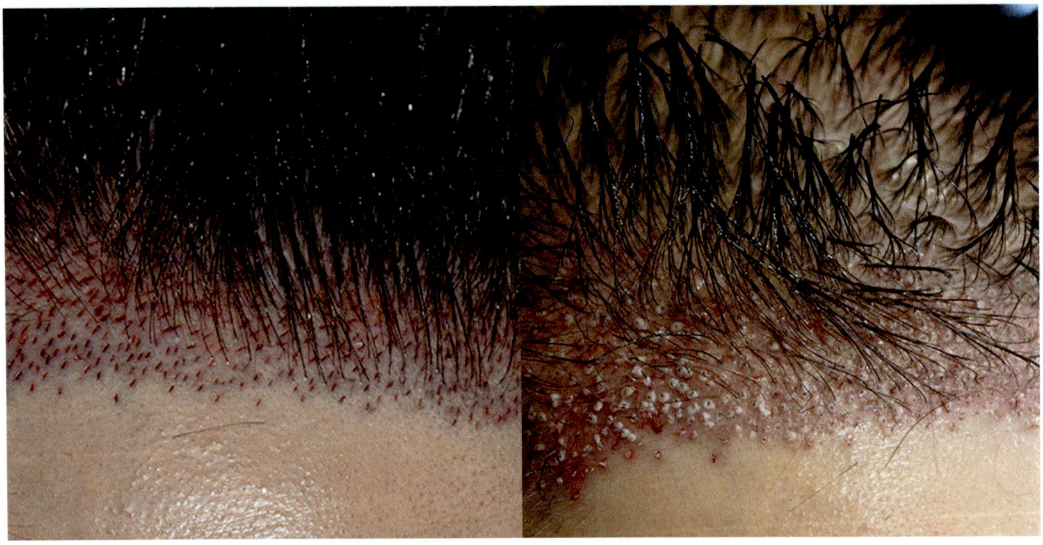

Fig. 39.10 Completed recipient sites and view of grafts in place

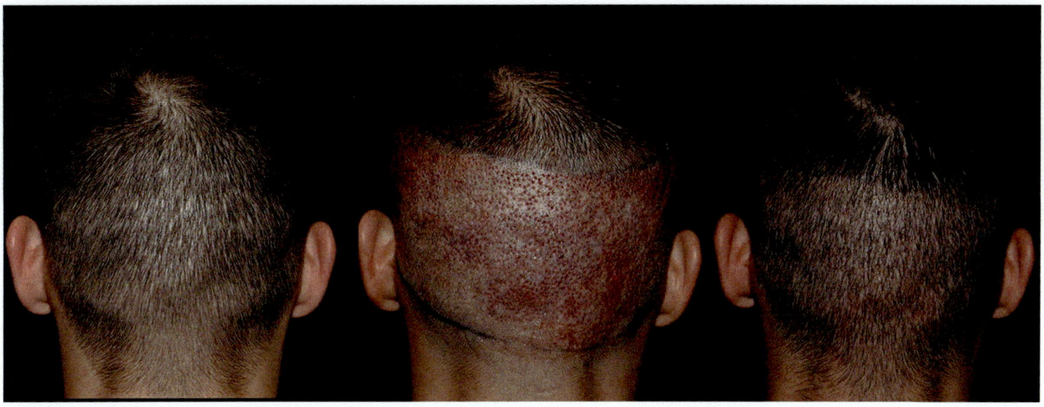

Fig. 39.12 Donor site views prior to, 3 days post, and 14 days post automated FUE harvest

the camouflage of the healing harvest sites in a timely fashion (Fig. 39.12).

In recent years, surgeons have introduced technology to automate the implanting process, similar to the extraction stage. There are several automated implanters on the market today. Many are equipped with a sharp tip so that graft sites can be created at the same moment that FUs are implanted. Since many physicians prefer the freedom to create their own graft sites, the sharp tips on the implanter may be sanded with 400–600 g to dull the implanter [20]. In this way, grafts can be placed into pre-made sites without additional damage to the skin or surrounding follicles.

39.5 Advantages to Automated Follicular Unit Extraction

Perhaps the most obvious advantages to automated FUE are that it allows the patient to restore hair loss without a scalpel incision with sutures, avoiding greater pain and numbness, and permanent linear scar visibility. For individuals who prefer a short hairstyle, the scar from FUT can be a significant burden. Some patients may experience emotional anxiety about the invasiveness of FUT, which minimally invasive FUE avoids. Tricophytic closure has been employed to reduce the scar of FUT [25] but poses a risk for burial of hair. FUT may also result in nerve injury and post-op hypo- or hyperesthesia [28]. Since automated FUE does not require a dissection of the posterior scalp, FUE patients routinely recover more quickly, with minimal discomfort. Therefore, employees and athletes are often able to return to full activity in a shorter time interval. It should also be noted that FUE harvest sites close over in 24–36 h and are well sealed in 4–5 days, whereas sutures in FUT would be placed for 7–14 days [24]. For individuals who experience a poor outcome from FUT due to the linear scar, automated FUE grafting of the scar can be performed to improve camouflage of the scar. Many patients who have undergone one or multiple strip harvestings remain undertreated for their hair loss but have exhausted the ability to harvest further grafts with FUT. These patients can routinely be treated further with automated FUE even if it requires a series of smaller sessions to harvest an adequate total of grafts needed for the restoration goals (Fig. 39.13). Automated FUE can also be used to effectively treat hair loss in regions of facial hair including the eyebrows, mustache, and beard and regions of surgical or scar alopecia (Figs. 39.14 and 39.15).

Donor site healing in patients following automated FUE harvest allows multiple subsequent procedures to be performed to serially treat ongoing hair loss needs and treat patients that present with very advanced loss in Norwood Class 5, 6,

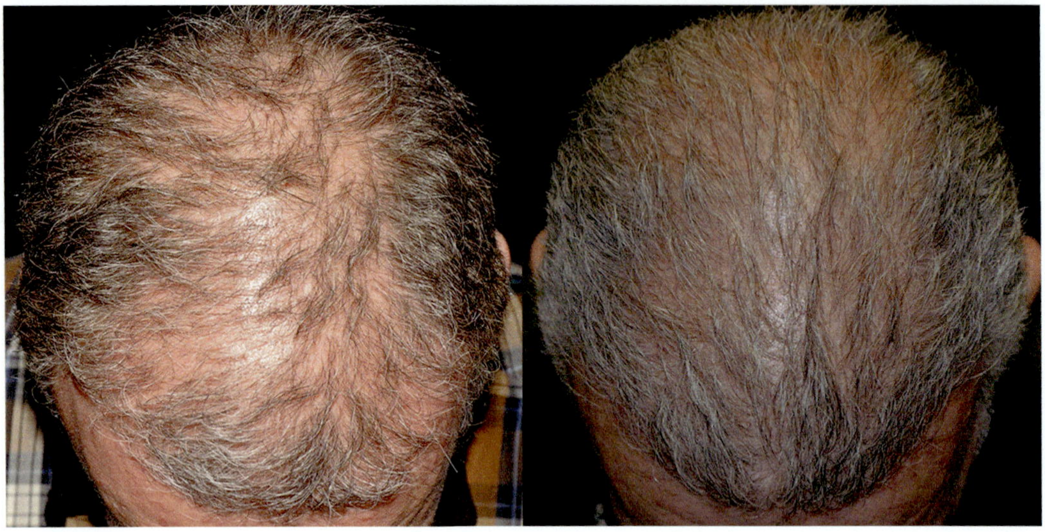

Fig. 39.13 Multistage restoration in patient status post six previous strip harvests (FUT), before and 1 year after three sessions of Neograft Automated FUE with 3631 grafts

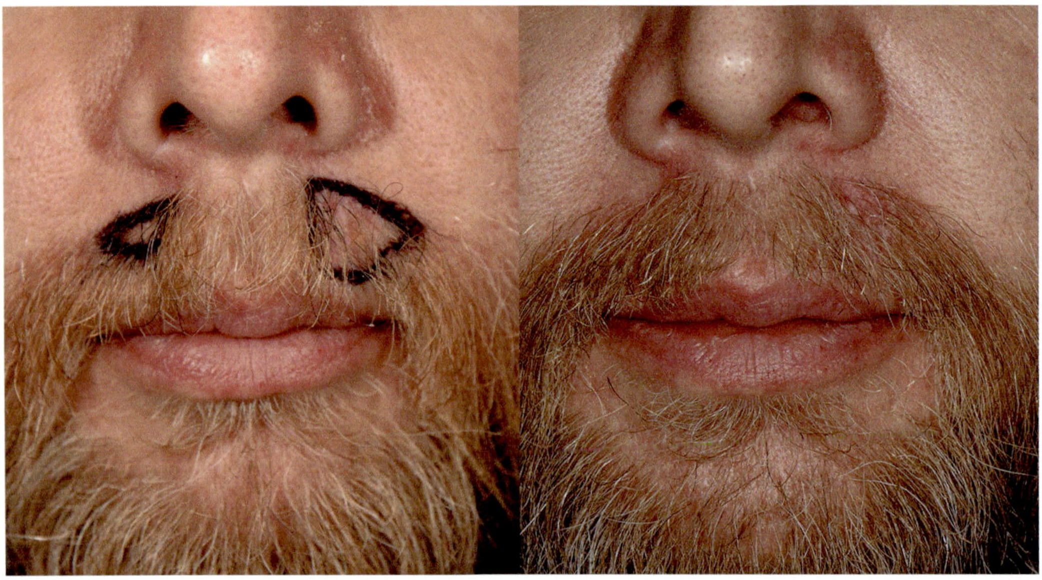

Fig. 39.14 Mustache reconstruction following scarring with previous CO2 laser treatments, before and 1 year after Neograft Automated FUE with 60 grafts

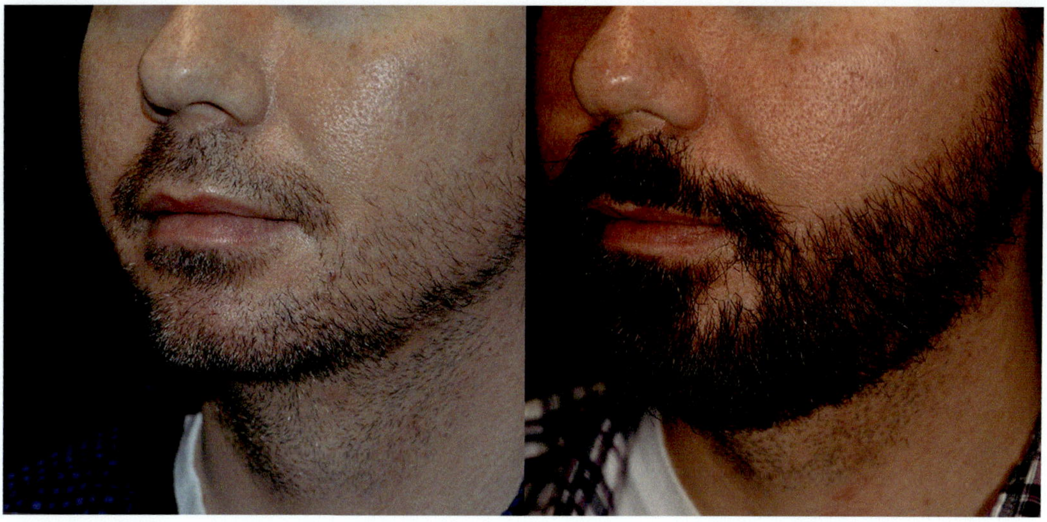

Fig. 39.15 Beard restoration with Neograft automated FUE with 2002 grafts, before and 18 months post transplantation

and 7. The multiple harvests are well tolerated by the donor region as long as a minimum hair density for remaining coverage is respected and maintained. This can allow the surgeon to achieve a very complete restoration for the patient over several sessions without increasing complications (Figs. 39.16, 39.17, 39.18, and 39.19).

Another advantage to follicular unit extraction is the ability to preferably select or "cherry-pick" grafts from the donor area. In automated FUE, the surgeon can pick and choose which grafts appear the healthiest, and most closely match the recipient hair characteristics, or select with a bias toward the graft caliber most desirable for the particular treatment zone. With the strip harvest method, surgeons are confined directly to the donor area. Furthermore, if the donor area is weak, or the site is not healthy enough for FUT, FUE offers the ability to choose grafts from the beard or body. This gives patients additional flexibility in terms of choosing their donor sites. For surgeons who choose to harvest body hair, additional planning should be done as it has been found that these hairs do not change color, curl, or shaft diameter post-transplantation. Thus, the site at which hairs are harvested from plays a significant role in the final outcome [29].

Additional advantages are conferred to physicians who choose to utilize automation for their follicular unit extraction. Automated FUE with motorized punches still requires significant dexterity and skill in harvest; however, it speeds operative times by turning harvest into a one-step procedure instead of the two- or three-step versions described previously. It also shortens the learning curve for novice surgeons by reducing the number of hand motions required for follicular unit collection. Automation may also be applied to the implantation stage to increase speed. It is important to remember that operative times under 6–8 h are advisable to maintain optimal health of extracted grafts. The speed of the harvest and implantation of manual FUE limits large sessions when several thousand follicular units are needed. Employing automation allows physicians to harvest and implant more quickly, which allows larger transplant sessions for the patient. Overall, this can translate into improved results for patients and a more productive and successful practice for surgeons. Aside from simply saving time and reducing graft manipulation and graft and donor site trauma, automation reduces the number of assistants required for FUE, which in turn reduces costs.

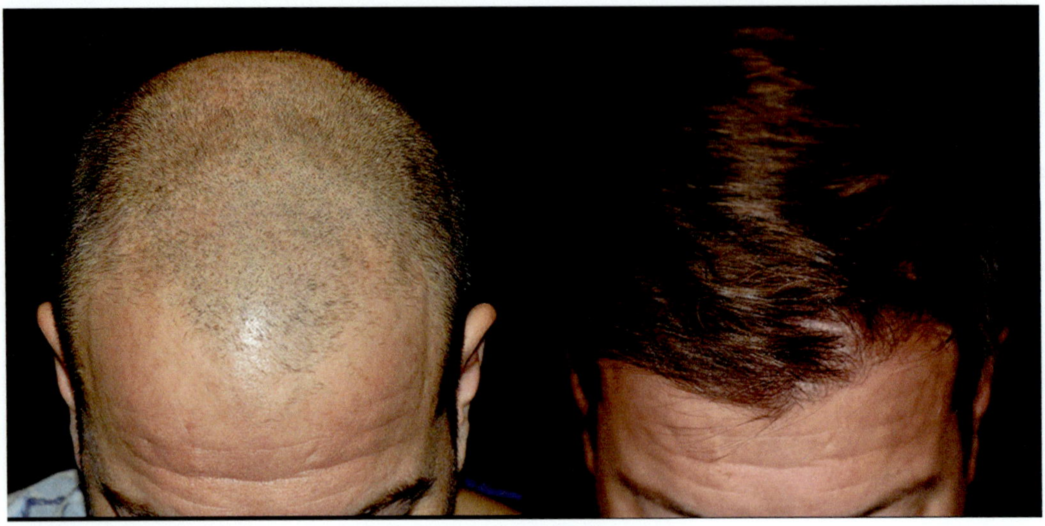

Fig. 39.16 Multistage restoration with three sessions of Neograft Automated FUE, frontal look-down view before and 2 years after third treatment (10,400 grafts total)

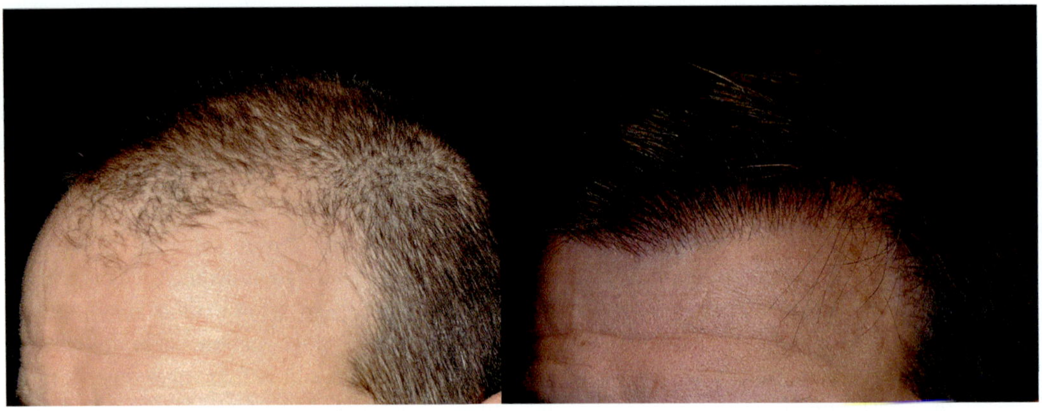

Fig. 39.17 Multistage restoration with three sessions of Neograft Automated FUE, oblique look-down view before and 2 years after third treatment (10,400 grafts total)

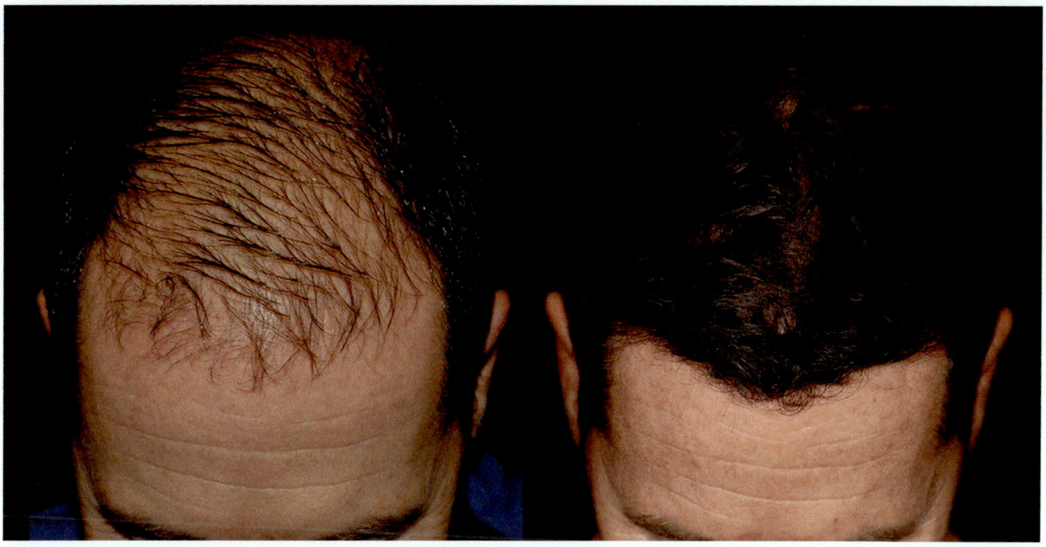

Fig. 39.18 Multistage restoration with four sessions of Neograft automated FUE, frontal look-down view before and 2 years after fourth treatment (7743 grafts total)

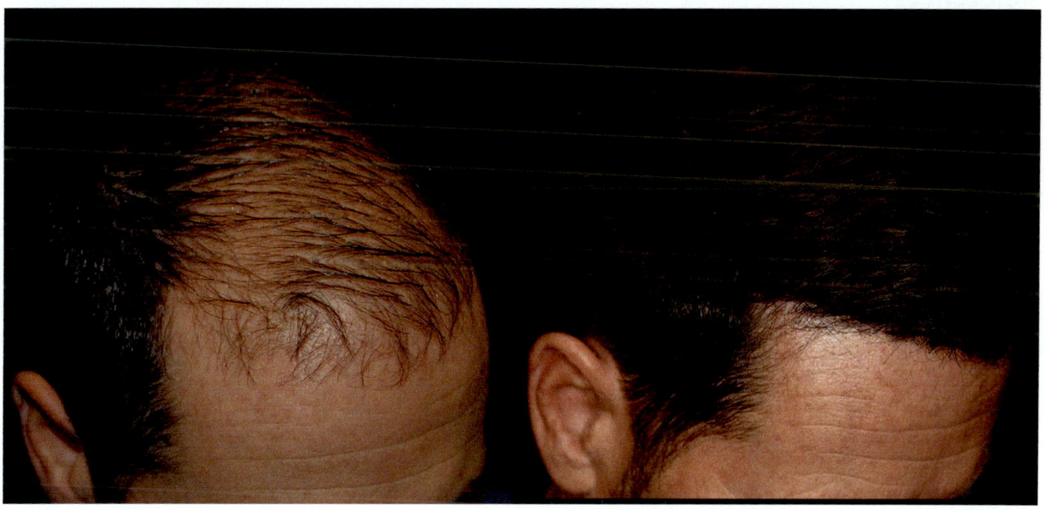

Fig. 39.19 Multistage restoration with four sessions of Neograft automated FUE, oblique look down view before and 2 years after fourth treatment (7743 grafts total)

39.6 Conclusions

In conclusion, automated FUE is an overwhelmingly successful operation which can be performed to correct cosmetic defects from alopecia. Advantages to the operation include absence of a linear surgical scar, versatility to correct small defects from previous trauma or dermatologic conditions, and the ability to choose grafts which most closely match the recipient characteristics. Additional advantages are seen in automated FUE including quicker harvest rates while maintaining a low rate of transection, allowing for procedures containing several thousand grafts. This translates to an optimal aesthetic outcome for the patient, while allowing for additional productivity in a busy practice setting.

References

1. Sigelman L, Dawson E, Nitz M, Whicker M. Hair loss and electability: the bald truth. J Nonverbal Behav. 1990;14:269–83.
2. Hamilton JB. Patterned loss of hair in man: types and incidence. Ann N Y Acad Sci. 1951;53:708–28.
3. Norwood OT. Male pattern baldness: classification and incidence. South Med J. 1975;68:1359–65.
4. Williamson D, Gonzalez M, Finlay AY. The effect of hair loss on quality of life. J Eur Acad Dermatol Venereol. 2001;15:137–9.
5. Wells P, Willmoth T, Russel R. Does fortune favour the bald? Psychological correlates of hair loss in males. Br J Psychol. 1995;86:337–44.
6. Passchier J. Quality of life issues in male pattern hair loss. Dermatology. 1998;197:217–8.
7. Kaufman KD, Olsen EA, Whiting D, Savin R, DeVillez R, Bergfeld W, Price VH, Van Neste D, Roberts JL, Hordinsky M, Shapiro J, Binkowitz B, Gormley GJ. Finasteride in the treatment of men with androgenetic alopecia. Finasteride male pattern hair loss study group. J Am Acad Dermatol. 1998;39:578–89.
8. Kreindler TG. Topical minoxidil in early androgenetic alopecia. J Am Acad Dermatol. 1987;16:718–24.
9. Bater K, Ishii M, Joseph A. Perception of hair transplant for androgenetic alopecia. JAMA Facial Plast Surg. 2016;18:413–8.
10. Pak JP, Gazoni P, Zeballos A, Rassman W. The history of hair transplantation. Am J Cosmet Surg. 2008;25(4):231–6.
11. Okuda S. Clinical and experimental studies on hair transplanting of living hair. Jpn J Dermatol Urol. 1939;46:537–87.
12. Dua K, Dua A. Follicular unit extraction hair transplant. J Cutan Aesthet Surg. 2010;3(2):76–81.
13. Rassman WR, Bernstein RM, McClellan R, Jones R, Worton E, Uttendaele H. Follicular unit extraction: minimally invasive surgery for hair transplantation. Dermatologic Surg. 2002;28(8):720–7.
14. Unger W, Unger R. Surgical treatment of hair loss. In: Blume-Peytavi U, Whiting DA, Trueb RA, editors. Hair growth and disorders. Berlin/Heidelberg: Springer-Verlag; 2008. p. 447–65.
15. Otberg N. Ethnic variation in hair. In: Baran R, Maibach H, editors. Textbook of cosmetic dermatology. CRC Press; 2010. p. 390–7.
16. Park JH, Na YC, Moh JS, Lee SY, You SH. Predicting the permanent safe donor area for hair transplantation in Koreans with male pattern baldness according to the position of the parietal whorl. Arch Plast Surg. 2014;41(3):277–84.
17. Unger W, Solish N, Giguere D, Bertucci V, Coleman W, Loukas M, Unger R. Delineating the "safe" donor area for hair transplanting. Am J Cosmet Surg. 1994;11(4):239–43.
18. Oguz O. The proportion of the face in younger adults using the thumb rule of Leonardo da Vinci. Surg Radiol Anat. 1996;18:111–4.
19. Vogel J. The aesthetics of hair restoration. Aesthet Surg J. 2004;24(6):561–4.
20. Rose PT. Hair restoration surgery: challenges and solutions. Clin Cosmet Investig Dermatol. 2015;8:361–70.
21. Bicknell L, Kash N, Kavaouspour C, Rashid RM. Follicular unit extraction hair transplant harvest: a review of current recommendations and future considerations. Dermatol Online J. 2014;20(3):doj_21754.
22. Harris JA. The SAFE system: new instrumentation and methodology to improve follicular unit extraction. Hair Transplant Forum Int. 2004;14:157–64.
23. Bernstein R, Rassman W. New instrumentation for three step follicular unit extraction. Hair Transplant Forum Int. 2006;16:236–9.
24. Rose P, Nusbaum B. Robotic hair restoration. Dermatol Clin. 2014;32(1):97–107.
25. Bunagan K, Banka N, Shapiro J. Hair transplantation update: procedural techniques, innovations, and applications. Dermatol Clin. 2013;31:141–53.
26. Krugluger W, Moser K, Moser C, Laciak K, Hugeneck J. Enhancement of in vitro hair shaft elongation in follicles stored in buffers that prevent follicle cell apoptosis. Dermatologic Surg. 2004;30:1–5.
27. Sirinturk S, Bagheri H, Govsa F, Pinar Y, Ozer MA. Study of frontal hairline patterns for natural design and restoration. Surg Radiol Anat. 2017;39:679–84.
28. Wesley CK, Unger RH, Rosenberg M, Unger MA, Unger WP. Factors influencing postoperative hyperesthesia in hair restoration surgery. Am J Cosmet Dermatol. 2011;10(4):301–6.
29. Poswal A. Use of body and beard donor hair in surgical treatment of androgenic alopecia. Indian J Plast Surg. 2013;46:117–20.

40 Beard and Eyebrow Restoration

Tim Neavin

40.1 Beard Transplantation

40.1.1 Background

The absence or a paucity of hair in the male beard distribution can be acquired through trauma or surgery, or it may be congenital. While techniques in the literature have been described to reconstruct hair-bearing regions with regional and free flaps, the use of hair follicle transplantation can often obviate the need for major surgery and its accompanied downtime while providing very natural-looking results [1–3].

As beards continue to dominate many of the covers of fashion and sport magazines, men more than ever are mimicking this trend by growing beards—or attempting to grow beards, ranging from the five o'clock shadow to the goatee to the lumberjack.

In fact, as one begins to fancy himself or herself with beard aesthetics, one may easily become overwhelmed with the plethora of patterns that exist and own their own unique names. It may be helpful to familiarize oneself with its nomenclature: jawline beard, chinstrap, neckbeard, circle beard and doorknocker, designer stubble, etc.

In many men, however, beard growth may be incomplete or sparse. Achieving particularly desired looks from facial hair can be difficult or impossible in certain men without hair transplantation from the scalp (or body) to the beard. Beard transplants, as it is commonly called, provide predictable and permanent solutions.

40.1.2 Technique

40.1.2.1 Preoperative Evaluation

Like any other cosmetic surgery procedure, clearly identifying desires and expectations of the patient is of prime importance. One must first consider if the desired beard can be created. Most men will show photos of beards that they wish to have. This is helpful, but it is important to ground patients with what is achievable with even the most advanced technology and skilled hands. Perfection, or completely matching an admired beard must never be the goal as it will yield failure in one hundred percent of cases. Limitations with hair transplantation exist, ranging from the density achievable to hair grow orientation. Goals to greatly improve existing beards or create beards that can look very natural should be the mark we set.

In addition, one must consider if enough donor site exists to fulfill the patient's goal; or, if one possesses enough donor sites for the procedure to be accomplished in one session.

In large transplants that may require over 3000 grafts, a second procedure may be indicated. And if this is the case, planning must carefully

T. Neavin (✉)
Private Practice, Plastic/Reconstructive Surgery, Beverly Hills, CA, USA

K. Jeffords et al. (eds.), *Aesthetic Surgery for Men*, https://doi.org/10.1007/978-3-032-03840-1_40

consider region and density for the first stage and subsequent stages to ensure natural intermediate growth between procedures. After all, the face cannot be as easily camouflaged as the head when one has a hair transplant. In large cases where the entire beard is to be considered, it may make most sense to begin with a narrow "strap" beard of proper hair density, then fill the remaining geography on a second session 1 year later.

For this reason as well, scarring potential for the face must be more carefully considered than the scalp. Importantly, patients with a history of forming large hypertrophic scars or keloids are likely poor candidates for beard transplantation, given difficulties in correcting or hiding visible scarring on the face if they happen to develop.

For men with curly hair, such as often is the case with men of African descent, beard transplant may still be considered. However, harvest can prove to be more difficult given the inherent curl sometimes existing within the follicle—the risk of transaction during extraction may be greater. And one must again consider scar visibility of donor and recipient sites. While the development of keloids is uncommon from the tools routinely used in harvesting and site placement, poor scarring (and the ability to conceal poor scarring) must be discussed in any person with dark skin. Test areas of 10–20 grafts can be considered safe first steps in this particular population.

Even in patients who have adequate donor for single-stage transplantation, it is always wise to explain to patients that, despite best efforts, secondary procedures may be necessary to correct any density discrepancies or to "touch up" areas for more robust beard growth.

Another consideration is donor scar. Linear scars resulting from scalp harvesting can be avoided with follicular unit extraction (FUE). While FUE is not innocent of leaving scars, the punches used generally range from 0.8 mm to 1.25 mm and often result in both less postoperative pain and potential healing complications, and a scar pattern that is not obvious with short hair. In men who enjoy sporting short hair in the back, FUE is the superior choice for harvesting (Fig. 40.1).

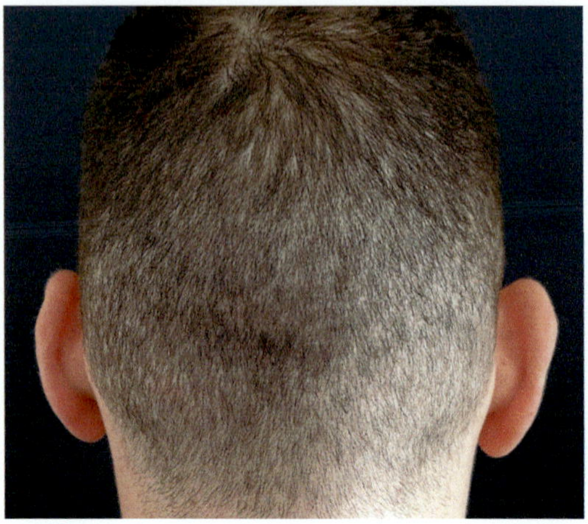

Fig. 40.1 Scalp one year after follicular unit extraction

40.1.2.2 Operative Considerations

The success of a beard transplantation will be dependent on a number of factors: proper markings, symmetry, graft survival and growth, donor site and recipient site scarring, hair growth orientation, proper follicle placement with respect to single or multiple unit follicles, and of course, meeting the expectations of the patient.

Even though the goal isn't to restore hair loss related to male pattern baldness, the donor site must be respected as it pertains to potential male pattern follicle death. Meaning, only hairs that are outside the potential zone of male pattern baldness should be considered for transplantation since the property of the follicle determines its fate regardless of where it lives within the body—not its dependence on the geographic location on the body. Thus, even in younger men that are currently displaying no evidence of hair loss, it is vitally important to be mindful that follicles on the posterior scalp approaching the vertex may succumb to DHT and become incapable of producing hair as one ages.

It is also wise to counsel patients that their resources of hair are not infinite. Younger men in particular who wish to have a beard and also a full head of hair their entire life may not be appropriate candidates for a beard (or hair transplant). Beard transplants can easily swallow up as many follicles as a hair transplant. That is, potential patients must weigh the value of having a full

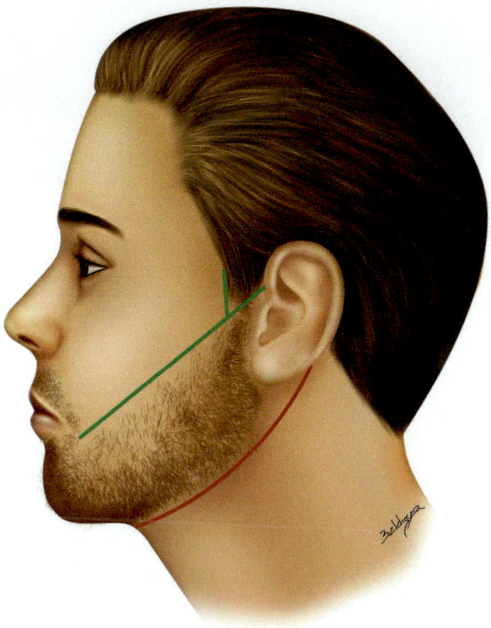

Fig. 40.2 Ideal modern grooming of the beard

beard versus a more robust head of hair if they are thinning or have a propensity to go bald, according to their current pattern and family history.

When it comes to making the sites for placement, there are a few things one should keep in mind to avoid unnatural beard appearances. Several different beard guide-shaping templates exist, but they are often unnecessary, particularly when patients already have beards and are just looking to add more fullness or camouflage a scar.

Most stylists recommend grooming the beard shaving hair above a line beginning from the most anterior point of the superior sideburn to the mustache as it connects to the corner of the mouth (Fig. 40.2).

Hair above this region is certainly commonly seen in men who are naturally endowed with full beards, but the density of hair in this region tapers off. And many styles eliminate this hair with razors while they groom.

40.1.2.3 The Procedure

There is little difference from a preparation and technical standpoint between hair transplants to the scalp and to the beard. One must take a good history and be aware of any medical conditions that may place a patient at risk for the procedure or impair healing. One must be off Accutane® (isotretinoin) for 6 months before surgery. Vitamin E and herbs as well as any medications, including aspirin, must be stopped at least 10 days prior to the procedure if approved by the patient's primary care doctor. Excessive bleeding is generally not life-threatening but poses as a real nuisance and slows down the procedure while making extraction and placement more difficult.

We generally prescribe an anxiolytic and narcotic for the patient to take 45 min prior to the start of the case, Diazepam 10 mg and Percocet® 5/325, respectively.

Both the harvest and donor site are marked. If follicular unit extraction is planned, the patient's back of the head is shaved with an electric razor. Care is taken to blend the haircut to the sides and crown to avoid a "surgical haircut." If a strip of scalp is to be harvested, then shaving of the back of the head becomes unnecessary.

Unlike a scalp hair transplant, the hair of the beard, regardless of extraction method, is trimmed with an electric razor.

If concerns for keloiding or poor scarring exist, it is advisable to do a test area in the most inconspicuous area possible of less than 20 grafts spread across the proposed transplant site. In some patients (particularly those with dark skin), caution must be exercised when considering grafting the region between lower lip and chin, given this area's propensity to develop small bumps which may be difficult to treat [4].

We prefer using automated follicular extraction with Neograft® (Venus Concept) with a 0.8–0.9 mm punch.

The donor site is marked with attention given to potential areas to avoid—namely, the crown, where male pattern hair loss can surface. This is an important consideration, particularly in younger men who may not have yet experienced male pattern hair loss to any discernible degree (Fig. 40.3).

Vibration is used when injecting local anesthesia to distract from pain. A number of vibration

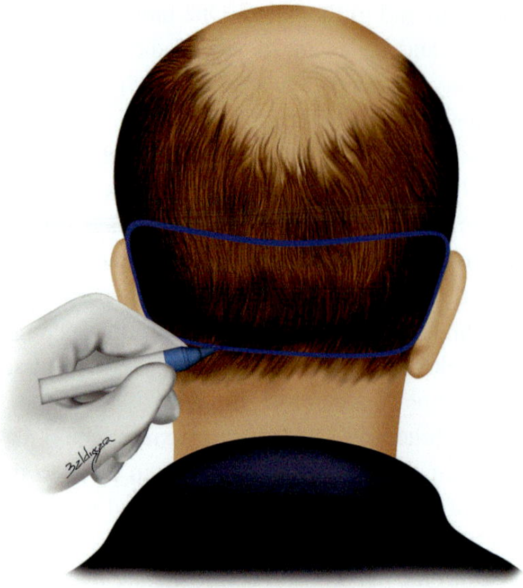

Fig. 40.3 The donor site must be considered to avoid potential hair loss with the transplanted grafts

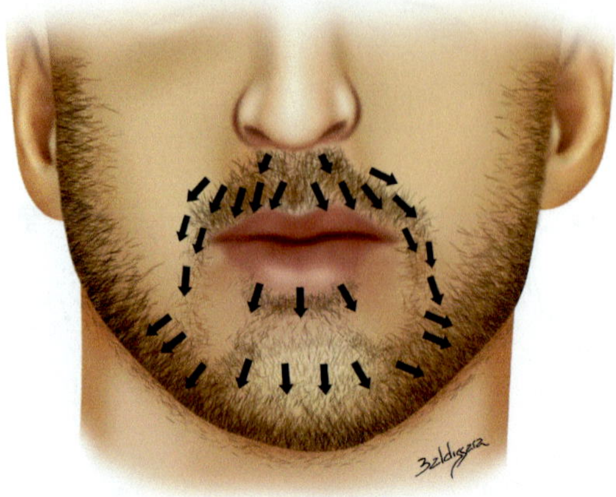

Fig. 40.4 Natural orientation of hair growth must be respected

devices are available that will suffice, including mini-massagers and even "erotic toys."

Three cc syringes with a 1-inch 30-gauge needle containing 0.5 of 8.4% sodium bicarbonate and 2.75 cc mixed with 1.25 cc 1% lidocaine with epinephrine and 1.25 cc of 25% Marcaine® (bupivacaine) are used to anesthetize the donor and recipient site.

The donor site is prepped with alcohol. Then, injections for the donor site begin at the most inferior portion of the posterior scalp and move cephalad, row by row. Approximately 4–5 cc syringes, or 15 cc of local anesthesia if placed properly, can adequately anesthetize the entire donor site for several hours.

Extraction is performed with the patient in the prone position. Extracted follicles are placed in petri dishes containing half normal saline and half HypoThermosol® (BioLife Solutions) and placed into a refrigerator at 34–36 degrees Celsius as the extraction progresses.

After complete extraction, the follicles are inspected under magnification (2–4× is generally adequate) and grouped into single unit follicles, double unit follicles, and more than double. The triple and quadruple unit follicles are split with a razor into single and double unit follicles on a back table while the face is injected. This is because triple unit follicles and quadruple unit follicles are generally not used for the beard.

It is a good idea to perform infraorbital nerve and mental nerve blocks, but these are usually insufficient to anesthetize the entire recipient site. Areas that remain sensitive should be injected with local anesthesia.

Site placement is created with a 19-gauge needle approximately 6 mm depth—shallow off the skin—mimicking the orientation of the native beard growth (if facial hair exists). If it doesn't, one must recognize that the angulation of site placement is rather acute off the skin at less than 15 degrees with parallel growth oriented mainly caudal in sideburns and main beard; some lateral growth exists within the mustache (Fig. 40.4).

Up to 20 hairs per square centimeter may be placed. The large majority of follicles should be single units.

40.1.2.4 Post-operative Care

Anticipate that the surgery will take up to 10 h in very large cases. The donor site is dressed with antimicrobial ointment and petroleum jelly-based impregnated gauze or Xeroform® covered by ABD pads. The head is wrapped with 2″ 3 M Coban®.

The recipient site is sprayed with normal saline.

Patients are instructed to remove the head wrap 24–36 h after surgery and to rinse their face with a mixture of baby shampoo and water in the

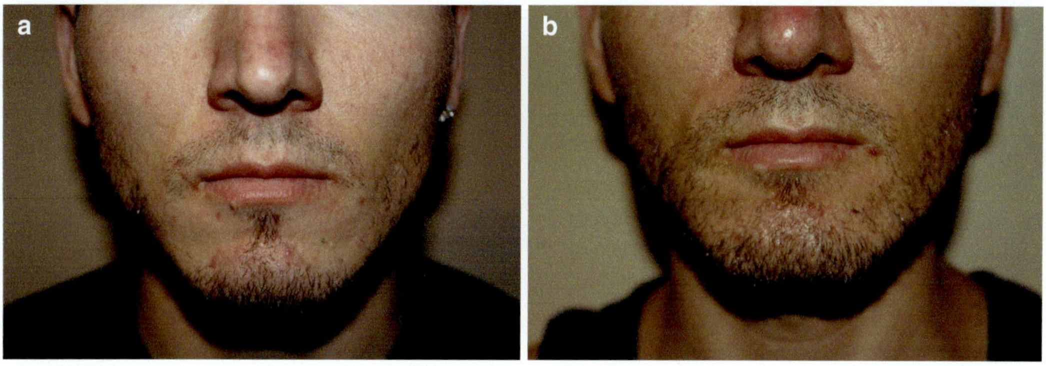

Fig. 40.5 Before (**a**) and after (**b**) 1600 follicles transplanted to the mustache and lower beard line to connect the goatee

tub. No direct shower stream should strike the face for at least 2 weeks after the procedure.

This author does not prescribe antibiotics. Patients are advised to take Percocet® or simply acetaminophen for pain. One can expect full growth of the new beard in approximately one year (Fig. 40.5).

40.1.3 Thoughts and Pearls

Unlike the scalp, the face is much more difficult to conceal scars or mistakes. Beard and mustache creation should not be performed without prior experience in hair transplantation.

Patients should know that scabs or redness on the face from the procedure may be evident for up to days and that growth may not be completed for up to a year or more.

The hair match between face and head is close, but not exact. Color variations must also be considered since the beard may gray more or less than the donor site. Similarly, the growth rate and growth potential are different.

One must approach darker-skinned patients with more caution, given greater propensity to form keloids or poor scarring.

40.2 Eyebrow Transplantation

40.2.1 Background

Many women have succumbed to trends in the 1990s and early 2000s of aggressive eyebrow plucking, leaving many hair-barren. The act of plucking can traumatize a follicle—so much that it dies, never to produce a hair again. For this reason, men should avoid plucking their "grays" as some tend to do. In fact, plucking should rarely be in the playbook for male brow grooming unless it is in the hands of a professional or if one understands the ideal eyebrow position and shape. Grooming eyebrows—often in addition to a good haircut—can transform even perfectly chiseled faces into ones that appear unkempt and tired-looking.

The eyebrow in males should not be ignored. Well-groomed and pleasantly shaped brows with proper density frame the eyes and heighten attraction in the periorbital area. Poorly groomed eyebrows or eyebrows with improper density and shape are, at best, distracting. Men's eyebrows tend to be thicker than women's, and this is particularly true as both sexes age. If a man is blessed with both ideal density and shape of the brows, then routine grooming with a mustache comb, trimming eyebrows with brow shaping scissors, tweezing out hairs outside ideal brow parameters, and even slicking thicker, longer brows with clear brow gel may do the trick. But for men who have distractingly thin brows, poor density of brows, large asymmetry between both brows, or simply a desire to thicken their brow and conform to the growing trend of "bushier," then an eyebrow transplantation may provide a useful tool.

40.2.2 Eyebrow Ideals in the Male

The ideal shape of eyebrows has been studied extensively in the literature. As it concerns men, this author subscribes mainly to the concepts described by Westmore with slight modifications as illustrated below [5, 6]. The ideal male eyebrow should begin at or slightly medial to an imaginary vertical line from the medial canthus (red line).

1. The eyebrow should end laterally at an oblique line drawn from the ala through the lateral canthus (blue line).
2. The eyebrow should sit at the supraorbital rim or up to 1 cm above it.
3. The medial and lateral ends of the brow should lie at the same imaginary horizontal line (yellow line).
4. The eyebrow should peak somewhere between the following two points: above a vertical line drawn from the lateral limbus (green line) to a point drawn from the ala through the lateral limbus (maroon line) (Fig. 40.6).

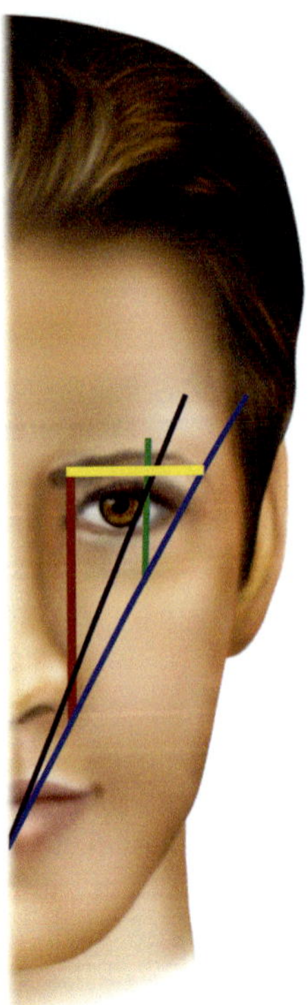

Fig. 40.6 Ideal shape and position of the male eyebrow

Of note, Westmore did not describe an ideal width of the male eyebrow. However, make-up artists do consider brow width in relation to the hairline and forehead and facial shape. For instance, longer faces in general benefit from thicker eyebrows. Conversely, wider faces often benefit from thinner eyebrows [3].

40.2.3 Ideal Brow Shape Pearls and Pitfalls

With the eyebrow starting more lateral to the vertical red line, the illusion of a wider (and often more attractive) face can be created. Male brows often tend to be more flat and less angled than women's. Gentle arches of angles greater than 140 degrees are often considered less feminine appearing.

Eyebrows that possess arches greater than 140 degrees may impart a surprised, feminine, or unintelligent appearance in the man.

Medial eyebrow that has descended lower than the orbital rim often imparts an angry appearance to the face.

40.2.4 Technique

40.2.4.1 Preoperative Evaluation and Considerations

The author generally asks men to show photos of men who possess what they consider the ideal eyebrow shape. However, all men should be counseled that perfect results should not be expected. Their final eyebrow will not be identical to any other man's shown in a photo. The idea of photos is to establish desired shape and thickness. Hair transplanted to the eyebrow will often not be the same exact density as native eyebrow hair. And its growth may not obey the precise direction the follicle was placed. Eyebrows may need to be trained, as described below.

One should also understand that the transplanted hair may grow at a different rate with the potential to grow much, much longer than native eyebrows. That is, the follicle transplanted will retain its inherent growth potential properties.

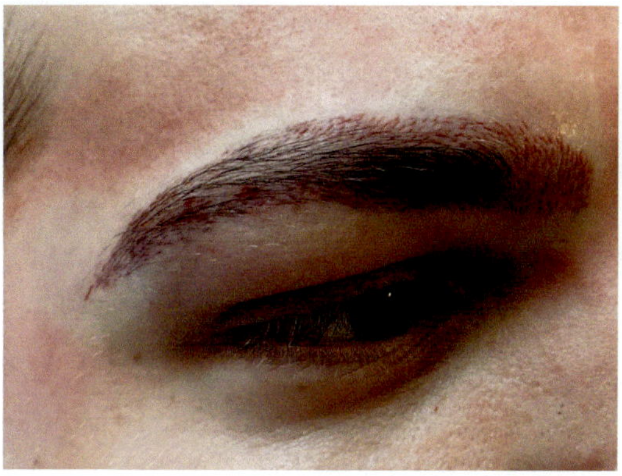

Fig. 40.7 Site placement for over 300 follicles for the brow. Note that sites are not placed within the hair-bearing region of the brow due to the great density; follicle damage can occur, resulting in shock loss

Thus, if one didn't groom before surgery, you can counsel him that his routine will have to change. Grooming will become an essential part of his life to maintain the new eyebrow properly.

In men with unnaturally thin brows or absent hair in scar, it is best to counsel patients that a secondary session may be required to obtain optimal density. It is wise to wait at least 1 year before performing a "touch up procedure," as we conveniently label this.

Some, but certainly not all, asymmetries can be improved with brow transplant. In cases where there is scar from either trauma or burn, the tissue should be assessed for mobility and thickness. And it must be stressed to the patient that there is no guarantee that the scar will accept one hundred percent of the grafts. To quickly assess the viability of a recipient site, the author sometimes pricks the tissue with a 25-gauge needle. If blood is visible in less than 5 s, it provides more confidence that the graft will do well once placed.

The donor site should be inspected for graft availability. Most male eyebrow transplantation cases use less than 800 grafts. In even most men who have had prior hair transplantation, donor site volume should not be an issue.

During the day of the procedure, the author often has his preferred make-up artist accompany the team to study the face of the patient in relation to their desired eyebrow shape and create or modify the plan as he and the patient see fit to amplify overall beauty. The artist, with input from the patient, draws the blueprints for the brow shape with his makeup pen. The markings are then replaced with a surgical marker.

40.2.4.2 The Procedure

The principles of extraction, including pre-procedure medication and the anesthetizing of tissue, mainly follow the same processes seen with beard transplantation described in this chapter. While the other prefers automated unit extraction, follicular unit transplant via the strip method will suffice.

One small difference one must consider when it comes to eyebrow transplant is the donor site. The hair that most closely resembles the eyebrow is generally found closer to the neck than to the vertex. However, grafts from the nape of the neck should be avoided since scars here may be too visible.

When it comes to site placement, local anesthesia using the same solution for harvesting (each 3 cc string will contain 0.5 cc 8.4% sodium bicarbonate, 1.25 cc 1% lidocaine and 1:100,000 with epinephrine, and 0.25% bupivacaine); a total of 3–6 cc of the solution is injected directly under the brow. The volume also serves to expand tissue to allow for greater density with placement.

All follicles harvested with the follicular unit extraction method are inspected under magnification. Any transected follicle or follicle with sparse tissue is discarded. Any three or four unit follicle is split with a razor blade under magnification into single or double unit follicles. No three or four unit follicles will be placed. And any double unit follicle will be placed in the medial fifth of the brow only.

Orientation must be considered in both direction of growth and angle off the skin. Site placement respecting these parameters is created with a 19- or 20-gauge needle, depending on hair thickness (Fig. 40.7).

The hair within the brow grows in a herring pattern, with very acute angles off the skin, which makes site placement more technically challenging than hair transplantation and is not advisable to perform with a novice technician team if technicians site place. Of importance, double unit follicles, if placed, should be placed in the medial aspect of the brow, which is highlighted yellow in (Fig. 40.8).

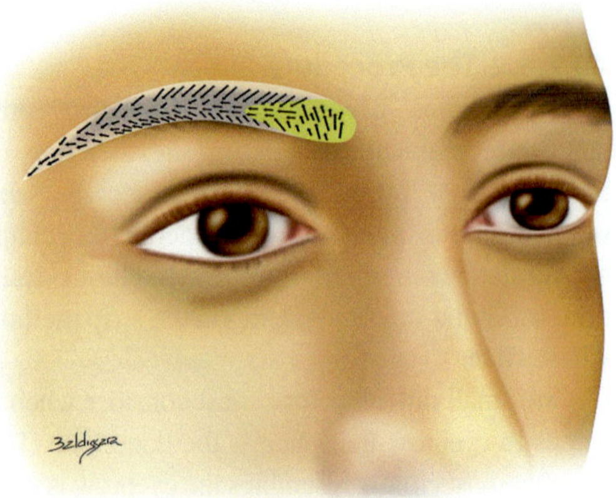

Fig. 40.8 Note the direction of hair growth, and hence, follicle site placement orientation. The yellow region represents where double unit follicles may be placed

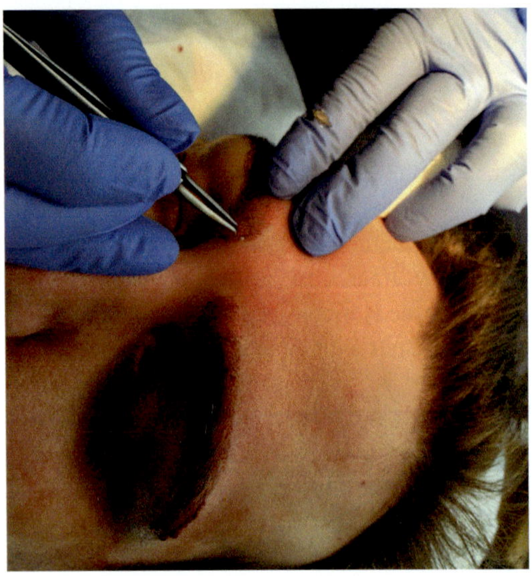

Fig. 40.9 Site placement for over 300 follicles for the brow. Note that sites are not placed within the hair-bearing region of the brow due to the great density; follicle damage can occur, resulting in shock loss

In brows that are already full of density and the goal is to either thicken or reshape, site placement should focus mainly on the area that is barren of hair or in areas with poor density. Damage to follicles can occur if too many sites are placed into dense, hair-bearing brow. Follicle injury can generate shock loss (or "shedding") of hairs. While this is usually temporary, permanent injury can occur.

With the tissue expanded from local anesthesia, up to 35 hairs per square centimeter density can be achieved (Fig. 40.9).

40.2.4.3 Postoperative Care

Most bilateral eyebrow transplant cases using automated follicular unit extraction take 4–6 h. After the procedure, the head is wrapped with Bacitracin®, Xeroform®, and 2″ or 4" Coban®. The patient is given a take-home kit that includes a plastic bowl, a small bottle of baby shampoo, and a spray bottle filled with normal saline.

Patients are to remove the head wrap and shower the following day, with care to not get direct stream of shower on the eyebrows. Half a tablespoon of baby shampoo can be mixed into the plastic bowl and brought into the shower to aid in raising the eyebrows.

Men must know that there will be scabs at the recipient site for up to 10 days. Periorbital edema should be expected to persist for no more than 72 h in general. Bruising is highly unlikely.

The author prescribes no antibiotics. While narcotics are prescribed, they are rarely required to combat post-procedural pain.

One should expect hair to grow and shed within the first month. Then, by 1 year to 18 months, all hair should be growing. As the new brows grow, they may not all grow in the planned orientation. As the brows do grow, they can be "trained" with clear eyebrow gels. As the hair develops an adequate length, the weight of gels can, to some degree, re-orient hair growth (Fig. 40.10).

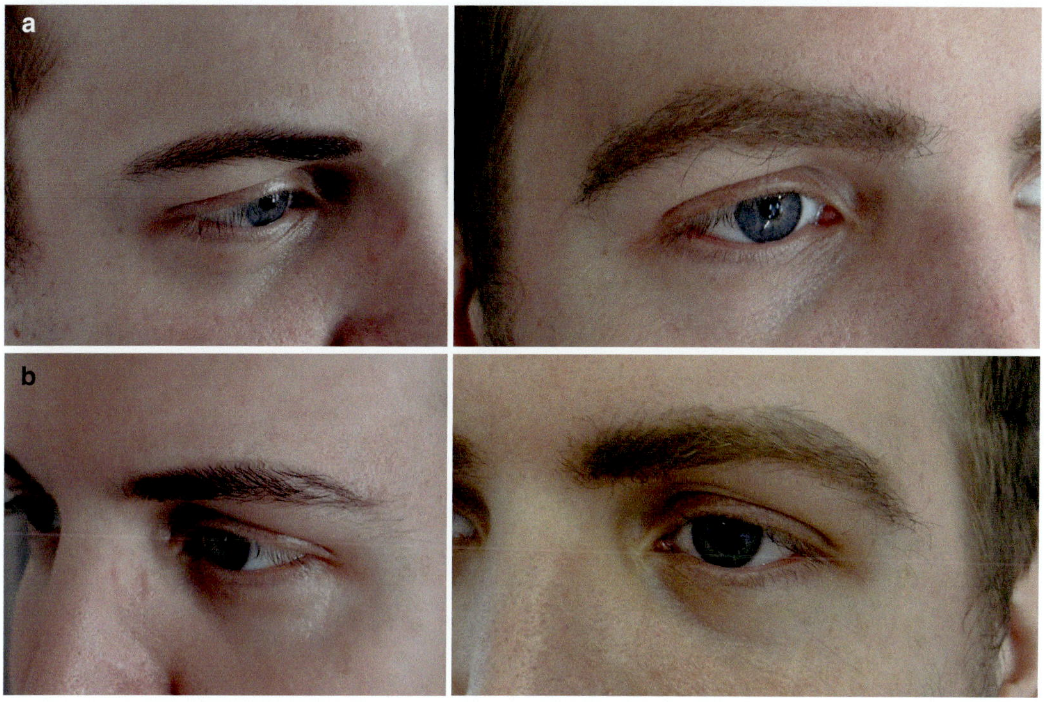

Fig. 40.10 Before and after 350 follicle transplant per eyebrow

References

1. Nordstrom RE. "Stretch-back" in scalp reductions for male pattern baldness. Plast Reconstr Surg. 1984;73(3):422–6.
2. Juri J. The use of the Juri Tempero-Parieto-occipital flap. Semin Plast Surg. 2005;19(2):128–36.
3. Norwood OT, Shiell RC, Morrison ID. Complications of scalp reductions. J Dermatol Surg Oncol. 1983;9(10):828–35.
4. Epstein JS. Transplantation to the beard, chest, and other areas. In: Lam SM, editor. Hair transplantation 360: advances, techniques, business development and global perspectives. New Delhi: Jaypee Brothers Medical Publishing; 2014. p. 223–33.
5. Baker SB, Dayan JH, Crane A, Kim S. The influence of brow shape on the perception of facial form and brow aesthetics. Plastic Reconstr Surg. 2007;99(7):1808–16.
6. Westmore MG. Facial cosmetics in conjunction with surgery. Paper presented at: Aesthetic Plastic Surgical Society Meeting May 7, 1974 Vancouver, British Columbia; Ellenbogen R. Transcoronal eyebrow lift with concomitant upper blepharoplasty. Plast Reconstr Surg. 1983;71:490–99.

Part VI

Non-surgical Aesthetics

Facial Rejuvenation/Sun Damage/ Resurfacing for Men (Including Ethnic Men)

41

Robert Jaroslaw Dabek, William G. Austen, Jr., and Branko Bojovic

41.1 Introduction

The face is one of the most complex regions in the human body. Inevitably, as we age, the appearance of our face and facial expression changes. Facial rejuvenation techniques aim to restore a more youthful appearance. A variety of surgical and nonsurgical options have become available to improve facial appearance by attempting to restore the various effected parts to their more youthful state. It is important to understand that these elective procedures come with inherent risks which must be carefully assessed and disclosed to patients considering any intervention.

The most recent data from the Cosmetic Surgery National Data Bank shows that men account for approximately 9.2% of nonsurgical cosmetic interventions performed in 2017 [1]. Of the approximately 300,000 procedures, roughly 10% were skin rejuvenation procedures, undoubtably the majority occurring on the facial skin. Photorejuvenation with intense pulsed light (IPL), chemical peels, fractional ablative laser resurfacing, and full field ablative laser resurfacing were the most commonly performed procedures. These figures demonstrate a steady increase in procedures over the last 15 years or more. Men may prefer noninvasive options when pursuing facial rejuvenation due to the limited downtime, reduced pain, and lesser social stigma than that of surgical cosmetic procedures.

R. J. Dabek
St. Agnes Hospital, Baltimore, MD, USA
e-mail: bbojovic@mgb.org

W. G. Austen, Jr.
Division of Plastic and Reconstructive Surgery, Massachusetts General Hospital, Boston, MA, USA
e-mail: wausten@mgh.harvard.edu

B. Bojovic (✉)
Division of Plastic and Reconstructive Surgery, Department of Surgery, Massachusetts General Hospital, Boston, MA, USA
e-mail: bbojovic@partners.org

41.2 Gender Differences of the Aging Face

Facial aging is attributed to a multifactorial process involving both intrinsic and extrinsic factors. Intrinsic factors are the hormonal, biochemical, and genetic processes affecting aging, while extrinsic factors refer to the environmental exposures such as pollution, sun exposure, repetitive movement, diet, and smoking which can lead to accelerated aging. The complex three-dimensional changes that occur affect the epidermis, dermis, subcutaneous adipose tissue, musculature, ligaments, and bone. The onset of age-related changes differs in the aforementioned structures and varies between individuals [2]. The culmination of these changes can be seen clinically as rhytids, dyschromia, dermatochalasis, volume loss, and alopecia. The noninvasive procedures that are discussed in this chapter

K. Jeffords et al. (eds.), *Aesthetic Surgery for Men*, https://doi.org/10.1007/978-3-032-03840-1_41

address changes occurring primarily in the skin, and to a lesser extent the subcutaneous adipose tissue. Knowledge of age-related facial anatomy is key for appropriate restoration of a youthful face.

41.2.1 Intrinsic Factors

One of the key changes occurring as we age is an overall reduction of sex hormone production. It has been shown that age-related changes in testosterone levels of males vary widely between individuals. In general, there is a decrease in testosterone levels of about 1% per year after the age of 30 [3]. Male skin is thicker than female skin at all ages [4]; however, the gradual decrease of testosterone leads to a decrease in skin thickness [5, 6]. The differences in thickness are thought to be due to differences in dermal hydroxyl-proline and collagen content [6]. The higher levels of androgens in males lead to the development of terminal hairs on the face, particularly in the chin and upper lip regions. Males also have increased levels of sebum and sweat production, and a decreased intraepidermal pH as compared to female skin [6]. Although sebum acts to maintain the flexibility of the skin and aids in waterproofing, excess sebum production has been associated with undesirable effects such as acne or enlarged pores. The adnexal skin structures are thought to be responsible for the larger dermal vascular plexus seen in males. The increased vascularity of the male face is thought to contribute to higher rates of post-procedural bleeding [7].

The bony skeleton and attached musculature lend a great deal to the dimorphism seen in facial anatomy. These elements have a substantial impact on craniofacial shape and aging appearance. Males generally have less subcutaneous adipose tissue and more muscle mass than females, leading to flat and angular facial features. Men have more prominent supraorbital ridges, wider and taller foreheads, greater glabellar projection, larger orbits, prominent flexure of the mandibular ramus, and larger, more forward-protruding chins. All of these factors contribute to the square appearance of the aging male face. The increase in mimetic musculature and greater capacity for facial muscle movement [8] in the face causes men to develop more deeply pronounced expressive rhytids.

41.2.2 Extrinsic Factors

Sun exposure (photoaging) and smoking are arguably the two most significant extrinsic factors for an aging facial appearance. Ultraviolet (UV) light exposure causes direct damage to DNA and induces inflammation suppression [9]. Clinically, photoaged skin is characterized by rhytids, lentigines, telangiectasias, coarseness, sallow color, laxity, decreased elasticity and turgor, impaired wound healing, and benign and malignant growths [10, 11]. Histologically apparent changes in photoaged skin include epidermal atrophy with loss of the rete ridges or epidermal thickening, loss of dermal extracellular matrix and collagen fiber breakdown, and loss of elastic fibers [12, 13]. The cumulative degree of exposure and skin type determines the severity of the clinical appearance. In general, individuals with higher Fitzpatrick skin types accumulate less photoaging damage. While both men and women are subject to photoaging and the effects of UV exposure, men usually accumulate more damage by the time they have reached the same age.

The effects of cigarette smoking on skin have been documented in the literature for over a hundred years. The effects of smoking on facial appearance are associated with a decrease in attractiveness [14] with clinically evident increases in rhytids, early hair loss, pale or grayish skin, yellow teeth, decreased skin perfusion, and impaired wound healing [15]. Specifically, upper eyelid skin redundancy, lower lid bags, malar bags, nasolabial folds, upper lip rhytids, lower lip vermillion rhytids, and jowls are predominant in smokers as compared to non-smoking counterparts [16].

In general, extrinsic factors affecting facial aging are more predominant in men. Historically, men have had occupations which involved greater sun exposure than women and often apply protective measures such as sunscreens less frequently [17, 18]. Due to social and psychological factors, men are more likely to smoke cigarettes than women, and consume more cigarettes per day among smokers [19, 20]. Additionally, as we age, reactive oxygen species (ROS) levels rise and antioxidant activity declines [21]. A number of studies have shown that men have higher levels of oxidative stress than women [22], likely due to decreased levels of native antioxidants in men [23, 24]. These factors put men at particularly high risk for facial aging due to environmental exposures.

41.3 Preventative Measures

Preventative measures primarily deal with our ability to minimize extrinsic exposures and enhance our physiologic ability to deal with intrinsic factors of aging. Sun protection, smoking cessation, and good skin care regimens are our primary tools for slowing the process of facial aging.

41.3.1 Sun Protection

Exposure to the sun's UV radiation is the predominant modifiable risk factor for facial aging. A discussion should be had with patients of every age and skin type regarding the use of sun protective measures. The American Academy of Dermatology (ADA) recommends that sunscreen is applied to all sun-exposed skin approximately 15 min before exposure [25]. The chosen sunscreen should be broad spectrum, waterproof, and rated with a SPF of at least 30. It is recommended that sunscreen is reapplied after bathing or sweating, or 2 h after the first application. Although the UV intensity is lower in winter months and cloudy days, the ADA recommends that sun protective measures be applied year-round and in cloudy weather. Additional sun protection with clothing to minimize exposed surfaces and wide-brimmed hats are recommended particularly for men with hair loss. Tanning beds should be avoided due to the intense UV exposure. Patients should be counseled on the use of daily facial moisturizing creams with SPF 15 or more to further protect against UV radiation.

41.3.2 Topical Skin Care Products

Topical cosmetic products constitute a multibillion-dollar industry in the United States. These products establish the first line of defense in the battle against aging facial appearance. Traditionally, these products were marketed toward women; however, men are expressing more interest in utilizing the anti-aging effects that they may provide. Knowledge regarding the multitude of ingredients available on the market is essential in advising patients on their efficacy and use. Many of these products' ingredients have been shown to be effective in reducing the appearance of facial aging. At a minimum, we recommend that men begin daily care in their 20s or 30s with high-quality vitamin A and C products.

41.3.2.1 Vitamin A

Topical vitamin A and its derivatives (retinoids) (Fig. 41.1) are available in many forms within skin care products and act as a standard for clinically effective aging products. This group constitutes the cornerstone of treatment for photodamaged skin. Regardless of the type, the retinoids all undergo conversion to retinoic acid within keratinocytes, which bind to the retinoic acid receptors which regulate over 500 genes [26, 27]. The most potent drugs in this class are the prescription retinoic acid products: Tretinoin, Tazarotene, and Adapalene. These products are marketed for the treatment of acne, psoriasis, and rhytids. They have been shown to be effective for the treatment of rhytids and improve the appearance of photodamaged skin. Some patients, particularly those naïve to vitamin A, will not tolerate the use of retinoic acid. It is suggested to start with a low dose, applied every other day, and work up to daily use. The ideal time to apply retinoic acid products is in the evening due to the increased risk of photosensitivity.

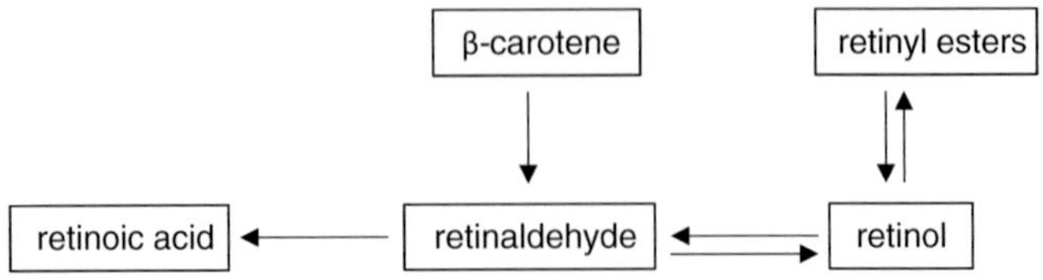

Fig. 41.1 Cellular pathway for vitamin A

The precursor to retinaldehyde and retinoic acid, retinol, is the most commonly used vitamin A derivative available in cosmetic products around the world [28]. A number of clinical studies have demonstrated that retinol is effective in treating both extrinsic and intrinsic causes of aging skin [29, 30]. The results are less pronounced than those seen with retinoic acids, but these products are well tolerated and cause significantly less skin irritation. The authors recommend that all men concerned with facial appearance use a nightly formulation of high-quality and potent retinol beginning in their 20s or 30s. Additionally, anecdotal evidence suggests that retinol may be used as a bridging agent to retinoic acid in patients with sensitive skin.

Retinaldehyde, another vitamin A derivative available in many cosmetic products globally, has been shown to reduce the appearance of deep and fine rhytids. Retinaldehyde is thought to fall between retinol and retinoic acid in potency, and much like retinol, its potential for skin irritation is blunted compared to retinoic acid.

Other vitamin A derivatives have demonstrated mixed results in clinical trials [31]. The vitamin A esters (retinyl-acetate and retinyl-palmitate) are often considered the weakest vitamin A derivatives and have not been shown to produce statistically significant results when compared to placebo [32, 33].

41.3.2.2 Vitamin C

Vitamin C has been used for many decades to combat the appearance of ageing skin. Concentrations of 5–10% of this powerful antioxidant have been shown to promote collagen synthesis and improve the appearance of hyperpigmentation and rhytids [34]. Vitamin C also protects the skin from free radical damage caused by UV light, and has been shown to improve a variety of inflammatory skin conditions [35]. Additionally, topical application of vitamin C following CO_2 laser resurfacing procedures has been shown to reduce postoperative erythema [36]. Due to the supporting evidence, we recommend that men begin using a daily vitamin C product in their 20s and 30s. Multitudes of these products are available over the counter. The ingredients within each product may vary substantially, so it is important to recommend a reputable source when advising patients to add vitamin C products to their daily skin care regimen.

41.3.2.3 Others

An endless and rapidly growing list of other topical skin care products is marketed in the United States and worldwide. There is mixed evidence (or a complete lack of data) to support many of these products' claims. We advise providers recommending these products to perform an unbiased analysis of the available evidence supporting them before advising patients to use them as part of their skin care armamentarium.

41.4 Introduction to Laser and Light Devices

Light Amplification by Stimulated Emission of Radiation (LASER) was first described by Albert Einstein who established a theoretical foundation for lasers in his 1917 paper, On the Quantum Theory of Radiation [37]. In 1960, the first laser device was developed using a ruby crystal and almost immediately after laser devices emerged into the field of medicine, initially in ophthalmology [38]. Within the next few years, Xenon, Argon, and Krypton lasers were devised with CO_2 lasers entering the picture in 1965. Laser skin resurfacing techniques have been employed as rejuvenative procedures since the late 1980s

[39]. The continuous wave lasers at this time would create too much thermal injury to the tissue and often cause excessive scarring and pigmentation changes. In the 1990s, pulsed lasers were developed which mitigated the collateral damage to neighboring and deep tissue. Fractional photothermolysis was later approved in the mid-2000s for skin resurfacing, further reducing the risks of complications associated with treatments.

The increasing trend of utilizing energy-based devices in facial rejuvenation can be attributed to their relative safety and accessibility. Many laser devices are available today for facial rejuvenation in male patients. Lentigines, acne scaring, telangiectasias, seborrheic keratosis, and rhytids can be addressed with laser devices. Although these technologies are identical to those used for women, there are subtle differences in the anatomy of male skin as well as male psyche and male patient intentions that warrant discussion. This is evident when examining gender differences in rates of the most commonly performed nonsurgical facial rejuvenation procedures (Table 41.1) [1] Men, more so than women, will often want minimal downtime, or contrastingly, an aggressive approach that does not require repeat procedures. This may be due to perceived social acceptance of cosmetic procedures among men. Additionally, due to anatomical differences in the skin, men may experience more severe post-procedural erythema, and are more reluctant to wear face makeup than women. The energy-based rejuvenating treatments are often "gateway procedures" for men, leading to subsequent, more invasive interventions [40]. As with other cosmetic procedures, a thorough discussion of risks, expectations, and pre- and post-treatment instructions must occur prior to choosing the appropriate intervention.

Table 41.1 Gender differences in most commonly performed facial rejuvenation procedures in men

Procedure	Rank	Males	Females
Photorejuvination (IPL)	5	8%	92%
Chemical peel	6	5.5%	94.5%
Fractional ablative resurfacing	8	7.3%	92.7%
Full-field ablative resurfacing	10	12.6%	87.4%
Nonsurgical skin tightening (Thermage, Pelleve, Ulthera, etc.)	12	5.7%	94.3%
Microdermabrasion	13	3.4%	96.6%
Dermabrasion (not including microdermabrasion)	15	4.9%	95.1%

The second column indicates the rank within total nonsurgical cosmetic procedures performed in men in 2017 in the United States. Other procedures omitted from the table include: neuromodulator injections, fillers, CoolSculpting, laser hair removal, tattoo removal, etc.

41.4.1 Fully Ablative Laser Resurfacing

Ablative laser resurfacing procedures are an effective tool for facial rejuvenation. The fully ablative CO_2 and erbium:yttrium-aluminum-garnet (Er:YAG) lasers have a target (chromophore) of water and remain as the gold standard for facial rejuvenation. These devices are an excellent choice for the treatment of deep rhytids, actinic keratosis, skin laxity, poikiloderma, and widespread acne scarring. Although these treatments are considered very effective, with visible results seen after a single treatment, many men will choose other interventions due to the associated risks and downtime [41]. Severe erythema which lasts several weeks after the procedure is typical. Other complications include crusting, bruising, edema, infections, scarring, changes in pigment, and activations of herpes (HSV). Pretreatment with antibiotics and antivirals may reduce the risks of infection or viral activation. Pretreatments with topical vitamin A and vitamin C, and proper post-procedural care may help reduce the risks of other complications. Postoperative vitamin C and a single application of corticosteroids may reduce erythema [36, 40, 42]. Application of sunscreen during the healing process may reduce the risk of hyperpigmentation; however, these procedures should be avoided in Fitzpatrick skin types IV to VI due to the increased risk of hyperpigmentation [43, 44]. If hyperpigmentation occurs, it may be treated with retinoic acid or glycolic acid. The Er:YAG and CO_2 lasers are effective in treating actinic keratosis (AK) and do so more reliably than photodynamic therapy. They have also been shown to prevent further development of AK and potentially reduce the risk of nonmelanoma skin cancer [45, 46]. Sun damage on the scalp is also amenable to intervention with CO_2 or Er:YAG laser. It is important to note that thicker scalp skin, as well as skin of the nose and glabella, may require multiple interventions due to the relative skin thickness and extent of sun damage. Patients may be concerned with hair loss following interventions on the scalp; however, the CO_2 and Er:YAG laser may actually stimulate hair growth, rather than cause alopecia [47]. An option to reduce the downtime is to offer therapy with lower energy levels as to cause more superficial destruction [48]. This will lead to less efficacy in rhytid reduction and will require multiple treatments. Another option is to employ a fractional ablative device.

41.4.2 Fractional Ablative Laser Resurfacing

Fractional ablative devices cause destruction of a defined percentage of the skin surface area while sparring the remaining epidermis by creating thousands of microthermal zones [49]. The advantage of these procedures is the reduction of downtime and a reduction of risks experienced with fully ablative treatments. The fractional ablative CO_2 and Er:YAG lasers are effective for the treatment of facial scarring, deep and fine rhytids, dyschromic lesions, contour irregularities, skin laxity, and rhinophyma. However, the results may be less dramatic than those seen with fully ablative procedures. Edema, erythema, pinpoint bleeding, and crusting are among some of the adverse effects of treatment. Most postoperative sequelae are resolved within 1 week. The wavelength emitted by the Er:YAG laser is more specific for water than the CO_2 laser, and therefore requires lower fluences. Due to the high absorption by water, the maximum depth of ablation is approximately 2.0–2.5 mm per pass, compared to the CO_2 laser's maximum depth of up to about 4.0 mm. It is important to note that given the same depth of penetration, the CO_2 laser will require higher energy settings than the Er:YAG laser. This additional energy used with the CO_2 laser may cause more thermal damage than that seen with the Er:YAG, and thus may increase healing time [50]. Patients who are particularly concerned with downtime may opt for lower energy and density settings. While this will substantially reduce the healing time, the number of procedures required to achieve a particular result will increase. The frequency of procedures will depend on need and healing time; at least 1 week between procedures as a rule-of-thumb. Energy settings should be adjusted based on the depth of the lesion or severity of rhytids that require treatment, with fine rhytids requiring approximately half the energy as deep rhytids. In general, thicker skin seen in men requires higher energy settings than those used in women. Ideal laser settings will vary widely based on the type, make, and model of the laser system used. It is important to consult manufacturer guidelines and seek guidance from an experienced operator when beginning to utilize laser treatments in practice. Although fractional devices may reduce the risk of postprocedural hyperpigmentation, care must be taken when treating patients with darker skin types. Proper pre- and post-treatment care may reduce these risks. Fractional ablative devices can be effective in the treatment of rhinophyma. High energy and density settings with multiple passes are typical while still causing less scarring than fully ablative devices [51].

41.4.3 Non-ablative Devices

The non-ablative lasers cause thermal injury to the dermis while preserving the stratum corneum and epidermis. As such, these lasers stimulate the production and remodeling of collagen with a shortened recovery time and reduced risk of complications. Clinical results are typically less profound than those seen with ablative procedures; however, they remain as a good option for appropriately selected patients. Men concerned with postoperative recovery time may be good candidates for multiple treatments with a combination of these non-ablative devices. Non-ablative lasers can be classified into three groups: infrared lasers, visible lasers, and intense pulsed light (IPL), which is not a true laser [52].

41.4.4 Infrared Lasers

The neodymium yttrium aluminum garnet (Nd:YAG) (1320 nm), diode (1450 nm), erbium:glass (1540 nm), and recently, thulium fiber laser (1927 nm) are the most frequently utilized infrared lasers. These lasers have all been shown to provide minimal to mild improvement in the appearance of facial rhytids and scars [53–56]. The downtime associated with these lasers is typically less than 1 week. These non-ablative lasers have been shown to be effective in the treatment of melasma, particularly in the Asian patient [57]. However, a risk of treatment is worsening of melasma and postoperative hyperpigmentation. Lower energy settings and longer duration between treatments may be an effective way to reduce the risk [57]. Melasma in Asians has also been successfully treated with the alexandrite laser which produced superior results to that of the Nd:YAG laser [58]. The thulium fiber laser has been shown to provide improvement for solar lentigines, fine rhytids, and keratosis of the male scalp [59] and has been effectively used for the treatment of melasma [60]. Similar to the fractional ablative lasers, patients may be hesitant to undergo scalp treatment due to a misconception that it may trigger hair loss. With the exception of the alexandrite and diode lasers (at the proper settings, these lasers are used for laser hair removal), many of these devices have been implicated in having a mild benefit in male androgenic alopecia [47]. Other broad-spectrum infrared devices (1100-1800 nm) are available for treatment of skin laxity [52]. These devices create widespread thermal damage to the dermal tissue causing contracture during healing. They have been shown to produce mild to drastic improvement in skin laxity, and may be safe options for Asian or dark skin types [61, 62]. Many of the newer devices employ cooling methods which limit pain and may decrease the risk of complications.

41.4.5 Visible Lasers

Several visible light-emitting lasers, including the pulsed dye laser (PDL) and the potassium titanyl phosphate (KTP) laser, can be used for facial rejuvenation. The PDL laser has been shown to improve striae, rhytids, acne scars, and telangiectasia. Studies have reported mild to moderate improvement in rhytids thought to be attributed to collagen induction [63–65], though the primary use of the PDL laser lies in its ability to destroy superficial dilated blood vessels. This makes it an excellent choice for treatment of vascular lesions such as telangiectasias, port-wine stains, and hemangiomas [66]. The less popular KTP laser has similar indications. When compared to the PDL laser, the KTP laser has been shown to have comparable results for the treatment of telangiectasias and facial redness, but may cause more edema and erythema [67, 68]. Alexandrite lasers, technically in the infrared range (755 nm), have also been effectively used for the treatment of facial erythema and telangiectasias [69]. More recently topical photosensitizing agents, such as aminolevulinic acid (ALA) or methyl aminolevulinate (MAL), have been used in combination with PDL therapy to treat actinic keratosis, lentigines, rhytids, and textural and contour abnormalities. The photodynamic therapy (PDT) works by the activation of a photosensitizing agent, which accumulates in target cells, with the laser light source. The cellular destruction occurs through an immune-mediated response or direct apoptosis. Studies suggest that PDL used in conjunction with PDT may be more effective than PDT alone [70, 71]. The use of PDT is not limited to the PDL; intense pulsed light (IPL) [72], blue light, and many other lasers and light sources can be used to activate photosensitizing agents and enhance [73].

41.4.6 Intense Pulsed Light

The spectrum of light emitted by the IPL devices (550–1200 nm) is capable of targeting both hemoglobin and melanin, which results in improvements to pigmentation and vascularity. The use of filters to block wavelengths up to or beyond a certain range can further improve results by selectively targeting one chromophore over the other. This makes IPL devices versatile tools in the armamentarium of facial rejuvenation professionals. IPL treatments have been shown to mildly reduce rhytids while having immense effects on pigment and vascular abnormalities [74–76]. IPL treatments are commonly paired with PDT [72] or other laser treatments to safely achieve excellent results often superior to those seen with monotherapy [77, 78].

41.5 Fully Ablative Laser Resurfacing

41.5.1 Indications and Patient Selection

Fully ablative laser treatments are more aggressive than other laser treatments and are useful for the treatment of a number of conditions. Photoaging, including treatment of rhytids, increased vascularity and erythema, solar elastosis, actinic keratosis (AK), and dyspigmentation, is the most common indication for use of ablative laser treatments. Acne, traumatic, and surgical scars are also amenable to ablative treatments. Candidates, particularly men who may have less social exposure to these procedures, should be realistic regarding expectations and fully understand the recovery course. These procedures are particularly effective for the treatment of fine rhytids in the periorbital, perioral, forehead, and cheek regions. The deeper creases are also improved after several treatments, likely due to a general tightening effect. The procedure can be performed after a face lift to target the unimproved perioral and periorbital rhytids. Superficial and deeper scars are responsive to treatment with more superficial and less aged scars demonstrating superior remodeling with fewer treatments. We recommend waiting approximately 6 weeks before attempting resurfacing of surgical scars. However, the most effective timing for the treatment of surgical scars has not yet been determined and some surgeons will perform treatment immediately following a procedure [79, 80]. Due to impaired wound healing, with potentially higher risks of skin necrosis, scarring, and infection [81], combination treatments are best saved for experienced surgeons [82]. In addition to rhytids and scarring, ablative lasers are well suited for the treatment of diffuse AK, solar elastosis, and other superficial lesions.

These procedures are appropriate for any age patient in good health with evidence of the above indications. The procedure should be avoided in skin types IV to VI due to the risk of hyperpigmentation. The importance of obtaining a pertinent history should not be overlooked prior to offering an ablative procedure.

A focused history should be obtained prior to any resurfacing procedure. In particular, it is important to note whether there have been any prior surgical or nonsurgical facial procedures performed. The results of any previous facial ablation or laser treatment should be noted along with complications that occurred. History of face lift and blepharoplasty is of particular importance. Face lift procedures may pull some of the thinner non-facial skin onto the face, whereas blepharoplasties can increase the risk of ectropion after resurfacing [83]. Knowledge of these prior procedures will affect your treatment plan and technique. Previous evidence of keloids or radiation therapy is a contraindication to use of ablative procedures. Candidates with connective tissue diseases are also best avoided, although there is some evidence to suggest that certain laser procedures may be appropriate for these individuals [84, 85]. Patients with vitiligo, psoriasis, verrucae, and molluscum contagiosum and other conditions which may undergo Koebnerization after ablative laser skin resurfacing should be identified and not be treated with these modalities due to the risk of disease progression to treated areas. Patients with recent isotretinoin therapy should be approached with caution. Due to prior reports of patients developing keloids and delayed wound healing, recommendations call for waiting at least 6 months prior to resurfacing procedures [86–88]. Although there have been challenges to this paradigm, we would recommend against using fully ablative procedures within 6 months of use of isotretinoin.

41.5.2 Preoperative Management

Patients should be optimized to minimize complications and increase response to the laser therapy. Preventative measures include antiviral and antibiotic agents. All patients should be treated with oral antivirals, such as valacyclovir, acyclovir, or famciclovir, regardless of prior history of herpes (HSV). Therapy should be initiated 1 day prior to the procedure and continue for 10–14 days postoperatively [89, 90]. Single or two-dose regimens have been shown to be less effective [91]. Laser resurfaced areas are vulnerable to bacterial cellulitis (*Staphylococcus aureus*, *Streptococcus pyogenes*, and *Pseudomonas aeruginosa*) and may be prevented with oral antibiotics. Some studies suggest that there is little difference in rates of infection between treated and untreated groups and that rather, meticulous wound care should be employed [92, 93]. Some providers will advocate for the use of antifungal medication such as oral fluconazole; however, we believe this is not necessary. Pretreatment with retinoic acid may have a benefit due to the positive effect on epithelization and decrease in depth of injury. The latest recommendations are to treat ablative laser candidates with 3 months of daily topical 0.1% tretinoin therapy, and to discontinue treatment 24 h prior to laser resurfacing (Fig. 41.2) [94]. Although, we are not aware of any studies demonstrating benefit to therapy being discontinued 24 h prior to the procedure. Retinoic acid therapy should not be started within 4 weeks of the procedure due to the initial exfoliative effect of the retinoic acid.

41.5.3 Anesthesia Concerns and Technique

Regardless of the laser type used, the procedure will be painful and require some form of pain control. In general, CO_2 laser procedures are more painful due to the more diffuse heating of tissue, as compared to the Er:YAG laser. Lidocaine cream or other topical agents may suffice for superficial Er:YAG treatments. Local infiltration of 2% lidocaine and epinephrine, as well as nerve blocks, can be used for both Er:YAG and CO_2 procedures. The addition of hyaluronidase and bicarbonate will improve diffusion into the tissue and decrease injection pain, respectively. Procedures targeting deeper tissue and more surface area are best performed in conjunction with intravenous anesthesia with propofol, fentanyl, and an LMA.

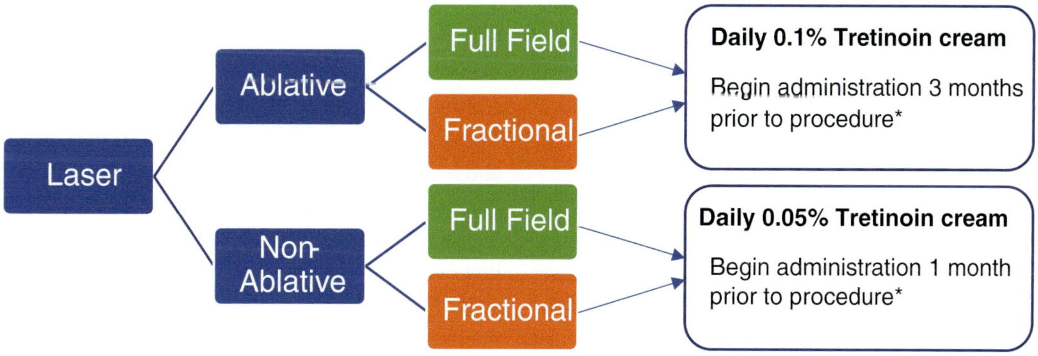

Fig. 41.2 Tretinoin pretreatment for laser facial procedures. *Treatment should not be initiated within a 4-week window of the procedure and should be discontinued 24 h prior to the procedure

The skin should be prepped with alcohol or other sterile manner. Appropriate protective eyewear must be utilized for both the patient and providers. The procedure then involves covering the entire treatment area with a single pass of the CO_2 or Er:YAG laser. The coagulated tissue should be wiped away with a wet sponge and dried with a gauze. A second pass is typically required for the CO_2 laser, with subsequent wiping and drying of the skin. Any areas of thicker scar tissue, or pronounced deep rhytids, may be "feathered" with a third or fourth pass with lower energy settings. The total depth of ablation is related to the energy settings and the number of passes performed. The ablative target depth should reach no further than the upper papillary dermis. The actual settings used will vary between devices, but in general CO_2 lasers will require much higher fluences than the Er:YAG laser to achieve the same depth per pass. When completing the last pass with a CO_2 laser, an Er:YAG laser may be used to remove the most superficial of the coagulated tissue, thereby reducing healing time. When performing ablation with an Er:YAG laser, 2–4 passes will typically be required to remove the epidermis and another 6–8 passes to reach the desired depth, again feathering the problem areas. It is not essential to wipe away debris after each pass, and not advised after the final pass due to the risk of bleeding. Scars will require deeper penetration and pronounced scars should be addressed prior to the entire facial resurfacing. This will eliminate any doubt as to their location. Non-fractional ablative procedures are best performed on the full face to decrease the demarcation between treated and untreated skin.

41.5.4 Postoperative Management

Patients should be thoroughly prepared for the recovery phase prior to beginning ablative laser treatments. This begins with a discussion of the postoperative course and possible complications which could occur and the steps to be taken to minimize the risk. Meticulous wound care in this period is essential. Edema is expected to occur postoperatively, peaking at 48–72 h. Oral nonsteroidal anti-inflammatory agents such as ibuprofen may be used alongside ice packs and head elevation. Oral corticosteroids may be used if the edema is severe or intolerable. Bio-occlusive or semi-occlusive dressings may be used in the first 3–7 days to facilitate re-epithelization and potentially reduce postoperative pain [95]. However, these closed systems generally come with a higher risk of infection [96, 97]. The other option is to apply a thick ointment to the skin surface to keep the surface moist and free of dry crust or scabs. Erythema may continue for many weeks following the procedure. The use of topical ascorbic acid at least 4 weeks following resurfacing may decrease the inflammation and erythema. Sunscreens, other topical drugs, and cosmetics should be avoided in the first several weeks until considerable reepithelialization and healing have occurred. UV exposure should be avoided and sunscreens should be applied after the reepithelialization phase to reduce risk of pigment changes and scarring.

41.6 Fractional Ablative Laser Resurfacing

41.6.1 Indications and Patient Selection

Fractional ablative laser treatments are less aggressive than their fully ablative counterparts and are useful for the treatment of many of the same conditions. The laser devices cause vaporization of columns known as microthermal zones. These zones typically cover 5–25% of the surface and heal more rapidly than fully ablated surfaces. As compared to fully ablative procedures, there is a reduction of complications and healing time; however, the typical results are also less impressive. Most patients will require multiple treatments (3–6) to achieve desirable results. Like fully ablative procedure, photoaging and scars are amenable to fractional ablative treatments and remain the most commonly treated conditions. Additionally, melasma is commonly treated with fractional ablative systems.

The ideal candidates for fractional ablative treatment are men who would like to see more pronounced results than those attained with non-ablative devices, but are not committed to the lengthy recovery period seen with fully ablative procedures. These procedures are also excellent choices for younger men with less accumulated sun damage due to the relatively fewer required treatments. Patients should be fully informed and expectations should be thoroughly addressed. Many of the same contraindications exist as with fully ablative devices; however, Fitzpatrick types IV and V may be treated with low density and energy settings, requiring a greater number of procedures. As with fully ablative procedures, a proper history regarding prior procedures, dermatologic or systemic illnesses, and medication use, particularly isotretinoin use, should be documented. The recommendations of waiting 6 months after discontinuation of isotretinoin holds for fractional procedures.

41.6.2 Preoperative Management

As with fully ablative procedures, patients should be optimized for greatest results and limited complications. Many of the same considerations for preoperative management seen with fully ablative procedures will hold true for fractional procedures. Topical Tretinoin 0.1% should be started 3 months prior to the procedure date and discontinued 24 h before the procedure. Again, Tretinoin should not be started within 4 weeks of the procedure. Vitamin C can also be used prior to the procedure and discontinued at the same time. Oral antiviral medication should be started 1 day prior to the procedure and continued for about 5 days, or until reepithelialization is complete. Oral antibiotics are generally not warranted unless there have been documented past bacterial infections of the facial skin. Antifungals and corticosteroids are not necessary.

41.6.3 Anesthesia Concerns and Technique

Fractional laser procedures commonly require topical pain control. In general, the fractional CO_2 laser procedures are more painful due to the more diffuse heating of tissue, as compared to the Er:YAG laser. Lidocaine cream or other topical agents may suffice for both CO_2 and Er:YAG laser treatments. In patients with severe pain, a local infiltration of 2% lidocaine and epinephrine may be used. Many of the newer fractional systems also have cold air cooling devices which are used to limit thermal damage and reduce pain.

The topical anesthetic should remain in place for about 60 min prior to the procedure and then wiped away using a dry gauze. The surface can be treated with a sterile prep solution and allowed to fully dry. Appropriate protective eyewear must be utilized for both the patient and providers. There are a variety of settings that can be used to achieve the targeted improvements. In general, density settings of about 10 or 15% are used with about 6–10 passes. The energy settings will depend on the system, the patient, and the provider. Less aggressive treatments can be done if there is greater concern for complications. Scars can be treated with higher energy settings, preferably with a CO_2 laser, either before or after the entire facial treatment is performed. Many surgeons now advocate for the use of both superficial and deep treatments with fractional systems to achieve results in fewer treatments. The number of required treatments will vary with sun damage and fine rhytids responding sooner than deeper rhytids and hypertrophic scars. The treatments should be spaced at 2–4-week intervals.

41.6.4 Postoperative Management

The face should be wiped and cleaned with a wet cloth immediately following the procedure. After drying, a moisturizing ointment should be applied. The postoperative care is much less complex than that seen with fully ablative laser procedures. The area should be kept clean and dry, or covered with a moisturizing balm. Patients should be educated on the importance of avoiding sun exposure and not applying any facial cosmetic products prior to reepithelization. After about 7 days, makeup and sunscreens can be used safely, and vitamin C may be used to help reduce persistent erythema. Edema and erythema are typically resolved within 1–2 weeks.

41.7 Non-ablative Laser Resurfacing and Other Energy Techniques

41.7.1 Indications and Patient Selection

The goal of non-ablative rejuvenation treatments are to improve rhytids, telangiectasias, lentigines, and overall skin texture. Ideal candidates for non-ablative techniques will be otherwise healthy men with mild to severe rhytids and evidence of photodamage. These patients are typically reluctant to accept the risks and recovery time associated with ablative procedures or want to pair them with ablative procedures for expedited results. Although these procedures are generally safer, darker skin types should be informed of the risk of dyspigmentation with many of these laser modalities. Test areas can be treated in unexposed skin to determine the likelihood of pigment changes. A history of facial surgery, nonsurgical procedures, systemic or dermatologic illnesses, and medication use should be obtained. Patients should discontinue use of isotretinoin at least 1 month prior to non-ablative procedures [88]. The use of radiofrequency devices with preexisting fillers may be contraindicated due to the increased inflammatory response and potential for developing nodularity [98].

41.7.2 Preoperative Management

Preoperative optimization should be done with all patients undergoing non-ablative rejuvenation procedures. Daily topical 0.05% tretinoin is recommended for at least 1 month prior to treatment and stopped the day prior to the procedure (Fig. 41.2) [94]. Bacterial prophylaxis or antiviral prophylaxis is reserved for patients with a history of bacterial facial skin infections or a history of recurrent HSV infections. In the authors' experience, these are rarely used in practice.

41.7.3 Anesthesia Concerns and Technique

Non-ablative procedures are relatively painless, particularly IPL, PDL, and KTP, which usually require no anesthetic use. Topical anesthetic such as lidocaine may be applied for other procedures or if pain is encountered. Many of the newer systems have cooling devices built into the handpieces and cryogen spray. Cold towels or cold packs can be applied if there is any pain or discomfort following the procedure. The most painful of the non-ablative procedures are some of the RF devices in which sedation may be used.

Each of the non-ablative devices are vastly different and as such the technique will vary greatly. Appropriate protective eyewear must be utilized for both the patient and providers. PDL, alexandrite, and KTP are used at sub-purpuric fluences and pulse durations in single passes. These treatments are performed at 3–4 weeks apart for a total of 3–8 treatments. Infrared lasers should be operated at high fluences in the treatment of rhytids as low fluences produce little or no results. Devices with built-in skin temperature monitoring systems allow for the surgeon to titrate the fluence to achieve a peak temperature not exceeding 108 degrees Fahrenheit (42 °C) [52]. The treatments are usually spaced at 2–4 weeks apart for a total of 5 or 6 treatments. The endpoint of minimal edema and erythema should be achieved during the treatment sessions. IPL treatments are performed usually in 1–4 passes with a cold aqueous gel applied after each pass. Usually, 4–8 treatments are required with IPL devices, spaced at 2–4 weeks apart. Radiofrequency devices vary greatly between types. A gel or fluid is applied to the skin to contact the treatment tips. Monopolar devices require the patient to be grounded using a grounding pad.

Bipolar and newer unipolar devices do not require grounding. Combination devices or combined treatments with non-ablative devices are common. Some sense needs to be used to ensure there is no overlapping damage to particular layers of the skin. Importantly, manufacturer guidelines should be followed, and less aggressive approaches are warranted for surgeons not familiar with the use of these devices.

41.7.4 Postoperative Management

After completion of treatment, ice packs can be applied to reduce edema and alleviate discomfort. The face should be gently cleansed with soap and water. A course of antibiotics can be prescribed if the patient has a history of acne breakouts after prior treatment. The edema will typically subside in several days and skin may have a light bronzing during this time. Superficial desquamation may occur for up to 2 weeks depending on the device, and patients should be instructed not to exfoliate.

41.8 Other Rejuvenation Techniques

There are numerous other techniques available when approaching facial rejuvenation. Chemical peels, microneedling, dermabrasion, and radiofrequency devices can be an effective means of addressing patient concerns.

41.8.1 Radiofrequency Devices

Radiofrequency devices operate at a variety of wavelengths which are designed to target the reticular dermis, inducing collagen destruction and remodeling. The devices operate by one of two means. The first devices sent a current through the tissue, changing polarity millions of times per second, causing any electrically charged particles within the field to change orientation. More recent devices act by generating electromagnetic waves within the radiofrequency spectrum which are applied directly to the skin. In either case, heat is generated at a target depth in the range of 2–30 mm. The overall effect is a tightening of the dermal skin causing a reduction of skin laxity. A number of recent clinical trials have shown efficacy of these treatments in reducing skin laxity and improving facial contour [99, 100]. However, early devices were unable to achieve reproducible results in all patients, with a minority experiencing drastic improvement, while the majority had little or no improvement after treatment. Older devices appeared to have little, no effect, or a negative effect on rhytids. Newer devices have been shown to improve rhytids, particularly in the periocular region [101, 102]. Results often require several treatments with improvements peaking several months following treatment and lasting over a year. As with other rejuvenation technologies, the radiofrequency devices are being developed at an exceptional rate. Additionally, much like other rejuvenation techniques, radiofrequency devices are now commonly employed in conjunction with one or more laser or light modalities to achieve a global improvement in facial aging. As with other less invasive modalities, the adverse effects of treatment are mild and limited to pain and edema. Due to the depth of thermal energy being delivered and epidermal temperature monitoring systems, radiofrequency devices are considered to be safe options for all skin types. This does not hold true for coblation devices which are based on bipolar radiofrequency technologies. These devices cause a destruction and exfoliation of the epidermis and may result in hyperpigmentation in darker skin types [103]. Like other ablative devices, coblation is effective in treating skin laxity, rhytids, telangiectasias, scarring, and dyschromia.

41.8.2 Microneedling

The modern use of microneedling, or percutaneous collagen induction (PCI), dates back to the mid-1990s and early 2000s where various microneedling devices and procedures were used in the treatment of scaring, tattoo removal, and facial rejuvenation [104–106]. These procedures have since gained popularity due to their simplicity and low rates of adverse events. Regardless of the type of device, these procedures create cutaneous microtrauma which results in activation of the wound healing response, triggering collagen remodeling of the underlying skin. There is little risk of hyperpigmentation, even in patients with darker skin types due to the lack of thermal injury and no specific melanocyte destruction [107]. Studies have demonstrated favorable results in the treatment of rhytids, skin laxity, scars, and melasma with rapid post-procedural recovery [108–110]. The result profile, paired with limited downtime, makes microneedling an excellent option when approaching male facial rejuvenation. Patients typically experience mild pain and bleeding. The relatively higher rate of bleeding compared to energy-based devices may deter some patients from undergoing repeat procedures. The utilization of topical drugs may have additive benefits to microneedling procedures due to enhanced dermal drug delivery.

41.8.3 Chemical Peels

The use of chemical peels has become increasingly popular among men with the American Society for Aesthetic Plastic Surgery listing them as the seventh most common non-surgical aesthetic procedure among men [1]. There are a variety of chemical agents employed as facial peels for the treatment of the aging face. The application of these agents (or combination of agents) causes keratolysis or keratocoagulation of the surface of the skin, resulting in a controlled destruction of parts of the epidermis or dermis [111]. These agents are typically classified by their depth of destruction, ranging from light superficial (destruction to the superficial epidermis but sparing the deeper epidermis) to deep (destruction up to the reticular dermis) [112]. The tissue damage causes regeneration and collagen remodeling, resulting in a reduction of many signs of facial aging. Chemical peels are useful for a variety of indications, including rhytids, scarring, actinic keratoses, melasma, and skin laxity. Adverse effects of treatment range from mild to severe depending on the agent and technique. As a general rule, practice caution when approaching chemical peels due to the risk of hypo- or hyper-pigmentation, particularly in darker skin types.

41.8.4 Dermabrasion

The popularity of dermabrasion has decreased in favor of other procedures [1]. Men accounted for approximately 4000 cosmetic dermabrasion procedures in 2017 [1]. Nonetheless, dermabrasion can be a useful tool to combat the appearance of facial aging. Scarring and rhytids are typically treated with dermabrasion. This method of facial rejuvenation can work best for select deep rhytids and pronounced small scars. This lies in the ability of the surgeon to focally control the depth of tissue destruction allowing for a very precise control not typically seen with other methods. Recovery times and adverse effects are similar to those seen for ablative procedures, and darker skin types should be avoided. Dermabrasion also remains a useful tool in the treatment of rhinophyma and could be used for pigment transfer to sites of severe scarring.

41.9 Conclusion

Nonsurgical facial rejuvenation has grown over the last three decades into a huge field. To that aim, numerous technologies exist today and continue to be developed at a rapid rate. Men have begun to pay closer attention to their facial appearance than they had previously. As such, they have begun to utilize nonsurgical means of facial rejuvenation in an aim to restore a youthful appearance. Subtle differences between male patients' goals, facial anatomy, and social reception require attention to these details when approaching male facial rejuvenation. Ultimately, knowledge of these devices and their proper use, as well as the development of new technology and techniques, will be increasingly important for the treatment of male patients.

References

1. American Society for Aesthetic Plastic Surgery Statistics. Available from: www.surgery.org/media/statistics. Accessed 25 Feb 2019.
2. Cotofana S, Fratila A, Schenck T, et al. The anatomy of the aging face: a review. Facial Plast Surg. 2016;32:253–60.
3. Matsumoto AM. Andropause: clinical implications of the decline in serum testosterone levels with aging in men. J Gerontol A Biol Sci Med Sci. 2002;57:M76–99.
4. Shuster S, Black MM, McVitie E. The influence of age and sex on skin thickness, skin collagen and density. Br J Dermatol. 1975;93:639–43.
5. Dao H, Kazin RA. Gender differences in skin: a review of the literature. Gend Med. 2007;4:308–28.
6. Giacomoni PU, Mammone T, Teri M. Gender-linked differences in human skin. J Dermatol Sci. 2009;55:144–9.
7. Baker DC, Stefani WA, Chiu ES. Reducing the incidence of hematoma requiring surgical evacuation following male rhytidectomy: a 30-year review of 985 cases. Plast Reconstr Surg. 2005;116:1973–85. discussion 1986–7
8. Houstis O, Kiliaridis S. Gender and age differences in facial expressions. Eur J Orthod. 2009;31:459–66.
9. Yaar M, Gilchrest BA. Photoageing: mechanism, prevention and therapy. Br J Dermatol. 2007;157:874–87.
10. Han A, Chien AL, Kang S. Photoaging. Dermatol Clin. 2014;32:291–9.
11. Farage MA, Miller KW, Elsner P, et al. Characteristics of the aging skin. Adv Wound Care. 2013;2:5–10.
12. Varani J, Warner RL, Gharaee-Kermani M, et al. Vitamin A antagonizes decreased cell growth and elevated collagen-degrading matrix metalloproteinases and stimulates collagen accumulation in naturally aged human skin. J Invest Dermatol. 2000;114:480–6.
13. Tsuji T. Loss of dermal elastic tissue in solar elastosis. Arch Dermatol. 1980;116:474–5.
14. Brinker TJ, Enk A, Gatzka M, et al. A dermatologist's ammunition in the war against smoking: a Photoaging app. J Med Internet Res. 2017;19:e326.
15. Just M, Ribera M, Monso E, et al. Effect of smoking on skin elastic fibres: morphometric and immunohistochemical analysis. Br J Dermatol. 2007;156:85–91.
16. Okada HC, Alleyne B, Varghai K, et al. Facial changes caused by smoking: a comparison between smoking and nonsmoking identical twins. Plast Reconstr Surg. 2013;132:1085–92.
17. Abroms L, Jorgensen CM, Southwell BG, et al. Gender differences in young adults' beliefs about sunscreen use. Health Educ Behav. 2003;30:29–43.
18. McCarthy EM, Ethridge KP, Wagner RF. Beach holiday sunburn: the sunscreen paradox and gender differences. Cutis. 1999;64:37–42.
19. Waldron I. Patterns and causes of gender differences in smoking. Soc Sci Med. 1991;32:989–1005.
20. Allen AM, Scheuermann TS, Nollen N, et al. Gender differences in smoking behavior and dependence motives among daily and nondaily smokers. Nicotine Tob Res. 2016;18:1408–13.
21. Hu HL, Forsey RJ, Blades TJ, et al. Antioxidants may contribute in the fight against ageing: an in vitro model. Mech Ageing Dev. 2000;121:217–30.
22. Ide T, Tsutsui H, Ohashi N, et al. Greater oxidative stress in healthy young men compared with premenopausal women. Arterioscler Thromb Vasc Biol. 2002;22:438–42.
23. Vina J, Borrás C, Gambini J, et al. Why females live longer than males: control of longevity by sex hormones. Sci Aging Knowl Environ. 2005;2005:pe17-pe17.
24. Katalinic V, Modun D, Music I, et al. Gender differences in antioxidant capacity of rat tissues determined by 2,2′-azinobis (3-ethylbenzothiazoline 6-sulfonate; ABTS) and ferric reducing antioxidant power (FRAP) assays. Comp Biochem Physiol C Toxicol Pharmacol. 2005;140:47–52.
25. How to apply sunscreen | American Academy of Dermatology. Available from: https://www.aad.org/public/spot-skin-cancer/learn-about-skin-cancer/prevent/how-to-apply-sunscreen. Accessed 4 Mar 2019.
26. Creidi P, Vienne MP, Ochonisky S, et al. Profilometric evaluation of photodamage after topical retinaldehyde and retinoic acid treatment. J Am Acad Dermatol. 1998;39:960–5.
27. Brun P-J, Wongsiriroj N, Blaner WS. Retinoids in the pancreas. Hepatobiliary Surg Nutr. 2016;5:1–14.
28. Ganceviciene R, Liakou AI, Theodoridis A, et al. Skin anti-aging strategies. Dermato-Endocrinology. 2012;4:308–19.
29. Bhawan J. Short- and long-term histologic effects of topical tretinoin on photodamaged skin. Int J Dermatol. 1998;37:286–92.
30. Varani J, Warner RL, Gharaee-Kermani M, et al. Vitamin a antagonizes decreased cell growth and elevated collagen-degrading matrix Metalloproteinases and stimulates collagen accumulation in naturally aged human Skin1. J Invest Dermatol. 2000;114:480–6.
31. Babamiri K, Nassab R. Cosmeceuticals: the evidence behind the Retinoids. Aesthetic Surg J. 2010;30:74–7.
32. Green C, Orchard G, Cerio R, et al. A clinicopathological study of the effects of topical retinyl propionate cream in skin photoageing. Clin Exp Dermatol. 1998;23:162–7.
33. Watson REB, Long SP, Bowden JJ, et al. Repair of photoaged dermal matrix by topical application of a cosmetic 'antiageing' product. Br J Dermatol. 2007;158:472–7.
34. Humbert PG, Haftek M, Creidi P, et al. Topical ascorbic acid on photoaged skin. Clinical, topographical

and ultrastructural evaluation: double-blind study vs. placebo. Exp Dermatol. 2003;12:237–44.
35. Farris PK. Topical vitamin C: a useful agent for treating photoaging and other dermatologic conditions. Dermatologic Surg. 2005;31:814–7; discussion 818.
36. Alster TS, West TB. Effect of topical vitamin C on postoperative carbon dioxide laser resurfacing erythema. Dermatologic Surg. 1998;24:331–4.
37. Einstein A. Zur Quantentheorie der Strahlung. Phys Zeitschrift, Band 18, Seite 121–28.;18 Available from: http://adsabs.harvard.edu/abs/1917PhyZ...18..121E. 1917. Accessed 29 Apr 2019.
38. Choy D. History of lasers in medicine. Thorac Cardiovasc Surg. 1988;36:114–7.
39. Spadoni D, Cain CL, Facial resurfacing. Using the carbon dioxide laser. AORN J. 1989;50(1007):1009–13.
40. Green JB, Metelitsa AI, Kaufman J, et al. Laser and light-based aesthetics in men. J Drugs Dermatol. 2015;14:1061–4.
41. Poore SO, Shama L, Marcus B. Facial resurfacing of the male patient. Facial Plast Surg Clin North Am. 2008;16:357–69.
42. Frucht CS, Ortiz AE. Nonsurgical cosmetic procedures for men: trends and technique considerations. J Clin Aesthet Dermatol. 2016;9:33–43.
43. Alam M, Warycha M. Complications of lasers and light treatments. Dermatol Ther. 2011;24:571–80.
44. Cole PD, Hatef DA, Kaufman Y, et al. Laser therapy in ethnic populations. Semin Plast Surg. 2009;23:173–7.
45. Hantash BM, Stewart DB, Cooper ZA, et al. Facial resurfacing for nonmelanoma skin cancer prophylaxis. Arch Dermatol. 2006;142:976–82.
46. Iyer S, Friedli A, Bowes L, et al. Full face laser resurfacing: therapy and prophylaxis for actinic keratoses and non-melanoma skin cancer. Lasers Surg Med. 2004;34:114–9.
47. Dabek RJ, Austen WG, Bojovic B. Laser-assisted hair regrowth: fractional laser modalities for the treatment of androgenic alopecia. Plast Reconstr Surg Glob Open. 2019;7:e2157.
48. Juhász M, Marmur E. Energy-based devices in male skin rejuvenation. Dermatol Clin. 2018;36:21–8.
49. Manstein D, Herron GS, Sink RK, et al. Fractional Photothermolysis: a new concept for cutaneous Remodeling using microscopic patterns of thermal injury. Lasers Surg Med. 2004;34:426–38.
50. Goldberg DJ. Erbium:YAG laser resurfacing: what is its role? Aesthet Surg J. 1998;18:255–60.
51. Crispin MK, Hruza GJ, Kilmer SL. Lasers and energy-based devices in men. Dermatologic Surg. 2017;43:S176–84.
52. Alexiades-Armenakas MR, Dover JS, Arndt KA. The spectrum of laser skin resurfacing: nonablative, fractional, and ablative laser resurfacing. J Am Acad Dermatol. 2008;58:719–37.
53. Doshi SN, Alster TS. 1450 nm long-pulsed diode laser for nonablative skin rejuvenation. Dermatologic Surg. 2005;31:1223–6. discussion 1226
54. Bhatia AC, Dover JS, Arndt KA, et al. Patient satisfaction and reported long-term therapeutic efficacy associated with 1,320 nm Nd:YAG laser treatment of acne scarring and photoaging. Dermatologic Surg. 2006;32:346–52.
55. Karabudak O, Dogan B, Baloglu H. Histologic evidence of new collagen formation using a Q-switched Nd:YAG laser in periorbital rhytids. J Dermatolog Treat. 2008;19:300–4.
56. de Sica RCP, Rodrigues CJ, Maria DA, et al. Study of 1550-nm Erbium glass laser fractional nonablative treatment of photoaging: comparative clinical effects, histopathology, electron microscopy, and immunohistochemistry. J Cosmet Laser Ther. 2016;18:193–203.
57. Wat H, Wu DC, Chan HHL. Fractional resurfacing in the Asian patient: current state of the art. Lasers Surg Med. 2017;49:45–59.
58. Lee M-C, Lin Y-F, Hu S, et al. A split-face study: comparison of picosecond alexandrite laser and Q-switched Nd:YAG laser in the treatment of melasma in Asians. Lasers Med Sci. 2018;33:1733–8.
59. Boen M, Wilson MJV, Goldman MP, et al. Rejuvenation of the male scalp using 1,927 nm nonablative fractional thulium fiber laser. Lasers Surg Med. 2017;49:475–9.
60. Lee HM, Haw S, Kim JK, et al. Split-face study using a 1,927-nm thulium Fiber fractional laser to treat Photoaging and Melasma in Asian skin. Dermatologic Surg. 2013;39:879–88.
61. Tanaka Y, Tsunemi Y, Kawashima M, et al. Objective assessment of skin tightening in Asians using a water-filtered near-infrared (1,000–1,800 nm) device with contact-cooling and freezer-stored gel. Clin Cosmet Investig Dermatol. 2013;6:167.
62. Goldberg DJ, Hussain M, Fazeli A, et al. Treatment of skin laxity of the lower face and neck in older individuals with a broad-spectrum infrared light device. J Cosmet Laser Ther. 2007;9:35–40.
63. Bjerring P, Clement M, Heickendorff L, et al. Selective non-ablative wrinkle reduction by laser. J Cutan Laser Ther. 2000;2:9–15.
64. Zelickson BD, Kilmer SL, Bernstein E, et al. Pulsed dye laser therapy for sun damaged skin. Lasers Surg Med. 1999;25:229–36.
65. Bernstein EF. The new-generation, high-energy, 595-nm, long pulse-duration pulsed-dye laser improves the appearance of photodamaged skin. Lasers Surg Med. 2007;39:157–63.
66. Liu A, Moy RL, Ross EV, et al. Pulsed dye laser and pulsed dye laser–mediated photodynamic therapy in the treatment of dermatologic disorders. Dermatologic Surg. 2012;38:351–66.
67. Uebelhoer NS, Bogle MA, Stewart B, et al. A split-face comparison study of pulsed 532-nm KTP laser and 595-nm pulsed dye laser in the treatment of facial telangiectasias and diffuse telangiectatic facial erythema. Dermatologic Surg. 2007;33:441–8.
68. McGill DJ, MacLaren W, Mackay IR. A direct comparison of pulsed dye, alexandrite, KTP and Nd:YAG lasers and IPL in patients with previously

treated capillary malformations. Lasers Surg Med. 2008;40:390–8.
69. Ross VE, Meehan KJ, Domankevitz Y, et al. Use of a variable long-pulse alexandrite laser in the treatment of facial telangiectasia. Dermatologic Surg. 2010;36:470–4.
70. Orringer JS, Hammerberg C, Hamilton T, et al. Molecular effects of photodynamic therapy for photoaging. Arch Dermatol. 2008;144:1296–302.
71. Kessels J, Nelemans P, Mosterd K, et al. Laser-mediated photodynamic therapy: an alternative treatment for actinic keratosis? Acta Derm Venereol. 2016;96:351–4.
72. Alster TS, Tanzi EL, Welsh EC. Photorejuvenation of facial skin with topical 20% 5-aminolevulinic acid and intense pulsed light treatment: a split-face comparison study. J Drugs Dermatol. 2005;4:35–8.
73. Wan MT, Lin JY. Current evidence and applications of photodynamic therapy in dermatology. Clin Cosmet Investig Dermatol. 2014;7:145–63.
74. Ping C, Xueliang D, Yongxuan L, et al. A retrospective study on the clinical efficacy of the intense pulsed light source for photodamage and skin rejuvenation. J Cosmet Laser Ther. 2016;18:217–24.
75. Jiang M, Yan F, Avram M, et al. A prospective study of the safety and efficacy of a combined bipolar radiofrequency, intense pulsed light, and infrared diode laser treatment for global facial photoaging. Lasers Med Sci. 2017;32:1051–61.
76. Knight JM, Kautz G. Sequential facial skin rejuvenation with intense pulsed light and non-ablative fractionated laser resurfacing in fitzpatrick skin type II-IV patients: a prospective multicenter analysis. Lasers Surg Med. 2019;51:141–9.
77. Tao L, Wu J, Qian H, et al. Intense pulsed light, near infrared pulsed light, and fractional laser combination therapy for skin rejuvenation in Asian subjects: a prospective multi-center study in China. Lasers Med Sci. 2015;30:1977–83.
78. Mei X-L, Wang L. Ablative fractional carbon dioxide laser combined with intense pulsed light for the treatment of photoaging skin in Chinese population. Medicine (Baltimore). 2018;97:e9494.
79. Archer KA, Perkins SW. Skin resurfacing in combination with facelift surgery. Facial Plast Surg. 2017;33:299–310.
80. Koch BB, Perkins SW. Simultaneous rhytidectomy and full-face carbon dioxide laser resurfacing: a case series and meta-analysis. Arch Facial Plast Surg. 2002;4:227–33.
81. Hayes DK, Berkland ME, Stambaugh KI. Dermal healing after local skin flaps and chemical peel. Arch Otolaryngol Head Neck Surg. 1990;116:794–7.
82. Mayl N, Felder DS. CO_2 laser resurfacingover facial flaps. Aesthet Surg J. 1997;17:285–92.
83. Blanco G, Clavero A, Soparkar CNS, et al. Periocular laser complications. Semin Plast Surg. 2007;21:74–9.
84. Byun YS, Son JH, Cho YS, et al. Intense pulsed light and Q-switched 1,064-nm neodymium-doped yttrium Aluminum garnet laser treatment for the scarring lesion of discoid lupus erythematosus. Ann Dermatol. 2017;29:331.
85. Brauer JA, Gordon Spratt EA, Geronemus RG. Laser therapy in the treatment of connective tissue diseases: a review. Dermatologic Surg. 2014;40:1–13.
86. Zachariae H. Delayed wound healing and keloid formation following argon laser treatment or dermabrasion during isotretinoin treatment. Br J Dermatol. 1988;118:703–6.
87. Bernestein LJ, Geronemus RG. Keloid formation with the 585-nm pulsed dye laser during isotretinoin treatment. Arch Dermatol. 1997;133:111–2.
88. Saluja SS, Walker ML, Summers EM, et al. Safety of non-ablative fractional laser for acne scars within 1 month after treatment with oral isotretinoin: a randomized split-face controlled trial. Lasers Surg Med. 2017;49:886–90.
89. Gilbert S. Improving the outcome of facial resurfacing–prevention of herpes simplex virus type 1 reactivation. J Antimicrob Chemother. 2001;47(Suppl T1):29–34.
90. Beeson WH, Rachel JD. Valacyclovir prophylaxis for herpes simplex virus infection or infection recurrence following laser skin resurfacing. Dermatologic Surg. 2002;28:331–6.
91. Alster TS, Nanni CA. Famciclovir prophylaxis of herpes simplex virus reactivation after laser skin resurfacing. Dermatologic Surg. 1999;25:242–6.
92. Walia S, Alster TS. Cutaneous CO_2 laser resurfacing infection rate with and without prophylactic antibiotics. Dermatologic Surg. 1999;25:857–61.
93. Gaspar Z, Vinciullo C, Elliott T, et al. Antibiotic prophylaxis for full-face laser resurfacing: is it necessary? Arch Dermatol. 2001;137:313–5.
94. Buchanan PJ, Gilman RH. Retinoids: literature review and suggested algorithm for use prior to Facial resurfacing procedures. J Cutan Aesthet Surg. 2016;9:139–44.
95. Batra RS, Ort RJ, Jacob C, et al. Evaluation of a silicone occlusive dressing after laser skin resurfacing. Arch Dermatol. 2001;137:1317–21.
96. McDaniel DH, Ash K, Lord J, et al. Accelerated laser resurfacing wound healing using a triad of topical antioxidants. Dermatologic Surg. 1998;24:661–4.
97. Fisher AA. Lasers and allergic contact dermatitis to topical antibiotics, with particular reference to bacitracin. Cutis. 1996;58:252–4.
98. Shumaker PR, England LJ, Dover JS, et al. Effect of monopolar radiofrequency treatment over soft-tissue fillers in an animal model: part 2. Lasers Surg Med. 2006;38:211–7.
99. Beasley KL, Weiss RA. Radiofrequency in cosmetic dermatology. Dermatol Clin. 2014;32:79–90.
100. Carruthers J, Fabi S, Weiss R. Monopolar radiofrequency for skin tightening. Dermatologic Surg. 2014;40:S168–73.
101. Javate RM, Grantoza CL, Buyucan KFN. Use of an imaging device after nonablative radiofrequency (Pellevé). Ophthalmic Plast Reconstr Surg. 2014;30:499–503.

102. Al-Muriesh M, Zhang X, Wang Q, et al. Efficacy of noninvasive multisource radiofrequency treatment on periorbital rhytids using an imaging device. Lasers Surg Med. 2019;51:251–5.
103. Mancini PF. A new system for skin resurfacing: preliminary clinical and histologic reports. Aesthet Surg J. 1999;19:459–64.
104. Orentreich DS, Orentreich N. Subcutaneous incisionless (subcision) surgery for the correction of depressed scars and wrinkles. Dermatologic Surg. 1995;21:543–9.
105. Camirand A, Doucet J. Needle dermabrasion. Aesthet Plast Surg. 1997;21:48–51.
106. Fernandes D. Percutaneous collagen induction: an alternative to laser resurfacing. Aesthet Surg J. 2002;22:307–9.
107. Cohen BE, Elbuluk N. Microneedling in skin of color: a review of uses and efficacy. J Am Acad Dermatol. 2016;74:348–55.
108. Ablon G. Safety and effectiveness of an automated microneedling device in improving the signs of aging skin. J Clin Aesthet Dermatol. 2018;11:29–34.
109. Iriarte C, Awosika O, Rengifo-Pardo M, et al. Review of applications of microneedling in dermatology. Clin Cosmet Investig Dermatol. 2017;10:289–98.
110. Alster TS, Graham PM. Microneedling. Dermatol Surg. 2017;44:1.
111. O'Connor AA, Lowe PM, Shumack S, et al. Chemical peels: a review of current practice. Australas J Dermatol. 2018;59:171–81.
112. Reserva J, Champlain A, Soon SL, et al. Chemical peels: indications and special considerations for the male patient. Dermatologic Surg. 2017;43:S163–73.

Genital Fillers

42

Denis Valente and Pedro Piccinini

42.1 Introduction

A man's perception of his genitalia significantly affects temperament and self-esteem. Looking down at the penis from above makes it appear narrower than how it looks straight on or from the side. Seeing one's own penis from this perspective and comparing it with other men's appendages from a different perspective may develop an erroneous belief about penis size [1, 2].

The emotional trauma triggered by dissatisfaction about one's genitalia sometimes originates in childhood, from comparing one's own penis with other persons of the same age or parents' anxiety concerning their children's phallus. With increased access to pornographic material, young men may reinforce false ideas that a penis of extreme girth or length is genuine and normal. Up to 45% of men believe they have a small penis [1, 3].

Therefore, most men seeking penile girth augmentation have physiologically normal penises but may suffer from severe preoccupation with phallus size, known as a penile dysmorphophobic disorder. Most patients who seek penile augmentation desire both penile shaft and glans penis augmentation. To date, the use of cosmetic interventions (surgical or non-surgical) for penis enlargement remains highly controversial. There is a lack of standardization between all the various procedures described in the literature, as well as indications and outcome measures [4].

Many scientific studies have tried to answer the question men—and women—worldwide want clear information about: What size is the average penis? This answer is vital to performing the correct patient selection. Across studies, the average flaccid circumference ranges from 3.5 to 3.9 in. The average erect girth is around 4.5 in [5, 6].

Penis enlargement with dermal fillers is indicated for patients with a flaccid penile girth less than or equal to 3 in. It is not necessary to perform circumcision before the procedure. Contraindications to the procedure are soft tissue infection at the genitalia, prior history of allergic reaction to dermal fillers or local anesthetic agents, bleeding diathesis, psychological disorders, uncooperative patients, autoimmune diseases, recent use of steroids, needlephobia, previous penile procedures using permanent fillers, and history of keloid or hypertrophic scars.

Patient expectations for treatment outcomes should be assessed prior to the procedure to ensure these are realistic to help prevent dissatisfaction. In addition, care should be taken to address both the physical and psychological aspects of the problem. Informed consent must be obtained from patients regarding the paucity of solid scientific studies on the procedure and

D. Valente (✉) · P. Piccinini
Plastic Surgery, Federal University of Medical Sciences of Porto Alegre,
Porto Alegre, Rio Grande do Sul, Brazil

K. Jeffords et al. (eds.), *Aesthetic Surgery for Men*, https://doi.org/10.1007/978-3-032-03840-1_42

that there is no dermal filler specifically approved for penile augmentation [6]. Some questions regarding filler's election should be discussed with the patient prior to the procedure: What is this dermal filler approved for? Are there other fillers or therapies that are approved to increase penile girth? Are scientific studies available to support using this filler to treat other medical conditions? Is it likely that this filler will work better to treat the penis than using other treatments? What are the potential benefits and risks of increasing penile girth with this filler?

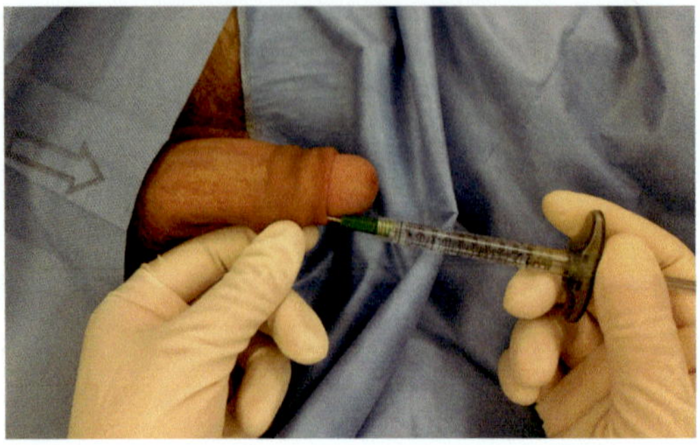

Fig. 42.1 Cannula inserted into the space between the superficial fascia and the deep fascia of the penis shaft at the 9 o'clock position

42.2 Technique

A dorsal penile nerve block is performed with a 22-G needle and 20 mL of ropivacaine 7.5%. After skin preparation with aqueous chlorhexidine and palpation of the arch of the lower border of the symphysis pubis, the phallus base is gently pulled down, and the needle is inserted on either side of the midline distal to the inferior ramus of the pubic bone. The needle is advanced slowly towards the center of the penile shaft until loss of resistance is felt as it penetrates the superficial fascia; the syringe is aspirated to ensure there is no flashback, indicating the needle tip lies in a vein or an artery. The local anesthetic is infiltrated equally on each side.

We prefer to perform the entire block through a midline approach and angle the needle to avoid midline structures and reach the right and left dorsal penile nerves. This technique is generally well tolerated by patients, provides safe and prompt onset of anesthesia, dispenses sedation, and allows penis enlargement in an office setting.

To increase the circumference of the penile shaft, two access points are created through the skin, reaching the superficial fascia using an 18 G × 1/2″ needle trying to avoid the superficial veins. To allow optimal 360-degree smooth coverage of the phallus, these points are created at the distal portion of the penis body laterally at the "9 o'clock" and "3 o'clock" positions. A blunt 20 G × 4″ disposable cannula is inserted through the access point and is utilized to retrogradely inject the filler into the space between the superficial fascia and the deep fascia of the penis using a fanning technique parallel to the corpora cavernosa between the distal shaft and the root of the penis (Fig. 42.1).

Some collagen fibrous septa can create some resistance when the blunt cannula is advancing. Multiple fanning movements are made with the cannula delivering a total volume ranging between 8 and 30 mL, depending on the dermal filler used, as well as the initial width and length of the patient's phallus. Caution must be taken when injecting the filler to avoid penetration along the deep fascia causing urethral occlusion, vascular injuries, or corpora cavernosa or corpus spongiosum trauma. Then, the patient is asked to manually massage his penis for 10 min to smooth any irregularities.

To increase the volume of the glans penis, dermal fillers are injected into the lamina propria layer (subcutaneous) of the glans using a fanning technique through a 22 G × 1/2″ needle. First, the injection needle is positioned at the 12 o'clock position on the corona of the glans (Fig. 42.2). Next, the needle is directed laterally and posteriorly, parallel to the glans penis, distributing the material as uniformly as possible by retrograde injection. To bring balance with the patient's shaft, multiple movements are made with the needle delivering a total volume ranging between 4 and 7 mL. Then, the patient is asked to manually massage his penile glans for 10 min to smooth any irregularities.

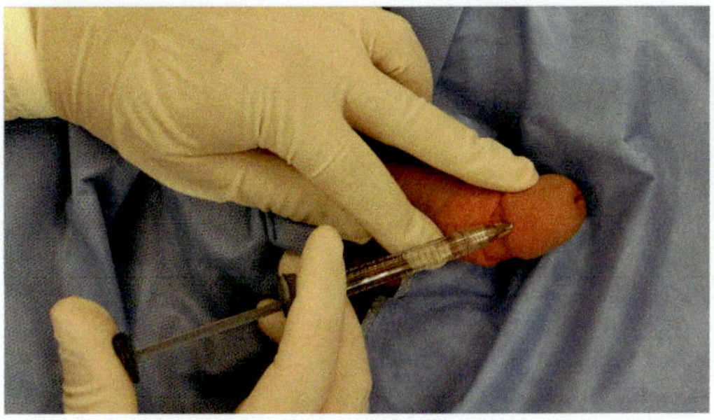

Fig. 42.2 Needle inserted into the lamina propria layer at the 12 o'clock position on the corona of the glans

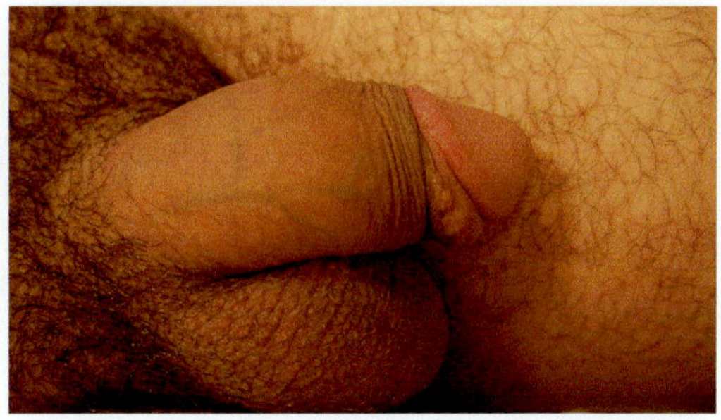

Fig. 42.3 Lumpiness 2 years after 31 mL of polymethylmethacrylate injected in the penis shaft

Aftercare following penile enlargement involves massages to smooth eventual irregularities twice per day and abstaining from masturbation or sexual intercourse for 4 weeks. No bandaging is required after the procedure.

42.3 Discussion

Patients seek out penile augmentation to boost their self-esteem and satisfy their partners. Interestingly, most patients consider the size of their penis in the flaccid state more important than its size when erect [7].

Penile augmentation surgery can result in major disabling complications. Cosmetic surgery of the penis is associated with a high risk of litigation. Phalloplasty for girth enhancement using multiple graft materials can result in up to 42% of patients developing infectious complications [8, 9].

Although dermal filler injections are minimally invasive compared to surgical cosmetic procedures, their safety has been the subject of significant debate. Liposuction with fat grafting to multiple body and face areas is a popular procedure worldwide, usually performed with few complications. However, various complications like infections, necrosis, penile curvature reabsorption, and pulmonary embolism have been reported with penile fat grafting [10].

Several penile injection materials have been introduced and used for penile shaft augmentation. Silicone injection for girth enhancement can result in granulomatous reactions, distant migration, drifting, swelling, and penile distortion.

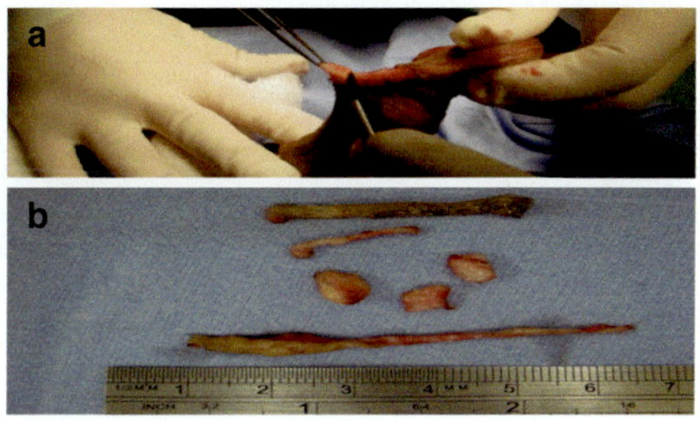

Fig. 42.4 Surgery for lumps removal 2 years after polymethylmethacrylate injection. (**a**) resection of a lump. (**b**) Skin and lumps resected

This material can damage blood vessels and nerves, resulting in decreased sensation and erectile dysfunction. The collagen products that were first used as dermal fillers also exhibited problems related to rapid degradation and hypersensitivity reactions [11].

Our personal experience with penis enlargement started in 2005 using polymethylmethacrylate; however, we have abandoned this filler due to a lumpiness rate of 22% (Fig. 42.3). Since then, hyaluronic acid has become our preferred filler for penis augmentation. From 2012 to 2014, we used calcium hydroxyapatite in some patients in an attempt to obtain longer-lasting results compared with hyaluronic acid. However, its nodule formation rate was 12%. This complication often requires surgical repair (Fig. 42.4).

After 11 years of using hyaluronic acid and 247 individuals treated, we have recorded a low complication rate: 1.2% lumpiness or nodules, 0.8% seroma, and 0.4% hematoma. We have not had any cases of skin necrosis or urological alter-

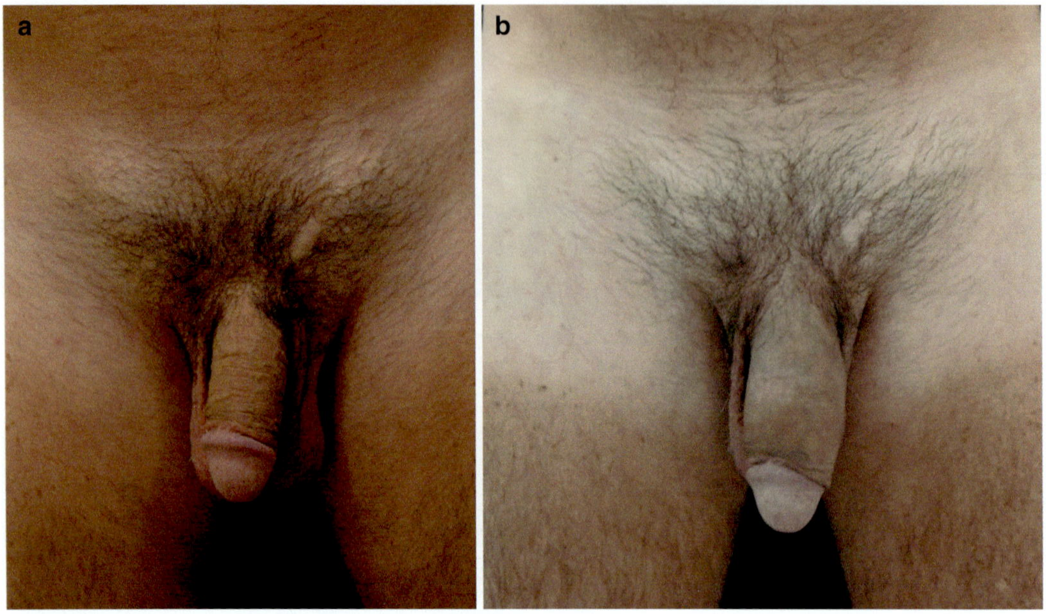

Fig. 42.5 Frontal view comparative photographs 11 months after 22 mL of hyaluronic acid injected in the penis shaft and 4 mL in the glans penis

Fig. 42.6 Lateral view comparative photographs 11 months after 22 mL of hyaluronic acid injected in the penis shaft and 4 mL in the glans penis

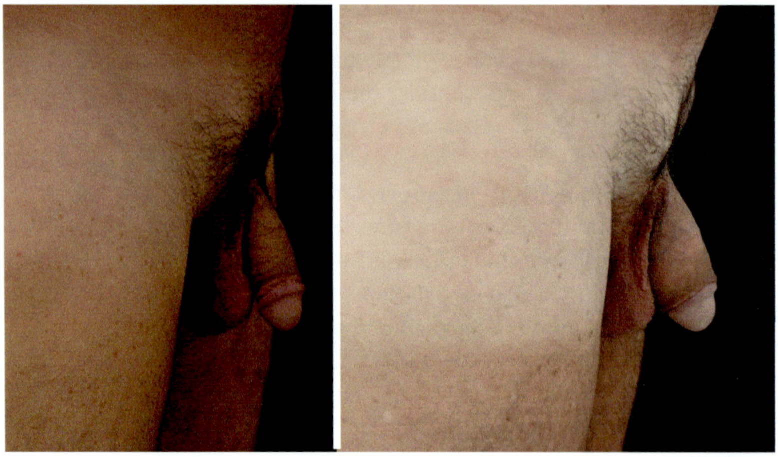

ations. Currently, hyaluronic acid-based gels are the gold standard for penis enlargement in our private practice. With this technique we observed an average of 1 in of penis girth enlargement (Fig. 42.5 and Fig. 42.6). In addition, hyaluronic acid offers the advantages of being wholly reabsorbed and rapid reversal using enzymatic degradation via hyaluronidase in case of vascular compromise or patient dissatisfaction. Thus, any irregularities can be readily corrected, or the entire procedure can be reversed.

42.4 Conclusion

Penile augmentation with hyaluronic acid is a minimally invasive, non-permanent technique that is safe and effective in increasing penile girth without the disadvantages of nodularities, which occur more frequently with other filler materials. In addition, patient satisfaction is high when adequate preoperative counseling and patient selection are performed.

References

1. Veale D, Miles S, Read J, Troglia A, Wylie K, Muir G. Sexual functioning and behavior of men with body dysmorphic disorder concerning penis size compared with men anxious about penis size and with controls: a cohort study. Sex Med. 2015;3(3):147–55.
2. Mondaini N, Ponchietti R, Gontero P, et al. Penile length is normal in most men seeking penile lengthening procedures. Int J Impot Res. 2002;14(4):283–6.
3. Hehemann MC, Towe M, Huynh LM, El-Khatib FM, Yafi FA. Penile girth enlargement strategies: what's the evidence? Sex Med Rev. 2019;7:535.
4. Ghanem H, Glina S, Assalian P, Buvat J. Position paper: management of men complaining of a small penis despite an actually normal size. J Sex Med. 2013,10(1):294 303.
5. Kayes O, Shabbir M, Ralph D, Minhas S. Therapeutic strategies for patients with micropenis or penile dysmorphic disorder. Nat Rev Urol. 2012;9(9):499–507.
6. Veale D, Miles S, Bramley S, Muir G, Hodsoll J. Am I normal? A systematic review and construction of nomograms for flaccid and erect penis length and circumference in up to 15,521 men. BJU Int. 2015;115(6):978–86.
7. Sharp G, Oates J. Nonsurgical medical penile girth augmentation: a retrospective study of psychological and psychosexual outcomes. Aesthet Surg J. 2019;39(3):306–16.
8. Solomon M, Komlo C, DeFrain M. Allograft materials in phalloplasty. Ann Plast Surg. 2013;71(3):297–9.
9. Chevrot A, Droupy S. Cosmetic surgery of the penis. Rev Prat. 2017;67(6):623–7.
10. Zilg B, Råsten-Almqvist P. Fatal fat embolism after penis enlargement by autologous fat transfer: a case report and review of the literature. J Forensic Sci. 2017;62(5):1383–5.
11. Vardi Y, Har-Shai Y, Gil T, Gruenwald I. A critical analysis of penile enhancement procedures for patients with normal penile size: surgical techniques, success, and complications. Eur Urol. 2008;54(5):1042–50.

Nails: The Care and Treatment of Nails of Hands and Feet

43

Zoe M. MacIsaac, Joseph C. English III, and Ernest K. Manders

43.1 Background

While the functional purpose of the nail is to protect the finger tip, increase finger sensibility, and improve fine dexterity, nails also perform an aesthetic function.

43.2 Anatomy

For such a small area, tissues of the distal fingertip include skin, connective tissue, bone, ligaments, tendons and tendon sheaths, associated vasculature, sensory receptors, lymphatic tissue, and fat. Specific to the nail unit are the *nail matrix, nail plate, nail bed, eponychium, paronychium,* and *hyponychium*. The *nail plate* refers to the "fingernail" itself and is comprised of keratin and flattened squamous cells which lose their nuclei as they migrate distally, contributing to the apparent translucent characteristic of the nail plate. The nail matrix consists of the nail plate germinal center in the dorsal and ventral matrix. The dorsal matrix makes a one-cell-layer "true" cuticle that is usually naked to the human eye. The ventral matrix consists of a proximal portion that forms the ventral portion of the nail plate and a distal portion makes the dorsal (belly) of the nail plate. The nail matrix correlates to the visible lunula. The *nail plate* rests upon the *nail bed,* which *is the epithelium that attaches the nail plate firmly*. The firm attachment between the nail bed and nail plate occurs secondary to the interlocking of ridges and furrows at their interface. The *eponychium* refers to the proximal fold of skin covering the nail plate (visible cuticle), the *paronychium* refers to the lateral nail folds, and the *hyponychium* refers to the confluence of the nail bed and fingertip epidermis and is the point of the free nail edge (the component of the nail plate trimmed). The eponychium, paronychium, and hyponychium seal the nail bed from the external environment, forming a protective barrier. Normal nail growth relies upon the integrity of these structures and occurs at a rate 1–3 millimeters per month for finger nails [1]. An entire fingernail requires approximately 6 months for full replacement. Toenails are replaced at one-third to one-half as fast as finger nails with a 12-month full replacement time.

Z. M. MacIsaac
City of Hope Cancer Center, Goodyear, AZ, USA

J. C. English III
Department of Dermatology, Medical Arts Building, Pittsburgh, PA, USA

E. K. Manders (✉)
Department of Plastic Surgery, University of Pittsburgh, Pittsburgh, PA, USA
e-mail: mandersek@upmc.edu

K. Jeffords et al. (eds.), *Aesthetic Surgery for Men*, https://doi.org/10.1007/978-3-032-03840-1_43

43.3 Nail Examination

The hands and nails provide a window into a patient's hobbies and vocation. In addition, the condition of the nails provides insight into general medical history and nail health. Softness/flexibility, nail shape and color, and surrounding skin should be examined. Hands should be compared with one another.

As with other medical examinations, assessment of the nails should be systematic. The nail folds, lunula, nail bed, hyponychium, and nail plate should each be separately examined for color and shape. Nail folds should be without breaks in the skin nor have drainage; ideally, there should be no hang nails (agnails) which are detached nail fold epithelium and the skin should be well hydrated. The lunula should be white, shaped like a crescent moon. Normally, the lunula is visible at the thumb and rarely at the ring finger and small finger. Visibility of the lunula at the index and long fingers is variable. The nail bed should be pink, owing to the robust vasculature of the nailbed, and blanch easily to light pressure. The transition of the hyponychium should be a smooth, curved line at the most distal aspect of the attachment of the nail plate to the nailbed. In general, the nail plate should appear transparent with a soft shine. Distal to the hyponychium, the nail plate should be white. Nails should be without clubbing and pitting, and without significant contour abnormalities such as koilonychia (spoon nails).

43.4 Nail Care

For most, standard personal nail trimming and moisturization with emollients are sufficient to maintain nail health. Biotin, an essential cofactor involved in metabolic pathways, may be taken as an oral supplement and has been demonstrated to improve nail firmness, hardness and thickness [2]. However recently biotin has been shown to cause laboratory anomalies for thyroid function tests and for heart attack screening lab troponin [3, 4]. Patients must let their physicians know if taking this supplement or avoid consumption. An alternative supplement recommended is choline-stabilized orthosilicic acid [5, 6]. Conditioners containing mandelic acid such as Derma Nail (Summer Laboratories Inc., Collegeville, PA, USA) may be applied to harden nails.

While men have not traditionally paid much attention to their nails compared to women, men seeking a "mani-pedi" are more common in larger metropolitan areas such as New York City, and a manicure and pedicure may be an enjoyable adjunct to routine nail care when performed correctly. Usually conducted in a quiet space with a trained aesthetician, it is a comfortable interlude in an often otherwise frenetic day. The manicure often begins with a short soaking in soapy water, after which there is a moisturizing hand massage and application of a cuticle hydrating lotion. Keratinized projections over the eponychial folds are carefully removed with a scissor or clipper. This removes the potential for troublesome hangnails. Excess cuticle is removed (although if done to aggressively can lead to nail disease) and the nails are trimmed and smoothed with an emery board. After this a clear lacquer is applied with a brush and allowed to dry. The result is lustrous nails with a pleasing shape and a smoothness to their edges so that their touch is soft and without the potential for scratching. Oftentimes nail lacquers are hardened with ultraviolet light and can cause a photo-onycholysis and this should be avoided in general. Of note, oral medications such as doxycycline and chemotherapeutic medications can also result in photo-oncycholysis. Onycholysis is the separation of the nail plate from the nail bed.

Performed similarly to a manicure, a pedicure can be important for health reasons, more so than the manicure. One does not have to be diabetic or have a vascular insufficiency to benefit, however. Particularly as we age, some among us lose the ability to reach our toes and to care for them. As examining physicians, we see the results of this all the time. Many patients have long, curved nails (onychogryphosis) which have not been trimmed in months or years. A pedicure can address the problem of nail hygiene in a positive way. However, as with a manicure, this must be performed in the appropriate setting with a trained aesthetician. Feet are often soaked in "thrones" or foot baths, which if inappropriately cleaned have led to atypical mycobacterial skin infections in patients whose legs have been shaved prior to the procedure [7, 8]. Fish pedicures by using *Gara rufa* fish have been reported to cause atypical mycobacterial infections and onychomadesis (proximal nail shedding) [9, 10].

While aesthetic nail care is seldom pursued by men, plastic surgeons in aesthetic practice should be acquainted with not only the range of nail additions and enhancement products, but also should be aware of some of the medical complications that can attend nail care. Surgeons should be aware that the chemicals and physical manipulations used in cosmetic nail care can cause thinning of the nails and actual onycholysis. A lack of proper hygiene can lead to infections, including mycobacterial infections. Occasionally patients will present with allergic contact dermatitis from components of their care. Ultraviolet light is used to cure nail gels, and skin exposed in the process should be shielded. It should be noted that these concerns can be encountered but that cosmetic nail care may be of benefit to patients with a variety of nail disorders [11].

43.5 Common Nail Pathologies

Here we review only several of the most common nail pathologies. This is not meant to be a comprehensive review. An excellent summary of how to diagnose and treat common nail maladies is in the chapter of M. Lorizzo entitled "Tips to Treat the 5 Most Common Nail Disorders" [12].

43.5.1 Onychomycosis

Some men are bothered by the discoloration and irregular shape of nails with onychomycosis (Fig. 43.1) [13]. The review article by Lipner and Scher discusses the current state of the art in medical and surgical management of onychomycosis. Nails grow slowly, and patients must be counselled that results will generally not be apparent overnight. Treatment courses are by in

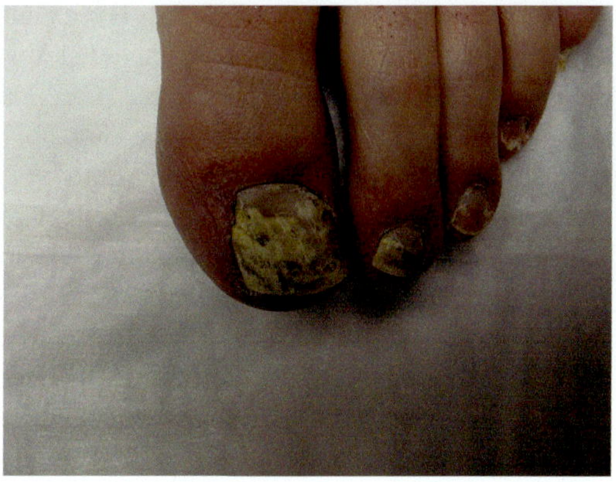

Fig. 43.1 Patient presenting with onychomycosis of the toenails

large lengthy and an initial response may be followed by recurrence. There is need for a broad knowledge of how to treat the problem, for strategies should be matched to particular patients for the best results [13]. If a patient raises this concern, the first order of business is to establish an accurate diagnosis with a careful examination and history. This is important because other disease states can present similarly such as psoriasis. It is important to obtain a culture specimen for fungi as it will confirm the diagnosis and direct most appropriate therapy. Scraping under the nail or clippings of nail plate will afford material for evaluation in a mycology laboratory. Hyphae and spores may be seen under the physician-performed microscopy in office, or nail clippings can be sent to pathology for PAS stain or PCR identification of fungal organisms, but ONLY culture will yield results identifying the genus and species of the dermatophyte (e.g., *Trichosporon*, *Epidermophyton*) or non-dermatophyte fungal organism (e.g., *Candidiasis*, *Fusarium*, *Scatylidium*). When the diagnosis is made, some discussion should follow to determine what sort of treatment the patient wishes to pursue (Table 43.1).

Prescription topical therapies consist of ciclopirox 8% lacquer, efinaconazole 10% solution, or Tavaborole 5% solution for dermatophyte infections. Although treatment success increases with duration of treatment, they have been demonstrated to be only up to 30–45% effective at

48 weeks of daily treatment [14, 15]. For extensively diseased nails, oral therapies include terbinafine (Dermatophyte sp.), fluconazole (Candida sp.), and Itraconazole (dermatophyte and non-dermatophyte species). These agents require several weeks of therapy, but the desired effect of returning the nail to normal may take up to 6 months for fingernails and 12 months for toenails in up to 80% of cases only [16]. These agents can have significant drug-drug interactions and side effects that the patient must be informed about. Nail plate avulsion +/− phenol matrixectomy can be used for onychomycosis with secondary severe onychauxis (thickened nails) and onychogryphosis. The procedure will require a digital block which can cause significant discomfort [17]. Rather than removing the nail surgically and if unable to utilize oral antifungal medications, an alternative is the application of 50% urea paste under occlusion with athletic tape q 48 hrs and repeat till the nail dissolves. This medication is only available at compounding pharmacies and should be used at a 50% concentration as 40% urea cream is not as effective. In 10 to 12 days, the nail will lift off the nail matrix and it can be trimmed back to its base. All the above can allow improvement which may not prove permanent, but it may be repeated as needed for recurrence. If no pain or disability results from the nail fungus, no therapy may be indicated. However, patients with history of diabetes, recurrent lower leg cellulitis, or *on long-term immunosuppression should be considered for these therapies.*

Table 43.1 Onychomycosis

Medication	Dosing	Side effects
Ciclopirox 8% nail lacquer (topical) [2]	Fingernails: Daily for 24 weeks Toenails: Daily for 48 weeks	Burning, itching, redness
Efinaconazole 10% solution (topical) [2]	Toenails: daily for 48 weeks	Burning, itching, redness
Tavaborole 5% solution (topical) [2]	Toenails: daily for 48 weeks	Burning, itching, redness
Terbinafine (systemic, po) [2]	Fingernails: 250 mg qd for 6 weeks Toenails: 250 mg qd for 12 weeks	Headache, gastrointestinal symptoms, rash, among others (rare—Liver injury/failure, neutropenia, thrombocytopenia, anemia, among others)
Itraconazole (systemic, po) [2]	Fingernails: 200 mg BID 1 week per month for 2 months Toenails: 200 mg qd for 12 weeks for toenails	Headache, rhinitis, upper respiratory tract infection, among others (Rare—Liver injury/failure, leukopenia, thrombocytopenia, congestive heart failure, among others)
Fluconazole (systemic, po) [28]	150 mg weekly for more than 6 months	Headache, nausea, abdominal pain, diarrhea (Rare—Seizures, Stevens-Johnson syndrome, liver failure)

43.5.2 Onychocryptosis

Onychocryptosis (ingrown nail) (Fig. 43.2) can often be addressed with the simple measure of packing cotton fiber from a Q-tip under the buried end of the offending nail. In most cases, maintaining the packing and slowly augmenting it when changed can reshape the nail and deliver it to a comfortable and safe position. This condition may be managed conservatively with gutter

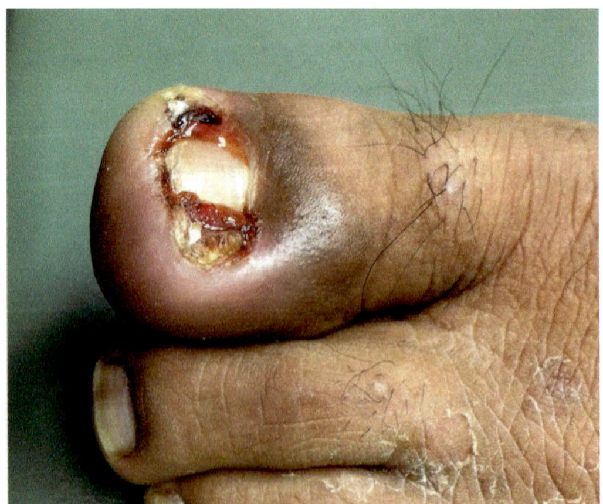

Fig. 43.2 Patient presenting with onychocryptosis. (Courtesy of Arthur Huen, MD, Pittsburgh VAMC, Department of Dermatology)

splint treatment, whereby a guard is placed between the lateral nail plate and fold and fixed in place; braces may also be used to open the curvature of the nail.

Surgical management for onychocryptosis involves either removal of soft tissue or reduction of nail plate width. A portion of the nail may be avulsed, allowing the nail to grow outward without pressure on the lateral nail folds [18]. A portion of the ipsilateral nail matrix may be excised, with narrowing of the resulting nail plate, and phenol may be applied for selective cauterization [18]. As an alternative, an ellipse of skin lateral to the lateral nail fold may be excised to pull the fold laterally from the nail, thereby relieving pressure.

Ingrown toenails are a frequent source of concern and even disability until the problem is solved. At times, a surgical solution is indicated. Studies have been conducted on the outcome of direct removal of the buried nail component and the nail matrix that gives rise to it. An alternative is lateral nail plate avulsion with chemomatricectomy using phenol, sodium hydroxide, or trichloroacetic acid. When the results of nail removal with subsequent surgical matricectomy versus phenol chemical matricectomy were compared, surgical matricectomy was more successful long term (around 5% recurrence rate) in patients, while phenol matricectomy was recurrent an average of 24% of the time. Despite the higher success rates associated with direct surgical excision of nail matrix, patient satisfaction with the post-treatment course was higher with the phenol treatment ($p = 0.028$). Ultimately, although the post-treatment course with phenol was easier to endure than the surgical course, both treatments had a high level of satisfaction when patients were queried [19]. Review of surgical procedures (Howard-Dubois and the super U techniques) is described by Di Chiacchio and Di Chiacchio [20].

43.5.3 Psoriatic Nails

An inflammatory disease affecting approximately 2% of the population, the majority of patients with psoriatic arthritis experience involvement of their nails and in some patients this may be the only manifestation of the disease [21]. Patients with nail psoriasis may experience distress, and traditionally, the condition has been challenging to treat. The changes usually affect several nails and include a variety of signs depending on whether the nail matrix, the nail bed, or both are involved (Fig. 43.3). Manifestations may include subungual hyperkeratosis, onycholysis, and pitting. Nail matrix involvement is characterized by nail pitting, surface ridging, and nail plate thickening. Nail bed disease presents with salmon patches, onycholysis, subungual hyperkeratosis, and rarely pustules [12]. Most specific for nail psoriasis are oil drops (a yellowish-orange discoloration), subungual hyperkeratosis, onycholysis, and pitting [22]. Psoriatic nails must be differentiated from onychomycosis and lichen planus, and cultures should be obtained to ensure appropriate treatment. Often pustular nail psoriasis is inappropriately diagnosed as an acute paronychia. Psoriatic arthritis should be suspected when a onychodystrophy is associate with bone pain and digital inflammation ("Sausage digit").

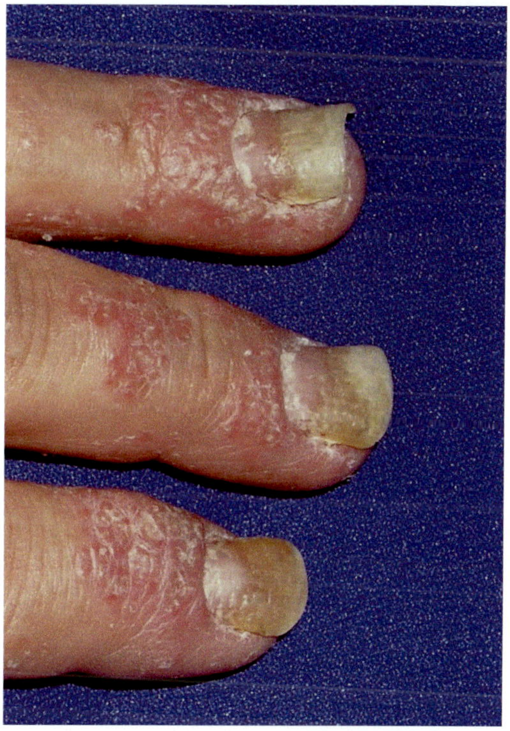

Fig. 43.3 Patient presenting with psoriatic nails

Adequate treatment duration corresponds to the duration of nail growth, with 6 months for fingers, and longer for toes, and initial approach depends on disease severity [22]. The challenge for the treating physician is to choose a therapy with a minimum of complications for the patient (Table 43.2). There is no definitive curative treatment, and treatment is directed at long-term control of the disorder. The exhaustive review by McClanahan and English [22] details the broad range of therapeutic options available, including treatments for lichen planus. The reader is directed there for detailed therapeutic strategies, including therapeutic ladders showing the escalation of treatment options as necessary. In brief, for mild disease, topical steroids may be first attempted, avoiding systematic side effects. Topical tazarotene and tacrolimus have also been utilized with success [22]. Intralesional injection with corticosteroids has also been described, albeit with a 36% discontinuation rate secondary to pain upon injection [18, 22]. For more severe cases, for recalcitrant disease, or when multiple nails are involved, systematic treatments, including methotrexate, cyclosporine, acitretin, apremilast, and biologics (e.g. adalimumab), may be prescribed [22].

Nail care is important, and reminding the patient that trauma will worsen the condition of the nails is crucial to limiting adverse progression. Topical therapy can make a difference but will generally be an addition to systemic care.

43.5.4 Lichen Planus

Lichen planus afflicts 0.5–1% of the population, with 10% of those with cutaneous manifestations also having nail involvement. Clinical features present in the nails include longitudinal ridging (onychorrhexis) (Fig. 43.4), fissuring (excessive brittleness), and erythronychia. Both nail bed and the nail matrix are affected. Nail matrix involvement produces splinter hemorrhages, onycholysis, and subungual hyperkeratosis. Approximately 20% of patients will progress to developing an end-stage dorsal pterygium with destruction of the nail matrix and a V-shaped extension of the proximal nail fold [22]. Therapeutic options are based on treatment of generalized lichen planus to include topical retinoids and steroids with or without oral methotrexate or acitretin.

Table 43.2 Psoriatic nails

Medication	Dosing	Side effects
Clobetasol nail lacquer 0.05% Or betamethasone dipropionate (0.05%) (topical) [29]	Daily or BID	Skin atrophy (Rare with prolonged use—atrophy of underlying distal phalanx, among others)
Methotrexate (systemic, po) [30]	Fingernails: 5 mg/week to 15 mg/week, not to exceed 22.5 mg/week, for 9 months Toenails: 5 mg/week to 15 mg/week, not to exceed 22.5 mg/week, for 13 months	Liver and kidney toxicity, bone marrow suppression
Cyclosporine (systemic, po) [31]	3 mg/kg/day for 48 weeks	Abdominal pain, nausea, vomiting, sore throat, hypertension, leukopenia, thrombocytopenia
Acitretin (systemic, po) [32]	0.2–0.3 mg/kg/day for 6 months	Dryness of skin and mucous membranes, hypertriglyceridemia, hepatitis
Apremilast (systemic, po) [33]	30 mg bid for 52 weeks	Diarrhea, nausea, headache, upper respiratory tract infection, nasopharyngitis
Adalimumab (systemic, po) [34]	40 mg every other week for 26 weeks	Redness, itching, infection (rare—Liver disease, seizures, chest pain)

43.5.5 Photoonycholysis

Photoonycholysis (Fig. 43.5) may be secondary to one of several conditions, and may rarely be spontaneous. Pain may precede the physical appearance. The nail then separates off of the central nail bed, leaving the lateral edges intact. There are several variations beyond this, some involving abnormalities of pigmentation, such as brownish or yellow staining, while bullae may also develop [23]. Common causative medications include NSAIDS, tetracyclines, isotretinoin and etretinate, 5-fluorouracil, amiodarone, cyclosporine, dapsone, pyridoxine, and sulfonylureas, chemotherapy, among others [23]. Photoonycholysis may also be associated with porphyria and pseudoporphyria [23, 24]. Ultraviolet light and medication exposure (e.g., naproxen) can cause a pseudoporphyria but does not exhibit the characteristic elevations in porphyrins. Treatment of photoonycholysis is limited, with the most effective management being eliminating the underlying cause.

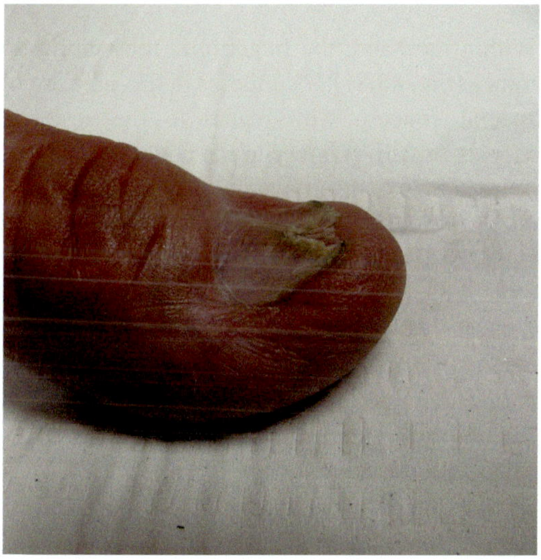

Fig. 43.4 Patient presenting with changes secondary to lichen planus

43.5.6 Paronychia

Paronychia refers to an infection of the eponychial folds and may be either acute (less than 6 weeks duration) or chronic [25]. Acute paronychia (Fig. 43.6) occurs secondary to bacterial infiltration of the nail fold following trauma, which may be as minor as picking a hangnail.

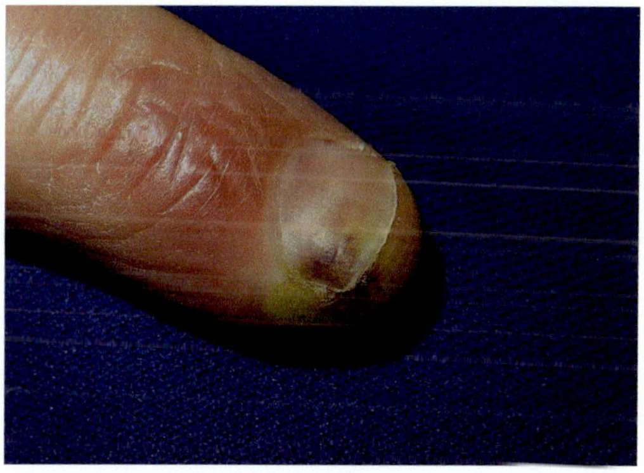

Fig. 43.6 Patient presenting with acute paronychia and purulence of the eponychial fold

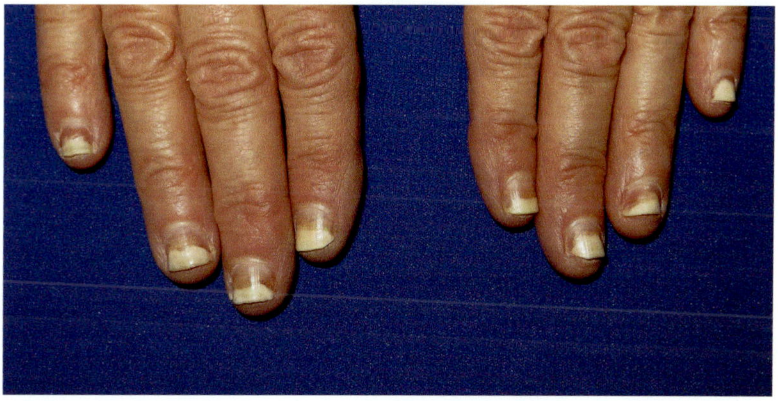

Fig. 43.5 Patient presenting with photoonycholysis

Paronychia is more likely to occur in patients with nail biting and poor nail hygiene. Should purulence be present, a quick incision and drainage is all that is often required, but if extensive, a digital block should be placed and the perionychial fold incised, sending cultures of drainage. *Staphylococcus aureus* is the most frequent infectious agent and antibiotics covering this organism should be prescribed. Unresponsive patients, or those at high risk such as patients with diabetes or those who are immunocompromised, may receive intravenous antibiotics, and cases of felon and flexor tenosynovitis *must* be differentiated, and these cases should be immediately referred to a surgeon trained in hand surgery. Felon will present with infection of the distal finger pulp and associated pain, erythema, and fullness over the volar distal phalanx, while flexor tenosynovitis will present with pain to palpation along the flexor tendon sheath, finger held in flexion, pain with passive extension and fusiform swelling. Warm soaks and elevation should be adhered to. Should acute paronychia be more extensive and involve the nail bed, or be unresponsive to incision and debridement and antibiotics, the nail plate should be removed in part or in its entirety, and the eponychial fold stented with iodiform gauze.

Chronic paronychia (Fig. 43.7) most frequently results from *Candida albicans*, although it may result from *Pseudomonas* ("green nail") or atypical mycobacteria (*M. marinum*). Patients exposed chronically to moisture and those with compromised immune systems are more likely to suffer from this condition. These patients have a longer duration of symptoms. High-dose topical steroids (e.g., Clobetasol solution 0.05%) applied under proximal nail fold have been demonstrated to allow regrowth of the cuticle and reduction of nail fold inflammation and swelling [26]. Failing this, eponychial marsupialization may be performed following a digital block and removing a strip of skin proximal to the eponychial fold, allowing the wound to close by secondary intention.

43.5.7 Nail Trauma

Within the hand, the fingertip is most prone to injury (Fig. 43.8) [27]. Injuries in this area are of special concern with regard to the aesthetic aspects of nail as injury to the nailbed, as, if left untreated, may result in deformity at which point correction may require surgical intervention and even so result in incomplete correction.

Upon presentation, fingertip injuries should be thoroughly irrigated and cleaned to allow for adequate inspection. History of tetanus vaccine should be taken and updated as appropriate. A digital block should be performed if pain interferes with the examination.

Subungual hematomas are a frequent pathology in the emergency department. Trephination, using either heated battery-powered cautery or a heated paper clip, may be performed for hemato-

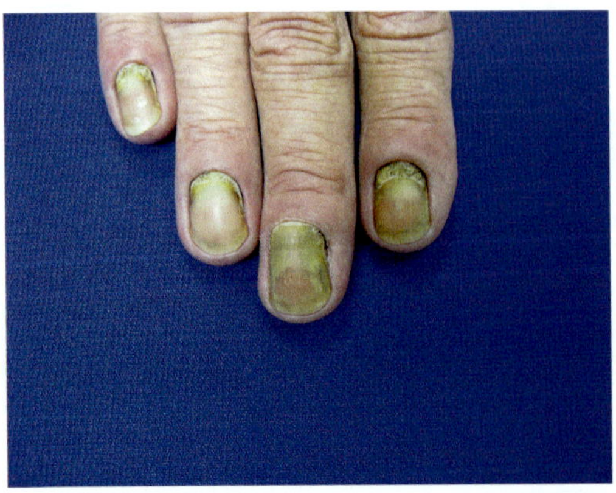

Fig. 43.7 Patient presenting with changes secondary to chronic paronychia

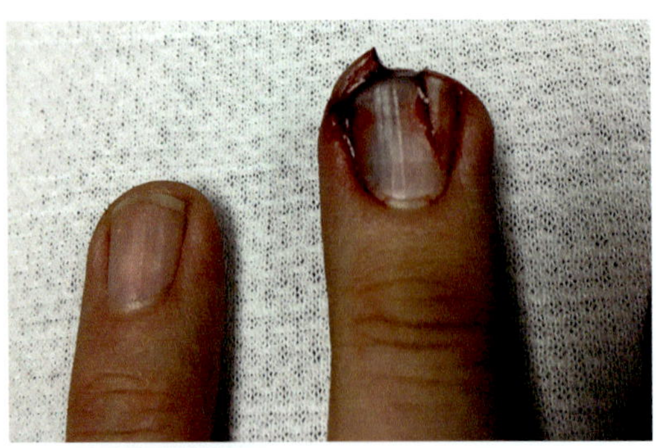

Fig. 43.8 Acute nail trauma, involving injury to the nailbed and surrounding soft tissues

mas smaller than 50% of the nail bed area. Subungual hematomas greater than 50% or those in association with distal phalanx fracture can benefit from nail plate removal and nail bed repair to prevent nail plate nonadherence. In these cases, a digital block is performed, and the nail plate is carefully elevated using a tool of choice, such as an elevator or scissors. The nail bed is then examined and repaired either with tissue glue or with absorbable suture. The avulsed nail or a substitute such as foil from a packet of suture should be placed within the eponychial fold in order to prevent formation of synechiae and resulting ridging. Should any nail bed be avulsed, it should be replaced as a graft when possible.

Patients should be counseled as to the length required for new nail growth, and any distal phalanx fractures should be splinted and treated with a course of oral antibiotics. Long-term deformities may result, even with appropriate management. Onychorrhexis (nail ridges/tenting) results from a scarred nail bed; split nails result from scar within the nail matrix. These may often be managed with scar excision and nail bed repair, but pending severity may require transfer from another anatomical area such as the great toe for adequate correction.

References

1. Bean WB. Nail growth. Thirty-five years of observation. Arch Internal Med. 1980;140(1):73–6. https://doi.org/10.1001/archinte.1980.00330130075019.
2. Lipner SR, Scher RK. Biotin for the treatment of nail disease: what is the evidence? J Dermatol Treat. 2018;29(4):411–4. https://doi.org/10.1080/09546634.2017.1395799.
3. Ylli D, Soldin SJ, Stolze B, et al. Biotin interference in assays for thyroid hormones, thyrotropin and thyroglobulin. Thyroid. 2021;31(8):1160–70. https://doi.org/10.1089/thy.2020.0866.
4. Sancar F. Update on biotin interference with troponin tests. JAMA. 2019;322(23):2277. https://doi.org/10.1001/jama.2019.20129.
5. Jurkic LM, Cepanec I, Pavelic SK, et al. Biological and therapeutic effects of ortho-silicic acid and some ortho-silicic acid-releasing compounds: new perspectives for therapy. Nutr Metab (Lond). 2013;10(1):2. https://doi.org/10.1186/1743-7075-10-2.
6. Barel A, Calomme M, Timchenko A, et al. Effect of oral intake of choline-stabilized orthosilicic acid on skin, nails and hair in women with photodamaged skin. Arch Dermatol Res. 2005;297(4):147–53. https://doi.org/10.1007/s00403-005-0584-6.
7. Winthrop KL, Abrams M, Yakrus M, Schwartz I, Ely J, Gilles D, Vugia DJ. An outbreak of mycobacterial furunculosis associated with footbaths at a nail salon. N Engl J Med. 2002;346(18):1366–71. https://doi.org/10.1056/NEJMoa012643.
8. Redbord KP, Shearer DA, Gloster H, Younger B, Connelly BL, Kindel SE, et al. Atypical mycobacterium furunculosis occurring after pedicures. J Am Acad Dermatol. 2006;54:520–4. https://doi.org/10.1016/j.jaad.2005.10.018.
9. Lipner SR. Onychomadesis following a fish pedicure. JAMA Dermatol. 2018;154:1091–2. https://doi.org/10.1001/jamadermatol.2018.1827.
10. Vanhooteghem O, Theate I. Fish pedicure-induced foot mycobacteriosis infection due to Mycobacterium marinum: a first case report. Eur J Dermatol. 2017;27:299–300. https://doi.org/10.1684/ejd.2017.2976.
11. Dinani N, George S. Nail cosmetics: a dermatological perspective. Clin Exp Dermatol. 2018; https://doi.org/10.1111/ced.13929.
12. Iorizzo M. Tips to treat the 5 most common nail disorders. Brittle nails, onycholysis, paronychia, psoriasis, onychomycosis. Dermatol Clin. 2015;33:175–83. https://doi.org/10.1016/j.det.2014.12.001.
13. Lipner SR, Scher RK. Onychomycosis. J Am Acad Dermatol. 2019;80:853–67. https://doi.org/10.1016/j.jaad.2018.05.1260.
14. Elewski BE, Vlahovic TC, Korotzer A. Treatment for Onchomycosis: is it more effective than the clinical data suggests? J Clin Aesthet Dermatol. 2016;9(11):34–9.
15. Epstein E. How often does oral treatment of toenail onchomycosis produce a disease free nail? An analysis of published data. Arch Dermatol. 1998;134(12):1551–4.
16. Kuokkanen K, Alava S. Fluconazole in the treatment of onychomycosis caused by dermatophytes. J Dermatol Treat. 1993;3:115–7. https://doi.org/10.3109/09546639209088703.
17. Romero-Perez D, Betloch-Mas I, Encabo-Duran B. Onychocryptosis: a long-term retrospective and comparative follow-up study of surgical and phenol chemical matricectomy in 520 procedures. Int J Dermatol. 2017;56:221–4. https://doi.org/10.1111/ijd.13406.
18. Grover C, Bansal S, Nanda S, et al. Efficacy of triamcinolone acetonide in various acquired nail dystrophies. J Dermatol. 2005;32(12):963–8.
19. Hassel JC, Hassel AJ, Loser C. Phenol chemical matricectomy is less painful, with shsorter recovery times but higher recurrence rates, than surgical matricectomy: a patient's view.

Dermatologic Surg. 2010;36:1294–9. https://doi.org/10.1111/j.1524-4725.2010.01625.x.
20. Di Chiacchio N, Di Chiacchio NG. Best way to treat an ingrown toenail. Dermatol Clin. 2015;33:277–82. https://doi.org/10.1016/j.det.2014.12.009.
21. Christophers E. Psoriasis – epidemiology and clinical spectrum. Clin Exp Dermatol. 2001;26:314–20.
22. McClanahan DR, English JC. Therapeutics for adult nail psoriasis and nail lichen planus: a guide for clinicians. Am J Clin Dermatol. 2018;19(4):559–84. https://doi.org/10.1007/s40257-018-0350-0.
23. Baran R, Juhlin L. Photoonycholysis. Photodermatol Photoimmunol Photomed. 2002;18:202–7. https://doi.org/10.5001/omj.2016.12.
24. Green JJ, Manders SM. Pseudoporphyria. J Am Acad Dermatol. 2001;44:100–8.
25. Leggit JC. Acute and chronic paronychia. Am Fam Physician. 2017;96:44–51.
26. Tosti A, Piraccini BM, Ghetti E, Colombo MD. Topical steroids versus systemic antifungals in the treatment of chronic paronychia: an open, randomized double-blind and double dummy study. J Am Acad Dermatol. 2002;47:73–6.
27. Sorock GS, Lombardi DA, Hauser RB, et al. Acute traumatic occupational hand injuries: type, location, and severity. J Occup Environ Med. 2002;44:345–51.
28. Gupta AK, Drummond-Main C, Paquet M. Evidence-based optimal fluconazole dosing regimen for onychomycosis treatment. J Dermatolog Treat. 2013;24(1):75–80. https://doi.org/10.3109/09546634.2012.70330.
29. Piraccini BM, Starace M. Optimal management of nail disease in patients with psoriasis. Psoriasis (Aukl). 2015;5:25–33. https://doi.org/10.2147/PTT/S55338.
30. Gumusel M, Ozdemir M, Mevlitoglu I, Bodur S. Evaluation of the efficacy of methotrexate and cyclosporine therapies on psoriatic nails: a one-blind, randomized study. J Eur Acad Dermatol Venereol. 2011;25(9):1080–4. https://doi.org/10.1111/j.1468-3083.2010.03927.x.
31. Syuto T, Abe M, Ishibuchi H, Ishikawa O. Successful treatment of psoriatic nails with low-dose cyclosporine administration. Eur J Dermatol. 2007;17(3):248–9. https://doi.org/10.1684/ejd.2007.0163.
32. Tosti A, Ricotti C, Romanelli P, Cameli N, Piraccini BM. Evaluation of the efficacy of acitretin therapy for nail psoriasis. Arch Dermatol. 2009;145(3):269–71. https://doi.org/10.1001/archdermatol.2008.600.
33. Rich P, Gooderham M, Bachelez H, et al. Apremilast, an oral phosphodiesterase 4 inhibitor, in patients with difficult-to-treat nail and scalp psoriasis: results of 2 phase III randomized, controlled trials (ESTEEM 1 and ESTEEM 2). J Am Acad Dermatol. 2015;74(1):134–42.
34. Elewski BE, Okun MM, Papp K, Baker CS, Crowley JJ, Guillet G, et al. Adalimumab for nail psoriasis: efficacy and safety from the first 26 weeks of a phase 3, randomized, placebo-controlled trial. J Am Acad Dermatol. 2018;78(1):90–9. https://doi.org/10.1016/j.jaad.2017.08.029.

Laser and IPL Treatments for Men in Aesthetic Medicine

44

Eric Fuller and Blake Fuller

44.1 CO_2 Laser Treatments for Men in Aesthetic Medicine

44.1.1 Introduction

Men are increasingly embracing aesthetic treatments as part of their grooming and self-care routines. However, they often seek subtle, natural results that enhance their appearance without looking overdone. CO_2 lasers have become a go-to tool in addressing male-specific aesthetic concerns, offering precise, effective treatments with minimal downtime. From skin resurfacing to scar revision, CO_2 lasers provide men with a solution to maintain a youthful and refreshed appearance, while aligning with their preference for low-maintenance, high-impact results.

In this chapter, we will explore how CO_2 lasers are uniquely suited to meet the aesthetic needs of men and the benefits they offer in achieving natural, masculine results.

44.1.2 Key Uses of CO_2 Lasers for Men

1. *Skin Resurfacing for Aging Skin.*

As men age, they tend to develop deep wrinkles, particularly around the eyes, forehead, and mouth, due to their typically thicker skin and prominent facial expressions. CO_2 lasers are ideal for skin resurfacing in men, as they can treat these deeper wrinkles while promoting collagen regeneration to tighten and smooth the skin.

Skin resurfacing is particularly appealing to men because it offers subtle improvements without altering their natural appearance. The goal is not to erase every line but to soften the visible signs of aging, giving a more refreshed and youthful look. The controlled precision of the CO_2 laser allows for a natural finish, maintaining the rugged features that many men prefer.

E. Fuller · B. Fuller (✉)
Emvera Technologies, Aragon, GA, USA
e-mail: blake@emvera.com

K. Jeffords et al. (eds.), *Aesthetic Surgery for Men*, https://doi.org/10.1007/978-3-032-03840-1_44

Popular Areas for Men:
- Forehead wrinkles
- Crow's feet around the eyes
- Lines around the mouth
- Sun damage and uneven skin tone

44.2 Scar Revision

Scars, whether from acne, injury, or surgery, can significantly impact a man's confidence. CO_2 lasers are highly effective in improving the appearance of scars by smoothing the skin and stimulating the production of new skin cells. Acne scars, in particular, are a common concern among men, and CO_2 laser treatments offer a noninvasive way to diminish their appearance and restore even skin texture.

Men often prefer a more understated improvement, avoiding overly smooth skin, which may seem unnatural. Fractional CO_2 lasers are well-suited for this, as they allow for controlled depth and targeting, leaving surrounding skin intact for a balanced outcome. For many mal clients, scar revision provides a confidence boost without the need for surgical intervention or extensive recovery time.

44.3 Surgical Scars

CO_2 laser treatment is also an effective option for improving the appearance of surgical scars. It works by using focused laser light to remove the outer layer of skin and promote collagen production in the deeper layers. This can help smooth the texture, reduce discoloration, and improve overall skin quality.

Benefits:
- *Precision:* Targets specific areas without affecting surrounding tissue
- *Minimal downtime:* Most patients experience some redness and swelling, but recovery is usually quick
- *Long-lasting results:* Many see significant improvements after a few sessions

This approach to scar revision, especially with fractional CO_2 lasers, is ideal for men who seek a balanced improvement without dramatic changes, enhancing their confidence with minimal interruption to their daily lives.

Popular Treatments:
- Acne scar revision
- Surgical scar improvement
- Trauma-related scars

44.4 Facial Rejuvenation and Skin Tightening

Men typically have thicker, more collagen-rich skin than women, which gives them a natural advantage in aging slower. However, as they age, men may experience sagging skin, especially around the jawline, cheeks, and neck. CO_2 lasers can be used for nonsurgical facial rejuvenation to tighten loose skin and reduce the appearance of enlarged pores, leaving the skin looking firmer and more youthful.

Male clients often seek treatments that provide gradual, subtle results. CO_2 lasers excel at delivering such improvements, enhancing the jawline definition, reducing laxity, and addressing sun damage without the need for downtime. For men who want to maintain a strong, masculine appearance, laser skin tightening is a preferred option.

Popular Treatment Areas:
- Jawline and neck tightening
- Enlarged pores reduction
- Overall skin texture improvement
- Reduction of fine lines

44.5 Sun Damage Repair

Men, especially those who spend a lot of time outdoors, are prone to sun damage, which can lead to hyperpigmentation, fine lines, and rough skin texture. CO_2 lasers are an excellent option for treating these issues, as they work by removing damaged skin layers and encouraging the growth of new, healthier skin. The result is smoother, clearer skin with fewer signs of sun damage.

Popular Treatments:
- Sunspots and pigmentation reduction
- Evening out skin tone
- Improving rough, sun-damaged skin

44.5.1 Advantages of CO_2 Lasers for Men

- *Subtle, Natural-Looking Results:* Men generally prefer treatments that yield subtle, natural results. CO_2 lasers can rejuvenate the skin without creating a "done" look, making them ideal for male clients who want to improve their appearance without drawing attention to the fact that they've had a cosmetic procedure.
- *Minimal Downtime and Discretion:* CO_2 laser treatments are minimally invasive, which is important to many men who prioritize quick recovery and discretion. Many men prefer treatments that allow them to return to work and daily activities with minimal interruption, and CO_2 laser treatments often fit these criteria.
- *Targeting Specific Concerns:* From wrinkles to scars, CO_2 lasers offer a tailored approach to each individual concern. Men appreciate the precision and control that CO_2 lasers provide, allowing them to address specific issues without the need for more extensive procedures.
- *Long-Term Benefits:* CO_2 lasers not only provide immediate improvements but also stimulate collagen production, leading to ongoing skin rejuvenation. This is particularly appealing to men who want to maintain youthful skin over the long term without frequent touch-ups.

44.5.2 Considerations for Male Patients

Men have distinct aesthetic goals and skin characteristics that must be considered when performing CO_2 laser treatments:

- *Thicker Skin:* Men typically have thicker skin and more sebaceous (oil-producing) glands than women, which can influence how the skin reacts to laser treatments. This often allows for more aggressive laser settings to achieve desired results.
- *Hair Density:* Facial and body hair, particularly around areas like the beard, must be considered when planning CO_2 laser treatments to avoid damage to hair follicles.
- *Masculine Features:* Men often want to maintain their masculine features, such as strong jawlines and defined facial structure. CO_2 lasers can be used to subtly improve the appearance of wrinkles and sagging skin without creating an overly smooth or "feminine" appearance.

44.5.3 Conclusion

CO_2 laser treatments are a powerful tool in male aesthetics, offering effective solutions for wrinkles, scars, sun damage, and skin laxity. By providing natural-looking results with minimal downtime, these treatments align with the needs of today's male clients. Whether it's rejuvenating aging skin or improving scars, CO_2 lasers offer men a discreet yet impactful way to enhance their appearance and maintain their confidence.

With a deeper understanding of male skin physiology and aesthetic preferences, practitioners can use CO_2 lasers to deliver tailored treatments that cater specifically to the goals of men, allowing them to look and feel their best.

44.6 Intense Pulsed Light (IPL) Systems for Men in Aesthetic Medicine

44.6.1 Introduction

As men increasingly seek noninvasive cosmetic treatments to enhance their appearance, Intense Pulsed Light (IPL) systems have become a popular option due to their versatility, effectiveness, and minimal downtime. IPL devices are especially well-suited for male clients who want to address common skin concerns such as sun damage, unwanted hair, acne, and uneven skin tone while maintaining a natural and masculine look.

This section explores how IPL systems are used for men's aesthetic treatments, focusing on the key areas that matter most to male clients and the specific benefits of IPL for this demographic.

44.6.2 Key Uses of IPL for Men

1. *Photorejuvenation for Sun Damage and Pigmentation*

Men are often exposed to more sun over their lifetime, leading to sun spots, age spots, and pigmentation irregularities, especially on the face, neck, and hands. IPL is highly effective for treating these issues by targeting melanin in the skin and breaking down pigmented cells. This treatment can restore a more even skin tone, reduce visible damage, and promote healthier-looking skin.

Popular Treatment Areas for Men:
- Face and forehead
- Neck and chest (especially for men who spend time outdoors)
- Hands and arms

For men, IPL photorejuvenation provides a subtle but noticeable improvement in skin tone without the need for extensive downtime, making it ideal for those with busy lifestyles.

2. *Hair Removal*

IPL is commonly used for long-term hair reduction, and for men, this is a particularly appealing treatment for areas with dense, coarse hair, such as the back, chest, shoulders, and neck. Unlike shaving or waxing, which can lead to ingrown hairs and irritation, IPL offers a more permanent solution by damaging hair follicles and inhibiting future growth.

Popular Hair Removal Areas:
- Back and shoulders
- Chest and abdomen
- Neck (for reducing beard shadow or treating irritation from shaving)

Men typically have thicker hair, which can require more sessions than women for optimal results. However, the long-lasting benefits of IPL hair removal make it an attractive option for those seeking a cleaner, more polished appearance.

3. *Vascular Treatments (Spider Veins and Rosacea)*

Vascular issues such as spider veins, facial redness, and rosacea are common concerns for men, particularly those with lighter skin types. IPL can effectively treat these vascular conditions by targeting the blood vessels beneath the skin's surface without damaging the surrounding tissue. For men who experience redness or visible veins, especially on the nose or cheeks, IPL treatments provide a noninvasive solution to improve complexion and boost confidence.

Popular Vascular Treatment Areas:
- Nose and cheeks (for rosacea and broken capillaries)
- Legs (for spider veins)
- Facial veins due to sun exposure or genetics

4. *Acne and Acne Scar Treatment*

Adult acne is a persistent issue for many men, and IPL can be an effective part of an acne treatment regimen. By targeting the bacteria that cause acne and reducing excess oil production from sebaceous glands, IPL helps to minimize breakouts and prevent future acne. In addition to treating active acne, IPL can also reduce the redness and inflammation associated with it.

IPL is also beneficial for improving the appearance of acne scars, as it stimulates collagen production, promoting smoother, healthier skin over time. For men dealing with acne or its aftermath, IPL offers a noninvasive, convenient way to manage these concerns.

5. *Improving Skin Texture and Tone*

Men who are looking to refresh their appearance without undergoing invasive procedures can benefit from IPL's ability to improve skin texture and tone. By stimulating collagen production and targeting pigmentation and vascular issues, IPL treatments help to even out skin tone, reduce fine lines, and promote a more youthful appearance. This is especially appealing to male clients who want subtle, natural enhancements without the risk of looking over-treated.

Common Skin Texture Concerns Treated by IPL:

- Fine lines and early signs of aging
- Enlarged pores
- Uneven skin tone due to sun exposure or pigmentation

44.6.3 Advantages of IPL Treatments for Men

- *Noninvasive and Minimal Downtime:* Men often prefer treatments that require little to no recovery time, and IPL fits this preference perfectly. Most men can resume their regular activities immediately after treatment, making it ideal for those with demanding schedules.
- *Versatility:* IPL systems can address a variety of skin concerns, from pigmentation to vascular issues, acne, and hair removal, offering men a comprehensive solution to improve their appearance in a single device.
- *Natural-Looking Results:* IPL treatments deliver gradual improvements that help men look refreshed and rejuvenated without appearing dramatically altered. This aligns with the preference for subtle, natural enhancements that maintain a masculine appearance.
- *Long-Term Benefits:* Regular IPL sessions can improve skin quality over time, thanks to the collagen stimulation and ongoing reduction in pigmentation and redness. Men looking for a long-term skincare solution will find IPL a reliable, nonsurgical option.

44.6.4 Considerations for Treating Male Clients

When using IPL systems for male clients, practitioners should consider the following:

- *Thicker Skin and Coarse Hair:* Men tend to have thicker skin and coarser hair, which may require stronger settings or more sessions to achieve optimal results, particularly in hair removal treatments.
- *Post-Treatment Care:* Men may need more guidance on skincare after IPL treatments, particularly regarding sun protection and post-treatment care, as many men are less familiar with cosmetic aftercare routines.
- *Masculine Aesthetic Goals:* Men typically seek improvements that enhance their appearance while maintaining a rugged, natural look. IPL treatments should be adjusted to avoid overly smoothing the skin, ensuring that results appear subtle and in line with masculine aesthetic preferences.

44.6.5 Conclusion

IPL systems offer an effective, versatile, and non-invasive option for men seeking aesthetic enhancements. Whether addressing pigmentation, vascular issues, acne, or unwanted hair, IPL provides men with a way to improve their appearance with minimal downtime and natural-looking results. As the demand for male cosmetic treatments continues to grow, IPL remains a valuable tool in any aesthetic practice, offering tailored treatments that cater to men's unique skin and aesthetic needs.

44.7 Laser Hair Removal for Men: A Guide to Effective and Lasting Results

44.7.1 Introduction

Laser hair removal has become a popular solution for men seeking to reduce or eliminate unwanted body hair in a long-lasting, noninvasive way. Whether for aesthetic reasons, hygiene, or sports performance, more men are turning to this procedure to achieve a cleaner, more streamlined look without the hassle of constant shaving or waxing. Laser hair removal is effective, efficient, and offers long-term results that appeal to men looking for low-maintenance grooming solutions.

This section discusses how laser hair removal works, the specific benefits for male clients, and how the procedure can be tailored to suit different hair types and body areas.

44.7.2 Key Points About Laser Hair Removal for Men

1. *Types of Lasers Used:* There are several types of lasers used in hair removal, each with its own strengths, depending on the client's skin tone and hair type. The most commonly used lasers for men include the following.
   - *Alexandrite Lasers:* These lasers are ideal for men with lighter skin and darker hair, providing fast and effective results, especially on larger areas like the back or chest.
   - *Diode Lasers:* Suitable for a broader range of skin types, diode lasers are frequently used for men with both lighter and medium skin tones, making them a versatile option for various body areas.
   - *Nd:YAG Lasers:* Best suited for men with darker skin tones, this laser penetrates deeper into the skin and is less likely to cause hyperpigmentation, making it safer for men with more melanin in their skin.
2. Understanding the right laser for each client is crucial in achieving optimal hair removal results and ensuring that the procedure is both safe and effective.
3. *Effectiveness Based on Skin and Hair Types:* Laser hair removal works by targeting the pigment (melanin) in the hair follicle, which absorbs the light energy, damaging the follicle and inhibiting future hair growth. Men with light skin and dark hair generally experience the best results because the contrast allows the laser to effectively target the hair follicle without affecting the surrounding skin.

   However, advancements in laser technology, such as the Nd:YAG and diode lasers, have made it possible for men with darker skin or lighter hair to also benefit from the procedure. It is important for men to consult with a knowledgeable provider who can select the appropriate laser for their specific skin and hair combination.
4. *Areas Commonly Treated in Men:* While laser hair removal can be applied to almost any area of the body, men typically focus on specific regions where hair growth is thicker and more persistent. The most popular treatment areas for men include:
   - *Back and Shoulders:* One of the most requested areas, particularly for men who want to achieve a smooth, hair-free back for aesthetic reasons or to reduce the discomfort of excess sweating and ingrown hairs.

- *Chest and Abdomen:* Many men choose to reduce or eliminate hair on their chest and stomach for a cleaner look or to enhance muscle definition.
- *Neck and Beard Line:* Laser hair removal on the neck helps men maintain a sharp, well-defined beard line and reduces the irritation caused by shaving, particularly for those prone to ingrown hairs.
- *Arms and Legs:* Some men, especially athletes, opt for hair removal on their arms and legs to improve their performance or for personal grooming preferences.

5. *Multiple Sessions for Best Results:* Hair grows in cycles, and laser hair removal is only effective on actively growing hair follicles. As a result, multiple sessions are required to achieve optimal results, typically spaced 4–6 weeks apart. On average, men may need between six to eight sessions to significantly reduce hair growth in a particular area.

   For large areas like the back or chest, the number of sessions may vary depending on the hair density and thickness, while smaller areas such as the neck or beard line can often be treated in fewer sessions.
6. *Precision and Speed:* One of the advantages of laser hair removal is its ability to target multiple hair follicles simultaneously, making it a relatively quick procedure, even for larger areas. A full back treatment, for example, can often be completed in under an hour, while smaller areas like the neck or beard line can take just a few minutes. The precision of the lasers also allows practitioners to target specific areas without affecting the surrounding skin.
7. *Comfort and Minimal Discomfort:* Most men report minimal discomfort during laser hair removal, often describing it as a mild snapping or tingling sensation. Many modern laser systems come equipped with cooling devices or the option of using a topical anesthetic to further enhance comfort during the procedure.

   The discomfort level can vary depending on the area being treated and the density of hair, with more sensitive areas such as the neck or chest being slightly more uncomfortable than areas like the back or shoulders.
8. *Long-Lasting Results:* While some hair may eventually regrow after treatment, it is typically finer, lighter, and less noticeable than before. For most men, laser hair removal offers long-term hair reduction, with many clients enjoying smooth skin for months or even years after completing their treatment sessions. Regular maintenance sessions may be required to maintain results over time, but the amount of hair regrowth is significantly reduced compared to shaving or waxing.

44.7.3 The Benefits of Laser Hair Removal for Men

- *Low Maintenance:* Men appreciate the long-term benefits of laser hair removal, which eliminates the need for daily shaving or frequent waxing. This is particularly valuable for those who have dense body hair and are tired of the time-consuming process of managing it.
- *Reduced Ingrown Hairs and Skin Irritation:* Shaving and waxing can lead to ingrown hairs, razor burn, and skin irritation—common issues for men, especially in areas like the neck and beard line. Laser hair removal helps to reduce these problems by targeting the hair at the follicle, preventing it from growing back in a way that leads to irritation.
- *Enhanced Athletic Performance:* For athletes, particularly swimmers, cyclists, and bodybuilders, reducing body hair can improve performance and enhance aesthetics. Smooth skin reduces drag in water sports and allows for better visibility of muscle definition.
- *Aesthetic Appeal and Confidence:* Many men seek laser hair removal to feel more confident in their appearance, whether it's removing unwanted back hair, achieving a smooth chest, or defining a clean beard line. This contributes to a more polished, groomed appearance, which can boost self-esteem in both personal and professional settings.

44.7.4 Conclusion

Laser hair removal is an excellent solution for men who want to reduce or eliminate unwanted hair with minimal effort and long-lasting results. Whether for aesthetic reasons, improved hygiene, or enhanced athletic performance, this noninvasive procedure offers men a convenient, effective way to achieve their grooming goals. With advancements in laser technology, virtually all skin and hair types can benefit from laser hair removal, making it a versatile and appealing option for men looking to simplify their hair care routine.

Tissue Micro-coring (Ellacor®) 45

Krishna Vyas and William G. Austen, Jr.

45.1 Introduction

With aging, changes to the skin and underlying structures disrupt ideal facial proportions associated with attractiveness and youthfulness. Aged skin is characterized by thinning epidermis and dermis, collagen loss, altered elastin organization, and flattened rete ridges, among other histologic and cellular changes. Thus, skin rejuvenation aims to restore the typical architecture of the skin, remove damaged collagen, and promote new collagen growth.

Perioral rhytids and skin laxity are hallmarks of facial aging, particularly in the lower face. Perioral aging is often accompanied by vertical lengthening of a deflated upper lip; less pronounced philtral columns; reduction of visible vermilion, white roll, and cupid's bow; thinning cutis from degradation of collagen and elastic; atrophy of the orbicularis oris; increase of perioral rhytids; and deepening of the nasolabial folds. Clinically, this presents as lengthening of the upper lip with thinning of the vermillion, decrease of incisor show, and loss of anterior projection. Facial rejuvenation techniques aim to restore a youthful appearance. Traditionally, skin laxity has been addressed with surgery; however, there is increasing demand for alternative treatments with less downtime, risk, and scarring.

Although various nonsurgical and surgical options exist to improve facial aesthetics, it is essential to understand that these elective procedures have inherent risks and limitations. For example, ablative lasers work by resurfacing the epidermis and upper dermis to improve the skin appearance but often require multiple treatments and involve thermal energy, which risks severe complications such as scarring or dyspigmentation, particularly in higher Fitzpatrick skin types. Fractional ablative lasers create microthermal islands of ablation and coagulation surrounded by undamaged tissue that promotes regeneration but still have risks of scarring, prolonged erythema, and dyspigmentation. Furthermore, these do not remove skin or address skin laxity. Surgical lip lifts can improve the perioral area but can be associated with long, noticeable scars and do not significantly improve perioral rhytids. Facelifts address facial skin laxity but require surgery, long scars, and prolonged recovery and do not address the perioral area.

Tissue micro-coring addresses a critical treatment gap in aesthetic technologies, removing full-thickness skin and improving rhytids on a microscale without surgery, energy, scarring, or prolonged downtime. The technology uses an array of hollow hypodermic needles to remove cores of skin (below the threshold for scarring); this incites a healing response that promotes

K. Vyas · W. G. Austen, Jr. (✉)
Division of Plastic and Reconstructive Surgery, Massachusetts General Hospital and Harvard Medical School, Boston, MA, USA
e-mail: wausten@mgh.harvard.edu

K. Jeffords et al. (eds.), *Aesthetic Surgery for Men*, https://doi.org/10.1007/978-3-032-03840-1_45

collagen production and skin rejuvenation (Fig. 45.1). Ellacor® (Cytrellis Biosystems, Inc., Woburn, MA) is the first and only FDA-approved commercial micro-coring device to treat moderate to severe rhytids on the mid-to-lower face. Other applications that have been investigated include skin rejuvenation and tightening, pore size reduction, acne scar treatment, and scar revision. Since micro-coring does not generate thermal coagulation, it theoretically results in faster healing and is safer in higher Fitzpatrick skin types versus other energy-based aesthetic technologies.

45.1.1 Development

Ideal aesthetic technologies should be minimally invasive, low-risk, and well-tolerated with minimal downtime. Lasers and radiofrequency microneedling induce thermal injury to remodel skin but may not achieve significant skin tightening. Micro-coring removes full-thickness micro-cores of dermal and epidermal tissue. Before the development of dermal micro-coring technology, there was no way to excise skin without leaving a visible scar. This disruptive technology provides clinicians with a unique solution to address skin laxity. Ellacor® is a minimally invasive procedure that fills a gap between noninvasive options and surgery by diminishing the appearance of fine lines and wrinkles, reducing the appearance of jowls, and removing excess, sagging skin without incisions or scarring with an office-based procedure. The procedure can be performed under local anesthesia with tumescent and takes less than 1 h. Treatments can be repeated monthly in one or more sessions. On average, recovery takes about 1 week.

Energy-based devices such as lasers achieve fractional resurfacing, in which microscopic columns of skin are ablated via heat coagulation and necrosis of the dermis, resulting in microepidermal necrotic debris (MEND) that may prevent early closure of micro-cores and limit skin surface tightening and reduction. Since lasers use heat, adverse effects such as burns, scars, hyper- or hypopigmentation, and vascular necrosis may ensue.

Microneedling is a procedure that uses small needles to uniformly penetrate the dermis and create a controlled skin injury, which subsequently stimulates collagen and elastin fiber production, resulting in skin remodeling. Microneedling is used as a tool for skin rejuvenation, scars, drug delivery, and other indications and is occasionally combined with radiofrequency, which is thought to enhance dermal remodeling and clinical outcomes. However, microneedling is not effective in removing tissue or skin tightening.

45.1.2 Technology

Ellacor® (Cytrellis Biosystems, Inc., Woburn, MA) is a commercial FDA-approved mechanical dermal micro-coring technology approved for the

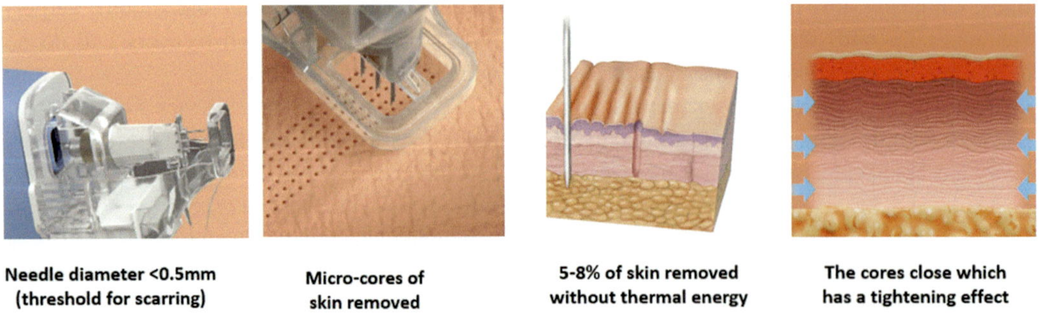

Fig. 45.1 **Micro-coring mechanism**. Up to 8% skin removal can be achieved in a single treatment, with depths of 3–5 mm. Micro-coring rejuvenates and tightens the skin, improves wrinkle and laxity, and creates new and increased collagen and elastin fibers without scarring

treatment of moderate to severe wrinkles in the mid to lower face of adults aged 22 and older with Fitzpatrick skin types I–IV. Invented at Massachusetts General Hospital and Harvard Medical School in Boston, MA, by William G. Austen, Jr., and Rox Anderson, MD, Ellacor® distinguishes itself from other nonsurgical and surgical skin rejuvenation methods by allowing scarless skin removal and healing without surgery or energy.

Most aesthetic modalities do not address skin redundancy, laxity, or wrinkling or are associated with prolonged recovery and the risk of scarring. Ellacor® is the first and only FDA-cleared procedure to remove skin excess by micro-coring using hollow hypodermic needles, thus allowing safe and scarless skin tightening and wrinkle improvement. Skin removal occurs within a 10 × 10 mm window of a triple-needle cartridge connected to a handpiece with suction. Each micro-core is an entire column of skin containing epidermis and dermis extracted by a 22-gauge core needle that removes 420-micrometer cores below the threshold that causes scar formation (<500 μm) [1]. This allows the skin to undergo a regenerative healing process that increases collagen and elastin content, epidermal and papillary dermal thickening, and restoration of rete ridges, resulting in rhytid improvement and skin-tightening. Up to 8% skin removal can be achieved in a single treatment, with depths of 3–4 mm [4]. Biomechanical remodeling results in the near-immediate closure of treatment cores and has been confirmed through optical coherence tomography. Micro-cores heal along the lines of relaxed skin tension.

Several multicenter clinical trials have shown safety and efficacy in skin tightness and wrinkle reduction. After micro-coring treatment, there are quantitative and directional reductions in the skin [8]. Micro-coring rejuvenates and tightens the skin, improves wrinkles and laxity, and creates new and increased collagen and elastin. Histology of treated areas in clinical trials showed no evidence of inflammation or scarring 90 days post-treatment [6].

45.1.3 Device

The system consists of a powered console (Fig. 45.2) with a reusable handpiece (Fig. 45.3), a foot switch, and a vacuum system (which includes a pump, filter, and suction tubing) to aspirate skin cores.

Console: Patient information is entered into the console; data include gender, age range, new or existing patient, and previous micro-coring treatments. The percentage of skin to be removed is selected or adjusted throughout the procedure. Selections include 1%, 3%, 5%, 7%, and 8%. A higher percentage of skin removal corresponds to more cores removed and a more aggressive treatment. Core penetration depth is customized for each patient in 0.5-mm increments from 0.0 mm to 4.0 mm.

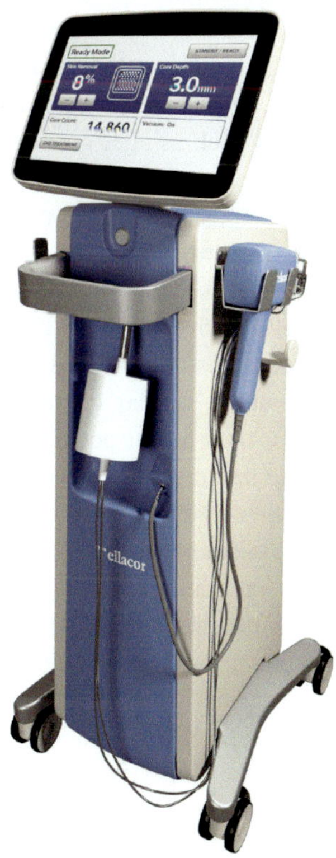

Fig. 45.2 **Ellacor Console**. Consists of interactive monitor, vacuum filter suction, and handheld coring apparatus

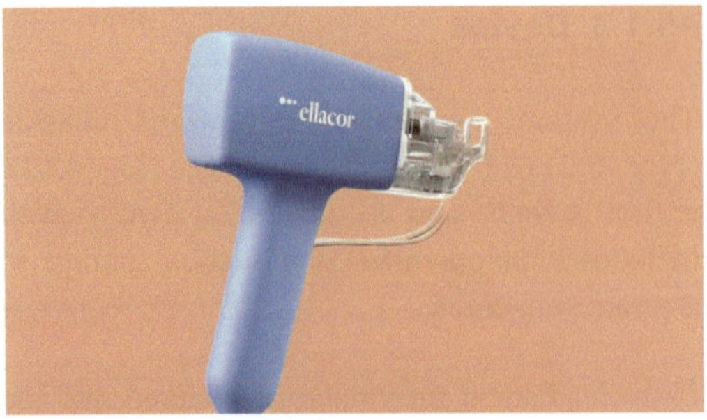

Fig. 45.3 **Handheld coring apparatus**. Ellacor is the first and only FDA-cleared procedure to remove skin excess by microcoring using hollow hypodermic needles, thus allowing safe and scarless skin tightening and wrinkle improvement. Skin removal occurs within a 10 × 10 mm window of a triple-needle cartridge connected to a handpiece with suction. Each micro-core is an entire column of skin containing epidermis and dermis extracted by a 22-gauge core needle that removes 420-micrometer cores, below the threshold that causes scar formation (<500 μm)

Initial settings should be based on patient assessment. Factors to consider include anatomic, skin laxity, quality, and texture; epidermal and dermal thickness; and patient demographics such as age, gender, BMI, and sun damage.

Handpiece: A disposable needle cartridge consisting of modified hollow stainless-steel hypodermic needles attaches to the handpiece. The needles remove 0.5 mm diameter full-thickness columns/micro-cores of skin in a fractional pattern, similar to punch biopsies. The operator uses a foot pedal to actuate the device at the treatment site. The needles penetrate the skin and extract tissue cores that are aspirated by vacuum suction.

Vacuum: The integrated suction stabilizes the skin while removing cores. During fractional laser treatment, defects are filled by microscopic epidermal necrotic debris (MEND), which limits contraction and skin tightening. The Ellacor® vacuum system allows for core aspiration, an essential component of skin tightening [5].

45.2 Technique

45.2.1 Patient Selection

Patient-specific factors to consider include patient expectations, age, gender, skin quality and texture, photodamage and exposure history, and relevant medical history (e.g., dermatologic, hematologic, or autoimmune conditions, immunosuppression, keloids or hypertrophic scars, or herpes simplex virus) and medications that could prolong healing or increase bleeding. History should also include prior treatments to the area (past or recent procedures or surgery, injectables, trauma, or scarring).

Patients should have moderate to severe skin laxity with or without rhytids. Patients with severe wrinkling or laxity are not ideal candidates. The procedure usually takes 30 min and is typically performed under local injectable anesthesia in the office. In our experience, many of our patients seek Ellacor® for skin rejuvenation with or without facelift procedures to address the perioral area that is otherwise not addressed with a facelift. If performed in combination with a facelift, Ellacor® is performed at the end of the procedure.

Careful assessment of the skin will help guide clinical decision-making and determine appropriate treatment settings.

45.2.1.1 Contraindications

Safety and efficacy have not been studied in several conditions. Ellacor® recommends against treating areas of skin with:

- Dermatosis (skin tumors, keloids or predisposition to keloids, solar keratosis, warts, or birthmarks)
- Dermatological or autoimmune conditions that may affect the treatment outcome, including but not limited to actinic keratosis, raised nevi, rosacea, melasma, active acne, cutaneous papules/nodules, active inflammatory

lesions, dermatitis, psoriasis, cellulitis, urticarial folliculitis, acute inflammatory phase of scleroderma, rheumatoid arthritis, eczema, psoriasis, allergic dermatitis, collagen disorders, or lupus
- Open wounds, sores, or irritated skin
- Areas within the bony orbital rim
- Mucous membranes
- Areas where silicone or synthetic material is implanted
- Pregnant or nursing individuals
- Systemic infections or acute local skin infections such as hepatitis or HIV
- Allergy to stainless steel or allergy to topical, oral, or injected medications or preparations that may be used during the procedure, such as local anesthetics)
- History of any clinically significant bleeding disorder
- High dose of anti-coagulants or blood-thinning substances (e.g., aspirin, nonsteroidal anti-inflammatory drugs, NSAIDs, warfarin, heparin, acetylsalicylic acid during the previous 2 weeks)
- High-dose chemotherapy, corticosteroid use, or radiation in the treatment area
- Scars less than 6 months old in the treatment area

Caution is warranted in patients with:

- History of hyperpigmentation
- Recent exposure to sun or tanning beds with red, peeling, or swollen skin
- Active, chronic, or recurrent infection, including bacterial or fungal infections
- History of active herpes simplex infection in the treatment area
- Use of topical or oral preparations/medications that may change the skin integrity or prolong healing
- Over-the-counter and herbal supplements that may increase the risk of bleeding or prolong healing, such as *Ginkgo biloba*, garlic, ginseng, dong quai, feverfew, and fish oil
- Other medications or medical conditions that may interfere with the treatment or that the treatment provider believes may compromise the patient's safety or the efficacy of the treatments.
- Recent trauma or surgery to the treatment area
- Injections of dermal fillers, fat, or botulinum toxin, or any minimally invasive/invasive skin treatment in the treatment area during the previous 6 months
- Undergone plastic surgery of the face within the last 12 months or have any facial surgical scars less than 12 months old

45.2.1.2 Imaging

All patients have standard and preoperative and postoperative two-dimensional and three-dimensional (3D) facial imaging with the VECTRA XT 3D Imaging System (Canfield Scientific, Inc., Fairfield, NJ) as part of the standard care for the senior author. VECTRA Imaging has been shown to provide validated and standardized stereophotogrammetry, and before/after photos are routinely shared with patients.

45.2.1.3 Consent

Discussing the risks, benefits, and alternatives of surgical facelifts, injectables, or energy devices is essential.

Patients with higher Fitzpatrick skin types are particularly susceptible to post-inflammatory hyperpigmentation and dyspigmentation with energy-based devices. Clinical studies evaluating micro-coring in Fitzpatrick IV to VI are lacking but should theoretically be safer. In our clinical experience and anecdotally, these patients with higher Fitzpatrick skin types have been successfully treated without prolonged erythema or dyspigmentation.

Patients must be willing to tolerate at least 3 days to 1 week of downtime with side effects such as ecchymoses, crusting, edema, erythema, burning, dryness, roughness, pain/discomfort, tenderness, tingling, bleeding, numbness, skin peeling, or circular marks on the skin. Other side effects not commonly observed with this procedure include itching, dyspigmentation, hematoma, infection, scarring, skin irregularities, skin necrosis, uneven appearance of the treated regions, or anesthesia toxicity (complications may include allergic reaction and death).

Patients are counseled and provided a printed copy of pre-procedure instructions (Table 45.1).

45.2.2 Preparation and Positioning

A Mayo prep stand is pre-prepared with all required supplies, including injectable anesthesia and 4 × 4 gauze. Patients are greeted and then taken to a procedure room, where they change into a gown. The patient is positioned comfortably in a reclining exam chair with the head elevated to 20–30 degrees and the hair secured in a net. Disposable medical absorbent chuck pads are placed on the patient's chest and shoulders and are secured with tape.

Table 45.1 Pre-procedure instructions for patients

After the consultation	Daily: Use sunscreen with SPF >30 Nightly: Start Tri-Luma (fluocinolone acetonide 0.01%, hydroquinone 4%, tretinoin 0.05%), Retin-A, or Differin cream to the face, particularly to the treatment areas Avoid contact with the eyes Reduce the frequency of application or discontinue if redness or irritation develops Avoid exposure to the sun or tanning beds that could result in red, peeling, or swollen skin If there is a concern for post-inflammatory hyperpigmentation, oral tranexamic acid (TXA) 650 mg once daily may be considered for 1 week prior to treatment and can be continued until redness resolves
Two weeks before the procedure	Avoid blood-thinning agents (such as NSAIDs, aspirin, vitamin E, fish oil, or over-the-counter supplements). If you are on a blood-thinning medication for a medical issue, please obtain approval from the prescriber before stopping Avoid skin treatments (such as exfoliants, lasers, chemical peels, etc.)
Day before the procedure	If within the treatment area, shave excessive facial hair, beard, or mustache Use an electric-powered shaver to minimize the potential for skin abrasions and cuts Patients with a history of herpes simplex virus (HSV) or cold sores should start valacyclovir 500 mg BID and continue for 1 week
Procedure day	Cleanse face with routine cleanser Do not apply makeup, lotion, or other skincare products Remove any jewelry

45.2.3 Local and Tumescence

In our experience, micro-coring is well-tolerated with minimal pain and a favorable healing and safety profile.

- Before the procedure, patients wash their face with a gentle skin cleanser.
- EMLA cream (2.5% lignocaine, 2.5% prilocaine) is applied to the treatment area about 30 min before the anticipated treatment time.
- 20% Benzocaine topical gel is applied with a cotton-tipped applicator to the anticipated intra-oral block needle entry sites.
- Infraorbital and mental nerve blocks are used to provide comfort to patients and to alleviate analgesia in the treatment area. Intraoral blocks are performed by injecting 1% lidocaine with 1:100,000 epinephrine into the mucobuccal fold above the second upper premolar superiorly (infraorbital nerve block) and between the lower first and second premolars inferiorly (mental nerve block) with approximately three cc to each site via a 27 or 30-gauge 1.5-inch needle.
- The EMLA is removed by gently wiping the face with a Vashe-soaked gauze.
- Tumescent local anesthesia is injected at the treatment site. Our mixture consists of:
  - Weight-based 0.25% lidocaine HCl with epinephrine injectable.
  - 1 amp (1 mg/cc) epinephrine
- Epinephrine-induced vasoconstriction (blanching) of the perioral region is often observed before beginning treatment.

45.2.4 Procedure

The patient turns their face away from the clinician, and the procedure ensues with the clinician's dominant hand. The clinician systematically addresses areas of the face, typically starting at the inferior marionettes and perioral area. Adequate tension and complete removal of cores are required to optimize results. The device should be positioned perpendicular to a taut skin surface. Some facial regions require counterpressure to create this tension, particularly the medial cheek or around the lips. A tongue depressor or gloved finger is used to achieve tension while treating the buccal area.

It is essential to set depth based on complete core extraction. Dental rolls may be used for the upper lip. For the lower lip and chin, a tongue depressor may be helpful. The process is repeated until the side is complete. The same process is repeated for the contralateral hemi-face. With the face positioned neutrally, the chin is addressed. Any gaps are identified and treated as needed; care is taken not to overlap core sites. After treatment, gentle compression with 4 × 4 gauze is applied to the face to control bleeding.

45.3 Clinical Tips on Micro-coring

- The procedure can be performed as a single treatment or over multiple sessions spaced at least 1 month apart.
- When treating areas of the face where the bone is close to the skin, such as the zygoma or chin, the coring depth should be reduced. Treatment at a lower density is recommended since these areas may be more susceptible to prolonged erythema.
- After a few serial core extractions, the senior author (W.G.A.) routinely wipes the treatment areas with a chilled sterile surgical towel and gauze soaked in epinephrine-saline solution to ensure that blood or debris does not clot the fresh core sites. We know from energy-based devices such as lasers that necrotic debris may prevent early closure of micro-cores and limit skin surface tightening and reduction. Sites should be cleansed thoroughly multiple times per day after the treatment to remove cores and blood products.
- We advise against using a lap pad or any material that can shed or deposit small fibers into the fresh core sites.

45.4 Postoperative Course

Post-procedure care is essential for optimizing outcomes. It is expected to encounter effects such as swelling, bruising, erythema, or skin irregularities for 1–2 weeks. In our experience, no patients had inclusion cysts, infections, scars, dyspigmentation, or refractory erythema.

45.4.1 Pain

Most patients do not have pain in the treatment area; however, if the patient does have pain, we recommend oral Tylenol as needed and the avoidance of NSAIDs (Aleve, Advil, Ibuprofen) for at least 5 days, since these can increase the risk of bleeding or bruising.

45.4.2 Diet

A regular diet can be resumed immediately.

45.4.3 Activity

Following the procedure, patients return to normal activities almost immediately with little to no downtime. Activities that result in excessive sweating, elevation of the heart rate or blood pressure, or dependent head positioning may increase swelling.

45.4.4 Wound Care

We advise against shaving, tanning beds, sun exposure, lasers, facials, waxing, harsh creams, or ointments until instructed further. We recommend that patients cleanse the treatment area twice daily with Vashe, normal saline, or a mild facial cleanser such as Cetaphil and pat dry with a clean towel. It is important to wipe away all clots from the cores to enhance healing. We recommend Vaseline topical emollient (free from lanolin) *only* for dryness or irritation. We recommend against Aquaphor, which can clog the micropores. Clobetasol propri-onate 0.05% ointment is applied to the face immediately after the treatment and can be applied twice daily for up to 2 weeks. After that, patients may resume and continue Tri-Luma or retinoids, moisturizer, sunscreen, and make-up. Tri-Luma or retinoids application frequency can be reduced if redness or irritation develops.

45.4.5 Erythema

Micro-coring treatments with a higher density can be more intense and may result in more extended downtime. Strict sun avoidance and use of sun protection factor (SPF) 30 or greater should be prioritized for at least 1 month and longer if there is erythema. Patients at high risk for prolonged erythema are often prescribed oral tranexamic acid (TXA) 1 week prior to the procedure and continue this medication until the redness resolves. Persistent erythema can be managed through treatments such as pulsed dye or long-pulse KTP if clinically indicated. This can be performed 30 days post-treatment, with additional treatments every 2–4 weeks.

45.4.6 Follow-Up

After the procedure, return for follow-up visits at 1 week and then again at 30, 60, and 90 days. We discuss additional treatments after swelling or erythema has resolved. In published studies, treatments are typically performed at least 1 month apart.

45.5 Evidence

Clinical trials performed with Ellacor® show an overall high subject improvement and satisfaction. Studies have typically included up to three procedures per patient with an average downtime of 3–5 days. There are a few reports of prolonged redness, but these usually resolve without further sequelae.

Preclinical animal studies have demonstrated biological skin-tightening mechanisms of micro-coring. Fernandes et al. published histologic studies of micro-coring in a swine animal model showing regeneration of new skin components with an 89% increase in newly organized collagen and elastin fibers at 3 months postoperatively. The study also reported fibroblast induction and rete-ridge formation, with a 196% increase in papillary dermal and epidermal thicknesses. Micro-cores are thought to undergo micro-contracture due to myofibroblast activation. Together, these mechanisms result in a skin-tightening effect with reduced fine lines [3]. Porcine skin treated at 10% coring density experienced a reduction in skin surface area by 9%, which was statistically significant when compared with baseline and control [9]. Ramot et al. tested robotic micro-coring in swine, demonstrating time-related elimination of necrotic tissue and fibroblastic replacement. These results suggest that the histologic effects of MCT are similar to those expected in humans [7].

Subsequent clinical trials demonstrated skin tightening and increased skin thickness with decreased skin surface area. Pozner et al. reported an increased facial thickness from 1856 um to 2097 um following MCT ($p < 0.05$) and reduced facial skin surface area by 9.4% at 30 days ($p < 0.01$) [6]. Dayan employed a micro-coring system to address skin laxity in the submental fat pad and enhance neck rejuvenation for 31 patients. Most patients experienced an improvement of at least one grade in skin laxity and lipodystrophy. Eighty-four percent expressed satisfaction with the appearance of their neck and jawline, and 97% were inclined to recommend the procedure to others [2].

Gfrerer et al. published a prospective, multi-center clinical trial of 51 patients who underwent mid and lower face micro-coring treatments. Subjects consisted of men and women between 40 and 70 years of age with grade 3 or 4 wrinkles at baseline and Fitzpatrick I to IV skin type. Endpoints included the Lemperle Wrinkle Severity Scale, Global Aesthetic Improvement Scale (GAIS), participant satisfaction, and evaluation of treatment outcome by independent reviewers at 1, 7, 30, 60, and 150 or 180 days after treatment. Bleeding, pain, and healing profiles were also assessed. Study results demonstrated a significant improvement in facial wrinkles with high patient satisfaction and fast recovery time. The mean Lemperle Wrinkle Severity Scale change was 1.3, with a mean improvement of 1.5 at the last follow-up, and 40% of patients improved >2 grades. The average improvement of GAIS was 1.5, with a near 89.7% improvement in GAIS. Patient-reported satisfaction was 85.6%. Patients experienced visible rhytide reduction and were aesthetically improved by subject and investigator GAIS at 90 days post-treatment. Procedure bleeding and pain were mild with good healing responses, and patients reported an average downtime of 3 days. No scarring or serious adverse events were reported. In this study, four minor adverse events were resolved without intervention (bruising, numbness, erythema, and circular marks).

In our experience, micro-coring has been well tolerated as an ala carte procedure or in combination with surgical procedures such as facelifts where the peri-oral area is not typically addressed. Patients with all Fitzpatrick skin types have been successfully treated without prolonged erythema or dyspigmentation. The technology has been shown to be safe for men, women, gender-neutral, and transitioning individuals. Many providers have used the device off-label for other indications, including scar treatment, brow lifts, and aesthetic improvements in other body areas.

Clinical pre-procedural and post-procedural photos are demonstrated in Figs. 45.4 and 45.5. Figure 45.5 demonstrates preprocedural (left) and 2-month postprocedural (right) photos in a male patient who underwent micro-coring alone. A “lip-lift” effect was noted, as confirmed by comparative measurements. Prior to the procedure, the nose-to-lip distance was 23.08 mm and after was 21.15 mm. With a 7% coring setting, a change of −8.4% was achieved. Softening of the left upper lip scar and improvement of the perioral rhytids were also noted.

45.5.1 Future Directions

Ellacor® is currently only FDA-approved for treating moderate to severe wrinkles in the mid to lower face of adults aged 22 and older with Fitzpatrick skin types I–IV. Micro-coring technology has generated interest in many off-label indications and research endeavors. Innovative applications in scar improvement, tattoo removal, wound healing, aesthetic improvements in other body areas, and diagnostic skin biopsies have been considered. Future applications could include tailored skincare and treatment protocols based on an individual’s skin health, genetic factors, and specific dermatological conditions and concerns. Micro-coring techniques for drug delivery are an area of interest for researchers aiming to improve the absorption and efficacy of topical medications, which may have implications for the treatment of dermatological conditions. Combinations of micro-coring procedures with other technologies also need to be explored to understand synergistic or antagonistic effects.

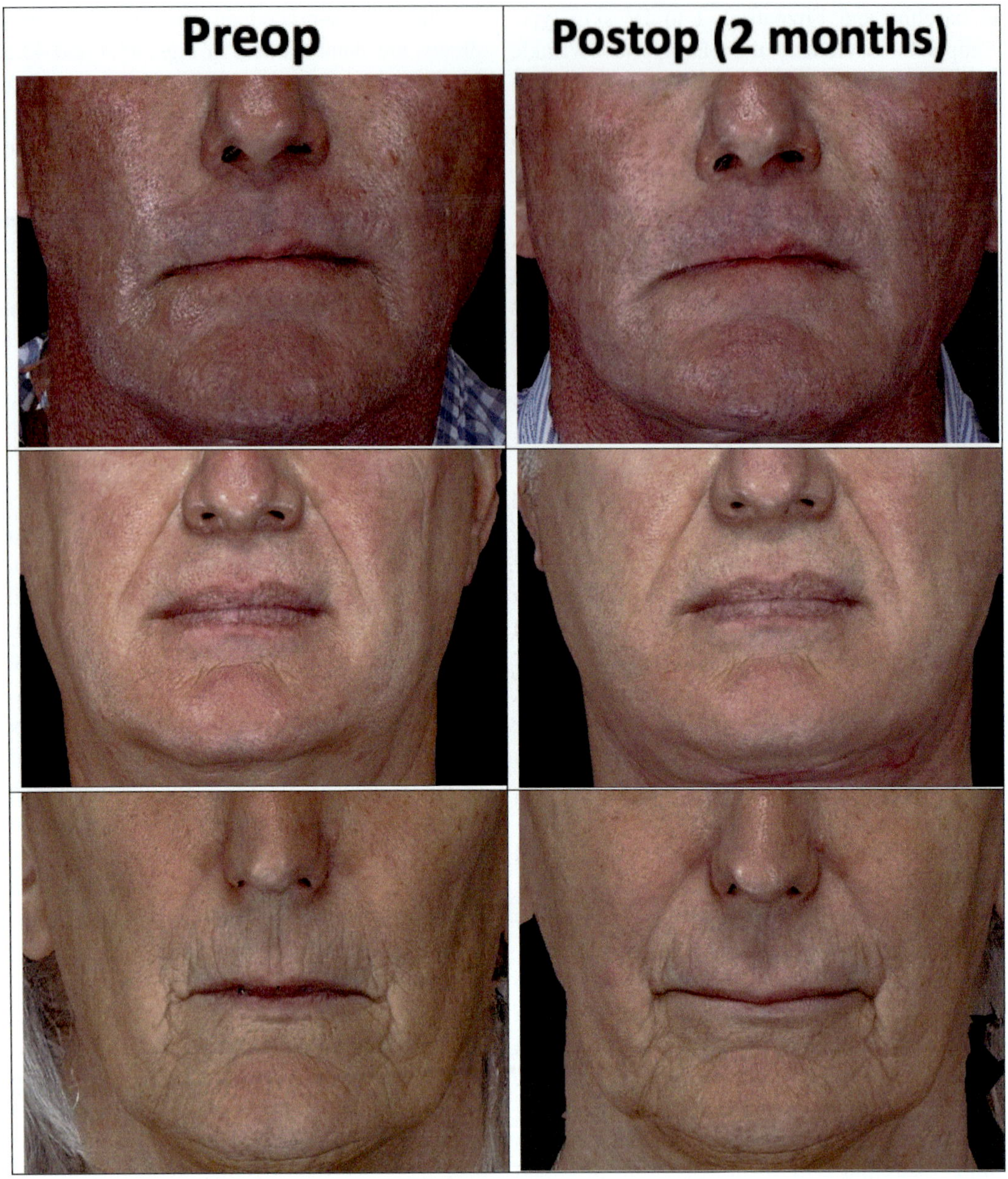

Fig. 45.4 Photos of three patients pre-Ellacor (left) and post-Ellacor (right) treatment. The bottom panel represents Ellacor performed on an individual undergoing gender affirmation

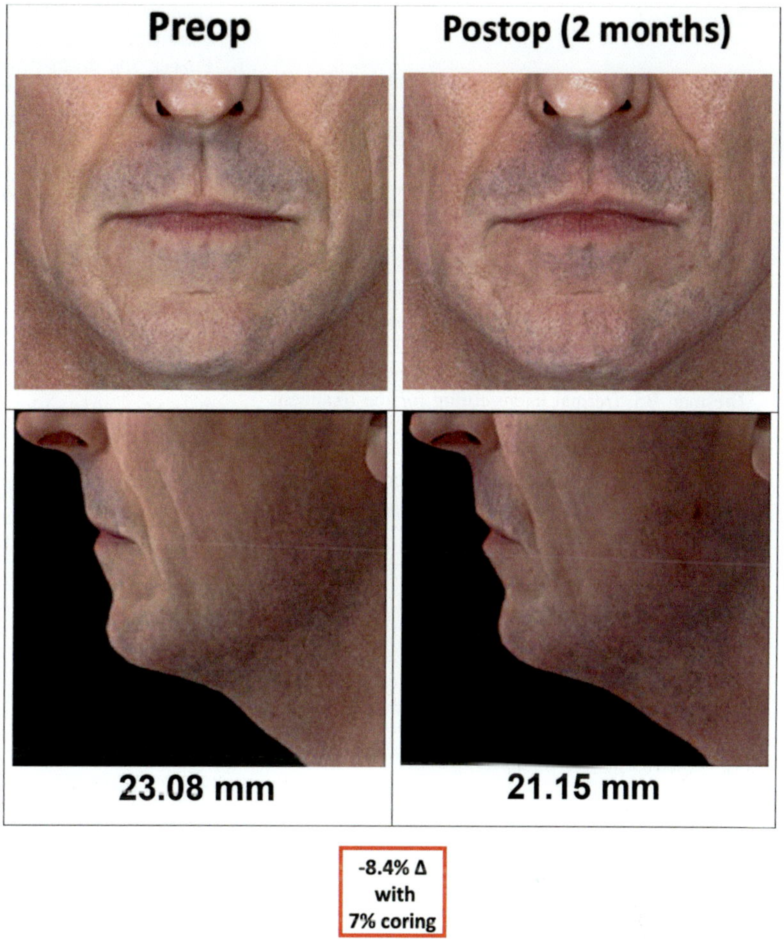

Fig. 45.5 Preprocedural (left) and two month postprocedural (right) photos in a male patient who underwent micro-coring alone. A "lip-lift" effect was noted, as confirmed by comparative measurements. Prior to the procedure, the nose-to-lip distance was 23.08 mm and after was 21.15 mm. With a 7% coring setting, a change of −8.4% was achieved. Softening of the left upper lip scar and improvement of the perioral rhytids were also noted

45.6 Summary

Dermal micro-coring is an effective treatment for moderate-to-severe facial wrinkles. The energy-free device can scarlessly remove up to 8% of skin surface area without scarring and rejuvenates the skin through neocollagenesis and elastinogenesis. Multiple clinical trials have demonstrated consistent and significant wrinkle improvement in treatment groups as well as high patient satisfaction.

Financial Disclosures This study was completed without supporting funds. The author, Krishna Vyas, M.D., Ph.D., M.H.S., has no commercial associations or financial disclosures that might pose or create a conflict of interest with the information presented in the attached manuscript. William G. Austen, Jr., M.D., receives royalties and is an advisor to Cytrellis Biosystems, Inc., Woburn, MA.

Disclaimer The information provided in this chapter is not intended to substitute for formal medical training or certification. Cytrellis makes no representations or warranties, either express or implied, of merchantability, fitness for a specific purpose, or of any other nature with respect to information or the product to which information is mentioned. Furthermore, Cytrellis makes no representations or warranties that the products/medications/treatments referred to in the presentations may be used without infringing the intellectual property rights of others. In no case should the information be considered a part of Cytrellis's terms and conditions of sale. Cytrellis does not take responsibility for services/education provided by the independent physicians/clinicians, nor does Cytrellis endorse any particular physician/clinician. Statements provided by physicians about the Ellacor® System with Micro-Coring® Technology are based on the individual experiences of the presenters. Individual experiences may vary.

References

1. Champlain AH, DiGiorgio CM, Zurakowski D, Sakamoto FH, Anderson RR. Wound healing after fractional skin harvesting. Dermatologic Surg. 2022;48(10):1083–8.
2. Dayan S. Aesthetic evolution drives birth of minimally invasive surgery subgroup. J Cosmet Dermatol. 2019;18(5):1182–5.
3. Fernandes JR, Samayoa JC, Broelsch GF, McCormack MC, Nicholls AM, Randolph MA, Mihm MC, Austen WG Jr. Micro-mechanical fractional skin rejuvenation. Plast Reconstr Surg. 2013;131(2):216–23.
4. Gfrerer L, Kilmer SL, Waibel JS, Geronemus RG, Biesman BS. Dermal micro-coring for the treatment of moderate to severe facial wrinkles. Plast Reconstr Surg Glob Open. 2022;10(10):e4547.
5. Manstein D, Herron GS, Sink RK, Tanner H, Anderson RR. Fractional photothermolysis: a new concept for cutaneous remodeling using microscopic patterns of thermal injury. Lasers Surg Med. 2004;34(5):426–38.
6. Pozner JN, Kilmer SL, Geronemus RG, Jack M, Burns JA, Kaminer MS. Cytrellis: a novel microcoring Technology for Scarless Skin Removal: summary of three prospective clinical trials. Plast Reconstr Surg Glob Open. 2021;9(10):e3905.
7. Ramot Y, Vazana U, Cacical O, Nyska A. Safety and efficacy of a novel robotic, fractional microcoring device in a swine model. J Toxicol Pathol. 2023;36(1):11–9.
8. Russe E, Purschke M, Farinelli WA, Wang Y, Doukas AG, Limpiangkanan W, Sakamoto FH, Tam J, Wechselberger G, Anderson RR. Micro-fractional, directional skin tightening: a porcine model. Lasers Surg Med. 2016a;48(3):264–9.
9. Russe E, Purschke M, Farinelli WA, Wang Y, Doukas AG, Limpiangkanan W, Sakamoto FH, Tam J, Wechselberger G, Anderson RR. Micro-fractional, directional skin tightening: a porcine model. Lasers Surg Med. 2016b;48(3):264–9.

46 Endocrine Support for the Aesthetic Patient

Alan A. Parsa and Fereydoun Don Parsa

46.1 Introduction

For centuries, performance-enhancing drugs have been used to gain an edge on opponents. While elite athletes continue to battle with ways to push their limits and gain an edge, others use similar therapies to improve physical form and sense of well-being. Of these, two common endocrine hormones in use are testosterone and growth hormone (GH). Some want men to believe that these hormones have magical properties and will suddenly morph them into optimal physical form while feeling younger with a strong sexual appetite. Advertisers and some practitioners have capitalized on this fantasy for monetary gain without fully understanding the true benefits or risks associated with these therapies. Here, we use published literature to help inform and guide the reader to the benefits and risks of both testosterone and growth hormone use in the aging male.

46.2 Testosterone

Exogenous testosterone is in increased use, not only by athletes but also by the aging male. This increase is driven by documented age-related testosterone decline [1–6] by approximately 30% in healthy males aged between 25 and 75 years [7]. These data suggest that all men lose testosterone levels similar to women undergoing menopause, a phenomenon referred to by some as andropause. Other studies have shown this to be a misrepresentation of the general population, where a significant number of men remain eugonadal with advanced age [8]. The Baltimore Longitudinal Study on Aging evaluated testosterone levels in 870 men and published that about 80% of men aged over 60, and 70% over 70 had normal biochemical testosterone levels [4]. This has not led to decreased testosterone prescriptions though. In the United States, anabolic steroids use in men aged 40 and older has increased by more than threefold from 2001 to 2011 [9]. Since a majority of men have preserved testosterone levels, much of the increase in use is likely related to improper workup and/or dosing based solely on perceived symptoms or desired results.

A. A. Parsa (✉)
University of Hawaii, John A. Burns School of Medicine, Department of Medicine, Honolulu, HI, USA
e-mail: aparsa@hawaii.edu

F. D. Parsa
Division of Plastic Surgery, Department of Surgery, John A. Burns School of Medicine, University of Hawaii, Honolulu, HI, USA

K. Jeffords et al. (eds.), *Aesthetic Surgery for Men*, https://doi.org/10.1007/978-3-032-03840-1_46

46.3 Testosterone Synthesis

In males, de novo testosterone production is dominated by the Leydig cells of the testes with minor assistance from the adrenal cortex of the adrenal glands and is regulated by the hypothalamo-pituitary-gonadal axis. Hormone production begins with gonadotropin-releasing hormone (GnRH), produced and secreted by the hypothalamus. GnRH targets the gonadotroph cells of the anterior pituitary gland, which in turn produces and secretes two hormones: follicular-stimulating hormone (FSH) and luteinizing hormone (LH). These peptide hormones target the testicles in males to initiate an enzymatically driven cascade to produce testosterone and sperm. Increased levels of testosterone and its metabolites, estradiol and dihydrotestosterone (DHT), negatively feed back to the hypothalamus and pituitary, inhibiting further production and secretion of GnRH, FSH, and LH [10]. Dehydroepiandrosterone (DHEA), its sulfate ester (DHEA-S), and androstenedione are weak-acting androgens produced by the zona reticularis of the adrenal glands capable of converting to testosterone by peripheral tissues [11, 12]. While we will not be reviewing DHEA in this text, it should be mentioned that in most cases, sustained oral supplementation of DHEA in men does not produce consistent beneficial effects [13, 14].

46.4 Muscle Mass/Strength

Physical performance-enhancing drugs are not a new concept. Ancient Greeks ate mushrooms and sesame seeds; Zulu warriors in South Africa used grape skin extract, Roman gladiators used stimulants to enhance endurance [15], and Olympic athletes use performance-enhancing drugs to gain a competitive advantage [16, 17]. The desire to increase athletic performance, increase muscle mass and strength, and improve physical appearance has been a major driving force for testosterone supplementation. Here we evaluate muscle mass and strength in the nonelite athlete.

Reports show an annual decline in muscle mass (sarcopenia) of around 1–2% per year after the age of 50 [18–20] with a suggested prevalence of sarcopenia between 6% and 15% in men aged 65 and older [21]. Much of this is related to obesity from a sedentary lifestyle [22, 23]. While muscle mass tends to decline with age, data regarding strength changes are inconsistent. A cross-sectional analysis of 847 subjects reported a general decline in male grip strength irrespective of muscle mass after the age of 40 [24] with a loss of muscular strength at a rate of 1.5–5% per year over the age of 50 [25, 26]. On the contrary, in comparing strength between younger (mean age 23 years) and older (mean age 62 years) males with similar activities of daily living (ADL), strength preservation was maintained in the upper body [27]. This suggests that decreased physical activity with age may be the leading force to loss of strength. A finding from two prospective studies equaling 1557 men, mean age of 75 years, did not show a 3-year decline in physical performance or muscular strength in hypogonadal males compared to eugonadal controls [28]. This is not consistent among all studies though. A systematic review and meta-analysis evaluated muscular response based on route of administration of testosterone (i.e., transdermal vs. intramuscular) [29] showing that intramuscular (IM) testosterone injections led to a 5.7% increase in fat-free mass compared to a 1.7% increase with transdermal formulations. Also, a 10–13% increase in total body strength was seen with IM injections with a 2–5% increase in transdermal, showing a dose-dependent manner response [30–34], while some studies suggest a less pronounced effect [35, 36]. A 2021 study noted that in those aged >50 with low/normal testosterone, transdermal testosterone therapy did not show a beneficial impact of exercise on vascular function and health compared to placebo [37]. Further studies are needed to determine who would best benefit from therapy. Experience shows that those who couple treatment with physical activity will have a better response than those who remain sedentary after therapy initiation.

In summary, muscle mass and strength decrease with age and is likely related, in part, to reduced physical activity. Testosterone therapy will increase fat-free mass and strength in a dose-dependent manner in both the hypogonadal and eugonadal male but should be coupled with physical activity for maximal benefits.

46.5 Obesity

The World Health Organization (WHO) estimates that the number of obese adults has tripled between 1975 and 2016, with 39% of adults being overweight and about 13% being obese in 2016 [38]. Adipokines, inflammatory and immune mediators, are thought to be a contributor to associated comorbidities, including cardiovascular disease, diabetes, and arthritis [39–41]. Obesity is related to reductions in testosterone levels that is noted particularly in the diabetic population. A study of approximately 2000 obese men in the United States aged 40 or older showed that 40% of nondiabetics and 50% of diabetics had subnormal free testosterone levels [42]. Although the pathogenesis of hypogonadism in obesity is poorly understood, data suggest that low testosterone in the moderately obese is related to insulin resistance associated with a reduction in sex hormone biding globulin leading to low levels of <u>total</u> serum testosterone, and in the more severe obese population, low testosterone is associated with reductions in both <u>total</u> and <u>free</u> testosterone levels related to suppression of the hypothalamic-pituitary-testicular axis [43, 44]. In other words, the moderately obese may show a low total testosterone level with normal free testosterone, while the severely obese will have both free and total testosterone levels low. While testosterone levels decrease in obesity, a linear relationship between measurements of total and free testosterone and severity of obesity is not well identified [45], and testosterone levels should not be used to determine the degree of obesity. Also, while testosterone deficiency increases with advancing age, the prevalence can be as high as 52–79% in the obese population as seen in a meta-analysis of 4546 obese males [46]. This is consistent with The European Male Aging Study showing that overweight and obese men have a three- to ninefold increase relative risk of developing secondary hypogonadism [47]. It appears that obesity-related low testosterone is a non-permanent state, which can be fully reversed with adequate weight loss [43, 48]. This is suggesting that obesity may lead to testosterone deficiency rather than low testosterone leading to obesity when other conditions are eliminated. Weight loss is paramount in normalizing testosterone levels but requires significant changes in lifestyle (i.e., diet, exercise) that many are unwilling or unable to accomplish. Studies have shown that testosterone therapy will modestly reduce fat mass while increasing muscle mass [49–52] with sustained effects [53, 54]. An 11-year study [55] administered testosterone to 428 normal weight, overweight, and obese men with a total testosterone levels <349 ng/dL comparing to 395 untreated men. The study showed sustained reductions in weight, waist circumference (WC), and body mass index (BMI) compared to the untreated men. While data have been supportive of testosterone therapy in obese males, therapy without adequate diet and exercise will unlikely produce the degree of weight loss that many hope to achieve.

In summary, while low testosterone levels are seen in the obese population, it is not permanent and is reversed with adequate weight loss. Testosterone therapy in the obese population is able to assist in weight control by reducing WC and BMI modestly but should be coupled with diet and exercise to maximize benefits.

46.6 Skin

Decreased levels of circulating testosterone have been suspected to decrease skin moisture retention, elasticity, and skin thickness. In men, we are not aware of studies evaluating effects of topical testosterone other than reports of skin irritation and contact dermatitis related to transdermal applications [56]. The skin irritation appears to be more associated with the delivery mechanism rather than the testosterone itself. Documented undesirable side effects of testosterone on skin include acne and androgenic alopecia, related to the conversion of testosterone to DHT [57]. Agents inhibiting enzyme 5-alpha reductase exist and prevent this conversion and may help minimize some of these effects. It is important to note that this block can lead to increased estrogen levels in males and the undesired gynecomastia.

Estrogens appear to have beneficial and protective roles in skin physiology [58]. In postmenopausal women, estrogen replacement has a positive effect on skin elasticity, skin hydration, as well as skin thickness [59, 60]. Studies using estrogens in men are lacking, likely due to the feminizing effects of estrogens (e.g., gynecomastia and possibly diminished libido). We are unaware of studies specifically evaluating the role of estrogens to improve skin health in men.

In summary, testosterone therapy is ineffective in improving skin health in men.

46.7 Sexual Function and Energy

Up to 35% of men with low circulating testosterone levels have erectile dysfunction (ED) [61–63]. Advertisers have capitalized on this by promising amazing results in sexual function with testosterone therapy. Several studies have evaluated the effects of testosterone replacement on sexual function in both the eugonadal [64, 65] and hypogonadal male [66–68] with varying results. In a meta-analysis in 2014, randomized controlled trials (RCT) showing significant improvement in erectile function and libido with testosterone thearpy as an add on to phosphodiesterase type 5 inhibitor (PDE5i) were in part or completely supported by pharaceutical companies (confidence interval [0.04-0.53] and [0.12; 0.52], respectively) [69] suggesting publication bias. The analysis further showed that while testosterone therapy has positive effects on hypogonadal males, the role is not clear in males not clearly hypogonadal.

Sexual desire and activity improved in a cohort of 470 men aged 65 or older with low libido and an average testosterone level <275 ng/dL when treated with testosterone gel compared to placebo, but no benefits were seen in erectile function [66]. Another randomized-placebo 12-week trial showed similar results of 715 men, mean age of 55 years, with low sex drive or decreased energy with testosterone levels <300 ng/dL [67]. “The Testosterone Trials” (TTrials), a 12-month evaluation of 788 males, mean age of 72 years, showed that testosterone gel therapy increased sexual activity and sexual desire, with a nonsignificant improvement in ED [95% CI: 1.06–4.02] [70]. This suggests that testosterone gel therapy appears to assist with sexual desire with little benefit to erectile function. Further support of this is seen when no further ED benefit was seen after adding testosterone therapy to males with ED after optimization with sildenafil citrate therapy, a phosphodiesterase type 5 inhibitor (PDE5i) [71]. A meta-analysis by Corona et al. suggests the degree of benefit is correlated with how low testosterone levels are, noting significant improvement in erectile function compared with placebo in patients with serum testosterone levels <231 ng/dL with milder improvement in those with serum testosterone <346 ng/dL) [72]. This supports the theory that “more is not always better” and targeting higher testosterone levels do not further improve erectile function. Keeping this in mind, it is important to evaluate the questioned dysfunction. Is it sexual desire? ED? What is the degree of ED? This will better assist in determining best treatment option.

In summary, treatrment with testosterone gel therapy has shown to improve sexual desire signiticanlty in those with low serum baseline testosterone levels (i.e., <250 ng/dL) but the effect is less pronounced in those with higher baseline testosterone level. There appears to be less of an effect on ED with testosterone therapy, and PDE5i such as sildenafil citrate therapy should be considered as first line in those with isolated ED issues.

46.8 Cardiac Function

There has been much debate between the effects of exogenous testosterone therapy and cardiac risks. Studies describe an inverse correlation between endogenous testosterone levels, cardiovascular disease (CVD), and all-cause mortality [73–76].

It is suggested that hypogonadal males have a 25% risk of coronary heart disease [77]. A prospective, population-based study of 794 men evaluated testosterone levels and mortality. They reported that men with total serum testosterone levels <241 ng/dL had a 40% higher risk of death over the following 20 years compared to those with higher endogenous testosterone levels [78]. Another report published that, men with lower endogenous testosterone levels are more likely to develop CVD during their lifetimes [76]. It has been suggested that low serum testosterone levels may be an overall indicator of poor health [74, 75], and other cardiometabolic risks such as metabolic syndrome, hypertension, obesity, type 2 diabetes (T2DM) may be present [79–81]. Thus, one should consider cardiometabolic risks in those with low testosterone prior to initiating therapy to minimize potential risks.

The question though remains: will replacement therapy lead to coronary events? A double blinded, placebo-controlled trial evaluated if testosterone gel replacement therapy could slow the progression of noncalcified coronary artery plaque [82]. While no events were recorded, among the 88 testosterone-treated males with symptomatic hypogonadism and serum testosterone levels <275 ng/dL, there was a significant increase in coronary artery noncalcified plaque volume compared to the 82 males in the placebo group when measured by coronary computed tomographic angiography (CTA). Similar results were also seen among 138 placebo-controlled males using testosterone gel [83]. On the contrary, a study of 308 males with serum testosterone levels between 100 and 400 ng/dL were randomized to testosterone gel compared to placebo [84]. This study, conducted over a 3-year period, did not result in significant differences in coronary calcium or common carotid artery intima-media thickness when targeting testosterone levels between 500 and 900 ng/dL [84]. A meta-analysis in 2005 evaluated 19 randomized placebo-controlled studies [85]. In the >90-day follow-up of 651 treated men and 417 placebo controls, the rate of cardiovascular events was similar in both groups (2.8% in treated and 3.7% in placebo). In a separate systematic review and meta-analysis, studies failed to show significant cardiac risks [86]. It should also be kept in mind that many of the reported studies used testosterone gels rather than intramuscular injections. This is an important distinction since peak testosterone levels in intramuscular injection are higher and remain at higher levels for longer duration than when using testosterone gel formulations. Whether this plays part in cardiovascular effects is yet to be seen and requires further long-term investigation.

In summary, reports suggest that low serum testosterone levels increase risks of CVD. It is likely that those with low testosterone levels may also have other cardiometabolic risks (i.e., diabetes, obesity, hypertension), and those conditions should be addressed. There is no clear evidence of increased cardiac risks with testosterone therapy. Testosterone gel, which appears to be more studied than injections, seems safe without significant increased risks. Long-term and dose-dependent studies are still needed.

46.9 Fertility

Testosterone therapy has been considered a potential form of male contraception for decades. Studies have shown that testosterone injections can lead to severe oligozoospermia or azoospermia [87–91] with suppression rates up to 100%. More recently, progesterone has been used in addition to testosterone to achieve sperm suppression [92, 93]. Investigators continue to evaluate different methods of male contraception, with many continuing to include testosterone therapy [94]. Keeping this in mind, long-term testosterone therapy may lead to infertility when fertility is desired. Most but not all men treated with injectable testosterone for 6–12 months recover fertility potential [88, 89, 93]. Personal experience has shown variable results when stopping testosterone therapy when fertility is desired.

In summary, use of testosterone therapy for male contraception has been shown to be effective but is not commonly used. This is likely from unclear long-term testosterone use on normalization of fertility potential to pre-treatment levels. This method of contraception should thus not be considered first-line treatment until studies have further elucidated long-term recovery.

46.10 Complications

An important treatment complication is related to long-term testosterone use in eugonadal males. Those who stop therapy after prolonged use, especially high dose, tend to undergo withdrawal symptoms, which can include sexual dysfunction, fatigue, depressed mood, depression, and potentially suicide [95, 96]. Some, when stopping therapy, will never regain normal testicular function [97] and require lifelong treatment to maintain normal testosterone levels. In fact, a substantial proportion of men requiring life-long testosterone therapy have a history of previous testosterone use [98, 99]. Thus, testosterone therapy has the potential to cause a permanent hypogonadal state when stopped. Also, tapering from therapy is important to avoid significant hypogonadal symptoms.

In the 1940s, testosterone levels were thought to be associated with increased risk of prostate Complications cancer [100]. Since then, studies have shown variable results regarding testosterone levels/therapy and prostate cancer risks [85, 101–108]. At this time, there are not adequate studies statistically powered to determine if testosterone therapy is associated with the development of prostate cancer. Alternatively, those with metastatic prostate cancer, testosterone therapy may promote prostatic neoplastic cells [109]. Since a prostate-specific antigen (PSA) level >4.0 ng/ml is an accepted indication for urological evaluation for prostate cancer [110], the Endocrine Society recommends avoidance of testosterone therapy until after the prostate has been adequately evaluated [95]. The use of testosterone in those with prostate cancer is beyond the scope of this review and can be found elsewhere.

Benign prostate hypertrophy (BPH) and prostate volume (PV) and their association with total testosterone levels has been controversial. Historically, it was thought that with increased testosterone levels, PV increases. This is a reason why the federal drug administration (FDA) issued a package insert (PI) warning that those with BPH treated with androgens "are at an increased risk for worsening of signs and symptoms of BPH" [111]. Data have shown that testosterone therapy has not resulted in increasing prostate size [30, 112, 113] but should be used in caution.

Lower urinary tract symptoms do not appear to worsen in those treated with testosterone therapy in those who did not have severe symptoms prior to treatment [108, 114, 115].

Erythrocytosis is a common complication to monitor for. Testosterone therapy increases erythropoietin (EPO) levels leading to increased hematocrit (Hct) and hemoglobin [116]. Hct increases more with injectable formulations than topical formulations [117] due to higher circulating testosterone levels with injectables [118]. There is a theoretical increased risk of cardiovascular and cerebrovascular events with elevated hematocrit. We are not aware of studies showing Hct cutoff levels where risks increase significantly. The Endocrine Society suggests against testosterone therapy with a baseline hematocrit above the upper limit of normal due to potential increased risks associated with erythrocytosis [95]. It is suggested that if Hct levels increase >54%, therapy should be stopped.

46.11 Growth Hormone

Growth hormone (GH), or somatotropin, is a peptide hormone secreted by the anterior pituitary gland. GH predominantly targets the liver driving hepatic expression of insulin-like growth factor-1 (IGF-1). IGF-1, an important postnatal linear growth factor, begins to decline along with GH when one attains full physical maturation and adult height [119–121].

The clinical syndrome of GH deficiency is described by non-specific features including reduced bone remodeling activity, decreased mood and sense of well-being, change in body fat distribution with increased central adiposity, decreased muscle mass and strength, hyperlipidemia, increased predisposition to cardiovascular diseases, and early mortality [122–125]. The estimated overall incidence rate of GH deficiency is approximately 2 per 100,000 population with adult-onset GH deficiency affecting about 1 per 100,000 population [126]. In the United States, approximately 6000 new cases of adult GH deficiency are diagnosed yearly with 20% continuation from childhood onset and 80% from damage to the hypothalamic-pituitary axis later in life [127, 128]. Treatment of GH deficiency subjects with recombinant human GH (rhGH) dramatically improves symptoms. A clear reduction of central adiposity and overall fat mass, increased lean body mass, reduction in cardiovascular risks, improved lipid profile, and increased bone density are seen [129]. Many practitioners feel that the same benefits will be seen in those without GH deficiency which brings us to our discussion as to its "aesthetic" benefits.

46.12 Adiposity

In 1990, a *New England Journal of Medicine* study reported that age-related decline in GH leads to loss of lean body mass, increased adiposity, and thinning of skin which can improve with GH therapy [130]. Since the 1960s, it has been shown that GH secretion is reduced in obese patients [131] and is reversible by weight loss [132, 133]. This recovery of the GH—IGF-1 axis suggests that decreased GH secretion is an effect, rather than a pre-existing disorder. The reason for GH reduction in obesity is currently poorly understood. A literature search by Rasmussen in 2010 [134] evaluated 19 randomized controlled studies that administered GH versus placebo to obese subjects. In those given GH, a reduction in visceral adipose tissue was seen ranging from 5% to 34% while weight loss interventions (i.e., caloric restriction or exercise) reduced visceral adiposity ranging between 9% and 49%. A meta-analysis [135] suggests that supratherapeutic doses of GH increase lean body mass with decreased visceral adiposity but with increased arthralgia and fluid retention. Studies in non-GH-deficient subjects have shown little to no improvements with untoward effects of therapy including: peripheral edema, carpal tunnel syndrome, insulin resistance, arthralgia, and paresthesia [136, 137]. Older and more obese individuals appear to be more susceptible to side effects from GH treatment [136, 138]. Individuals most likely to benefit from GH replacement therapy include those with severe GH deficiency defined by GH provocative testing.

In summary, GH levels decrease in obese subjects related to obesity rather than pre existing GH deficiency, and levels return to normal with adequate weight loss. GH therapy will reduce visceral adiposity with long-term therapy but comes with undesired complications (e.g., arthralgia, fluid retention). Until further studies are completed, risks associated with GH therapy outweigh benefits in non-GH-deficient males in respect to body composition.

46.13 Life Expectancy

Studies have clearly shown that elevated IGF-1 levels, as seen in acromegaly or gigantism, lead to a shortened lifespan with increased mortality due to its association with diabetes, cardiovascular disease, and malignancy [139, 140]. Transgenic mice models expressing prolonged elevated GH secretion result in drastically shortened life span [141]. On the other hand, GH-deficient transgenic mice show increased longevity by 25% to 60% compared to wild-type [142–144]. It has been suggested that low detectable levels of GH along with lower circulating IGF-1 levels account for the apparent longer lifespan [145]. This is also the suspected mechanism of the longer lifespan in those with Laron syndrome (inactive GH receptor resulting in IGF-1 deficiency) [146–148]. This is contrary to popular belief that GH replacement is anti-aging and leads to a longer lifespan.

In summary, the use of GH, at this time, has not been shown to extend life expectancy.

46.14 GH and Skin

Overproduction of GH is commonly associated with "oily skin." Reports show the presence of GH receptors on the skin as well as sebaceous glands [149, 150]. In those with GH excess, as in acromegaly, skin is observed to be thick, rough, oily, develop pigmented skin tags, acanthosis nigricans, and psoriasis [151]. IGF-1 has been shown to increase inflammatory biomarkers and sebum production and is implicated in the pathogenesis of acne [152–154], and inhibition of IGF-1 has been mentioned as a potential acne treatment [155, 156]. Recent data do not support the use of GH to improve skin health.

In summary, there is no apparent benefit to skin care with the administration of GH.

46.15 GH and Wound Healing

While wound healing is beyond the scope of this chapter, it is important to note the existence of benefits with GH therapy. For instance, the role of GH in wound healing of burn victims has been emerging with promising data [157] potentially related to GH ability to promote cell proliferation, angiogenesis, and synthesis of extracellular matrix [158] especially in burn victims. A 2014 Cochrane Review found that in those with burns covering more than 40% of total body surface, rhGH results in more rapid healing of burned wounds and donor sites in adults and children without increased incidence of mortality or scarring [157]. Studies have also been evaluating the role of topical GH to promote wound healing [159, 160]. Further studies will show other potential roles of GH therapy.

46.16 Conclusion

In our continual pursuit to identify hormones which may assist in halting or reversing the aging process, we must remember that there is much we do not yet understand. For the most part, testosterone and growth hormone levels decline normally with age and in most cases do not require replacement therapy. Testosterone therapy, in some cases, can improve overall physical appearance, sense of well-being, and libido but not without effort from the patient (i.e., exercise, diet, weight control). We must be cognizant that low testosterone may be a marker of other underlying conditions likely needing to be addressed (i.e., hypertension, obesity, type 2 diabetes). At this time, adverse events, related to testosterone therapy, appear to be minimal. The most important of these being fertility potential in the short term and potential loss of normal gonadal function upon cessation of therapy in the long term. Growth hormone does not appear to have any significant benefits in the aging male and risks currently outweighing its benefits.

References

1. Rudman D, Mattson DE, Nagraj HS, Feller AG, Jackson DL, Rudman IW. Plasma testosterone in nursing home men. J Clin Epidemiol. 1988;41:231–6.
2. Kosasih JB, Abbasi AA, Rudman D. Serum insulin-like growth factor-I and serum testosterone status of elderly men in an inpatient rehabilitation unit. Am J Med Sci. 1996;311:169–73.
3. Ferrini RL, Barrett-Connor E. Sex hormones and age: a cross-sectional study of testosterone and estradiol and their bioavailable fractions in community-dwelling men. Am J Epidemiol. 1998;147(8):750–4.
4. Harman SM, Metter EJ, Tobin JD, Pearson J, Baltimore Longitudinal Study of Aging. Longitudinal effects of aging on serum total and free testosterone levels in healthy men. Baltimore Longitudinal Study of Aging. J Clin Endocrinol Metab. 2001;86(2):724–31.
5. Gray A, Berlin JA, McKinlay JB, Longcope C. An examination of research design effects on the association of testosterone and male aging: results of a meta-analysis. J Clin Epidemiol. 1991;44:671–84.
6. Golan R, Scovell JM. Age-related testosterone decline is due to waning of both testicular and hypothalamic-pituitary function. Aging Male. 2015;18(3):201–4.
7. Morley JE, Kaiser FE, Perry HM III, Patrick P, Morley PM, Stauber PM, et al. Longitudinal changes in testosterone, luteinizing hormone, and follicle-stimulating hormone in healthy older men. Metabolism. 1997;46:410–3.

8. Feldman HA, Longcope C, Derby CA, Johannes CB, Araujo AB, Coviello AB, et al. Age trends in the level of serum testosterone and other hormones in middle-aged men: longitudinal results from the Massachusetts male aging study. J Clin Endocrinol Metab. 2002;87:589–98.
9. Baillargeon J, Urban R, Ottenbacher K, Pierson K, Goodwin J. Trends in androgen prescribing in the United States, 2001 to 2011. JAMA Intern Med. 2013;173(15):1465–6.
10. Corradi P, Corradi R, Greene L. Physiology of the hypothalamic pituitary gonadal axis in the male. Urol Clin North Am. 2016;43(2):151–62.
11. Clark B, Prough P, Klinge C. Mechanisms of action of dehydroepiandrosterone. Vitam Horm. 2018;108:29–73.
12. Labrie F, Bélanger A, Simard J, Luu-The V, Labrie C. DHEA and peripheral androgen and estrogen formation: intracrinology. Ann N Y Acad Sci. 1995;774:16–28.
13. Buvat J. Androgen therapy with dehydroepiandrosterone. World J Urol. 2003;21(5):346–55.
14. Morales AJ, Haubrich RH, Hwang JY, Asakura H, Yen SS. The effect of six months treatment with a 100 mg daily dose of dehydroepiandrosterone (DHEA) on circulating sex steroids, body composition and muscle strength in age-advanced men and women. Clin Endocrinol. 1998;49(4):421–32.
15. Prokop L. The struggle against doping and its history. J Sports Med Phys Fitness. 1970,10(1):45 8.
16. Prendergast HM, Bannen T, Erickson TB, Honore KR. The toxic torch of the modern Olympic Games. Vet Hum Toxicol. 2003;45(2):97–102.
17. Fitch KD. Blood doping at the Olympic Games. J Sports Med Phys Fitness. 2017;57(11):1526–32.
18. von Haehling S, Morley JE, Anker SD An overview of sarcopenia: facts and numbers on prevalence and clinical impact. J Cachexia Sarcopenia Muscle. 2010;1(2):129–33.
19. Baumgartner R, Waters D, Gallagher D, Morley J, Garry P. Predictors of skeletal muscle mass in elderly men and women. Mech Ageing Dev. 1999;107(2):123–36.
20. Saad F, Gooren LJ. Late onset hypogonadism of men is not equivalent to the menopause. Maturitas. 2014;79(1):52–7.
21. Melton LJ 3rd, Khosla S, Crowson CS, O'Connor MK, O'Fallon WM, Riggs BL. Epidemiology of sarcopenia. J Am Geriatr Soc. 2000;48(6):625–30.
22. Marcus RL, Brixner DI, Ghate S, Lastayo P. Fat modulates the relationship between sarcopenia and physical function in nonobese older adults. Curr Gerontol Geriatr Res. 2012;2012(1):216185.
23. Sternfeld B, Ngo L, Satariano WA, Tager IB. Associations of body composition with physical performance and self-reported functional limitation in elderly men and women. Am J Epidemiol. 2002;156(2):110–21.
24. Kallman DA, Plato CC, Tobin JD. The role of muscle loss in the age-related decline of grip strength: cross-sectional and longitudinal perspectives. J Gerontol. 1990;45(3):M82–8.
25. Marcell TJ, Hawkins SA, Wiswell RA. Leg strength declines with advancing age despite habitual endurance exercise in active older adults. J Strength Cond Res. 2014;28(2):504–13.
26. Frontera WR, Hughes VA, Fielding RA, Fiatarone MA, Evans WJ, Roubenoff R. Aging of skeletal muscle: a 12-yr longitudinal study. J Appl Physiol (1985). 2000;88(4):1321–6.
27. Nogueira FR, Libardi CA, Vechin FC, Lixandrão ME, de Barros Berton RP, de Souza TM, et al. Comparison of maximal muscle strength of elbow flexors and knee extensors between younger and older men with the same level of daily activity. Clin Interv Aging. 2013;8:401–7.
28. Schaap LA, Pluijm SM, Deeg DJ, Penninx BW, Nicklas BJ, Harris TB, et al. Low testosterone levels and decline in physical performance and muscle strength in older men: findings from two prospective cohort studies. Clin Endocrinol. 2008;68(1):42–50.
29. Skinner JW, Otzel DM, Bowser A, Nargi D, Agarwal S, Peterson MD, et al. Muscular responses to testosterone replacement vary by administration route: a systematic review and meta-analysis. J Cachexia Sarcopenia Muscle. 2018;9(3):465–81.
30. Bhasin S, Woodhouse L, Casaburi R, Singh A, Bhasin D, Berman N, et al. Testosterone dose-response relationships in healthy young men. Am J Physiol Endocrinol Metab. 2001;281(6):e1172–81.
31. Forbes GB. The effect of anabolic steroids on lean body mass: the dose response curve. Metabolism. 1985;34(6):571–3.
32. Bhasin S, Tenover J. Age-associated sarcopenia—issues in the use of testosterone as an anabolic agent in older men. J Clin Endocrinol Metab. 1997;82(6):1659–60.
33. Sih R, Morley JE, Kaiser FE, Perry HM 3rd, Patrick P, Ross C. Testosterone replacement in older hypogonadal men: a 12-month randomized controlled trial. J Clin Endocrinol Metab. 1997;82(6):1661–7.
34. Urban RJ, Bodenburg YH, Gilkison C, Foxworth J, Coggan AR, Wolfe RR, et al. Testosterone administration to elderly men increases skeletal muscle strength and protein synthesis. Am J Phys. 1995;269:E820–6.
35. Nam YS, Lee G, Yun JM, Cho B. Testosterone replacement, muscle strength, and physical function. World J Mens Health. 2018;36(2):110–22.
36. Storer TW, Basaria S, Traustadottir T, Harman SM, Pencina K, Li Z, et al. Effects of testosterone supplementation for 3 years on muscle performance and physical function in older men. J Clin Endocrinol Metab. 2017;102(2):583–93.
37. Chasland L, Naylor L, Yeap B, Maiorana A, Green D. Testosterone and exercise in middle-to-older aged men: combined and independent effects on vascular function. Hypertension. 2021;77(4):1095–105.
38. WHO. World Health Organization. [Online]; updated June 2021. Acceso 12 de Junede 2022.

Disponible en: https://www.who.int/en/news-room/fact-sheets/detail/obesity-and-overweight.
39. Kershaw EE, Flier JS. Adipose tissue as an endocrine organ. J Clin Endocrinol Metab. 2004;89(6):2548–56.
40. Fischer-Posovszky P, Wabitsch M, Hochberg Z. Endocrinology of adipose tissue—an update. Horm Metab Res. 2007;39(5):314–21.
41. Poulos SP, Hausman DB, Hausman GJ. The development and endocrine functions of adipose tissue. Mol Cell Endocrinol. 2010;323(1):20–34.
42. Dhindsa S, Miller MG, McWhirter CL, Mager DE, Ghanim H, Chaudhuri A, et al. Testosterone concentrations in diabetic and nondiabetic obese men. Diabetes Care. 2010;33(6):1186–92.
43. Fui MN, Dupuis P, Grossmann M. Lowered testosterone in male obesity: mechanisms, morbidity and management. Asian J Androl. 2014;16(2):223231.
44. Saboor Aftab SA, Kumar S, Barber TM. The role of obesity and type 2 diabetes mellitus in the development of male obesity-associated secondary hypogonadism. Clin Endocrinol. 2013;78(3):330–7.
45. Allan C, McLachlan R. Androgens and obesity. Curr Opin Endocrinol Diabetes Obes. 2010;17(3):224–32.
46. van Hulsteijn LT, Pasquali R, Casanueva F, Haluzik M, Ledoux S, Monteiro MP, et al. Prevalence of endocrine disorders in obese patients: systematic review and meta-analysis. Eur J Endocrinol. 2020;182(1):11–21.
47. Wu FC, Tajar A, Pye SR, Silman AJ, Finn JD, O'Neill TW, et al. Hypothalamic-pituitary-testicular axis disruptions in older men are differentially linked to age and modifiable risk factors: the European Male Aging Study. J Clin Endocrinol Metab. 2008;93(7):2737–45.
48. Corona G, Rastrelli G, Monami M, Saad F, Luconi M, Lucchese M, et al. Body weight loss reverts obesity-associated hypogonadotropic hypogonadism: a systematic review and meta-analysis. Eur J Endocrinol. 2013;168(6):829–43.
49. Grossmann M. Hypogonadism and male obesity: focus on unresolved questions. Clin Endocrinol. 2018;89(1):11–21.
50. Lovejoy JC, Bray GA, Greeson CS, Klemperer M, Morris J, Partington C, et al. Oral anabolic steroid treatment, but not parenteral androgen treatment, decreases abdominal fat in obese, older men. Int J Obes Relat Metab Disord. 1995;19(9):614–24.
51. Rebuffé-Scrive M, Mårin P, Björntorp P. Effect of testosterone on abdominal adipose tissue in men. Int J Obes. 1991;15(11):791–5.
52. Mårin P, Krotkiewski M, Björntorp P. Androgen treatment of middle-aged, obese men: effects on metabolism, muscle and adipose tissues. Eur J Med. 1992;1(6):329–36.
53. Traish AM. Testosterone and weight loss: the evidence. Curr Opin Endocrinol Diabetes Obes. 2014;21(5):313–22.
54. Saad F, Yassin A, Doros G, Haider A. Effects of long-term treatment with testosterone on weight and waist size in 411 hypogonadal men with obesity classes I-III: observational data from two registry studies. Int J Obes. 2016;40(1):162–70.
55. Saad F, Doros G, Haider KS, Haider A. Differential effects of 11 years of long-term injectable testosterone undecanoate therapy on anthropometric and metabolic parameters in hypogonadal men with normal weight, overweight and obesity in comparison with untreated controls: real-world data from. Int J Obes. 2020;44(6):1264–78.
56. Ta V, Chin WK, White AA. Allergic contact dermatitis to testosterone and estrogen in transdermal therapeutic systems. Dermatitis. 2014;25(5):279.
57. Inui S, Itami S. Molecular basis of androgenetic alopecia: from androgen to paracrine mediators through dermal papilla. J Dermatol Sci. 2011;61(1):1–6.
58. Thornton MJ. Oestrogen functions in skin and skin appendages. Expert Opin Ther Targets. 2005;9(3):617–29.
59. Sator PG, Sator MO, Schmidt JB, Nahavandi H, Radakovic S, Huber JC, et al. A prospective, randomized, double-blind, placebo-controlled study on the influence of a hormone replacement therapy on skin aging in postmenopausal women. Climacteric. 2007;10(4):320–34.
60. Brincat M, Baron Y, Galea R. Estrogens and the skin. Climacteric. 2005;8(2):110–23.
61. Korenman SG, Morley JE, Mooradian AD, Davis SS, Kaiser FE, Silver AJ, et al. Secondary hypogonadism in older men: its relation to impotence. J Clin Endocrinol Metab. 1990;71(4):963–9.
62. Luo Y, Zhang H, Liao M, Tang Q, Huang Y, Xie J, et al. Sex hormones predict the incidence of erectile dysfunction: from a population-based prospective cohort study (FAMHES). J Sex Med. 2015;12(5):1165–74.
63. O'Connor DB, Lee DM, Corona G, Forti G, Tajar A, O'Neill TW, et al. European Male Ageing Study Group. The relationships between sex hormones and sexual function in middle-aged and older European men. J Clin Endocrinol Metab. 2011;96(10):E1577–87.
64. Anderson R, Bancroft J, Wu F. The effects of exogenous testosterone on sexuality and mood of normal men. J Clin Endocrinol Metab. 1992;75(6):1503–7.
65. Schiavi RC, White D, Mandeli J, Levine AC. Effect of testosterone administration on sexual behavior and mood in men with erectile dysfunction. Arch Sex Behav. 1997;26(3):231–41.
66. Cunningham GR, Stephens-Shields AJ, Rosen RC, Wang C, Bhasin S, Matsumoto AM, et al. Testosterone treatment and sexual function in older men with low testosterone levels. J Clin Endocrinol Metab. 2016;101(8):3096–104.
67. Brock G, Heiselman D, Maggi M, Kim S, Rodríguez Vallejo J, Behre H, et al. Effect of testosterone solution 2% on testosterone concentration, sex drive and energy in hypogonadal men: results of a placebo controlled study. J Urol. 2016;195(3):699–705.

68. Jain P, Rademaker AW, McVary KT. Testosterone supplementation for erectile dysfunction: results of a meta-analysis. J Urol. 2000;164(2):371–5.
69. Corona G, Isidori A, Buvat J, Aversa A, Rastrelli G, Hackett G, et al. Testosterone supplementation and sexual function: a meta-analysis study. J Sex Med. 2014;11(6):1577–92.
70. Snyder PJ, Bhasin S, Cunningham GR, Matsumoto AM, Stephens-Shields AJ, Cauley JA, et al. Lessons from the testosterone trials. Endocr Rev. 2018;39(3):369–86.
71. Spitzer M, Basaria S, Travison TG, Davda MN, Paley A, Cohen B, et al. Effect of testosterone replacement on response to sildenafil citrate in men with erectile dysfunction: a parallel, randomized trial. Ann Intern Med. 2012;157(10):681–91.
72. Corona G, Rastrelli G, Morgentaler A, Sforza A, Mannucci E, Maggi M. Meta-analysis of results of testosterone therapy on sexual function based on international index of erectile function scores. Eur Urol. 2017;72(6):1000–11.
73. Kaur H, Werstuck GH. The effect of testosterone on cardiovascular disease and cardiovascular risk factors in men: a review of clinical and preclinical data. CJC Open. 2021;3(10):1238–48.
74. Araujo A, Dixon J, Suarez E, Murad M, Guey L. Clinical review: endogenous testosterone and mortality in men: a systematic review and meta-analysis. J Clin Endocrinol Metab. 2011;96(10):3007–19.
75. Ruige JB, Mahmoud AM, De Bacquer D, Kaufman JM. Endogenous testosterone and cardiovascular disease in healthy men: a meta-analysis. Heart. 2011;97(11):870–5.
76. Oskui PM, French WJ, Herring MJ, Mayeda GS, Burstein S, Kloner RA. Testosterone and the cardiovascular system: a comprehensive review of the clinical literature. J Am Heart Assoc. 2013;2(6):e000272.
77. Jones RD, Nettleship JE, Kapoor D, Jones HT, Channer S. Testosterone and atherosclerosis in aging men: purported association and clinical implications. Am J Cardiovasc Drugs. 2005;5(3):141–54.
78. Laughlin GA, Barrett-Connor E, Bergstrom J. Low serum testosterone and mortality in older men. J Clin Endocrinol Metab. 2008;93(1):68–75.
79. Ding EL, Song Y, Malik VS, Liu S. Sex differences of endogenous sex hormones and risk of type 2 diabetes. JAMA. 2006;295:1288/1299.
80. Yao QM, Wang B, An XF, Zhang JA, Ding L. Testosterone level and risk of type 2 diabetes in men: a systematic review and meta-analysis. Endocr Connect. 2018;7(1):220–31.
81. Tsai EC, Matsumoto AM, Fujimoto WY, Boyko EJ. Association of bioavailable, free, and total testosterone with insulin resistance: influence of sex hormone-binding globulin and body fat. Diabetes Care. 2004;27(4):861–8.
82. Budoff M, Ellenberg S, Lewis C, Mohler E 3rd, Wenger N, Bhasin S, et al. Testosterone treatment and coronary artery plaque volume in older men with low testosterone. JAMA. 2017;317(7):708–16.
83. Shaikh K, Ellenberg SS, Nakanishi R, Snyder PJ, Lee J, Wenger NK, et al. Biomarkers and noncalcified coronary artery plaque progression in older men treated with testosterone. J Clin Endocrinol Metab. 2020;105(7):2142–9.
84. Basaria S, Harman S, Travison T, Hodis H, Tsitouras P, Budoff M, et al. Effects of testosterone administration for 3 years on subclinical atherosclerosis progression in older men with low or low-normal testosterone levels: a randomized clinical trial. JAMA. 2015;314(6):570–81.
85. Calof OM, Singh AB, Lee ML, Kenny AM, Urban RJ, Tenover JL, et al. Adverse events associated with testosterone replacement in middle-aged and older men: a meta-analysis of randomized, placebo-controlled trials. J Gerontol A Biol Sci Med Sci. 2005;60(11):1451–7.
86. Haddad RM, Kennedy CC, Caples SM, Tracz MJ, Sideras K, Uraga MV, et al. Testosterone and cardiovascular risk in men: a systematic review and meta-analysis of randomized placebo-controlled trials. Mayo Clin Proc. 2007;82(1):29–39.
87. Gava G, Meriggiola MC. Update on male hormonal contraception. Ther Adv Endocrinol Metab. 2019;10.
88. Contraceptive efficacy of testosterone-induced azoospermia in normal men. World Health Organization Task Force on methods for the regulation of male fertility. Lancet. 1990;336(8721):955–9.
89. Turner L, Conway AJ, Jimenez M, Liu PY, Forbes E, McLachlan RI, et al. Contraceptive efficacy of a depot progestin and androgen combination in men. J Clin Endocrinol Metab. 2003;88(10):4659–67.
90. Gu Y, Liang X, Wu W, Liu M, Song S, Cheng L, et al. Multicenter contraceptive efficacy trial of injectable testosterone undecanoate in Chinese men. J Clin Endocrinol Metab. 2009;94(6):1910–5.
91. Corona G, Rastrelli G, Marchiani S, Filippi S, Morelli A, Sarchielli E, et al. Consequences of anabolic-androgenic steroid abuse in males; sexual and reproductive perspective. World J Mens Health. 2022;40(2):165–78.
92. Meriggiola MC, Costantino A, Cerpolini S, Bremner WJ, Huebler D, Morselli-Labate AM, et al. Testosterone undecanoate maintains spermatogenic suppression induced by cyproterone acetate plus testosterone undecanoate in normal men. J Clin Endocrinol Metab. 2003;88(12):5818–26.
93. Gu YQ, Tong JS, Ma DZ, Wang XH, Yuan D, Tang WH, et al. Male hormonal contraception: effects of injections of testosterone undecanoate and depot medroxyprogesterone acetate at eight-week intervals in chinese men. J Clin Endocrinol Metab. 2004;89(5):2254–62.
94. Long JE, Lee MS, Blithe DL. Update on novel hormonal and nonhormonal male contraceptive development. J Clin Endocrinol Metab. 2021;106(6):e2381–92.
95. Bhasin S, Brito J, Cunningham G, Hayes F, Hodis H, Matsumoto A, et al. Testosterone therapy in men with hypogonadism: an Endocrine Society Clinical

Practice Guideline. J Clin Endocrinol Metab. 2018;103(5):1715–44.
96. Pope HG Jr, Wood RI, Rogol A, Nyberg F, Bowers L, Bhasin S. Adverse health consequences of performance-enhancing drugs: an Endocrine Society scientific statement. Endocr Rev. 2014;35(3):341–75.
97. Kanayama G, Hudson JI, DeLuca J, Isaacs S, Baggish A, Weiner R, et al. Prolonged hypogonadism in males following withdrawal from anabolic-androgenic steroids: an under-recognized problem. Addiction. 2015;110(5):823–31.
98. Rasmussen JJ, Selmer C, Østergren PB, Pedersen KB, Schou M, Gustafsson F, et al. Former abusers of anabolic androgenic steroids exhibit decreased testosterone levels and hypogonadal symptoms years after cessation: a case-control study. PLoS One. 2016;11(8):e0161208.
99. Coward RM, Rajanahally S, Kovac JR, Smith RP, PastuszaK AW, Lipshultz LI. Anabolic steroid induced hypogonadism in young men. J Urol. 2013;190(6):2200–5.
100. Huggins C, Hodges CV. Studies on Prostatic Cancer. I. The effect of castration, of estrogen and of androgen injection on serum phosphatases in metastatic carcinoma of the prostate. J Urol. 1941;167:948–51.
101. Muller RL, Gerber L, Moreira DM, Andriole G, Castro-Santamaria R, Freedland SJ. Serum testosterone and dihydrotestosterone and prostate cancer risk in the placebo arm of the Reduction by Dutasteride of Prostate Cancer Events trial. Eur Urol. 2012;62(5):757–64.
102. Ano M, Imamoto T, Suzuki H, Fukasawa S, Kojima S. The clinical potential of pretreatment serum testosterone level to improve the efficiency of prostate cancer screening. Eur Urol. 2007;51(2):375–80.
103. Shin BS, Hwang EC, Im CM, Kim SO, Jung SI, Kang TW, et al. Is a decreased serum testosterone level a risk factor for prostate cancer? A cohort study of korean men. Korean J Urol. 2010;51(12):819–23.
104. Morote J, Ramirez C, Gómez E, Planas J, Raventós C. The relationship between total and free serum testosterone and the risk of prostate cancer and tumour aggressiveness. BJU Int. 2009;104(4):486–9.
105. Xia BW, Zhao SC, Chen ZP, Chen C, Liu TS, Yang F, et al. Relationship between serum total testosterone and prostate volume in aging men. Sci Rep. 2021;11(1):14122.
106. Baas W, Köhler T. Testosterone replacement therapy and BPH/LUTS. What is the evidence? Curr Urol Rep. 2016;17(6):46.
107. Koo JM, Shim BS. Significance of serum testosterone for prostate-specific antigen (PSA) elevation and prediction of prostate cancer in patients with PSA above 10 ng/ml. Korean J Urol. 2010;51(12):831–5.
108. Debruyne FM, Behre HM, Roehrborn CG, Maggi M, Wu FC, Schröder FH, et al. Testosterone treatment is not associated with increased risk of prostate cancer or worsening of lower urinary tract symptoms: prostate health outcomes in the Registry of Hypogonadism in Men. BJU. 2017;119(2):216–24.
109. Fowler JE Jr, Whitmore WF Jr. The response of metastatic adenocarcinoma of the prostate to exogenous testosterone. J Urol. 1981;126(3):372–5.
110. Thompson IM, Pauler DK, Goodman PJ, Tangen CM, Lucia MS, Parnes HL, et al. Prevalence of prostate cancer among men with a prostate-specific antigen level >.
111. AndroGel (testosterone gel) 1.62% Product Insert. [Online]. Acceso 12 de June de 2022. Disponible en: http://www.rxabbvie.com/pdf/androgel1_62_PI.pdf.
112. Cooper C, Perry P, Sparks A, MacIndoe J, Yates W, Williams R. Effect of exogenous testosterone on prostate volume, serum and semen prostate specific antigen levels in healthy young men. J Urol. 1998;159(2):441–3.
113. Rastrelli G, Vignozzi L, Corona G, Maggi M. Testosterone and benign prostatic hyperplasia. Sex Med Rev. 2019;7(2):259–71.
114. Kohn TP, Mata DA, Ramasamy R, Lipshultz LI. Effects of testosterone replacement therapy on lower urinary tract symptoms: a systematic review and meta-analysis. Eur Urol. 2016;69(6):1083–90.
115. Pearl JA, Berhanu D, François N, Masson P, Zargaroff S, Cashy J, et al. Testosterone supplementation does not worsen lower urinary tract symptoms. J Urol. 2013;190(5):1828–33.
116. Bachman E, Travison T, Basaria S, Davda M, Guo W, Li M, et al. Testosterone induces erythrocytosis via increased erythropoietin and suppressed hepcidin: evidence for a new erythropoietin/hemoglobin set point. J Gerontol A Biol Sci Med Sci. 2014;69(6):725–35.
117. Jones SD Jr, Dukovac T, Sangkum P, Yafi FA, Hellstrom WJ. Erythrocytosis and polycythemia secondary to testosterone replacement therapy in the aging male. Sex Med Rev. 2015;3(2):101–12.
118. Coviello AD, Kaplan B, Lakshman KM, Chen T, Singh AB, Bhasin S. Effects of graded doses of testosterone on erythropoiesis in healthy young and older men. J Clin Endocrinol Metab. 2008;93(3):914–9.
119. Corpas E, Harman S, Blackman M. Human growth hormone and human aging. Endocr Rev. 1993;14(1):20–39.
120. Veldhuis JD. Aging and hormones of the hypothalamo-pituitary axis: gonadotropic axis in men and somatotropic axes in men and women. Ageing Res Rev. 2008;7(3):189–208.
121. Maggio M, Ble A, Ceda GP, Metter EJ. Decline in insulin-like growth factor-I levels across adult life span in two large population studies. J Gerontol A Biol Sci Med Sci. 2006;61(2):182–3.
122. Rosén T, Bengtsson BA. Premature mortality due to cardiovascular disease in hypopituitarism. Lancet. 1990;336(8710):285–8.
123. Hazem A, Elamin MB, Bancos I, Malaga G, Prutsky G, Domecq JP, et al. Body composition and qual-

ity of life in adults treated with GH therapy: a systematic review and meta-analysis. Eur J Endocrinol. 2012;166(1):13–20.
124. Jørgensen JO, Müller J, Møller J, Wolthers T, Vahl N, Juul A, et al. Adult growth hormone deficiency. Horm Res. 1994;42(4–5):235–41.
125. Rosén T, Bosaeus I, Tölli J, Lindstedt G, Bengtsson RA. Increased body fat mass and decreased extracellular fluid volume in adults with growth hormone deficiency. Clin Endocrinol. 1993;38(1):63–71.
126. Stochholm K, Gravholt CH, Laursen T, Jørgensen JO, Laurberg P, Andersen M, et al. Incidence of GH deficiency—a nationwide study. Eur J Endocrinol. 2006;155(1):61–71.
127. Gharib H, Cook DM, Saenger PH, Bengtsson BA, Feld S, Nippoldt TB, et al. American Association of Clinical Endocrinologists medical guidelines for clinical practice for growth hormone use in adults and children—2003 update. Endocr Pract. 2003;9(1):64–76.
128. Feldt-Rasmussen U, Abs R, Bengtsson BA, Bennmarker H, Bramnert M, Hernberg-Ståhl E, et al. Growth hormone deficiency and replacement in hypopituitary patients previously treated for acromegaly or Cushing's disease. Eur J Endocrinol. 2002;146(1):67–74.
129. Reed ML, Merriam GR, Kargi AY. Adult growth hormone deficiency—benefits, side effects, and risks of growth hormone replacement. Front Endocrinol (Lausanne). 2013;4:64.
130. Rudman D, Feller AG, Nagraj HS, Gergans GA, Lalitha PY, Goldberg AF, et al. Effects of human growth hormone in men over 60 years old. N Engl J Med. 1990;323(1):1–6.
131. Beck P, Koumans J, Winterling C, Stein M, Daughaday W, Kipris D. Studies of insulin and growth hormone secretion in human obesity. J Lab Clin Med. 1964;64:654–67.
132. Rasmussen MH, Hvidberg A, Juul A, Main KM, Gotfredsen A, Skakkebaek NE, et al. Massive weight loss restores 24-hour growth hormone release profiles and serum insulin-like growth factor-I levels in obese subjects. J Clin Endocrinol Metab. 1995;80(4):1407–15.
133. Williams T, Berelowitz M, Joffe SN, Thorner MO, Rivier J, Vale W, et al. Impaired growth hormone responses to growth hormone-releasing factor in obesity. A pituitary defect reversed with weight reduction. N Engl J Med. 1984;311(22):1403–7.
134. Rasmussen MH. Obesity, growth hormone and weight loss. Mol Cell Endocrinol. 2010;316(2):147–53.
135. Mekala KC, Tritos NA. Effects of recombinant human growth hormone therapy in obesity in adults: a metaanalysis. J Clin Endocrinol Metab. 2009;94(1):130–7.
136. Blackman M, Sorkin J, Münzer T, Bellantoni M, Busby-Whitehead J, Stevens T, et al. Growth hormone and sex steroid administration in healthy aged women and men: a randomized controlled trial. JAMA. 2002;288(18):2282–92.
137. Liu H, Bravata DM, Olkin I, Nayak S, Roberts B, Garber AM, et al. Systematic review: the safety and efficacy of growth hormone in the healthy elderly. Ann Intern Med. 2007;146(2):104–15.
138. Hoffman AR, Strasburger CJ, Zagar A, Blum WF, Kehely A, Hartman ML, et al. Efficacy and tolerability of an individualized dosing regimen for adult growth hormone replacement therapy in comparison with fixed body weight-based dosing. J Clin Endocrinol Metab. 2004;89(7):3224–33.
139. Colao A, Ferone D, Marzullo P, Lombardi G. Systemic complications of acromegaly: epidemiology, pathogenesis, and management. Endocr Rev. 2004;25(1):102–52.
140. Pivonello R, Auriemma RS, Grasso LF, Pivonello C, Simeoli C, Patalano R, et al. Complications of acromegaly: cardiovascular, respiratory and metabolic comorbidities. Pituitary. 2017;20(1):46–62.
141. Bartke A. Can growth hormone (GH) accelerate aging? Evidence from GH-transgenic mice. Neuroendocrinology. 2003;78(4):210–06.
142. Bartke A, Coschigano K, Kopchick J, Chandrashekar V, Mattison J, Kinney B, et al. Genes that prolong life: relationships of growth hormone and growth to aging and life span. J Gerontol A Biol Sci Med Sci. 2001;56(8):B340–9.
143. Bartke A, Brown-Borg H. Life extension in the dwarf mouse. Curr Top Dev Biol. 2004;63:189–225.
144. Coschigano KT, Holland AN, Riders ME, List EO, Flyvbjerg A, Kopchick JJ. Deletion, but not antagonism, of the mouse growth hormone receptor results in severely decreased body weights, insulin, and insulin-like growth factor I levels and increased life span. Endocrinology. 2003;144(9):3799–810.
145. Aguiar-Oliveira M, Bartke A. Growth hormone deficiency: health and longevity. Endocr Rev. 2019;40(2):575–601.
146. Laron Z. The GH-IGF1 axis and longevity. The paradigm of IGF1 deficiency. Hormones. 2008;7(1):24–7.
147. Yaron-Saminsky D, Nagaraj K, Sarfstein R, Laron Z, Pasmanik-Chor M, Werner H. MicroRNA 132-3p is upregulated in Laron syndrome patients and controls longevity gene expression. Int J Mol Sci. 2021;22(21):11861.
148. Laron Z, Kauli R, Lapkina L, Werner H. IGF-I deficiency, longevity and cancer protection of patients with Laron syndrome. Mutat Res Rev Mutat Res. 2017;772:123–33.
149. Slominski A, Malarkey WB, Wortsman J, Asa SL, Carlson A. Human skin expresses growth hormone but not the prolactin gene. J Lab Clin Med. 2000;136(6):476–81.
150. Oakes SR, Haynes KM, Waters MJ, Herington AC, Werther GA. Demonstration and localization of growth hormone receptor in human skin and skin fibroblasts. J Clin Endocrinol Metab. 1992;75(5):1368–73.
151. Ben-Shlomo A, Melmed S. Skin manifestations in acromegaly. Clin Dermatol. 2006;24(4):256–9.

152. Kim H, Moon SY, Sohn MY, Lee WJ. Insulin-like growth factor-1 increases the expression of inflammatory biomarkers and sebum production in cultured sebocytes. Ann Dermatol. 2017;29(1):20–5.
153. Cappel M, Mauger D, Thiboutot D. Correlation between serum levels of insulin-like growth factor 1, dehydroepiandrosterone sulfate, and dihydrotestosterone and acne lesion counts in adult women. Arch Dermatol. 2005;141(3):333–8.
154. Assaf H, Abdel-Maged W, Elsadek B, Hassan M. Survivin as a novel biomarker in the pathogenesis of acne vulgaris and its correlation to insulin-like growth factor-I. Dis Markers. 2016;2016:1.
155. Hwang YL, Im M, Lee MH, Roh SS, Choi BW, Kim SJ, et al. Inhibitory effect of imperatorin on insulin-like growth factor-1-induced sebum production in human sebocytes cultured in vitro. Life Sci. 2016;144:49–53.
156. Wang C, Hwang YL, Li XM, Kim SJ, Zhu MJ, Lee JH, et al. Inhibition of insulin-like growth factor-1-induced sebum production by bilobetin in cultured human sebocytes. Ann Dermatol. 2019;31(3):294–9.
157. Breederveld R, Tuinebreijer W. Recombinant human growth hormone for treating burns and donor sites. Cochrane Database Syst Rev. 2014;9:CD008990.
158. Bitar MS. Insulin-like growth factor-1 reverses diabetes-induced wound healing impairment in rats. Horm Metab Res. 1997;29(8):383–6.
159. Kim SH, Heo EJ, Lee SW. The effect of topically applied recombinant human growth hormone on wound healing in pigs. Wounds. 2009;21(6):158–63.
160. Cristóbal L, de Los RN, Ortega MA, Álvarez-Mon M, García-Honduvilla N, Buján J, et al. Local growth hormone therapy for pressure ulcer healing on a human skin mouse model. Int J Mol Sci. 2019;20(17):4157.

47 Noninvasive Body Contouring Options for the Male Patient: A Guide to Cryolipolysis and HIFEM with Radiofrequency

Zakery Austin Koban and Brian Vassar Heil

47.1 Introduction

Various factors affecting men contribute to the lifetime risk of developing surplus adiposity, muscular atrophy, musculoskeletal injury, and eventual morbidity and mortality. The pursuit of physical fitness among modern men is challenged by powerful external factors: sedentary occupations, socioeconomic demands, and the widespread availability of inexpensive, high-calorie foods. These influences, compounded by the time restrictions of career-driven lifestyles, work against maintaining health, injury resistance, and aesthetic muscular development. The association between poor dietary habits, sedentary behavior, and physical inactivity on obesity and overall mortality has been well established. Income inequality also appears to play a role, with a significant association between income and obesity in middle and higher-income men [26]. Lack of time is a common self-reported reason for avoiding regular exercise, particularly strength training [7]. In addition, limited knowledge of proper form, training volume and frequency, caloric requirements for anabolism or catabolism, and nutrient timing often creates further barriers to achieving optimal muscular development in men.

Intrinsic influences are biological and, to some extent, hereditary. Research has revealed a substantial age-independent population-level decline in testosterone levels in recent years, possibly due to undocumented health-related or environmental phenomena. Low serum testosterone in men results in physiological manifestations of lower overall muscle mass, decreased bone density, higher body fat percentage, and aberrations in sexual function [23]. Elevation in body mass index (BMI) has been identified as an independent predictor of declining testosterone levels, and increasing BMI is found among young adult males over time [18]. Genetic predispositions related to bone structure and somatotype (i.e., ectomorphic and endomorphic body types) impose inherited restrictions on many men, both active and sedentary, by hereditarily affecting the ability to gain lean muscle mass or lose stubborn body fat through natural means. Senescent reduction in basal metabolic rate and the subsequent effect on total daily energy expenditure present additional weight loss challenges for the aging male (Fig. 47.1).

While healthy eating, proper sleeping, and androgen-boosting exercise should remain the primary standard for improving overall health and physical appearance, noninvasive body contouring (NIBC) modalities such as cryolipolysis offer an attractive option for men seeking to efficiently reduce *targeted* regions of excess adiposity while avoiding surgery and subsequent recovery, interruption of exercise, and disruption of familial, social, and work-related activities.

Z. A. Koban (✉) · B. V. Heil
Premier Plastic Surgery, PC, Wexford, PA, USA

K. Jeffords et al. (eds.), *Aesthetic Surgery for Men*, https://doi.org/10.1007/978-3-032-03840-1_47

Fig. 47.1 Extrinsic and intrinsic factors adversely affecting the male physique

Extrinsic	Intrinsic
Sedentary job status	Population-level serum testosterone
Socioeconomic status (middle and high income classes)	Somatotype (ectomorphic and endomorphic body types)
Poor nutritional intake	Senescent decline in basal metabolic rate
Lack of time for exercise	

Recent advances in high-intensity focused electromagnetic (HIFEM) and radiofrequency (RF) technology now reduce subcutaneous body fat with concurrent stimulation of underlying myocyte hyperplasia. The importance of *targeted* therapy here should not be understated. Transformation in overall body composition and reduction in the prevalence of preventable disease can only be achieved through regular resistance exercises, cardiovascular training, and proper nutrient intake. However, "spot-reduction" of stubborn body fat, once deemed impossible in the absence of surgery (i.e., liposuction), is now achievable using noninvasive body contouring modalities. Contouring systems such as CoolSculpting® (cryolipolysis) and EMSculpt® Neo (HIFEM with synchronized RF) enable plastic surgeons to circumvent *some* of the influences acting in detriment to the male physique, thus empowering the patient with greater proximity to his aesthetic goals.

47.2 Criteria for Optimization of Care Using NIBC

The clinical application of noninvasive body contouring is relatively simple, time-efficient, and can be carried out by medical support staff without requiring direct physician or advanced practice provider supervision in most instances. These systems are user-friendly and require minimal to moderate training to employ safely and efficaciously. Treatment delivery can therefore be carried out as a direct order with proper adherence to treatment guidelines and routine safety protocols. These systems are equipped with automatic safety interruption algorithms in the event of treatment anomaly or violation of manufacturer-set safety limits. Patient-prompted alert systems and emergency stop features allow for greater control and enhanced safety profile. It should be recognized that these integrated features, although helpful, do not replace a competent operator under indirect supervision. The degree of required supervision may also vary depending on local regulations, institutional policies, and scope-of-practice laws, and should always be aligned with governing standards of care.

Because noninvasive body contouring treatments do not require an advanced practitioner for treatment delivery, the initial patient encounter or clinical consultation should ideally be performed by either the plastic surgeon or mid-level provider. A thorough history and physical examination are critical to determining patient candidacy and selecting the best mode of treatment. A complete historical review will unveil the presence of absolute and relative contraindications to therapy and elicit patient goals and expectations regarding the outcome. Physical examination should include data collection such as height, weight, BMI, and circumferential measurements of the targeted treatment regions. This data serves as a valuable baseline for later comparative analysis and can be particularly useful when treating noncompliant patients. An initial standard photographic series should be taken before proceeding with any NIBC. This should become practice policy, without exception, and treatment should not continue if the patient declines to participate. Time-series photographic analysis provides the best evidence for treatment efficacy and (with formal patient consent) can be later used as a marketing resource (Fig. 47.2). Three-dimensional imaging systems (VECTRA® M3;

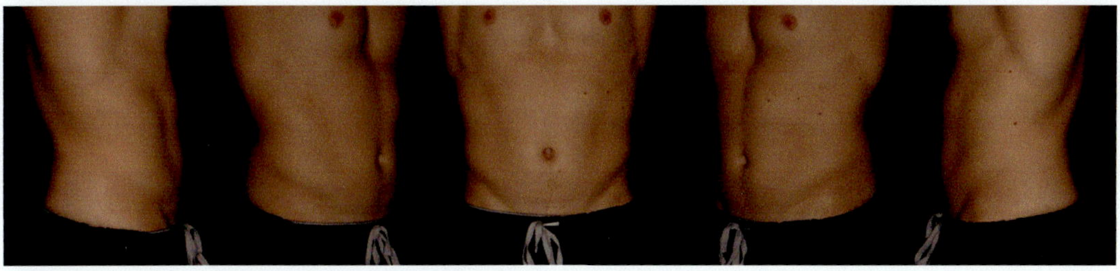

Fig. 47.2 Example of a Pretreatment Standard Photographic Series

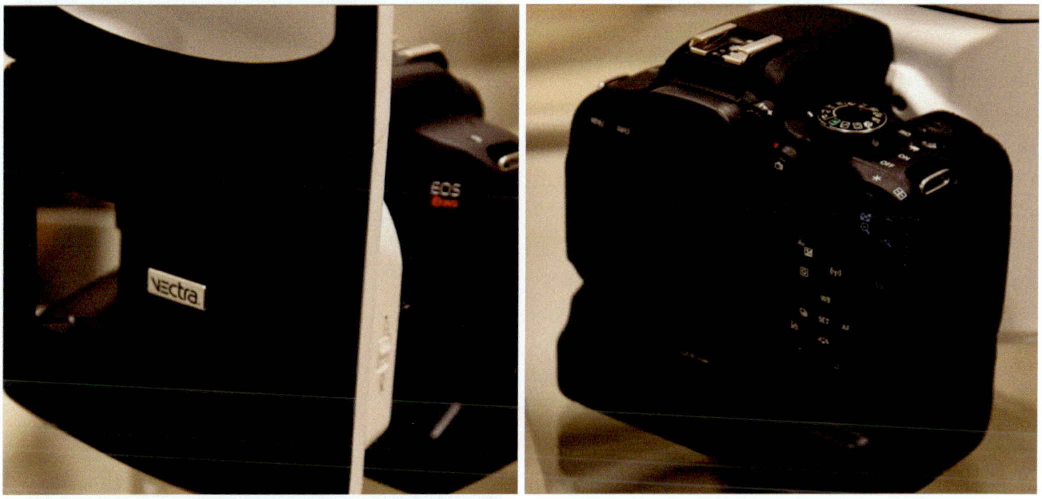

Fig. 47.3 Three-dimensional imaging systems like the hand-held VECTRA® lens and accompanying software can provide analyses (VECTRA® M3; Canfield Scientific, Inc., Fairfield, NJ)

Canfield Scientific, Inc., Fairfield, NJ) are recommended, as they can provide high-quality volumetric analyses [4] (Fig. 47.3).

Proper patient counseling should be centered on reasonable post-treatment expectations, lifestyle modifications, and risk of adverse events. Therefore, the surgeon (or physician-delegated mid-level provider) is responsible for making educated clinical decisions regarding patient candidacy and formulating an optimal treatment plan to be carried out by support staff. The criteria for optimization of care using NIBC modalities are fourfold; (1) proper patient selection, (2) choosing the most appropriate treatment modality, (3) patient education and expectation management, and (4) implementation of lifestyle or behavioral modifications (Fig. 47.4). We will explore each criterion in turn, but it is impossible to do so without first examining the necessary tools for the task.

Fig. 47.4 The criteria for optimization of care using NIBC

Four Criteria for Optimization of Care Using NIBC	
1	Proper patient selection
2	Selecting the most appropriate treatment modality
3	Patient education and expectation management
4	Lifestyle or behavioral modifications

47.3 Tools for the Task: Cryolipolysis

Numerous NIBC treatment systems are currently at the disposal of plastic surgeons. Several techniques, such as low-level laser therapy, focused ultrasound, and radiofrequency therapy, can reduce subcutaneous fat via adipocyte apoptosis or necrosis [1]. We will focus our attention on two types of NIBC systems of heightened interest: (1) cryolipolysis and (2) HIFEM with synchronized radiofrequency.

Cryolipolysis is a noninvasive body contouring treatment modality for localized adipocyte destruction achieved by employing controlled cooling [17]. CoolSculpting® (ZELTIQ Aesthetics, Inc., Pleasanton, CA) is an FDA-cleared Class II cryolipolytic device that exploits the temperature-sensitive nature of adipocytes with limited effects on surrounding tissue (Fig. 47.5). CoolSculpting® treatments are performed by placing protective gel and a vacuum or surface applicator device on the patient's skin. Vacuum applicators draw the skin and adipose tissue away from the body, filling the applicator and holding the tissue against the cooling surfaces of the device. The operator then initiates heat extraction, and sensors in the cooling surfaces of the applicator monitor the skin surface. Surface applicators function in the same fashion in the absence of suction (Figs. 47.6 and 47.7). Treatment duration varies by applicator and body region, ranging from 35 to 75 minutes. The system was cleared in 2010 by the FDA for the treatment of flank and abdominal fat and subcutaneous adiposity of the inner and outer thighs in 2014 [15]. The FDA later cleared this system for the treatment of other regions of subcutaneous adiposity, namely the upper arms, mid-back, infra-gluteal zones, and the submental and submandibular areas.

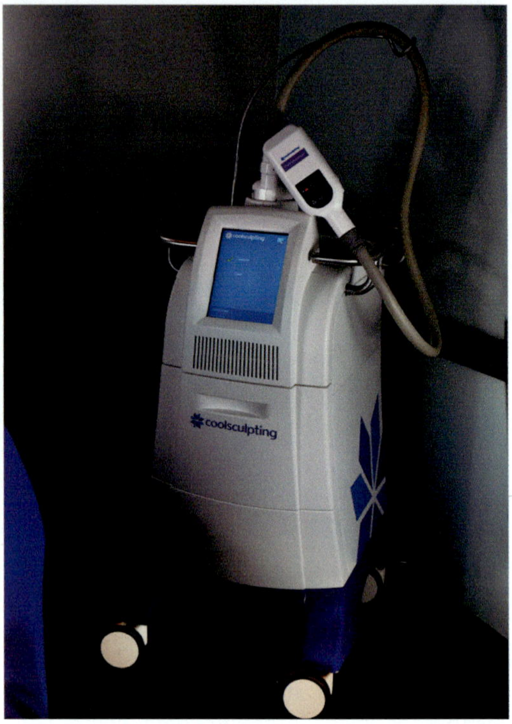

Fig. 47.5 The CoolSculpting® Cryolipolysis system

Cryolipolysis targets the physical properties of adipocytes that differentiate the fat layer from the overlying skin, resulting in selective adipocyte destruction [6]. Clinical findings of cold-induced panniculitis and transient fat necrosis in the cheeks of infants were first described in 1970 by Epstein and Oren [3]. These findings, paired with similar observations in adults, revealed increased lipid susceptibility to cold-induced injury relative to surrounding water-based tissues. In 2007, Manstein et al. undertook an animal study investigating the effects of cold

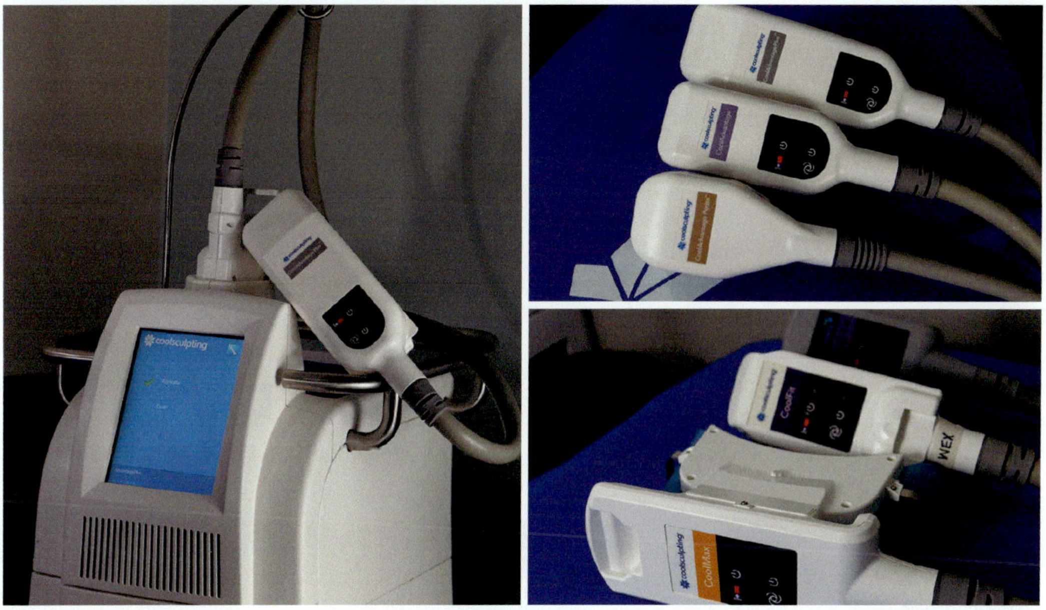

Fig. 47.6 CoolSculpting® vacuum applicators

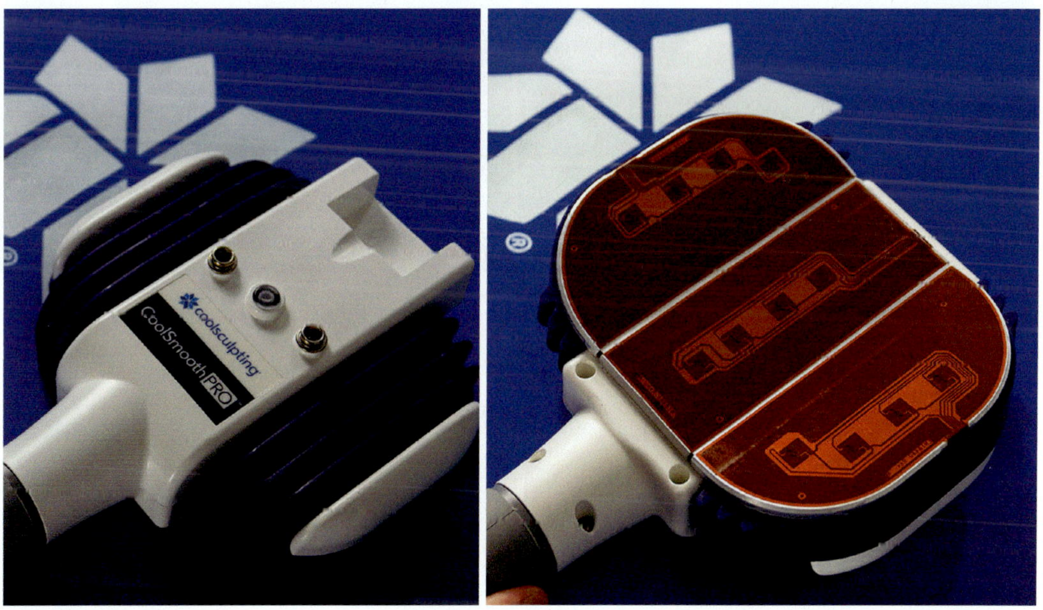

Fig. 47.7 CoolSmooth® surface applicator

exposure on subcutaneous fat in a porcine model, introducing the noninvasive method for fat reduction by freezing [6, 19]. The primary proposed mechanism of cryolipolysis suggests that the precise application of cold temperature induces adipocyte apoptosis and subsequent phagocytosis by macrophages within the targeted region of adiposity. It is hypothesized that vacuum suction and controlled heat extraction impede vascular perfusion, resulting in the crystallization of the targeted adipocytes without adversely affecting the overlying dermis and epidermis. Another mechanism proposes that the initial injury induced by adipocyte crystallization is further exacerbated by reperfusion injury [6]. An influx of inflammatory cells is observed at three days following exposure, reaching a maximum at day 14 as adipocytes are flooded by histiocytes, neutrophils, lymphocytes, and other mononuclear cells. At 14–30 days, macrophages engulf, digest, and remove lipid cells from the treatment site as part of the body's programmed response to the injury. At four weeks, inflammation and adipocyte volume are decreased. Inflammation progressively diminishes from 2 to 3 months following treatment, and adipose volume decreases to an appreciable level visually [15] (Figs. 47.8, 47.9, 47.10, and 47.11).

Recent years of research support the premise of enhanced cryolipolysis efficacy with multiple treatment applications in the same anatomical area [6, 17]. Loap et al. propose that the reduction in fat mass following cryolipolysis may be due to the adaptation of white tissue adipocytes to the phenomena of cold-induced thermogenesis, the repetitive applications of cryotherapy within a reasonably short time interval, rather than adipocyte apoptosis [17]. Additionally, the treatment of neighboring areas may help improve patient satisfaction and prevent unnatural outcomes [16].

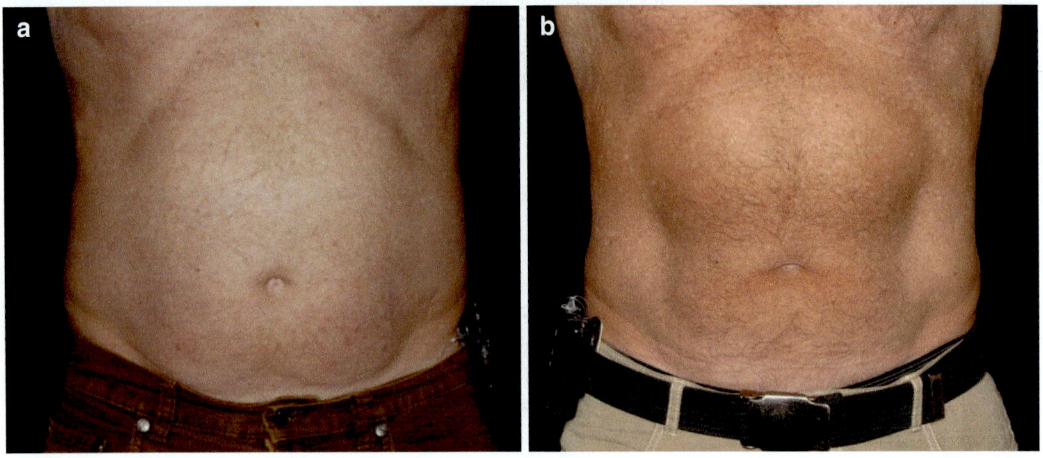

Fig. 47.8 CoolSculpting® (**a**) before and (**b**) after following treatment of the upper and lower abdomen; anterior view

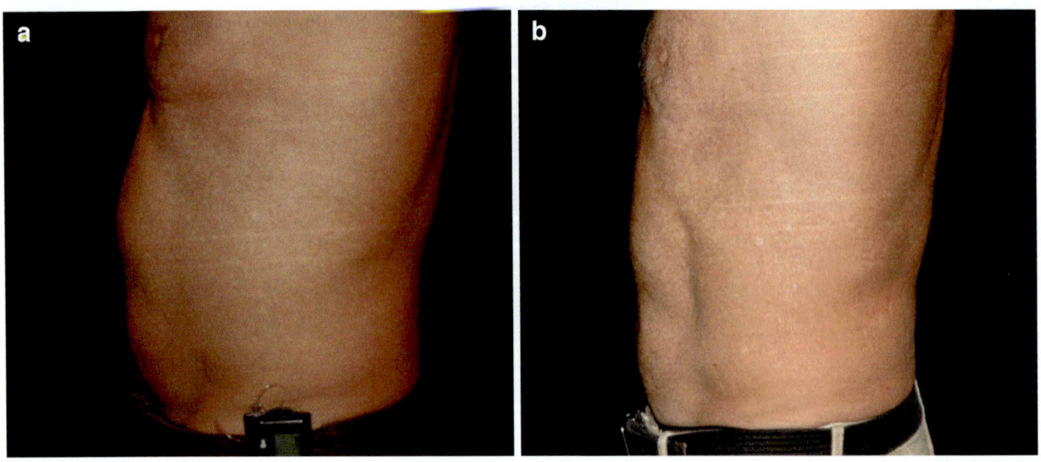

Fig. 47.9 CoolSculpting® (**a**) before and (**b**) after following treatment of the upper and lower abdomen; lateral view

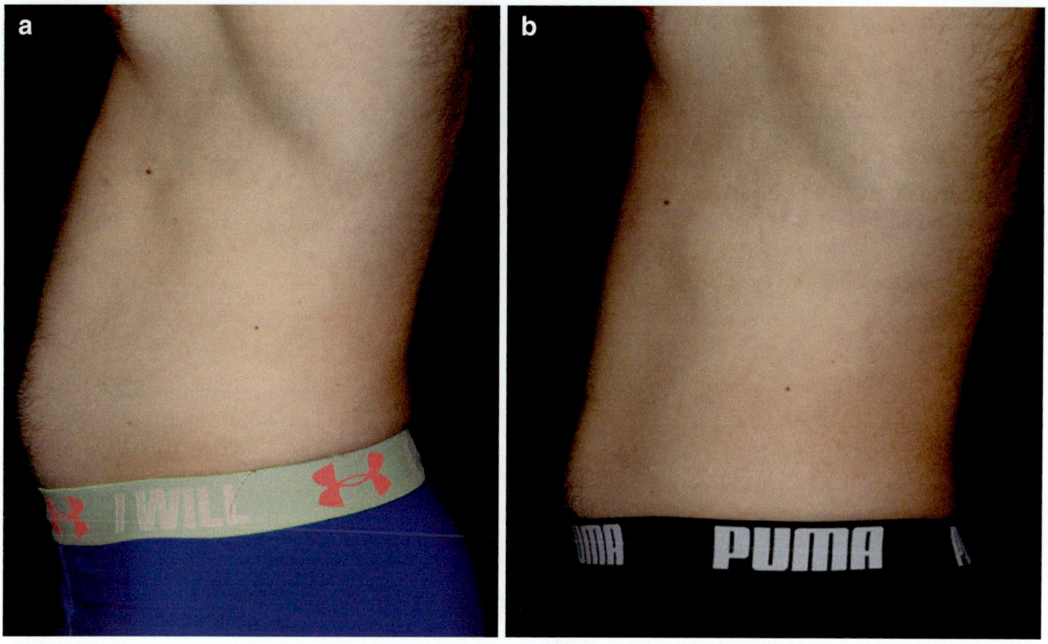

Fig. 47.10 CoolSculpting® (**a**) before and (**b**) after following treatment of refractory body fat in the upper and lower abdomen; lateral view

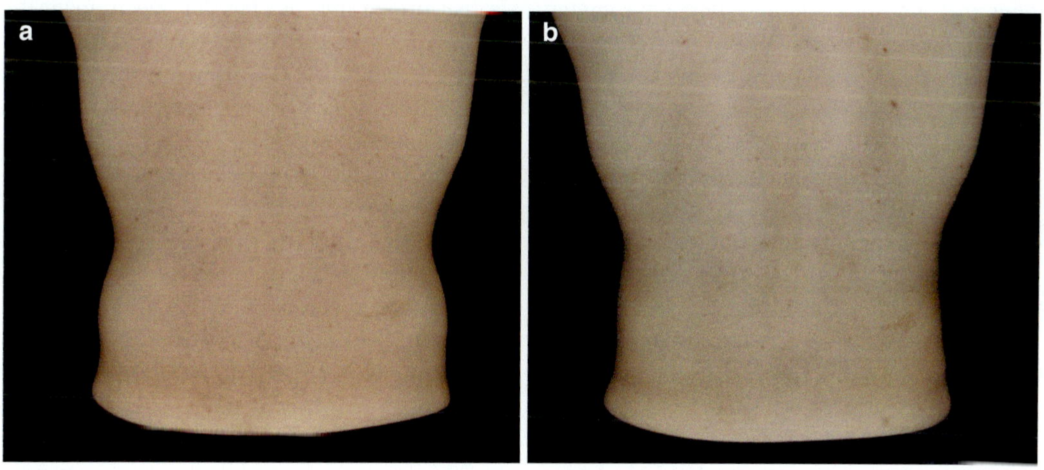

Fig. 47.11 CoolSculpting® (**a**) before and (**b**) after following of refractory body fat in the bilateral flanks; posterior view

Reasonable concerns for the systemic impact of adipocyte apoptosis and the processing of freed lipids have been addressed. Multiple studies have demonstrated that values for C-reactive protein, serum cholesterol, triglycerides, free fatty acids, liver enzymes, total bilirubin, albumin, and glucose remain within normal limits during and after therapy [6, 14, 17]. Consistency in the adverse events profile of cryolipolysis has been established, and it is generally regarded as an effective and well-tolerated method of NIBC [16]. Potential adverse effects and their associated mechanisms will be addressed later.

47.4 Tools for the Task: HIFEM with Synchronized RF

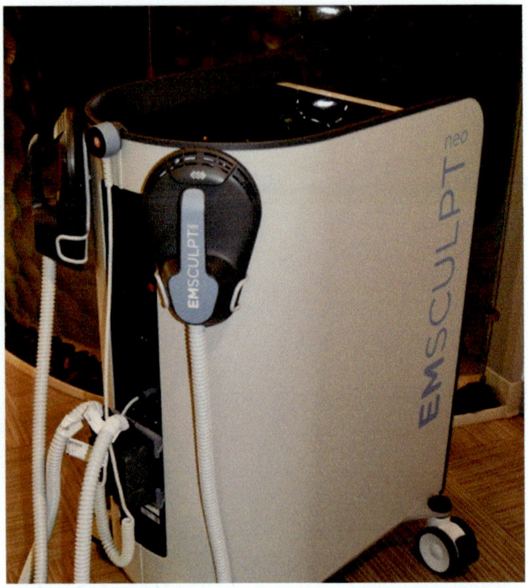

Fig. 47.12 The EMSculpt® Neo - HIFEM with synchronized RF device

EMSculpt® is an FDA-cleared, Class II powered muscle stimulator (BTL Industries, LTD, Waltham, MA). The device uses a High-Intensity Focused Electromagnetic Field (HIFEM) to stimulate powerful and prolonged muscle contractions that are not achievable through voluntary skeletal muscle control. HIFEM uses alternating magnetic fields to induce electrical currents, depolarizing neuromuscular tissue and resulting in contraction [5]. The HIFEM device produces a focused electromagnetic force with various frequency and pulse-amplitude algorithms designed to provide hyper-maximal muscle contraction and control lactic acid accumulation, thus preventing fatigue and delayed-onset muscle soreness. Recent device reports describe intensities of approximately 2–2.5 Tesla, depending on applicator design and treatment zone, highlighting the variability across clinical settings [13]. Magnetic field intensities delivered by HIFEM devices have been shown to reach up to 2.5 Tesla, supporting these observations [8]. This extreme muscle time-under-tension results in muscular hypertrophy and hyperplasia of the targeted region after a series of treatments. Electromagnetic stimulation of the targeted muscle is induced at an intensity level tolerable to the patient for 30 minutes (typically between 0.9 and 1.7 Tesla depending upon the muscle). HIFEM is FDA cleared for treating abdominal, gluteal, quadriceps, medial thigh, biceps, triceps, gastrocnemius, and soleus muscle groups. The treatment is performed by placing an electromagnetic applicator over the treatment zone and securing it with a fixation belt. The operator then initiates therapy and adjusts the intensity level based on patient comfort (Figs. 47.12 and 47.13).

HIFEM induces approximately 20,000 supramaximal muscle contractions within a 30-minute time frame. This degree of muscular training cannot be achieved voluntarily, as the power of muscle contraction is limited by the firing rates and conductivity of neural pathways [2]. The histological effects of HIFEM on skeletal muscle were evaluated in an in vivo porcine model in 2018. In treated animals, muscle mass density increased by 20.56% on average, while the average area per single muscle fiber increased by 12.15%, indicating muscular hypertrophy (volumetric growth of individual muscle fibers) [2]. The average number of muscle fibers increased in the study by 8.0%, representing muscular hyperplasia [2]. Human studies on the abdomen revealed a concurrent reduction of subcutaneous adiposity with simultaneous hypertrophy of the abdominal musculature. A 15.8% increase in abdominal muscle thickness was observed via computed tomogra-

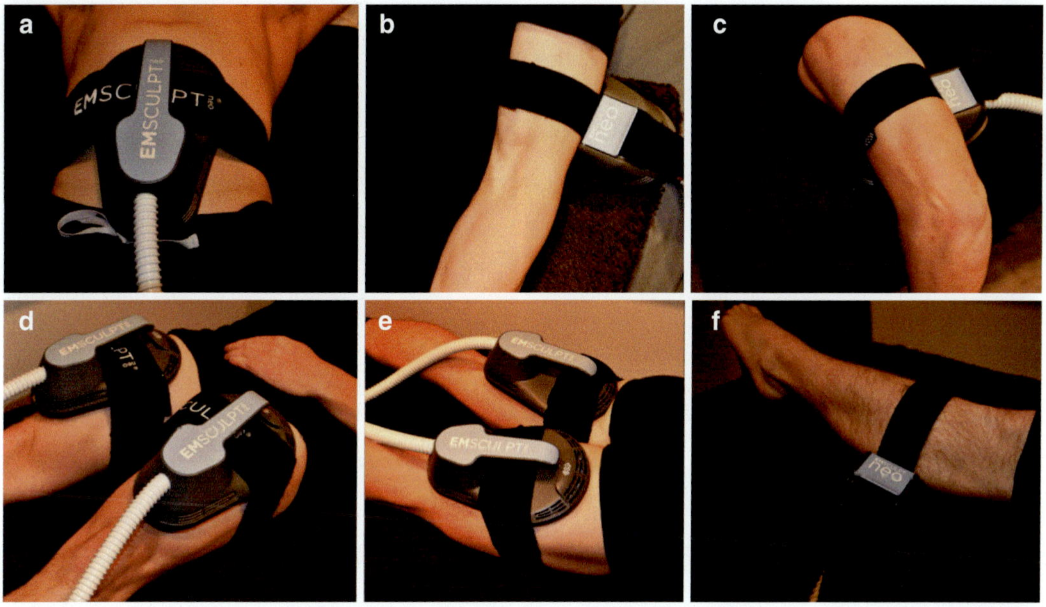

Fig. 47.13 The EMSculpt® Neo applicators in various treatment positions: (**a**) abdomen, (**b**) biceps, (**c**) triceps, (**d**) quadriceps, (**e**) hamstrings, (**f**) calves. Gluteal treatment not depicted

phy, with a 10.8% reduction in diastasis recti. This was accompanied by a mean reduction in subcutaneous abdominal fat by 19.2% and a 1.2-inch reduction in waist circumference [11]. Additional studies report consistent efficacy with a mean reduction of the abdominal fat thickness of 18.6%, concurrent increase in rectus abdominis thickness of 15.4%, 10.4% reduction in diastasis recti, and a 1.4-inch reduction in waist circumference [12]. EMSculpt® was initially intended to be the first and only noninvasive treatment modality to stimulate muscle growth; however, concurrent fat reduction appeared as a fortuitous side effect. Histological studies in a porcine model revealed a 92% increase in average apoptotic activity levels in adipocytes from 18.75% at baseline to 35.95% 8 hours following a single treatment. Researchers hypothesize a link between adipocyte apoptosis and free fatty acids released during hyper-maximal muscle contractions induced by the focused electromagnetic field [24].

EMSculpt Neo® (BTL Industries, LTD, Waltham, MA) was introduced in 2020 as an improved NIBC system. This device delivers synchronized radiofrequency *and* simultaneous HIFEM treatment to the target muscle to potentiate the lipolytic effects of HIFEM alone. Radiofrequency has been used for some time and in various forms to elevate subcutaneous adipose temperature, causing thermal lipolysis and visible fat reduction [20]. When delivered simultaneously, the potential for further RF or HIFEM-induced fat loss is increased [5]. Histological study of subcutaneous adipocytes treated with synchronized HIFEM and RF shows reduced adipocyte size, a substantial indicator of lipolysis [5]. The treated cells lose intracellular content due to the degradation of triglycerides into glycerol and free fatty acids. These FFA supply the considerable amount of energy required to sustain HIFEM-stimulated supra-maximal contractions [5]. Additionally, apoptotic changes such as pyknotic nuclei, distortions of cellular shape, and the relative absence of inflammation are strong indicators of adipocyte deletion following therapy [5]. Previous research supports the efficacy of the simultaneous application of HIFEM and synchronized RF, showing a 39.8% reduction in the subcutaneous fat layer [5] (Fig. 47.14, 47.15, and 47.16).

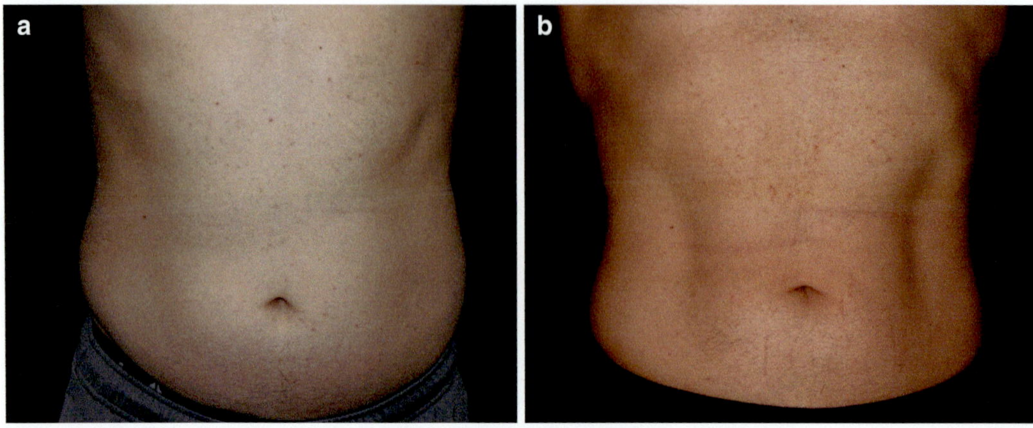

Fig. 47.14 EMSculpt® Neo (**a**) before and (**b**) after abdominal treatment series; anterior view

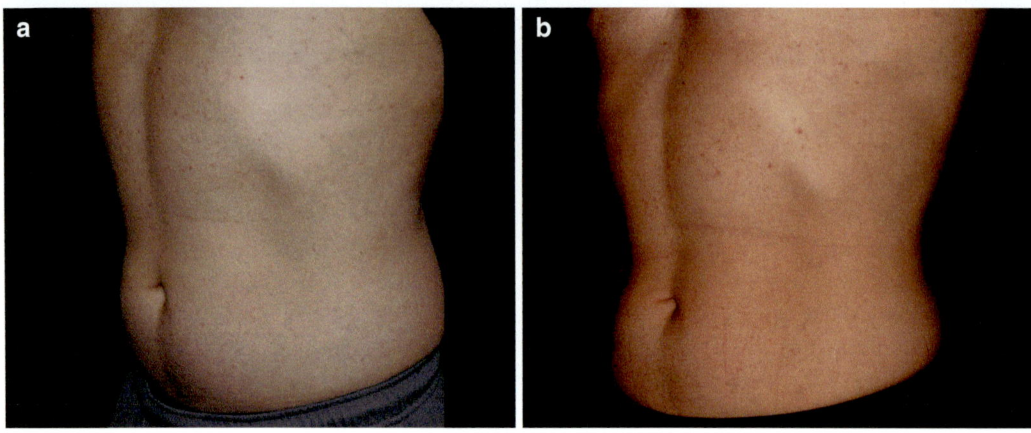

Fig. 47.15 EMSculpt® Neo (**a**) before and (**b**) after abdominal treatment series; oblique view

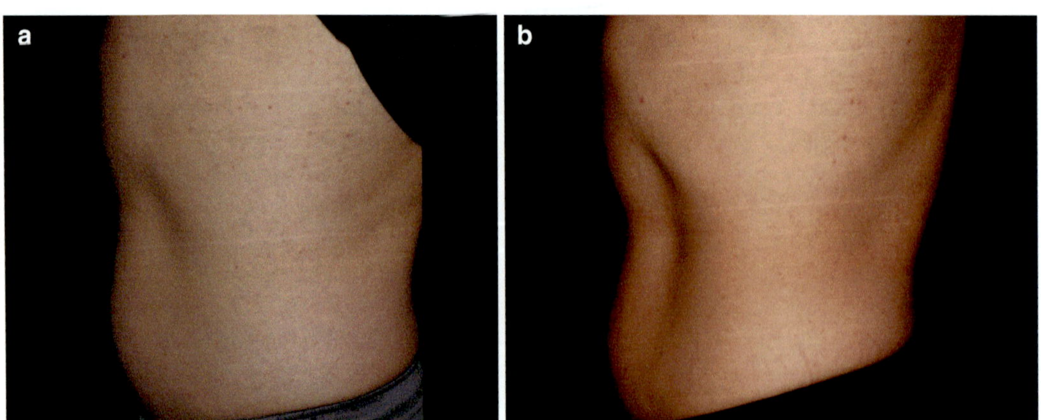

Fig. 47.16 EMSculpt® Neo (**a**) before and (**b**) after abdominal treatment series; lateral view

47.5 Patient Selection

Proper patient selection offers the most significant challenge in implementing NIBC treatments, requiring the surgeon's or consultation delegate's medical and anatomical expertise. The consultant should be able to identify any contraindications to treatment, perform a physical examination, make ethical and educated decisions regarding the most appropriate treatment modality, be able to discuss proper lifestyle and behavior modifications, elicit the patient's specific goals of treatment, and set reasonable expectations regarding patient outcome without making promises, guarantees, or predictions about the final result.

Proper patient selection is crucial to maximize safety and outcomes in noninvasive body contouring. Ideal cryolipolysis candidates tend to be individuals with moderate BMI profiles and localized adiposity in difficult-to-lose areas. Patients should be within 30 lbs of their goal body weight. CoolSculpting® is FDA cleared for patients with a BMI of 30 or less for body applications and 46.2 or less for submental treatments. It is important to note that the BMI ≤46.2 threshold applies only to submental and submandibular treatments, while all other body applications remain limited to BMI ≤30 as per FDA clearance [15]. Morbidly obese patients are unlikely to benefit from cryolipolysis and can be more effectively managed with diet, regular exercise, and bariatric surgery when indicated. In addition, patients with significant skin laxity present as poor candidates for cryolipolysis, as further reduction in subcutaneous fat volume can exacerbate the problem. These patients should receive surgical counseling. Very thin patients can also present a challenge, as inadequate baseline fat volume may present technical difficulty in treatment delivery and may not result in an appreciable reduction of fat. Absolute contraindications to cryolipolysis include a history of cryoglobinemia, paroxysmal cold hemoglobinuria, and cold agglutinin disease. Caution should be taken in treating patients with a history of cold urticaria or Raynaud's disease, pernio or Chilblains, known sensitivity to isopropyl alcohol and propylene glycol, impaired peripheral circulation in the treatment zone, post-herpetic neuralgia, diabetic neuropathy, impaired skin sensation, open or infected wounds, bleeding dyscrasia or antiplatelet therapy, recent surgery, scar tissue, skin conditions or hernia in or adjacent to the treatment area, active implanted devices such as a pacemaker or defibrillator, and history of chronic pain and anxiety disorder.

Nearly all patients may benefit from synchronized RF and HIFEM® therapy, although it is unlikely to induce a clinically significant change in the morbidly obese (greater than 100 lbs over ideal body weight or BMI profile >40.0). Deficiency in muscle mass is not required for treatment, and HIFEM® technology can be used to further enhance muscle tone and size in muscularly developed or physically fit individuals. Heavier patients may benefit from improving muscle tone and core stability, but reasonable expectations should be discussed in regard to the aesthetic outcome. Contraindications to EMSculpt Neo® treatment include the presence of cardiac pacemakers, implanted defibrillators, neurostimulators, electronic implants, pulmonary insufficiency, metal implants, drug pumps, malignant tumor, impaired or otherwise injured muscles, fever, cardiovascular disease, hemorrhagic conditions, septic conditions and empyema, acute inflammations, systemic or local infections such as osteomyelitis and tuberculosis, contagious skin disease, Basedow's disease, and sensitivity or allergy to latex.

47.6 Selecting the Appropriate Treatment

Selecting the appropriate method of NIBC is dependent upon the presence (or absence) of relative and absolute contraindications. Patient goals (muscle building versus fat reduction, or both) need to be considered as well. While both technologies can reduce subcutaneous adiposity, HIFEM is the only technology capable of inducing skeletal muscle hypertrophy. Patients who elect cryolipolysis treatment may need to consider a consultation with a qualified fitness trainer if an increase in muscle mass is desired. Additionally, the timing and frequency of treatments require consideration. CoolSculpting® can be performed as a single session with the option of additional treatments if a greater reduction in adiposity is desired. EMSculpt® Neo requires a series of treatments; one session weekly for four to six total treatments per body area. Cryolipolysis results in a greater degree of post-treatment inflammation, bruising, swelling, and tenderness at the treatment zone. HIFEM with RF treatment is without appreciable downtime, although mild sensitivity and transient erythema of the skin are possible following the application of radiofrequency. A physical examination will determine which treatment best suits the patient's anatomical concerns. Cryolipolysis candidates require at least one inch of pinch thickness adiposity to allow for proper vacuum suction applications. Surface applicators can be used on regions of greater fat layer adhesion, such as the inner and outer thighs. Finally, financial considerations may be necessary as newer technologies (i.e., EMSculpt® Neo) are generally more cost prohibitive than NIBC systems with a longer track record.

47.7 Patient Education and Expectation Management

While the physiologic mechanisms provide the scientific foundation, patient expectations and counseling ultimately determine satisfaction with treatment outcomes. The setting of reasonable patient expectations is critical in the application of NIBC treatments. All patients should be counseled regarding the pertinent risks, benefits, alternatives, and the potential recovery of any proposed treatment plan. Serious adverse effects, such as paradoxical adipose hyperplasia associated with cryolipolysis, should be directly addressed. All patients should be instructed that NIBC outcomes are modest and that the potential reduction in subcutaneous fat volume or increases in targeted muscle mass are relative to the patient's body habitus at baseline. Proper consultation regarding the possible need for subsequent treatments (the same or adjacent body regions) can prevent patient misconceptions and establish a realistic outcome mindset. Education on the mechanism and efficacy of the chosen treatment, patient obligations to lifestyle modifications and follow-up schedule, and informed consent documents should be provided at the time of consultation and reinforced throughout the treatment (or treatment series) by the device operator.

47.8 Lifestyle or Behavioral Modifications

While the surgeon or physician delegate is *directly* responsible for the first three elements above, he or she is *indirectly* responsible for the fourth. All patients require education regarding lifestyle modifications and result maintenance. The patient should clearly understand his agreement to maintain a regular treatment and follow-up schedule, a healthy, goal-oriented diet, and engagement in regular exercise. Patients should verbalize understanding that NIBC treatments are not suitable substitutes for the lifestyle modifications required to stimulate universal change in body composition and overall well-being. While patients do not have to "lose weight" to see positive NIBC treatment outcomes, treatment failure is much more likely in the absence of these practices. Thus, it is necessary to restate the importance of baseline body measurements and photographic documentation before proceeding with therapy. Noncompliant patients may not benefit from treatment and can be easily identified by inversely proportional changes in body weight and circumferential measurements. Referral sources such as certified fitness trainers and dieticians can be excellent resources for both struggling and motivated patients seeking to enhance their potential outcomes.

47.9 Potential NIBC Complications

Complications after cryolipolysis commonly include erythema, ecchymosis, numbness, paresthesia, swelling, cramping, pruritis, skin sensitivity, and transient neuralgia [6]. These side effects are generally self-resolving within a few days to 2 weeks after treatment. Numbness can persist for several weeks in some instances, and few patients require post-treatment pain management. Acetaminophen is the recommended drug of choice and may be taken as needed following cryolipolysis. Although some clinicians avoid NSAIDs post-treatment due to theoretical concerns of blunting the inflammatory response, direct clinical evidence is limited, and analgesic choice should be individualized [9]. Patients should be educated about the possibility of post-treatment delayed onset pain. Delayed onset pain is self-limited, typically occurring on day three and resolving by 11 days without long-term sequelae. Discomfort can be managed with low-dose Neurontin® (gabapentin), acetaminophen with codeine, transdermal anesthetic patches, and adequate compression. Early intervention of delayed onset pain can potentially reduce duration [9]. Possible side effects associated with HIFEM with synchronized RF include muscular pain, intramuscular fat decrease, temporary muscle spasm, temporary joint or tendon pain, local erythema, and panniculitis.

47.10 Paradoxical Adipose Hyperplasia (PAH)

Paradoxical adipose hyperplasia (PAH) is a rare adverse event following cryolipolysis in which the patient experiences a paradoxical growth of the treated soft tissue months following treatment. The precise mechanism of PAH is poorly understood, and the increased mass of PAH may be due to fibrosis of the adipose tissue in which the extracellular matrix is expanding [22]. Others have proposed hypertrophy of preexisting adipocytes, recruitment of stem-cell populations, changes in expression of receptors or soluble factors associated with adipocyte metabolism, hypoxic injury, reduction in sympathetic innervation, and reparative rebound hypertrophy in adipocytes, fibrous cells, and vasculature [21]. Physical examination findings reveal visible tissue enlargement where the applicator was used. This presents as a visible bulge that extends beyond the plane of the surrounding skin. The skin tone and texture are unchanged. The affected adipose tissue is firm and well-demarcated on palpation. The onset of PAH is typically 2 to 3 months after treatment, and enlargement is typically stabilized by 4 to 5 months (Fig. 47.17).

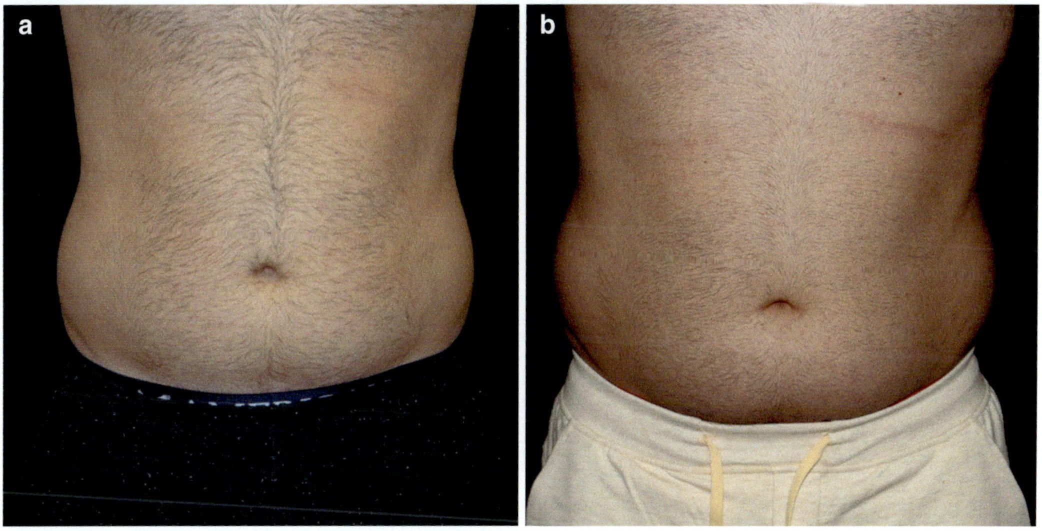

Fig. 47.17 (**a**) Baseline pretreatment anterior view of the abdomen prior to cryolipolysis. (**b**) Post-treatment complication of paradoxical adipose hyperplasia (PAH)

The manufacturer reports an incidence of one case of PAH for every 4000 treatment cycles (0.025%), although this may be understated [10]. Independent multicenter studies have reported a higher incidence of 0.05%–0.39%, suggesting that the true occurrence of PAH may exceed manufacturer estimates [25]. In reported cases, spontaneous regression has not been known to occur, and surgical intervention is required for correction [10]. Patients should be counseled on the possibility of PAH after cryolipolysis. Cases should be reported to the device manufacturer, and a clinical event form should be completed on behalf of the patient. Following the proper application process, the CoolSculpting® manufacturer (ZELTIQ Aesthetics, Inc., Pleasanton, CA) may provide financial reimbursement to cover costs associated with surgical correction. The device manufacturer recommends the use of ultrasonic-assisted liposuction for surgical correction of PAH (Figs. 47.18 and 47.19).

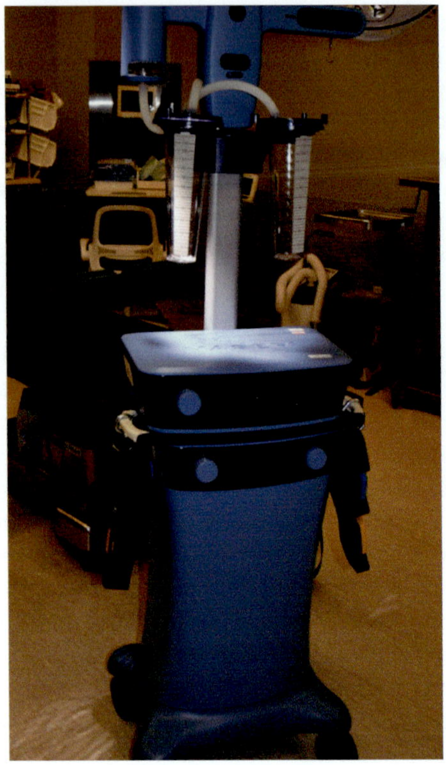

Fig. 47.18 VASER® Ultrasonic System (Solta Medical, Bothell, WA)

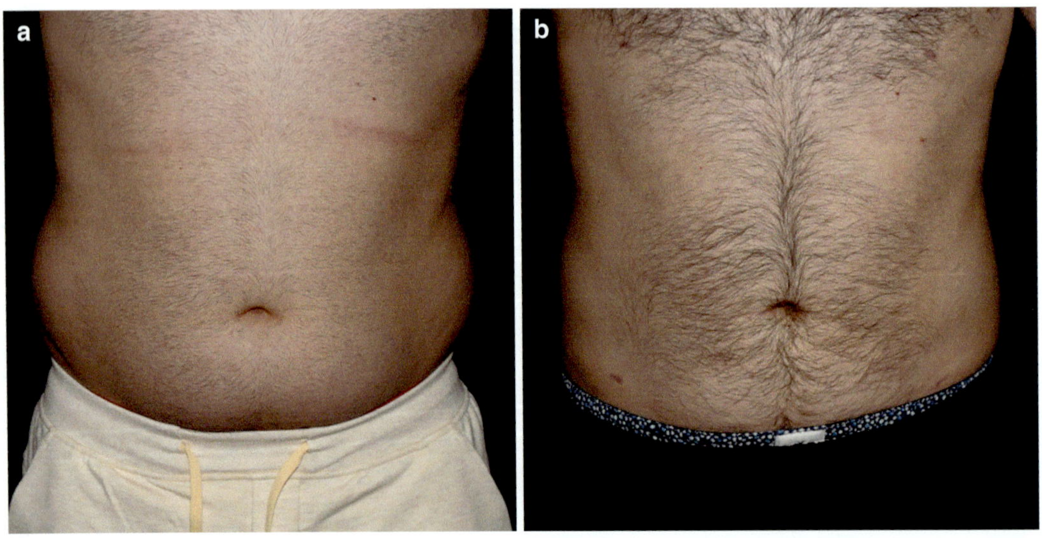

Fig. 47.19 The same patient following surgical correction of PAH using VASER® ultrasonic-assisted liposuction. (**a**) Preoperative anterior view. (**b**) Anterior view status post correction of PAH using ultrasonic liposuction

47.11 Conclusion

The inclusion of NIBC treatment systems such as CoolSculpting® and EMSculpt® Neo into the plastic surgery toolbox supplies the modern man with simple, safe, and efficacious ways to better meet his aesthetic goals. These systems should be intended to supplement regular diet and exercise routines required to transform body composition and overall health and wellness. The initial patient encounter or clinical consultation should be performed by either the plastic surgeon or a mid-level provider. A thorough history and physical examination are critical to determining patient candidacy and selecting the best mode of treatment. Optimization of care using NIBC treatment systems can be achieved through proper patient selection, careful consideration of the most suitable treatment modality, thorough patient education and expectation management, and implementing lifestyle or behavioral modifications. Cryolipolysis and HIFEM with synchronized RF are generally considered safe, simple, and effective noninvasive modalities to reduce stubborn adiposity and increase lean muscle mass in targeted body areas.

Works Cited

1. Adjadj ML, SidAhmed-Mezi PM, Mondoloni MM, Meningaud MP, Hersant MB. Assessment of efficacy of cryolipolysis on saddlebags: a prospective study of 53 patients. Plast Reconstr Surg. 2016:50–7.
2. Duncan MD, Dinev DP. Noninvasive induction of muscle fiber hypertrophy and hyperplasia: effects of high-intensity focused electromagnetic field evaluated in an in-vivo porcine model: a pilot study. Aesthet Surg J. 2020;40:568–74.
3. Epstein E, Oren M. Popsicle Panniculitis. N Engl J Med. 1970;282:966–7.
4. Garibyan L, Sipprell W, Jalian HR, Sakamoto FH, Avram M, Anderson RR. Three-dimensional volumetric quantification of fat loss following cryolipolysis. Lasers Surg Med. 2014;46:75–80.
5. Goldberg MJ. Deletion of adipocytes induced by a novel device simultaneously delivering synchronized radiofrequency and HIFEM: human histological study. J Cosmet Dermatol. 2021;20:1104–9.
6. Ingargiola MJ, Motakef S, Chung M, Vasconez H, Sasaki GH. Cryolipolysis for fat reduction and body contouring: safety and efficacy of current treatment paradigms. The American Society of Plastic Surgeons; 2014. p. 1581–90.
7. Iverson VM, Norum M, Schoenfeld BJ, Fimland MS. No time to lift? Designing time-efficient training programs for strength and hypertrophy: a narrative review. Sports Med. 2021;51:2079–95.
8. Jacob CI, Paskova K, Kinney BM, Duncan DI. High-intensity focused electromagnetic field (HIFEM) devices in dermatology. J Drugs Dermatol. 2019;18(12):1088–92.
9. Keaney TC, Gudas AT-C, Alster TS. Delayed onset pain associated with cryolipolysis treatment: a retrospective study with treatment recommendations. Dermatologic Surg. 2015;41(11):1296–9.
10. Kelly MM, Rodriguez-Feliz M, Torres MC, Kelly BE. Treatment of paradoxical adipose hyperplasia following cryolipolysis: a single-center experience. Plast Reconstr Surg. 2018;142:17e–22e.
11. Kent DE, Jacob CI. Computed tomography (CT) based evidence of simultaneous changes in human adipose and muscle tissues following a high intensity focused electromagnetic field (HIFEM) application: a new method for non-invasive body sculpting. Dallas: The Annual Meeting of the American Society for Laser Medicine and Surgery; 2018.
12. Kinney BM, Lozanova P. High intensity focused electro-magnetic therapy (HIFEM) evaluated by magnetic resonance imaging (MRI): safety and efficacy study of dual tissue effect based non invasive abdominal body shaping. Dallas: The Annual Meeting of the American Society for Laser Medicine and Surgery, 2018.
13. Kinney BM, Lozanova P. High intensity focused electromagnetic therapy evaluated by magnetic resonance imaging: Safety and efficacy study of a dual tissue effect based non-invasive abdominal body shaping. Lasers Surg Med. 2018;51(1):40–6. https://doi.org/10.1002/lsm.23024.
14. Klein KB, Zelickson B, Riopelle J, Okamoto E, Bachelor EP, Harry RS, Preciado JA. Non-invasive cryolipolysis for subcutaneous fat reduction does not affect serum lipid levels or liver function tests. Lasers Surg Med. 2009;41:785–90.
15. Krueger N, Mai SV, Luebberding S, Sadick NS. Cryolipolysis for noninvasive body contouring: clinical efficacy and patient satisfaction. Clin Cosmet Investig Dermatol. 2014;7:201–5.
16. Liam T, Ding SW, Chua CH, Moey HX. Enhancing the appearance of the "six-pack" muscles using cryolipolysis: a safe and effective method. Plast Reconstr Surg. 2021;148:775–9.
17. Loap MS, SidAhmed-Mezi PM, Meningaud MP, Hersant MP. A prospective, comparative study (before and after) for the evaluation of cryothermogenesis' efficacy in body contouring: abdomen and saddlebags. Plast Reconstr Surg. 2021:425e–8e.
18. Lokeshwar SD, Patel P, Fantus RJ, Halpern J, Chang C, Kargi AY, Ramasamy R. Decline in serum testosterone levels among adolescent and young adult men in the USA. Eur Urol Focus. 2021;7:886–9.

19. Nassab R. The evidence behind noninvasive body contouring. Aesthet Surg J. 2015;35(3):279–93.
20. Samuels JB, Katz B, Weiss RA. Radiofrequency heating and high-intensity focused electromagnetic treatment delivered simultaneously: the first sham-controlled randomized trial. Plast Reconstr Surg J. 2020;149:893e–900e.
21. Sasaki MG. Reply: cryolipolysis for fat reduction and body contouring: safety and efficacy of current treatment paradigms. Plast Reconstr Surg. 2016:640–641e.
22. Seaman S, Tannan S, Cao Y, Peirce S, Gammper T. Paradoxical adipose hyperplasia and cellular effects after cryolipolysis. Aesthet Surg J. 2016;36(1):6–13.
23. Travison TG, Araujo AB, O'Donnell AB, Kupelian V, McKinlay JB. A population-level decline in serum testosterone levels in American men. J Clin Endocrinol Metabol. 2007;92(1):196–202. Retrieved July 15, 2019, from https://academic.oup.com/jecm/article/92/1/196/2598434.
24. Weiss R, Bernardy J. Induction of fat apoptosis by a non-thermal device: safety and mechanism of action of non-invasive HIFEM technology evaluated in a histological porcine model. Dallas: The Annual Meeting of the American Society for Laser Medicine and Surgery; 2018.
25. Zakhary B, Aksu AE, Borman H, Nahai F. A multicenter evaluation of paradoxical adipose hyperplasia following cryolipolysis for fat reduction and body contouring: a review of 8,658 cycles in 2,114 patients. Aesthet Surg J. 2021;41(7):NP994–NP1002. https://doi.org/10.1093/asj/sjaa246.
26. Zare H, Gaskin D, Thorpe JR. Income inequality and obesity among US adults 1999-2016: does sex matter? Int J Environ Res Public Health. 2021; Retrieved September 16, 2022, from https://doi.org/10.3390/ijerph18137079.

Index

K. Jeffords et al. (eds.), *Aesthetic Surgery for Men*, https://doi.org/10.1007/978-3-032-03840-1

F

Q

R

MIX
Papier aus verantwortungsvollen Quellen
Paper from responsible sources
FSC® C105338

If you have any concerns about our products,
you can contact us on
ProductSafety@springernature.com

In case Publisher is established outside the EU,
the EU authorized representative is:
Springer Nature Customer Service Center GmbH
Europaplatz 3, 69115 Heidelberg, Germany

Printed by Libri Plureos GmbH
in Hamburg, Germany